YOUR FAMILY DOCTOR

Volume Two: Practical Volume
Guide to First Aid, Safety, Care of the Sick,
Pregnancy, Childbirth and Child Care, and Fitness

Your Family Doctor

Volume One: Reference Volume
Guide to Current Medical Practice

How your body works
Index of symptoms
Understanding medical terms
A–Z Medical Reference Guide

Volume Two: Practical Volume
Guide to First Aid, Safety, Care of the Sick,
Pregnancy, Childbirth and Child Care, and Fitness

First Aid
Family safety
Care of the sick at home
Professional care for the sick
Pregnancy and childbirth
The healthy child
Age-by-age charts
Taking care of your own body
Physical fitness and exercises
Mental fitness

GUILD PUBLISHING

The Home Medical Encyclopaedia

YOUR FAMILY DOCTOR

DR JAMES BEVAN

With a Foreword by Lord Hunt of Fawley, Past President
The Royal College of General Practitioners

Volume Two: Practical Volume
Guide to First Aid, Safety, Care of
the Sick, Pregnancy, Childbirth and
Child Care, and Fitness

Your Family Doctor

This edition published 1981 by Guild Publishing.
By arrangement with Mitchell Beazley Limited.

Filmset in Great Britain by Filmtype Services Ltd,
Scarborough
ISBN 085533 295 6
(Library of Congress Catalog Number 79-56907)
Printed and bound in Spain
by TONSA, San Sebastian
Dep. Leg. S.S. 360-80

Contents – Volume Two

First Aid

Section contents

For EMERGENCY treatment
see
Index of Emergencies p.504

For common injuries and disorders that are
not life-threatening, but that need attention
and treatment, *see* **Treating minor injuries
and disorders,** p.574

Introduction

It is absolutely essential to take no action in
assisting in an emergency unless you are
certain of what you are doing. The aim of this
section is to help you take the correct action
at the right time when faced with such an
emergency.

In an emergency situation, the **Index of
Emergencies** is designed to show the reader
immediately which page or pages to consult.
Look there first, and then refer to the
appropriate first aid procedure.

Emergency first aid uses words, pictures
and easy-to-read charts to explain clearly
how to (1) identify what is wrong, if it is not
already obvious; and (2) treat the condition
correctly – and above all, safely – until skilled
help arrives.

When the question is not so much what
treatment to give, but – more dramatically –
what can be *done*, **What to do in an
emergency** comes into its own. Confronted
by a scene of emergency, such as a road
accident, a person shouting for help after
falling through an iced-over pond, or a
person stuck half-way up a cliff, the most
effective actions arc quickly outlined as a
sequence of instructions to bring relief or
rescue.

But it is not only with emergencies that this
section is concerned. After all, it may be
necessary to administer first aid in other
circumstances.

For minor injuries, like those that occur
from time to time around the house, at
school or in the garden, **Treating minor
injuries and disorders** gives equally clear and
easy-to-follow advice. As the title suggests,
minor disorders are also discussed, with
appropriate treatment. For the reader's
convenience, the **Index of Emergencies**
contains references to both **Emergency first
aid** and **Treating minor injuries and
disorders.**

There may even be times when you suspect
that there could be something wrong with
your own body: a strange pain, perhaps, or a
disturbance in vision, or sudden vomiting. At
times like these, **What could be wrong?** may
be able to help, by indicating which first aid
procedures (if any) are immediately valuable
for self-administration, or whether to seek a
doctor's diagnosis. Further information on
how to use **What could be wrong?** is
contained in its own introduction, p.598.

Index of Emergencies

What to do in an emergency

For

Bleeding *see* First Aid page 516
Burns and scalds *see* First Aid page 524
Fractures *see* First Aid pages 546 to 553

If a person

has a head injury *see* page 511
has swallowed a poison or a chemical *see* page 511
is becoming overheated *see* page 511
is becoming too chilled *see* page 511
is drowning *see* page 510
is in a state of confusion *see* page 511
is in contact with an electric current *see* page 510
is lying inert in a gas-filled room *see* page 510
is lying still surrounded by fire *see* page 510
is stuck at a dangerous height *see* page 510
is wedged fast *see* page 510

General advice

1	Remain calm. Do not shout unless it is essential.
2	Obtain professional help at once.
3	Once you have made a decision, carry it out.
4	Tell others clearly and concisely what to do.
5	Prevent further accidents to victims or rescuers.

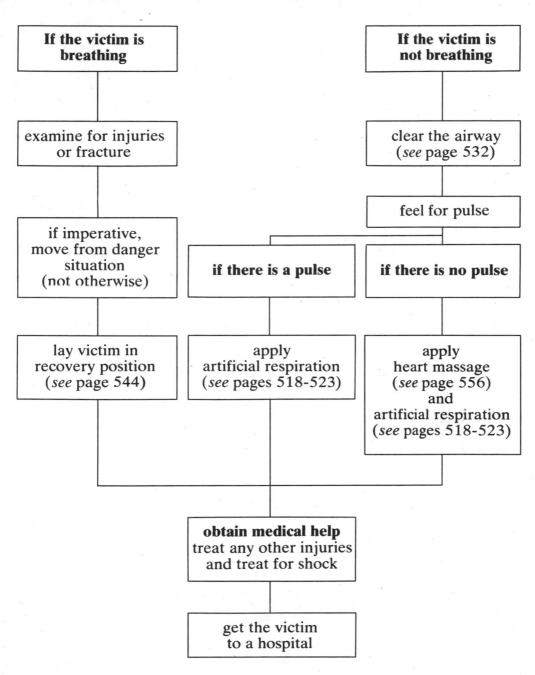

If the victim is lying on the ground

Do not move the victim
if there is any possibility of a fractured neck or spine

If the victim is breathing

examine for injuries or fracture

if imperative, move from danger situation (not otherwise)

lay victim in recovery position (*see* page 544)

If the victim is not breathing

clear the airway (*see* page 532)

feel for pulse

if there is a pulse

if there is no pulse

apply artificial respiration (*see* pages 518-523)

apply heart massage (*see* page 556) and artificial respiration (*see* pages 518-523)

obtain medical help treat any other injuries and treat for shock

get the victim to a hospital

Emergency situations

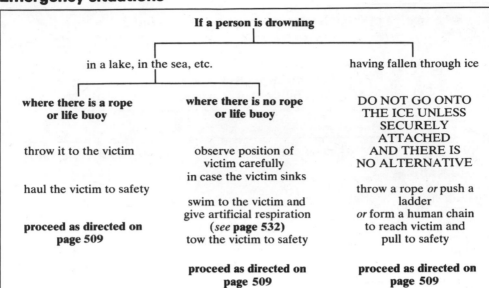

If a person is drowning

in a lake, in the sea, etc.   having fallen through ice

where there is a rope or life buoy

throw it to the victim

haul the victim to safety

proceed as directed on page 509

where there is no rope or life buoy

observe position of victim carefully in case the victim sinks

swim to the victim and give artificial respiration (*see* **page 532**) tow the victim to safety

proceed as directed on page 509

DO NOT GO ONTO THE ICE UNLESS SECURELY ATTACHED AND THERE IS NO ALTERNATIVE

throw a rope *or* push a ladder *or* form a human chain to reach victim and pull to safety

proceed as directed on page 509

If a person is wedged fast

DO NOT TRY TO MOVE THE VICTIM

shout for assistance

protect victim from any possible further injury as much as possible

proceed as directed on page 509

If a person is stuck at a dangerous height

reassure the victim by talking slowly and calmly

DO NOT ATTEMPT A RESCUE ON YOUR OWN

if you are alone, explain to the victim that you must go and get help

---

If a person is lying inert in a gas-filled room

DO NOT ENTER THE ROOM

see that professional assistance is called

obtain a rope and, if possible, breathing apparatus

tie the rope around your waist leaving the other end in the hands of assistants

enter the room (with breathing apparatus, if possible)

open the doors and windows

remove the victim

proceed as directed on page 509

(If you yourself are overcome by the gas, the rope will enable you to be hauled out immediately.)

If a person is in contact with an electric current

DO NOT TOUCH THE VICTIM

turn off the electric current *or* remove the fuse *or* if the victim is blocking the means of turning off the current, push the victim away, using a **wooden** chair or **dry** stick, and, standing on a dry surface, turn off

proceed as directed on page 509

If a person is lying inert surrounded by fire

wet a cloth

if the heat is too much, cover your nose and mouth with the cloth and crawl along the floor to the victim pull the victim to safety

proceed as directed on page 509

Emergency conditions

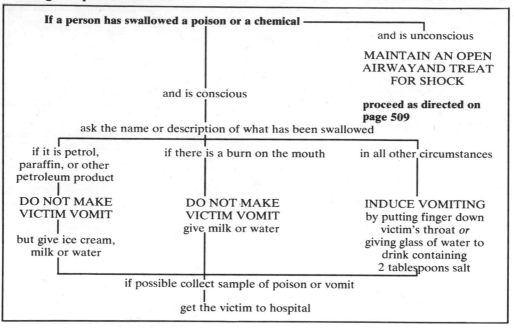

If a person has swallowed a poison or a chemical —————

and is unconscious

MAINTAIN AN OPEN AIRWAY AND TREAT FOR SHOCK

proceed as directed on page 509

and is conscious

ask the name or description of what has been swallowed

if it is petrol, paraffin, or other petroleum product	if there is a burn on the mouth	in all other circumstances
DO NOT MAKE VICTIM VOMIT	**DO NOT MAKE VICTIM VOMIT**	**INDUCE VOMITING**
but give ice cream, milk or water	give milk or water	by putting finger down victim's throat *or* giving glass of water to drink containing 2 tablespoons salt

if possible collect sample of poison or vomit

get the victim to hospital

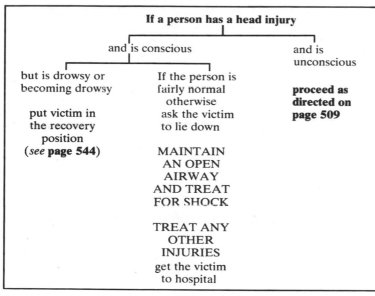

If a person has a head injury

and is conscious

but is drowsy or becoming drowsy

put victim in the recovery position (*see* **page 544**)

If the person is fairly normal otherwise ask the victim to lie down

MAINTAIN AN OPEN AIRWAY AND TREAT FOR SHOCK

TREAT ANY OTHER INJURIES get the victim to hospital

and is unconscious

proceed as directed on page 509

If a person is becoming overheated

move to shade or cool place

remove the victim's clothing

sponge all over with cool or tepid water

fan the victim

if the victim is still too hot, give a cold bath

If a person is in a state of confusion

DO NOT TRY TO RESTRAIN ANY ACTION, EVEN IF VIOLENT, EXCEPT TO PROTECT OTHERS, AND THEN ONLY WITH ASSISTANCE

try to persuade the person to sit or lie down

try to obtain professional assistance

If a person is becoming too chilled

find shelter and take off wet clothing

wrap in layered, warm, dry clothing

give warm drinks and food (not alcohol)

if the victim is still too cold, give a warm bath

At a road accident

1 Prevent further accidents

Turn off your engine, and ensure other drivers do the same;
ensure that the engine of any vehicle involved in the accident is turned off

Put out cigarettes

Place a warning signal (such as a red triangle) at least fifty metres (yards)
back down the road

Switch on your hazard warning lights

Shine your dimmed headlights either at oncoming traffic
or at the accident scene

Check around the accident scene for anyone who may have been thrown
clear of the crash, and who may be lying where he or she could be hit
by moving traffic

Remove debris from road

2 Carry out first aid procedures

Quickly check each victim and then tend to the most seriously injured

Undo all motorcycle crash helmet straps and remove helmet in order
to assess injury and to prevent suffocation
Do not do this if neck or back injuries are suspected

Do not move any victim unless there is serious danger of fire or fumes,
or of being run over

Treat victims with appropriate first aid (*see* following pages)

3 Alert the rescue and hospital services

The information they will require is:

the exact location

the nature of the accident

the number of victims

the type of injuries sustained

whether there are any victims trapped

whether there are any special hazards, such as fire, acid, gas, etc.

Emergency first aid

For EMERGENCY treatment see Index of Emergencies p.504

For common injuries and disorders that are not life-threatening, but that need attention and treatment, *see* Treating minor injuries and disorders, p.574.

Introduction

If only everyone had the natural ability to memorise a complete first aid course. If only everyone was then level-headed enough in an emergency to be able to make use of the knowledge promptly and correctly. All too often, as many people have discovered, the mind becomes completely blank when suddenly confronted with an accident or emergency victim. In spite of a real desire to be of assistance, many people are as helpless as the unfortunate victim. They may easily take the wrong action and endanger the victim's life by relying on panic-reduced half-memories and instinct.

When giving first aid, the first lesson is to do nothing unless you are certain both of what you are doing and of what the result should be. It is the particular aim of this section to help you to take the correct action at the right time, and to give you the confidence that you are doing everything that can be done for the victim.

In an emergency situation, the **Index of Emergencies** is designed to show the reader immediately which page or pages to consult. Look there first, and then refer to the appropriate first aid procedure. In general, the section has been arranged in alphabetical order itself, and should not be difficult to use even without prior research.

The information is presented for the most part visually – with clear, numbered illustrations – together with a corresponding text consisting of instructions and advice. The instructions are clear and easy to follow; as well as telling the reader what to do, the advice given also includes the important addition of what *not* to do. There may also be cross-references to other pages where alternative methods of treatment, or more urgent means of assistance, are described.

All the instructions contained in this section have been approved by some of the most authoritative first aid organisations. The advice has been checked to be consistent with their own.

Bites and stings

Although bites and stings are not usually dangerous, the more serious ones should be examined by a doctor to prevent infection or poisoning.

Rarely, anaphylactic shock may occur after a sting, causing faintness, pallor, nausea, vomiting, difficulty in breathing, and rapid heart-beat. It can be fatal. If the victim is suffering from anaphylactic shock, put in the recovery position and remain with the victim while emergency medical aid is summoned.

If the victim stops breathing, give artificial respiration. *See* **Breathing stoppage: the kiss of life,** p.518.

If the victim's heart stops, give external cardiac massage. *See* **Heart attack 2,** p.556.

Poisonous bites and stings are comparatively rare. The different poisons from various poisonous creatures require appropriate medical treatment; so it is important to identify the creature, or preferably kill or capture it for expert identification.

If you have identified the creature as being poisonous, or if you only suspect it, summon emergency medical aid.

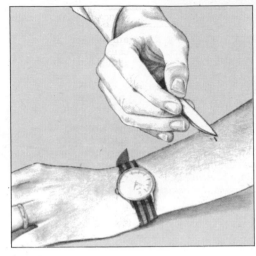

2
If an insect has left its sting in the skin, the sting may be removed by gently scraping it out. This is preferable to using tweezers, which often results in the injection of additional venom.

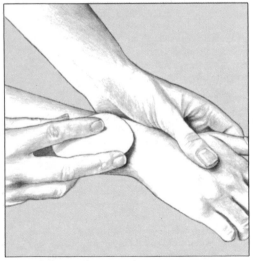

1
If the victim has been bitten or scratched by an animal, wash the wound with soap and water. Control any bleeding by pressing firmly on a dressing over the wound until the bleeding stops. Then dress and bandage the wound. The victim should have immediate medical attention if the wound is severe.

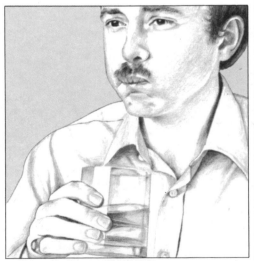

3
If the victim has been stung in the mouth, give the victim ice to suck and mouthwashes of sodium bicarbonate solution. Use about one teaspoon of sodium bicarbonate dissolved in a glass of water. This will help to reduce the swelling.

Summon emergency medical aid.

NAME	TOXIC SUBSTANCES	SYMPTOMS	TREATMENT
Horsefly Genus: *Tabanus.*	animal disease-causing organisms in saliva	Sharp stinging pain; female insects suck blood.	1. Antihistamine cream or calamine lotion relieves irritation. 2. Insect repellents. 3. Do not scratch. 4. Wash carefully.
Bee For example: honey-bee; bumble-bee. Genus: *Apis; Bombus; Halictus.*	acidic venom; enzymes; haemolytic agents; neurotoxin; vasodilator	Local pain; burning sensation; whiteness at site of sting; swelling and redness; multiple stings may cause generalised swelling, respiratory distress, and shock; rarely, death.	1. Identify insect. 2. Remove sting. 3. Apply anti-histamine cream. 4. Sodium bicarbonate neutralises poison. 5. Multiple stings require immediate hospitalisation.
Wasp or **hornet** Genus: *Polestes; Sceliphron; Vespa; Vespula.*	alkaline venom; enzymes; haemolytic agents; neurotoxin; vasodilator	Similar to the signs and symptoms of a bee sting.	1, 2, 3, and 5. Treat as a bee sting. 4. Vinegar or lemon neutralises poison.
Mosquito Genus: *Aedes; Anopheles; Culex.*	anticoagulant in saliva; disease-causing organisms in saliva of some tropical mosquito species	Slight local pain; swelling; itching. Organisms in mosquito bite may cause a variety of diseases, including malaria and yellow fever.	1. Antihistamine cream relieves irritation. 2. Do not scratch. 3. Antimalaria drugs, and insect repellents, if in malarial region.
Adder Genus: *Vipera*	enzymes	Shock; local pain; swelling; vomiting; abdominal pain; rarely, death.	1. Lay the victim down. 2. Do not give anything to eat or drink. 3. Take the victim to hospital for treatment with anti-venin and antitetanus injection.
Tick Genus: *Dermacentor; Ixodes; Ornithodoros.*	not known	Itching; local skin irritation. Poisonous species cause pain; redness; swelling; muscle cramps. Some species carry typhus.	1. Apply petroleum jelly, alcohol, or petrol to tick, to loosen its jaws. 2. Use tweezers to remove tick. Do not leave jaws embedded. 3. Wash carefully.
Jellyfish For example: Portuguese man-of-war. Genus: *Physalia.* Other species have less serious effect.	sea anemone toxin; vasoconstrictor	Acute stinging or burning sensation; rash; blistering; shock; rarely causes death, unless from drowning as a result of shock.	1. Remove all tentacles. 2. Wash area with sea-water, then with alcohol or ammonia. 3. Take victim to a hospital.

Bleeding

Bleeding from an artery can be recognised by the pumping of the blood from the wound and its bright scarlet colour.

When bleeding is from a vein, the blood is much darker and flows smoothly.

With internal bleeding it is important to recognise the general signs (which apply to both external and internal bleeding): pallor; cold, clammy skin; a weak, rapid pulse; and fast, shallow breathing. The victim may also feel faint or even pass out.

Internal bleeding is extremely serious. It is imperative to get medical help urgently.

Do not give a person suspected of internal bleeding any food or drink.

Action

The aim of first aid is to stop the bleeding quickly and to get medical assistance as soon as possible.

If internal bleeding is suspected, summon medical assistance; hospital treatment will be necessary.

If unconscious, the victim should be turned to the recovery position. *See* **Fainting,** p.544.

If conscious, the victim's legs should be raised to reduce the effects of shock.

Watch the victim's pulse and breathing. If the victim has stopped breathing, give artificial respiration. *See* **Breathing stoppage: the kiss of life,** p.518.

If an object has penetrated the victim's chest and is still in the wound, **do not** remove the object. If the victim has an open wound in the chest, cover it to prevent air entering the chest, and treat for a complicated rib fracture. *See* **Fractures: the spine or ribs,** p.551.

Bleeding from the womb may be due to several factors: particularly heavy menstruation; as a result of a miscarriage or abortion; during pregnancy; or during or after childbirth.

Lay the victim down with legs raised.

Keep the victim warm and comfortable but **do not** overheat.

Summon medical assistance immediately.

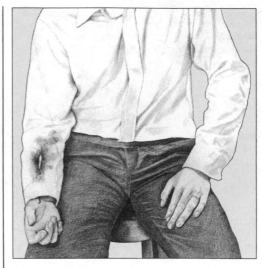

1
If the victim is bleeding from a vein, find the bleeding point.

Apply continuous pressure for at least ten minutes so that the blood has time to clot.

If a clean dressing is available, use this to help stop the bleeding.

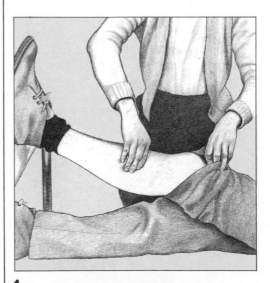

4
If the victim is bleeding from a varicose vein, raise the affected leg as high as possible.

Apply pressure to the bleeding point.

When the bleeding stops, cover the area with a clean dressing, bandage the whole leg, and get medical help.

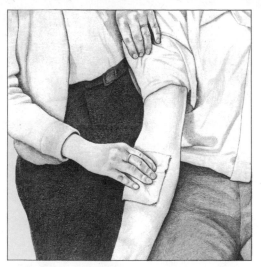

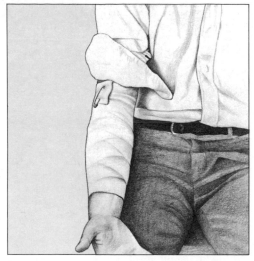

2

Continue to apply pressure over the dressing until the bleeding stops.

Raise the injured part if possible while continuing to apply pressure.

Lay the victim down with the legs raised, to reduce the effects of shock. If the victim goes into shock, *see* **Shock,** p.566.

3

Wash the wound and remove any foreign body that comes out easily. **Do not** remove a foreign body that is deeply embedded.

Apply a clean dressing and a firm bandage. **Do not** bandage too tightly.

Keep the injured part raised and summon medical help as soon as possible.

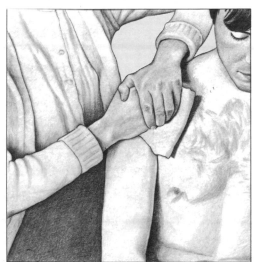

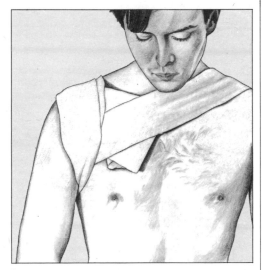

5

If the victim is bleeding from a deep wound, cover the wound with a clean dressing: a handkerchief would be suitable.

Apply firm pressure for at least ten minutes, or until the bleeding has stopped.

6

When the bleeding has stopped, apply a firm bandage to keep the dressing in place.

Do not remove the dressing or the bandage as this may re-open the wound.

Get medical help as soon as possible.

Breathing stoppage: the kiss of life

Mouth-to-mouth resuscitation is the most effective method of artificial respiration. When a person stops breathing, oxygenation of the blood ceases and brain damage may occur after 4-6 minutes or less, leading to death. If the victim's heart has stopped, *see* **Heart attack 2,** p.556.

If breathing has stopped, the victim will be unconscious and immobile, there will be no chest movement and the skin will be pale, possibly a slightly bluish colour.

Resuscitation may take a long time. Once resuscitated, the victim should be carefully observed until medical assistance arrives. The victim must be seen by a doctor.

Action
Before giving mouth-to-mouth resuscitation, tilt back the victim's head and check that breathing really has ceased by listening at the victim's mouth and nose and by looking for movement of the chest.

It is important to ensure that the victim's air passage is clear.

If the victim's mouth is damaged, a mouth-to-nose method can be used. This method is the same as mouth-to-mouth except that the victim's lips must be held together instead of the nose being pinched. Air is blown into the victim's nose.

Do not use mouth-to-mouth resuscitation:
If the victim's mouth and face are damaged. In this case *see* the **Holger Nielsen method,** p.520.

If the air passage is blocked. *See* **Choking and coughing,** p.526.

Follow the instructions carefully but as swiftly as possible
Keep calm. Your own breathing must be regular.

Be careful not to blow too hard, or air may be blown into the stomach and press on the victim's diaphragm, reducing the effectiveness of the method.

Try to indicate to others that medical assistance is required urgently.

Treat the victim for shock. *See* **Shock,** p.566.

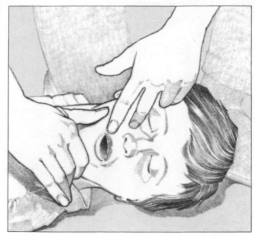

1
Lay the victim face upwards, if possible, but do not delay if the victim cannot be turned.

Loosen clothing around the neck.

Turn the head to one side. Use your fingers to remove any obstructions to breathing, including loosened false teeth.

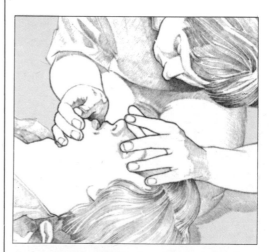

4
When you have filled the victim's lungs, remove your mouth and watch the chest deflate as you take another deep breath.

Check for breathing and check the victim's pulse. If there is no pulse, *see* **Heart attack 2**, p.556.

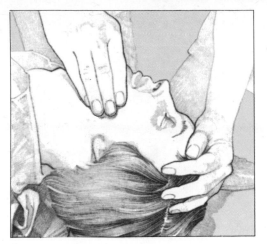

2
Turn the victim's head upwards.

Tilt the head backwards and support the shoulders with a piece of folded clothing or with your lower hand.

This position of the head opens the throat and allows the free passage of air to the victim's lungs.

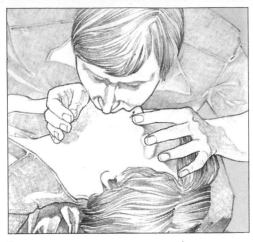

3
Pinch the victim's nostrils firmly.

Take a deep breath and place your mouth over the victim's mouth.

Give four quick, full breaths into the victim's lungs.

If the chest does not rise immediately, there is an obstruction to the air flow. *See* **Choking and coughing,** p.526.

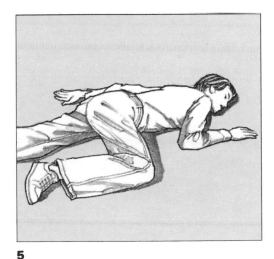

5
Continue the sequence every five seconds until independent breathing starts again.

When breathing has restarted, turn the victim over to the recovery position.

Observe the victim's pulse and breathing until medical help arrives.

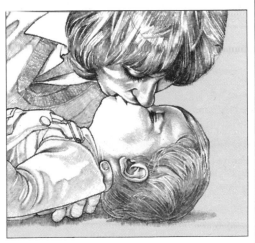

6
If the victim is a baby or a small child follow the same preliminary procedures as for an adult (stages 1 and 2). Now cover the victim's mouth and nose with your mouth. Breathe in through your nose, fill your cheeks with air, and puff the air gently into the child. Finish breathing out through your nose. Watch the victim's chest deflate as you take another small breath.

Breathing stoppage: the Holger Nielsen method

The Holger Nielsen method of artificial respiration is used if facial injuries prevent mouth-to-mouth resuscitation (*see* p.518) and when the victim can be placed face downwards. If the victim's heart has also stopped, *see* **Heart attack 2,** p.556.

It is important to check that the victim's mouth is not obstructed before artificial respiration begins. *See* **Choking and coughing,** p.526.

The Holger Nielsen method is not suitable for treating babies or small children. Nor is it suitable for a victim with major chest or arm injuries.

Action

Before using the Holger Nielsen method: Check that breathing really has ceased by listening at the victim's mouth and nose and by feeling for movement of the chest.

Place the victim face downwards on a hard, flat surface, such as the floor.

Turn the victim's head to one side.

Bend the victim's arms in front of the head so that the two hands support the forehead.

If there is an obvious obstruction to breathing (such as mud in the victim's mouth), remove it with your fingers.

Kneel with one knee at the victim's head and keep the other knee off the ground. This enables you to rock backwards and forwards more easily. It also allows you to exert more pressure on the victim's back.

Do not use the Holger Nielsen method:
If the victim's mouth or nose are undamaged and mouth-to-mouth resuscitation can be given.

If the victim has suffered major chest or arm injuries.

If the victim is a baby or a small child.

Follow the instructions carefully but as quickly as possible.
Keep calm. Concentrate on regular and continuous movements. Avoid sudden pressure. Keep the victim's airway clear at all times.

Get someone to summon medical assistance.

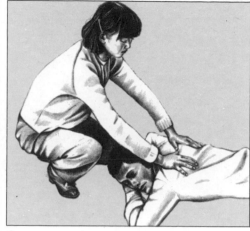

1
Kneel at the victim's head with one knee raised.

Lean forwards.

Place both hands, palms down and fingers spread, on the victim's shoulder blades.

Your arms should remain straight and your body should move with a rocking motion.

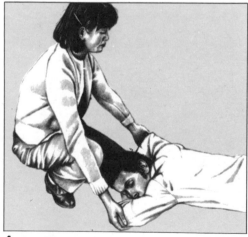

4
Keep a firm hold of the victim's elbows.

Lean backwards.

You should lean backwards until the victim's elbows have been raised about six or eight inches from the ground.

This movement expands the victim's chest, allowing air to be pumped into the lungs.

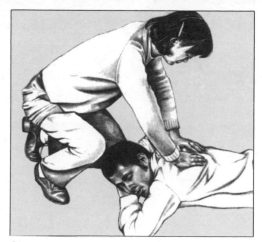

2

Rock forwards over the victim's head.

Your arms must remain straight.

The weight of your body will compress the victim's chest and will force air out of the lungs.

You should press on the victim's back for about one second.

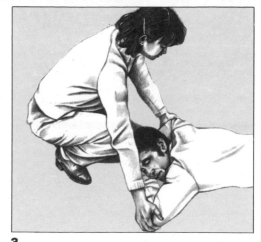

3

Release your pressure on the victim's back.

Slide your hands from the victim's shoulder blades to the upper arms and along to the elbows.

Take a firm hold of the victim's elbows.

Rock backwards as you prepare to lift the elbows from the ground.

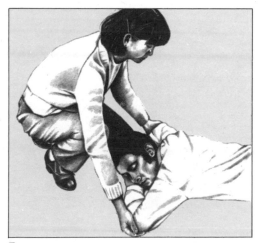

5

Replace the victim's elbows on the ground.

Return your hands to the victim's shoulder blades as soon as the elbows are on the ground. Do not waste time.

This concludes the sequence of movements of Holger Nielsen artificial respiration.

Each sequence takes about five seconds.

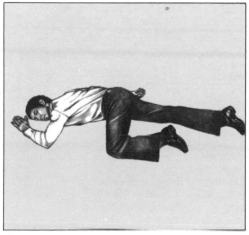

6

When independent breathing starts again, the victim should be placed in the recovery position. The airway must be kept clear if the victim starts to vomit. *See* **Choking and coughing,** p.526.

The victim's head is turned to one side.

The arm and leg on that side are bent. The other arm and leg remain straight.

521

Breathing stoppage: the Silvester method

The Silvester method of artificial respiration is used if facial injuries prevent mouth-to-mouth resuscitation (*see* p.518).

If external cardiac compression (heart massage) is also required, first aid is best given by two persons. One performs the Silvester method at the same time as the other gives cardiac compression. *See* **Heart attack 2,** p.556.

Maintain a clear airway throughout the procedure. Vomiting may occur as the victim recovers, and the victim's mouth must be kept clear of vomit at all times.

Get someone to summon medical assistance.

Action
Before using the Silvester method, check that breathing really has ceased by listening at the victim's mouth and nose and by looking for movement of the chest.

Check the victim's pulse by feeling the neck between the angle of the jaw and the windpipe. If no pulse can be felt, call for help immediately and *see* **Heart attack 2,** p.556.

Lay the victim face upwards on a hard, flat surface, such as the floor.

If you are alone and external cardiac compression is needed, you must give five firm presses over the victim's heart with the heel of your hand for each sequence of the Silvester method.

Press firmly on the victim's chest over the middle of the breastbone, but avoid sudden movements. The chest will compress as you lean on it and you will feel it expand again naturally as you remove your weight.

Do not use the Silvester method:
If the victim's mouth or nose is clear and you can use mouth-to-mouth resuscitation. *See* **The kiss of life,** p.518.

Follow the instructions carefully. Act as quickly as possible.

Keep calm. Concentrate on regular movements.

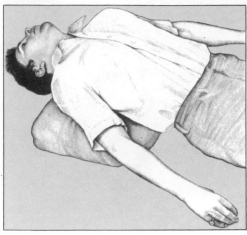

1
Lay the victim face upwards.

Turn the head to one side and remove obvious obstructions to the airflow through the nose and mouth. When the air passages are clear, turn the head face-upwards again.

Support the victim's shoulders with a soft object, such as a folded coat, so that the neck is extended and the head tilted back.

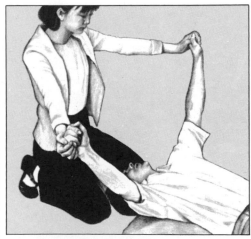

4
Lean backwards. Draw the victim's arms towards you in a sweeping movement, taking them outwards and down by your sides.

Observe the victim's chest as you bring the arms backwards. The chest should rise and you should notice air passing in through the victim's mouth or nose.

If this does not happen, check the airway.

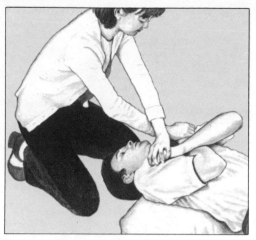

2
Kneel at the victim's head.

Grasp both wrists with your hands.

Place the victim's hands on the middle of the chest, over the breastbone.

Lean forwards so that your weight on the victim's hands compresses the chest. This pressure forces air out of the lungs.

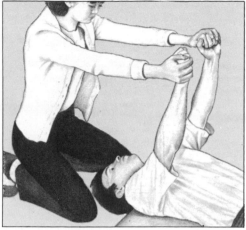

3
Release your pressure on the victim's chest and rock back to an upright position, raising the victim's arms in front of you.

This is the first of three movements which expand the victim's rib-cage and admit air into the lungs.

It is important to perform the three movements in a smooth sequence.

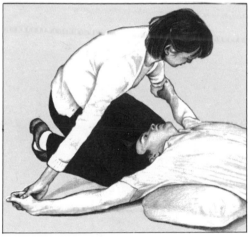

5
Stretch the victim's arms backwards so that they are held on the floor at your sides.

Take the victim's arms from this position in a smooth movement back again on to the victim's lower chest, over the breastbone, in order to begin the cycle again.

Each cycle of movements should be repeated every five seconds.

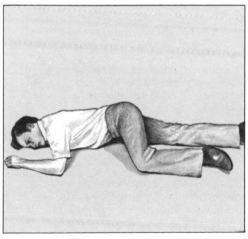

6
This sequence should be continued until medical help arrives or until the victim starts to breathe again unaided.

When breathing starts and the heart is beating unaided, place the victim in the recovery position (*see* p.544) if possible, with one arm and one leg bent, with the head turned to the side, and with the other arm and leg straight.

Burns and scalds

Burns are caused by contact with dry heat. Scalds result from contact with moist heat.

The effects of burns and scalds are similar.

In first-degree burns, the damage is limited to the outer layer of the skin, resulting in redness, warmth, an occasional blister, and tenderness. Mild sunburn is an example of a first-degree burn.

In second-degree burns, the injury goes through the outer layer and involves the deeper layers of skin, causing blisters.

In third-degree burns, the full thickness of skin is destroyed and a charred layer of seared tissue is exposed.

The seriousness of a burn depends on the surface area burned as well as on the depth of the burn.

Action

The aims of first aid are to reduce the effect of heat on the skin; to relieve pain; to prevent fluid loss; to prevent infection; to treat for shock; and to summon emergency medical aid. Correct first aid is essential for rapid recovery.

If the victim's clothing is alight, push the victim to the ground and move him or her away from the flames immediately.

When smothering the clothing, do not use highly inflammable material such as nylon. If necessary, roll the victim over to smother burning clothing.

If the victim's clothing has not caught alight but is smouldering, remove it at once and extinguish the smouldering.

Do not remove burned clothing once the flames have been extinguished. The burned clothing helps to protect against infection and prevents fluid loss. Also, the burned clothing may adhere to the wound. Its removal is painful and requires expert medical supervision.

If the victim's clothing is saturated with hot liquid, remove the clothes quickly but carefully.

The victim will be in a state of shock. *See* **Shock,** p.556.

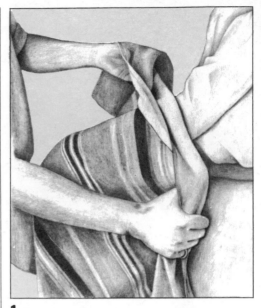

1
If the victim's clothing is on fire, push the victim to the ground. Use a large piece of material, such as a blanket, rug, or coat, to smother the flames.

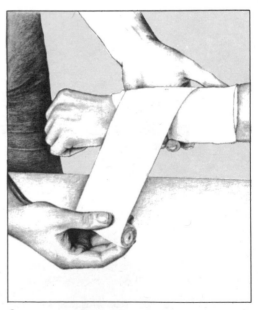

4
Cover the burned area with a sterile dressing. If none is available, use a clean dry sheet.

Touch the burned area as little as possible. **Do not** apply any lotions or ointments.

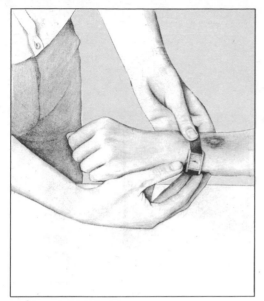

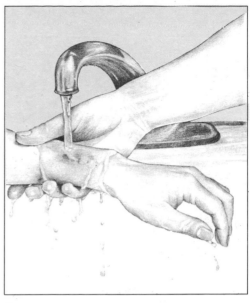

2
If possible, remove any restrictive items, such as rings, bracelets, belts, and shoes.

The burned area may swell later, and it may then be impossible to remove such items.

3
For first-degree burns, keep the burned area under cold, running water for at least ten minutes or until the pain has subsided. **Do not** immerse second-degree or third-degree burns in water.

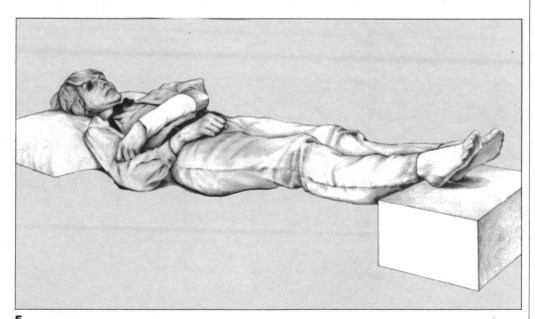

5
If the victim is conscious, administer small, cold drinks at frequent intervals. **Do not** give alcohol.

If unconscious, the victim should be placed in such a position as to maintain a clear airway. If possible, raise the burned area and the victim's legs above the level of the head to reduce the effects of shock. Summon emergency medical aid.

Choking and coughing

Choking is the interruption of breathing caused by an obstruction in the airway. The most common cause is food lodged in the windpipe. When this happens, fatal asphyxiation can occur in less than four minutes.

Another cause of choking is muscle spasms that result from inhaling poisonous fumes.

Many of the signs of choking resemble those of a heart attack. The unmistakable sign of choking is the inability to speak. The victim may also be coughing, and obviously struggling for breath. Lack of sufficient oxygen causes the victim's face to turn purple and then blue in colour.

An acute asthmatic attack may also cause the victim to choke and cough.

Action

If choking is caused by poisonous fumes or smoke, remove the victim to fresh air immediately.

If the victim is in an enclosed space, get additional help if possible. Before entering breathe in and out several times, then take a deep breath and hold it.

Go in and get the victim out. If the victim can not be removed at once, cut off the source of danger; open all windows and doors and get out. Do not take a breath until it is safe to do so. Return to remove the victim as soon as it is safe to do so.

Ensure that the victim's airway is clear.

Loosen all clothing around the victim's neck, chest, and waist.

If the victim has stopped breathing, give artificial respiration. *See* **Breathing stoppage: the kiss of life,** p.518.

If the victim's heart has stopped, use cardiac massage. *See* **Heart attack 2,** p.556.

If choking is caused by an asthmatic attack: get the victim to clasp the hands together, and with the palms outwards brace the arms against a table or a wall so that the rib-cage is expanded.

Allow the victim to use an inhaler or to take any tablets that a doctor has prescribed.

Summon emergency medical help if the inhaler or tablets do not relieve the symptoms.

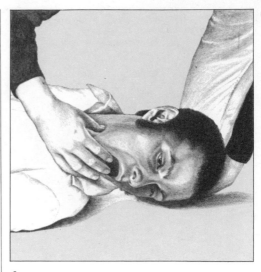

1
To clear the airway turn the victim's head to one side.

Using your fingers, remove any obvious obstructions, such as dentures or food.

If an obstruction cannot be removed by hand, it must be forced out.

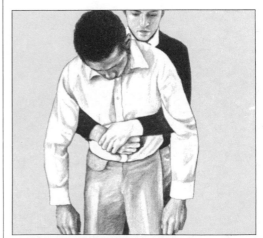

4
To remove an obstruction from an adult, try slapping the victim hard on the back two or three times. If this does not work, stand behind the victim with the arms firmly around the lower part of the victim's chest.

Make a fist with one hand and grasp it firmly with the other hand. Both hands should be placed centrally just below the victim's ribs.

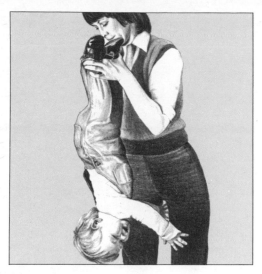

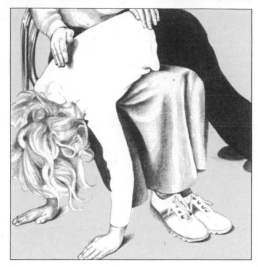

2
To remove an obstruction from a baby, hold the baby upside down.

Give the baby four sharp blows between the shoulders, using the heel of the hand.

When the obstruction is out, give artificial respiration if the baby is not breathing.

3
To remove an obstruction from a child, sit down and hold the child over the knees.

Strike the child smartly between the shoulders three or four times, using the heel of the hand.

When the obstruction is out, give artificial respiration if the child is not breathing.

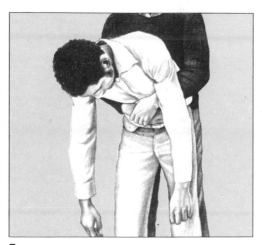

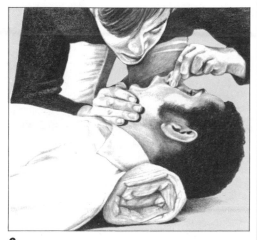

5
The victim should be leaning forwards with the head and arms hanging down.

Give a firm, inward and upward thrust against the victim's abdomen.

It may be necessary to repeat this manoeuvre a few times in order to force the victim to cough up the obstruction.

6
When the obstruction is out, give artificial respiration if the victim is not breathing.

When choking has been relieved and normal breathing has been restored, lay the victim in the recovery position. *See* **Fainting,** p.544.

Summon emergency medical aid or take the victim to hospital.

Convulsions

A convulsion is a sudden, usually violent, involuntary muscle contraction. A convulsive seizure is a series of such contractions.

Convulsions may be caused by a high fever, particularly in children under the age of two; head injury; drug overdose, poisoning; low blood sugar in diabetics; alcohol withdrawal; infection; or grand mal epilepsy.

Convulsive seizures resemble epileptic seizures and are treated in the same way, except convulsions caused by a head injury. With head injury, treat the victim as for shock, and summon emergency medical aid. *See* **Shock and heatstroke** p.566.

If the convulsions are caused by poisoning, drug overdose, diabetes, or a head injury, the victim may not recover consciousness after the convulsion. Summon emergency medical aid immediately.

Action

Before an epileptic seizure the victim may have a brief premonition of it, called an "aura". If possible, help the victim to lie down before he or she collapses.

The violent muscular actions usually begin after a brief period of rigidity. Move away any furniture that the victim could hurt himself or herself on.

An epileptic seizure lasts for about a minute. Then the victim relaxes and may go into a trance-like state, or fall asleep. **Do not** restrain the victim during the seizure.

When the movements have stopped, examine the victim for any injuries that may have been sustained during the seizure. Stay with the victim, who may be distressed and confused. Ask bystanders to keep away.

Allow the victim to sleep. When the victim wakes, advise him or her to consult a doctor.

If the victim is not breathing when the convulsions have stopped, check that the tongue is not blocking the airway. If the airway is clear and the victim is still not breathing, give artificial resuscitation. *See* **Breathing stoppage: the kiss of life,** p.518.

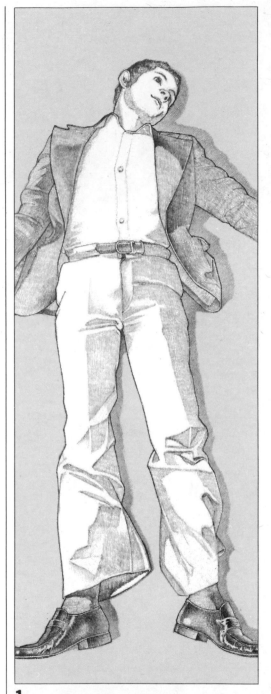

1
At the beginning of an epileptic attack, the victim loses consciousness and falls down, sometimes with a cry as air is forced out of the lungs. The victim may then become rigid for a few seconds. This is usually followed by convulsions, and noisy breathing.

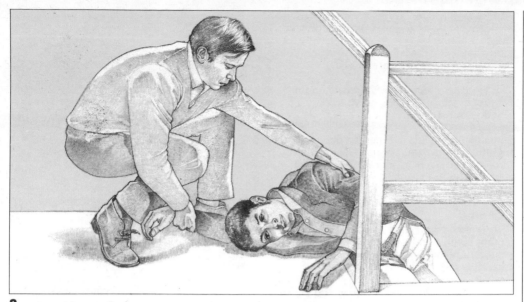

2

Lower the victim to the ground before he or she falls down.

Do not attempt to stop the convulsions by forcibly restraining the victim, because this may injure the victim.

Guide the victim away from any hazards so that the victim will not injure himself or herself. The jaw may be clenched and bloodstained froth may appear in the mouth. **Do not** attempt to force open the mouth of a person who is having convulsions.

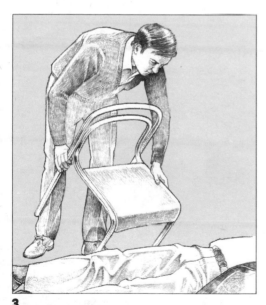

3

Remove any dangeous objects.

When the convulsions have finished, loosen the victim's clothing around the neck, chest, and waist, and place the victim in the recovery position. *See* **Fainting,** p.544.

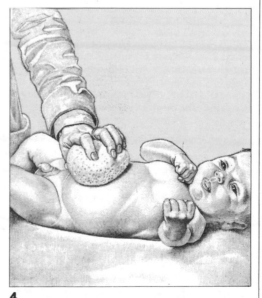

4

If a fever causes a child to have convulsions, follow the same procedure outlined on these pages. When the convulsions have stopped, sponge the child's body with tepid water.

Consult a doctor as soon as possible.

Dangerous plants

Although only a few plants are dangerous, no plant should be eaten unless you are certain that it is harmless. This applies especially to mushrooms and toadstools, because harmless and poisonous varieties are similar.

The symptoms of poisoning depend on the amount eaten and on the individual's reaction to the poison.

Some plants contain substances that are harmful only to those who are sensitive to them. Other plants irritate the skin. Initial contact does not give immunity but instead increases susceptibility.

Action

If the victim has been in contact with an irritant plant, ensure that your hands are protected before removing the victim's contaminated clothing.

Do not touch other parts of the victim's body, especially the eyes.

Wash the affected area several times with soap and water and apply calamine lotion.

If the victim has eaten a poisonous plant or mushroom, summon emergency medical aid.

If the victim is conscious:
Ask which plant was eaten.

Induce vomiting by making the victim drink a glass of salt water, or mustard and water. Tickling the throat will also cause vomiting. Save any specimen of vomit for medical analysis. **Do not** induce vomiting if the victim is having fits. *See* **Convulsions, p.528.**

Give milk or water to drink, to dilute the substance.

If the victim is unconscious:
Place the victim in the recovery position. **Do not** leave the victim alone. **Do not** give any food or drink. **Do not** induce vomiting.

If the victim stops breathing, give artificial resuscitation. *See* **Breathing stoppage: the kiss of life, p.518.**

If the victim's heart stops, get a trained person to apply external cardiac massage. *See* **Heart attack 2, p.556.**

If the victim starts to have fits, *see* **Convulsions, p.528.**

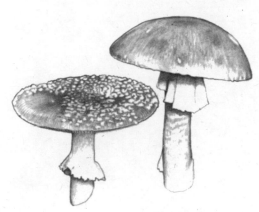

Death cap
Amanita phalloides
All parts are poisonous.
Symptoms of poisoning
Abdominal pain; nausea; vomiting; excessive thirst; jaundice; convulsions.

Fly agaric
Amanita muscaria
All parts are poisonous.
Symptoms of poisoning
Diarrhoea; vomiting; delirium; convulsions.

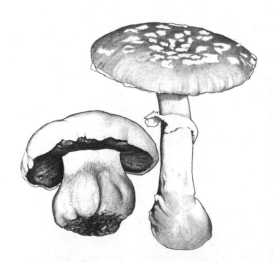

Devil's boletus
Boletus satanus
All parts are poisonous.
Symptoms of poisoning
Nausea; vomiting; diarrhoea.

Panther cap
Amanita pantherina
All parts are poisonous.
Symptoms of poisoning
Abdominal pain; nausea; vomiting; diarrhoea.

Table of dangerous plants

NAME	POISONOUS PARTS	SYMPTOMS OF POISONING
Aconite (monkshood)	Roots; leaves; seeds.	Nausea; vomiting; slow pulse; burning sensation in the mouth, throat, and skin; collapse.
Baneberry	Roots; sap; berries.	Vomiting; rapid pulse; diarrhoea.
Berberis	Berries.	Nausea; vomiting; diarrhoea.
Broom	All parts are poisonous, but only in large amounts.	Burning sensation in the mouth; nausea; vomiting; diarrhoea.
Cherry	Stones if broken and swallowed.	Headache; difficulty in breathing; vomiting; lack of co-ordination; dilation of the pupils; unconsciousness.
Daffodil	Bulbs.	Nausea; vomiting; diarrhoea.
Daphne	Bark; leaves; berries.	Burning sensation in the mouth and stomach; severe cramp.
Deadly nightshade (belladonna)	Roots; leaves; seeds.	Dry mouth; dilation of the pupils; irregular heart-beat; nausea; vomiting; coma.
Elderberry	Leaves; bark.	Headache; difficulty in breathing; vomiting; lack of co-ordination; dilation of the pupils; unconsciousness.
Foxglove	Leaves; seeds.	Dizziness; nausea; vomiting; slow pulse.
Hellebore	Roots; leaves; seeds.	Salivation; abdominal pain; clammy skin; coma.
Hemlock	Leaves; fruit.	Burning sensation in the mouth; slow pulse; paralysis; coma.
Holly	Berries.	Nausea; vomiting; diarrhoea; drowsiness.
Hydrangea	All parts are poisonous.	Headache; difficulty in breathing; vomiting; lack of co-ordination; dilation of the pupils; unconsciousness.
Laburnum	All parts are poisonous.	Burning sensation in the mouth; nausea; continual vomiting; diarrhoea; collapse; delirium; convulsions; coma.
Larkspur	Leaves; seeds.	Tingling sensation in the mouth; agitation; severe depression.
Lily of the valley	Roots; leaves; fruit.	Irregular pulse; nausea; vomiting; dizziness.
Lupin	Seeds.	Difficulty in breathing; paralysis; convulsions; collapse.
Mistletoe	All parts are poisonous.	Nausea; vomiting; diarrhoea; slow pulse.
Yew	All parts are poisonous.	Abdominal pain; nausea; vomiting; diarrhoea; difficulty in breathing.

Drowning

Drowning is suffocation in water or some other liquid. It occurs when liquid prevents air from reaching the lungs and entering the blood.

Many deaths are caused every year by drowning. It can happen in a swimming pool or bath as easily as in the sea, especially to small children.

Do not leave young children unattended near any body of water.

Even expert swimmers can get into difficulty while swimming. **Do not** go swimming alone.

A drowning person may be blue around the lips and cheeks, and there may be froth coming out of the mouth and nose.

The victim may be gasping for breath, or may have stopped breathing completely.

Action

A drowning person may be in a state of panic and may endanger the rescuer's life.

Do not attempt to rescue a drowning person if you are alone, unless you are trained in water rescue and life-saving techniques.

Ask someone to contact the coastguard, the inshore rescue service or the police while you keep the victim's position pinpointed.

If emergency help is not available, throw a line or extend a pole or branch toward the victim. If the water is of standing depth and there are other people in the vicinity, summon their help to make a human chain out to the victim.

Do not attempt to drain water out of the victim's lungs.

The victim may be suffering from shock. *See* **Shock,** p.566.

Keep the victim warm with blankets or clothing.

Do not give the victim alcohol to drink. Expert medical attention is necessary, even if the victim seems to have made a complete recovery, because near-drowning may lead to serious complications, such as pneumonia and heart problems.

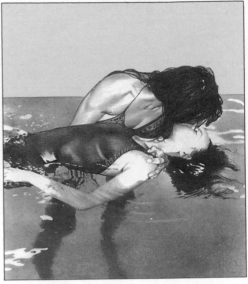

1

It is important to begin artificial respiration as soon as possible. *See* **Breathing stoppage: the kiss of life,** p.518.

Continue to resuscitate the victim while wading ashore.

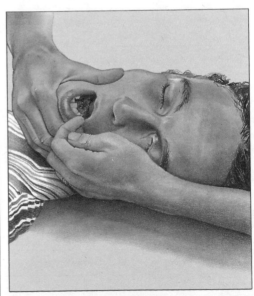

3

When ashore, clear the victim's airway of any obvious obstruction, using two fingers. *See* **Choking and coughing,** p.526.

Lift the victim's neck and tilt the head back so the tongue does not block the throat.

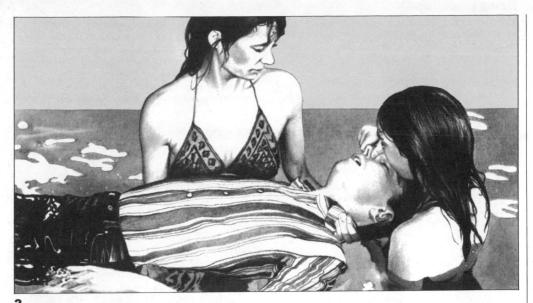

2
If other people are available, give artificial respiration once you are in shallow water. One person should support the victim's head and body while another gives mouth-to-mouth resuscitation. *See* **Breathing stoppage: the kiss of life,** p.518.

If you are alone, it is best to get the victim ashore as quickly as possible and begin artificial respiration there.

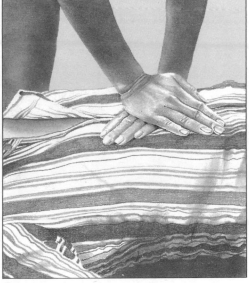

4
If the victim's heart has stopped, give heart massage. *See* **Heart attack 2,** p.556.

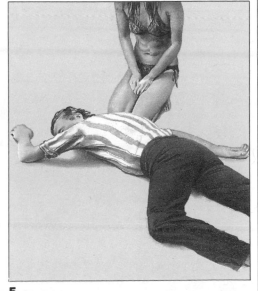

5
When the victim's heart-beat and breathing have been restored but are still weak, place him or her in the recovery position.

Do not leave the victim alone: the breathing may stop again.

Drug overdose

Many drugs cause extreme drowsiness or even unconsciousness if too much is taken at one time. An overdose may also result from taking small doses too frequently.

In many cases, the initial signs of a drug overdose are vomiting, restlessness, and lack of co-ordination. These symptoms are often followed by unconsciousness.

If a single large dose has been taken at one time, the symptoms usually appear rapidly.

If an overdose has been caused by taking small doses too frequently, the symptoms are likely to appear gradually over a longer period, and may be more difficult to recognise.

Action

The first aid treatment of a drug overdose is the same for all drugs.

Act swiftly. If time is wasted, more of the drug will be absorbed.

Do not leave the victim alone. Ask somebody else to summon emergency medical aid.

If the victim is conscious, ask what happened.

Try to keep the victim conscious. If the victim is a child only give milk or water to drink. Watch that the child does not choke if vomiting occurs.

If the victim is unconscious, place in the recovery position. *See* **Fainting,** p.544.

If the victim vomits while unconscious, check that the victim's air passage is clear. *See* **Choking and coughing,** p.526.

An overdose of some drugs may cause convulsions. *See* **Convulsions,** p.528.

Look for evidence to determine whether the victim has taken a drug.

There may be pills in the victim's mouth, or empty pill containers nearby. Drug addicts may have a hypodermic syringe; they may also have needle marks on their skin, usually on the inside of the forearm.

Keep pill containers, pills, and specimens of the victim's vomit. These will help in finding out which drug has been taken.

An overdose of diuretics will cause the victim to lose a large amount of water in the urine.

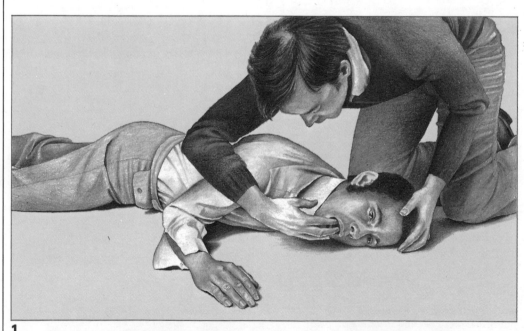

1
If the victim is conscious, induce vomiting by putting your fingers down the victim's throat. **Do not** give salt water to drink. This may be positively harmful.

Do not attempt to induce vomiting if the victim is unconscious, nor if the victim has taken a drug overdose by either injection or by inhalation.

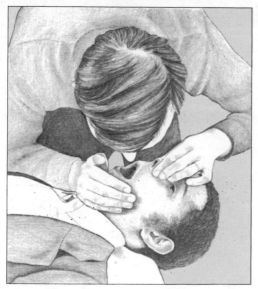

2
Keep a close check on the victim's breathing and pulse at all times.

If the victim stops breathing, give artificial resuscitation. *See* **Breathing stoppage: the kiss of life,** p.518.

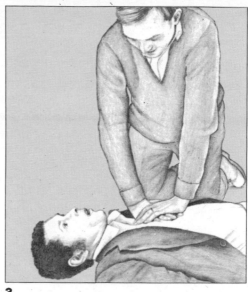

3
If the victim's heart stops, give heart massage. *See* **Heart attack 2,** p.556. If the victim has also stopped breathing and help is unavailable, you will have to alternate between heart massage and resuscitation.

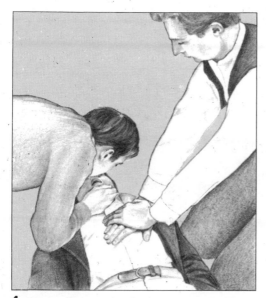

4
If the victim's heart and breathing have both stopped and help is available, one person should kneel at the victim's shoulder and give heart massage; another person should kneel at the victim's other side and give mouth-to-mouth resuscitation.

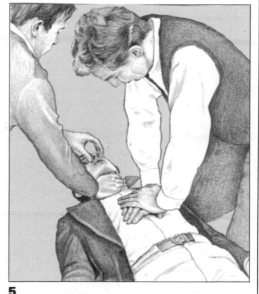

5
The person giving heart massage should press the victim's chest at a rate of 15 times in 11 seconds. Only a trained person should use this method. The person giving resuscitation should ventilate twice within 15 seconds.

Drug overdose 2

NAME	EXAMPLES	SIGNS AND SYMPTOMS OF OVERDOSAGE
Alcohol	Beers; wines; spirits.	Changes of mood; lack of co-ordination; slurred speech; sweating; rapid pulse; vomiting; drowsiness; and unconsciousness.
Amphetamines	Durophet*.	Excitement; dilated pupils; talkativeness; insomnia; tremors; exaggerated reflexes; bad breath; vomiting; diarrhoea; fever; irregular, rapid heart rate; hallucinations; delirium; convulsions; and unconsciousness.
Anticoagulants	Marevan*; Tromexan*; Dindevan*.	Nosebleeds; pallor; bleeding gums; bruising; blood in the urine and faeces; shock; and coma.
Antidepressants	1) Tricyclic compounds – Tofranil*; Tryptizol* 2) MAO inhibitors – Nardil*; Parnate*; Marsilid*.	1) Dry mouth; dilated pupils; vomiting; irregular heart rate; retention of urine; hallucinations; lack of co-ordination; exaggerated reflexes; agitation; convulsions and unconsciousness. 2) Agitation; hallucinations; exaggerated reflexes; irregular heart rate; sweating; retention of urine; convulsions; and muscular rigidity.
Antihistamines	Piriton*; Phenergan*; Histryl*.	Excitement or depression; drowsiness; headache; irregular heart rate; nervousness; disorientation; lack of co-ordination; high fever; hallucinations; fixed, dilated pupils; delirium; convulsions; and coma.
Atropine	Hyoscyamine; scopolamine.	Dry mouth; hot, dry skin; flushing; high fever; dilated pupils; irregular heart rate; excitement; confusion; convulsions; delirium; and unconsciousness.
Barbiturates	Amytal*; Nembutal*; Seconal*; phenobarbitone.	Drowsiness; headache; confusion; lack of co-ordination; slurred speech; lack of reflexes; slow breathing rate; and coma.
Benzodiazepines	Librium*; Valium*; Mogadon*.	Drowsiness; dizziness; lack of co-ordination; and, in rare cases, coma.
Caffeine	Coffee; tea.	Restlessness; excitement; frequent urination; rapid pulse; nausea; vomiting; fever; tremors; delirium; convulsions; and coma.
Cannabis		Overdosage usually causes only sleepiness.
Chloral hydrate	Noctec*.	An overdose of chloral hydrate produces symptoms similar to those of a barbiturate overdose, but chloral hydrate may also cause vomiting.
Cocaine		Stimulation followed by depression; nausea; vomiting; anxiety; hallucinations; sweating; difficulty breathing; and convulsions.

536   *= trade-name*

NAME	EXAMPLES	SIGNS AND SYMPTOMS OF OVERDOSAGE
Contraceptive pill		Overdose may cause nausea and vomiting. It does not usually require emergency medical aid, but it is advisable to consult a doctor.
Digitalis	Lanoxin*; Digoxin.	Vomiting; excessive salivation; diarrhoea; drowsiness; confusion; irregular heart rate; delirium; hallucinations; and unconsciousness.
Diuretics	Hygroton*; Lasix*; Edecrin*; thiazides.	Massive urine output and irregular heart rate. Rarely there may also be skin rashes and abnormal sensitivity to light.
Glutethimide	Doriden*.	Drowsiness; lack of reflexes; pupil dilation; slow breathing rate; and coma.
Hallucinogens	LSD; psilocybin; STP; DMT; mescaline.	The symptoms of an overdose are not readily distinguishable from the normal effects of these drugs, which vary between individuals. The effects include hallucinations; nausea; and lack of co-ordination. In some cases, there may be extreme anxiety and delusions.
Heroin and related drugs	Opium; morphine; methadone; pethidine.	Pinpoint pupils; drowsiness; shallow breathing; muscular relaxation; coma; slow pulse and respiratory arrest.
Ipecacuanha	Ipecac syrup.	Nausea; vomiting, sometimes bloodstained; diarrhoea; abdominal cramps; irregular heart rate; and cardiac arrest.
Iron		Nausea; vomiting, sometimes bloodstained; abdominal pain; pallor; headache; confusion; convulsions; and unconsciousness.
Meprobamate	Equanil*; Miltown*.	Drowsiness; relaxation and muscular weakness; sleep; lack of reflexes; and coma.
Paracetamol	Panadol*; Calpol*.	Nausea; vomiting; pallor; sweating; kidney failure; jaundice; difficulty breathing; delirium; and unconsciousness.
Phenothiazines	Chlorpromazine; prochlorperazine; trifluoperazine.	Sleepiness; dry mouth; lack of co-ordination; muscular rigidity; tremors; uncontrollable facial grimacing; low body temperature; irregular heart rate; convulsions; and coma.
Quinine	Antimalarial drugs.	Vomiting; deafness; blurred vision; dilated pupils; headache; dizziness; rapid breathing; irregular heart rate; and unconsciousness.
Rauwolfia alkaloids	Reserpine; Serpasil*.	Flushing; dry mouth; abdominal cramps; diarrhoea; irregular heart rate; tremors; muscular rigidity; and unconsciousness.
Salicylates	Aspirin and many aspirin-containing pain-killers.	Abdominal pain; nausea; vomiting; restlessness; noises in the ears; deafness; deep, rapid breathing; fever; sweating; irritability; confusion; delirium; convulsions; and coma.

Electric shock

The effects of an electric shock can be extremely severe. A high voltage electric shock may cause irregular beating of the heart, or may stop the heart completely. The victim may also stop breathing, and suffer burns.

A high voltage electric shock may also cause a sudden muscle spasm that may throw the victim away from the power source with extreme force, resulting in further injuries, such as fractures.

Lightning causes similar injuries to those of a high voltage electric current.

Do not attempt to rescue the victim if he or she is still in contact with, or is close to a high voltage electric current. Insulating material, such as rubber or dry wood, will not protect you against such high voltages.

Summon the police and emergency medical aid.

Remain at least 18 metres (60ft) from the victim. Wait until having been officially informed that it is safe before giving first-aid.

Action

Check whether the victim is in contact with a low or a high voltage current. The domestic power supply is a low voltage current. It is generally safe to attempt to rescue the victim provided the correct precautions are taken.

Summon emergency medical aid.

If the victim is not breathing, give mouth-to-mouth resuscitation. *See* **Breathing stoppage: the kiss of life,** p.518.

If the victim's heart has stopped, give heart massage. *See* **Heart attack 2,** p.556.

If the victim is unconscious, turn into the recovery position. *See* **Fainting,** p.544.

Control any serious bleeding. *See* **Bleeding,** p. 516.

Treat any burns that the victim may have sustained. *See* **Burns,** p.524.

Examine the victim for other injuries, and give the appropriate first-aid treatment.

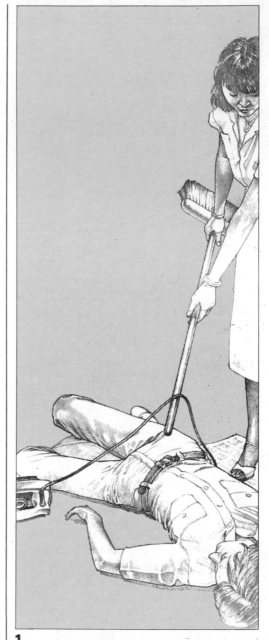

1
Do not touch a victim who is still in contact with the power supply. Switch off the current; remove the plug or fuse; or tear the cable free. If this is impossible, stand on some dry insulating material, such as wood or newspaper. Break the electrical contact by using dry wood, a piece of rubber or plastic, or a folded newspaper.

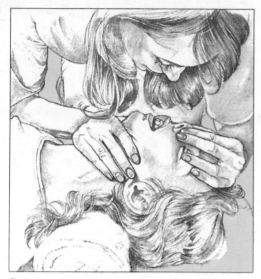

2
Keep a close check on the victim's breathing and heart-beat.

If the victim is not breathing, give artificial resuscitation. *See* **Breathing stoppage: the kiss of life,** p.518.

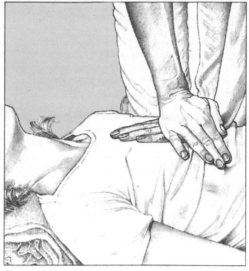

3
If the victim's heart has stopped, give heart massage. *See* **Heart attack 2,** p.556. If the victim has also stopped breathing and help is unavailable, you will have to alternate between heart massage and mouth-to-mouth resuscitation.

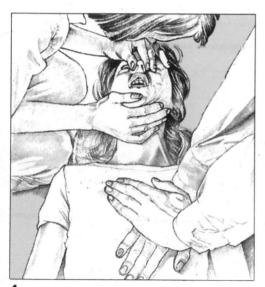

4
If the victim's heart and breathing have both stopped and help is available, one person should kneel at the victim's left shoulder and give heart massage; the other person should kneel at the victim's other side and give mouth-to-mouth resuscitation.

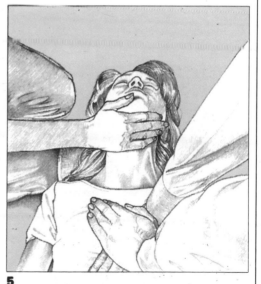

5
The person giving heart massage should press the victim's chest over the area of the heart at a rate slightly faster than once a second. The person giving artificial resuscitation should ventilate the victim's lungs once every five seconds.

Emergency delivery of a baby 1

Labour is divided into three stages.
During the first stage regular abdominal
pains begin, becoming longer and stronger
as labour progresses. There may be a low
backache and a discharge of bloodstained
mucus. The "breaking of waters" may also
occur during this stage when clear fluid
(the amniotic fluid) is expelled. This first
stage may last several hours, but is usually
shorter if the mother has had children
previously. The second stage is the birth
of the baby. The third stage is the delivery of
the afterbirth (placenta).

Action

Keep calm, there is usually ample time to
prepare for the birth. Summon medical
assistance. If medical help is on its way,
collect the mother's belongings ready for
transfer to hospital. If aid is unlikely to
arrive in time, prepare to help with the birth.

If in a public place, find somewhere which
provides privacy and is quiet and warm. It
is essential that everything is scrupulously
clean. Nobody with a cold or any other
infection should help. Scrub your hands
thoroughly, preferably under running water.
If they become dirty later, wash them again.

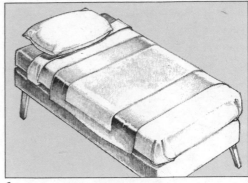

1

Prepare a clean surface, preferably a bed,
for the mother to lie on.

Protect the surface with a sheet of plastic
or newspapers covered with a clean towel
or sheet.

Ask the mother to empty her bladder; if it
is full, labour will be impeded. Do not
allow her to use the lavatory because the
birth may occur suddenly.

Assist the mother to the bed.

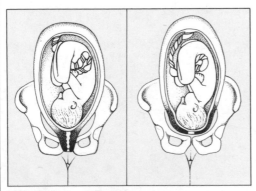

What the contractions mean

The abdominal pains during labour are
caused by regular contractions of the
womb. In all mothers these contractions
become more frequent as labour
progresses, occurring two minutes or less
apart when a birth is imminent. But there
are many exceptions and the frequency of
contractions is not a reliable indication of
the imminence of childbirth.
    The effect of the contractions is to
gradually dilate the birth canal until it is
wide enough to allow the baby's head to
pass through. The contractions also push
the baby downwards.

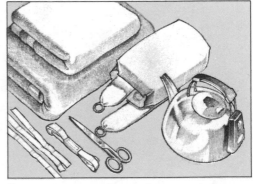

3

There should now be plenty of time to
gather the things you will need for the
birth and after delivery.

Blankets or towels to wrap the baby in.

Swabs or clean handkerchiefs.

Sanitary towels.

Scissors and three pieces of cloth tape.

Boiling water in which to sterilise the tape
and scissors.

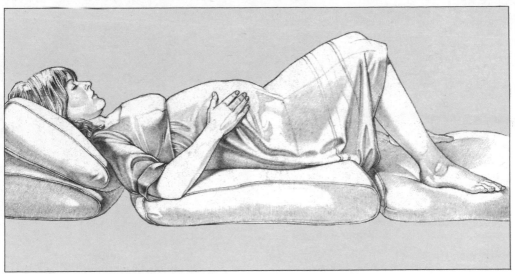

2

During the first stage of labour, the amnion (a sac surrounding the baby) may rupture, resulting in a sudden flow of clear fluid. Do not be alarmed, this is quite normal. Lay the mother on her back in the position shown, and remove all her clothing from the waist downwards.

Cover the mother with a blanket.

Ask the mother to bend her knees and let them fall apart.

Encourage the mother to relax between each contraction.

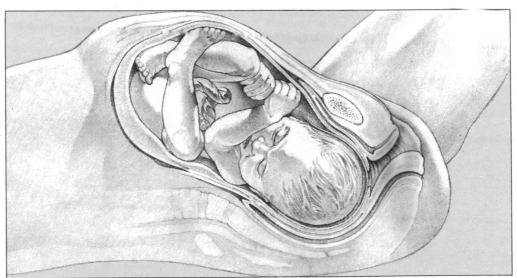

4

Contractions will now last longer and be stronger; the mother will want to bear down with each contraction.

Tell the mother to push with each contraction and to relax in between.

She may have a bowel movement during a contraction. If so, wipe it away from the front backwards. Do not dirty the birth canal.

Remember your hands must be clean; if they get dirty, wash them again.

Emergency delivery of a baby 2

By the start of the second stage of labour the birth canal is fully dilated and the top of the baby's head is soon visible. Tell the mother to continue to push. When most of the baby's head has emerged, the mother should not bear down and should not hold her breath during the contractions. Ask the mother to pant; this allows the rest of the baby's head to emerge slowly. The head of a newborn baby may be misshapen. Do not be alarmed, the head has been temporarily deformed by its passage through the birth canal and it eventually reverts to normal shape.

The contractions recommence shortly after the delivery of the baby; this is the third stage of labour: the delivery of the afterbirth (placenta). **Do not** try to speed up this process by pulling on the umbilical cord.

Action

Do not interfere with the progress of the birth by attempting to pull the baby out.

If a membrane is covering the baby's face, it must be carefully torn.

If the baby emerges with the umbilical cord around the neck, try to ease the cord over the head. Take great care not to stretch or break the cord.

Rarely the baby's buttocks, foot, or arm may emerge first. If so, do not interfere. If any part other than the head emerges first, make arrangements for immediate careful transportation to hospital.

Sometimes the labour continues. This may mean that the mother is having twins. If the placenta has already been delivered, the newborn baby should be wrapped and left, with the cord uncut, while the second baby is born. If the placenta has not been delivered, the appearance of the second baby, either head or buttocks first, means that the twins share the same placenta and are identical. Treat the second delivery as a normal labour and, in the third stage, deliver the placenta, which will have two cords, in the usual way. When both babies and placentas have been delivered, the cords can be tied and cut.

If there is much bleeding after childbirth, place a sanitary towel in position, raise the mother's legs and gently massage her abdomen just below the navel. This stimulates the womb to contract and should stop the bleeding. If the bleeding does not stop, urgent medical assistance is required.

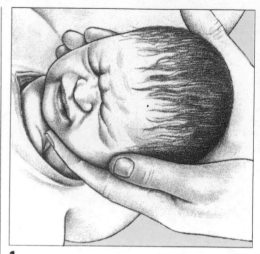

1

The baby is usually born head-first. As the head emerges ask the mother to stop bearing down and to start panting. This allows the head to emerge slowly.

Do not interfere with the baby's head, only support it gently with cupped hands.

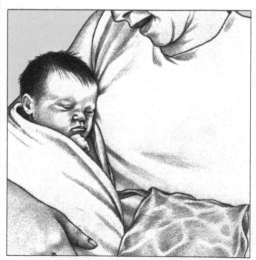

4

The baby can now be wrapped in a blanket, and placed by the mother's side. Remember, the baby is still attached to the mother by the cord.

When the placenta has been delivered, wrap it and place it next to the baby. The placenta must be inspected by a doctor.

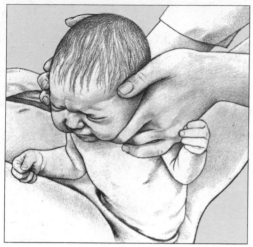

2
The shoulders and body will emerge quickly.
Do not try to pull the baby out.

Hold the baby gently under the armpits and
lift toward the mother's abdomen. The baby
will be slippery, so hold him or her firmly.

Do not pull or stretch the cord.

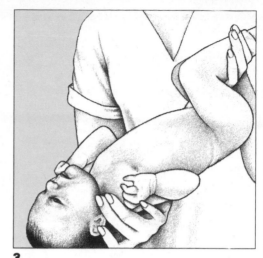

3
Cradle the baby carefully in your arms, with
the head positioned low to allow any fluid to
drain from the nose and mouth.

If the baby does not start to breathe immediately, wipe out the nose and mouth and begin
artificial respiration. *See* **Breathing stoppage:
the kiss of life,** p.518.

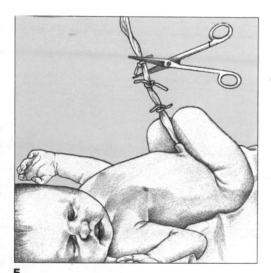

5
Do not cut the cord unless medical help is
unavailable. Wait until the placenta has been
delivered and sterilize a pair of scissors and
three pieces of cloth tape.

Tie the tapes very firmly around the cord at
three places: one 4 inches, one 6 inches, and
one 8 inches from the baby's navel.

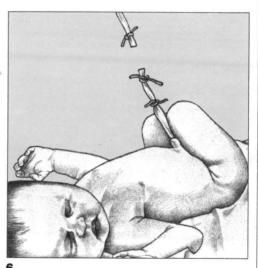

6
Cut the cord between the two ties that are
furthest from the baby's navel.

Inspect the cord at regular intervals to ensure
that no bleeding has occurred.

Wash the mother, wiping her front to back.
Fix a sanitary towel in position.

Fainting

Fainting is a temporary loss of consciousness that occurs when there is an inadequate supply of blood to the brain. A faint may begin with a feeling of giddiness or dizziness, or it may occur as a sudden collapse.

There are many causes of fainting, but although most of them are relatively minor, fainting may be a symptom of an underlying illness. If the victim has not regained consciousness within a few minutes, and completely recovered within fifteen minutes, summon medical help and treat for unconsciousness. *See* **Unconsciousness,** p.573.

If a faint lasts longer than three minutes, its cause may be an underlying illness, and the victim should seek medical advice on recovery.

Action

The aim of first aid is to restore an adequate supply of blood to the brain.

If the person is conscious, ask whether he or she is a diabetic. If so, give the person sugar or any sugar-containing substance; artificial sweeteners will not help.

There may be some warning before a faint. The person may feel unsteady and giddy; the face becomes pale with beads of perspiration appearing; the skin becomes cold and clammy; the pulse feels weak and erratic; and there may be attacks of nausea.

If fainting is imminent: 1) place the person in a sitting or lying position in a current of fresh air.

2) loosen any clothing around the person's neck and waist.

3) instruct the person to lower the head between the knees, to take slow, deep breaths, and to flex the thigh and leg muscles.

If the person is unconscious, 1) lay him or her down in the recovery position and loosen any clothing around the neck and waist.

2) treat any injury which may have been sustained during the faint.

3) when consciousness has been regained, do not allow the victim to stand up immediately. Gradually raise the victim to a sitting position and give sips of water.

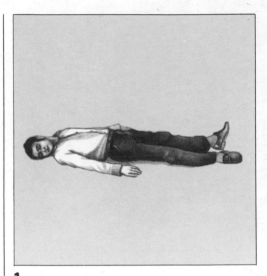

1
To turn the victim into the recovery position, first lay the victim face-up on the ground.

Loosen clothing, especially around the neck and waist. Place the victim's arms beside the body.

Turn the victim's head toward the right side.

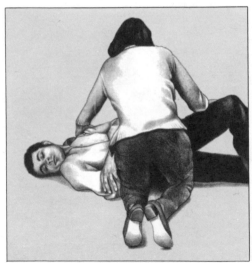

4
Kneel at the victim's right side.

Place your hands on the victim's left thigh and shoulder.

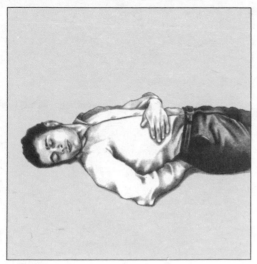

2

Tuck the right arm under the victim's buttock.

Place the victim's left arm across the chest.

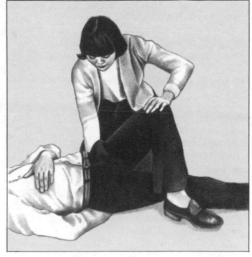

3

Bend the victim's left leg at the knee and cross the left leg over the right leg so that the thigh makes a right angle with the body.

Gently pull the right arm under the victim's body.

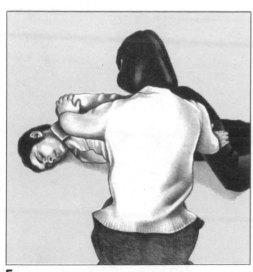

5

Gently pull the victim toward you.

Ensure that the victim's air passage remains free from obstruction throughout the procedure.

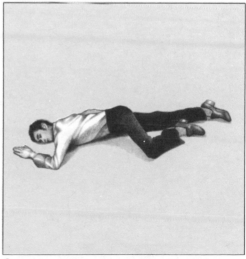

6

For the recovery position, place the victim's left arm on the ground, palm downwards and with the arm bent at the elbow.

Gently lift the victim's head upwards and backwards. With the victim's head turned to one side the air passage should remain clear even if the victim vomits.

Fractures: the arm or elbow

Fractures can be open or closed. Open fractures have wounds from the skin surface to the site of the fracture, or the fractured ends of the bone stick through the skin. With closed fractures, the skin is not broken.

Do not bandage directly over open fractures.

A dislocation is the displacement of the bones at a joint. The signs of both a fracture and a dislocation are similar; deformity of the limb and numbness immediately around the injured area, with pain and tenderness.

Do not give the victim food or drink, in case a general anaesthetic is needed later.

Treat bleeding before treating the fracture. *See* **Bleeding,** p.516.

Action

If there is uncertainty as to whether the injury is a fracture or a dislocation, always treat for a fracture.

Lay the victim down and treat for shock. *See* **Shock,** p.566.

Summon medical help as soon as possible.

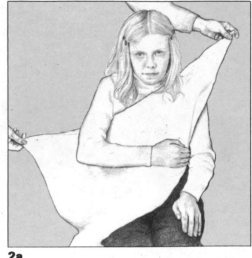

2a

If the arm is found in the bent position or if the elbow can be bent, use a triangular bandage or scarf to make a sling.

Place the bandage with the apex at the victim's elbow, one tip over the opposite shoulder and with the longest edge along the length of the body. Carefully fold the injured arm across the chest.

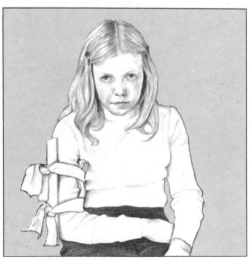

1

Immobilise the fracture by tying a splint on the outside of the victim's injured arm. Use two bandages; one above the fracture, and one below it. The splint should be long enough to extend from above the fracture to well below it. Tie the bandages over the splint on the outside of the victim's arm. Place padding between the arm and the chest.

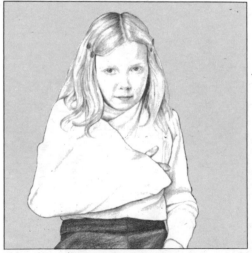

2b

Bring the lowest corner up to the neck and tie the ends on the injured side. Pin the corner at the elbow edge to give more support to the arm.

If the victim has an open fracture, follow the same procedure but apply a clean dressing over any open wound.

Fractures: the hand or finger

When the lower end of the forearm is fractured, there is often little or no deformity. It is a common fracture and may be mistaken for a sprained wrist.

Fractures of the hand and fingers may be complicated by bleeding into the tissues which causes swelling.

Do not bandage over the injury site if the victim has an open fracture. Apply a clean dressing gently over any open wound.

Do not attempt to straighten the injured limb if it is deformed.

Treat bleeding before treating the fracture. *See* **Bleeding,** p.516.

Action

Move the injured arm as little as possible.

Treat any suspected dislocation as a fracture.

Remove jewellery, such as rings, provided this does not aggravate the injury.

If the fracture is closed, an ice pack may be used to prevent further swelling. Do not let ice come into contact with the skin.

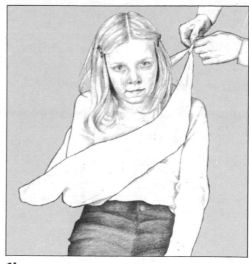

1b

Take the lower corner of the bandage behind the back and over the shoulder.

Pin the corner at the elbow edge to give more support to the arm.

Tie the two ends at the shoulder.

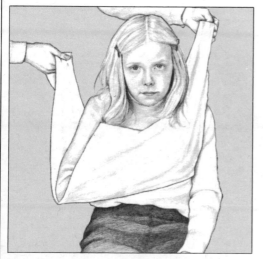

1a

Protect the hand by gently placing it in a fold of soft padding. Fold the injured arm across the chest. Place a triangular bandage over the arm with the apex at the elbow or mid-forearm and the longest side down the length of the body. While supporting the arm, turn the lower part of the bandage under the hand, arm, and elbow.

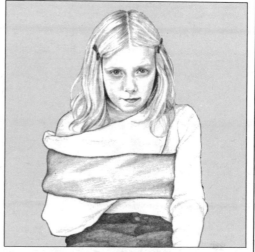

1c

Provide further support for the injured arm by using a broad bandage.

Place the bandage over the sling, around the chest and injured arm, and under the other armpit.

Tie the bandage at the back.

Fractures: the hip, thigh, or knee

Fractures of the hip may be complicated by injury to the organs of the pelvis. **Do not** move the victim, because there may also be injuries to the spine. *See* **Fractures: the spine or ribs,** p.551.

Tell the victim **not** to urinate.

Fractures of the thigh often cause severe internal bleeding. The broken bone may also be protruding through the skin.

Do not try to straighten the fractured bone. **Do not** raise the victim's legs.

Do not give the victim food or drink, in case a general anaesthetic is needed later.

Treat suspected dislocations as fractures.

Action

Treat bleeding before treating the fracture. *See* **Bleeding,** p.516.

Keep the victim lying down and observe the pulse and breathing. If breathing stops, give mouth-to-mouth resuscitation (*see* p.518).

Summon medical aid as soon as possible.

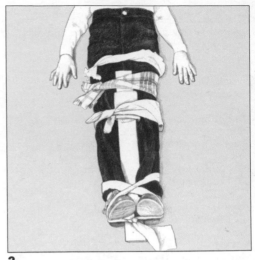

2
With a suspected fracture of the thigh, gently put the victim's legs together with padding between the thighs, knees, and ankles. If a splint is available, pad it and put it between the legs. Using the method described in 1, put broad bandages above and below the fracture and around the knees. Bandage the feet together.

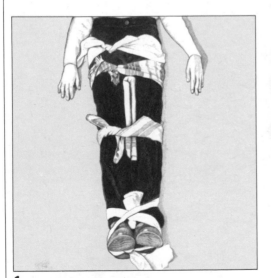

1
With a suspected hip fracture, gently put the victim's legs together with padding between the thighs, knees, and ankles.

Put two broad bandages around the hips, overlapping on the injured side, and one broad bandage around the knees. Wind a narrow bandage around the feet.

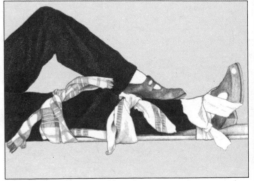

3
With a suspected knee fracture, place a long, padded splint behind the knee. The splint should be long enough to extend from the buttock to beyond the heel. The splint must also be rigid; a length of wood is ideal.

Place further padding between the knee and the splint, and between the ankle and the splint.

To secure the splint, use a broad bandage around the thigh, a broad bandage below the knee, and a narrow bandage around the foot and ankle.

Fractures: the foot, ankle, or toe

Fractures of the foot, ankle, and toe are common injuries, often caused by a fall. They are also relatively minor, so before treating them, make a check for and treat other more serious injuries.

It is often impossible to distinguish between fractures, dislocations, and bad sprains, the obvious sign in all three being swelling. If in doubt, always treat the injury as a fracture.

Do not move the injured limb to test for a possible fracture.

Do not allow the victim to attempt standing on the injured limb.

Treat any bleeding before treating the fracture. *See* **Bleeding,** p.516.

Action
Do not bandage directly over the injury if it is an open fracture.

Summon medical assistance. If it is necessary to transport the victim, a stretcher should be used. For methods of transportation, *see* **Transporting an injured person,** p.568.

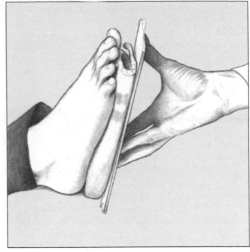

2a

With a suspected fracture of the foot or toe, carefully remove the victim's footwear. Raise the injured foot.

Place a broad padded splint against the sole of the foot. (A pillow could be used or a folded newspaper with a scarf as the padding.)

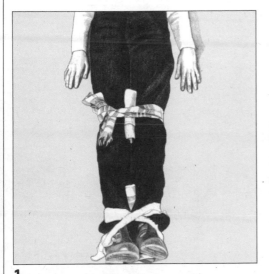

1

With a suspected fracture of the leg, lay the victim down, with both legs straight, and the uninjured leg beside the injured leg.

Place padding between the thighs, knees, and ankles; tie a broad bandage at the knees.

Tie a narrow bandage around the feet.

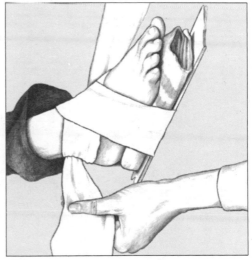

2b

Tie a narrow bandage around the foot in a figure-of-eight, to secure the splint.

If only one or two toes are fractured, an alternative is to use an uninjured toe as a splint. Place padding between the toes and tie a narrow bandage around the injured and uninjured toes.

549

Fractures: the shoulder or collar-bone

A fracture of the collar-bone is usually caused by a fall on the outstretched hand or on the point of the shoulder. This injury is relatively easy to recognise; the arm on the injured side is partly helpless, and swelling or deformity can be felt or seen over the fracture.

Do not try to straighten the fractured bone.

Do not bandage directly over the fracture site if the victim has an open fracture.

Do not give the victim food or drink, in case a general anaesthetic is needed later.

Move the arm on the fractured side as little as possible. Treat unconsciousness before treating the fracture. *See* **Unconsciousness,** p.573.

Action
Treat any bleeding before treating the fracture (*see* p.516).

Tilt the victim's head towards the injured side to relieve pain.

Try to indicate to others that medical assistance is required.

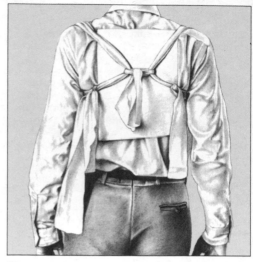

1b
Put padding between the shoulder blades.

Use a third bandage to hold together the two bandages encircling each shoulder.

The third bandage must be tight because it is necessary that the shoulders are braced well back and kept in this position.

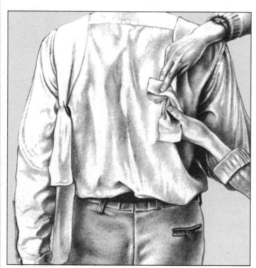

1a
Sit the victim down.

Fold two triangular bandages into narrow bandages.

Pass each bandage under the armpit and around the shoulder and tie the bandages just below the shoulder blade.

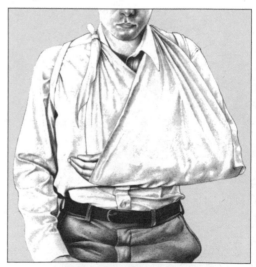

1c
Fold the arm on the injured side across the chest. Place a triangular bandage with the apex at the victim's elbow and one tip over the shoulder on the injured side. Fold the bandage under the arm, bring the tip up to the shoulder on the uninjured side, and tie the two ends. Pin the corner to provide support for the elbow.

Fractures: the spine or ribs

A fractured spine is an extremely serious injury. If the victim is incorrectly handled the spinal cord may be permanently damaged, resulting in paralysis.

Signs of a fractured spine include severe pain in the back, loss of limb sensation, and loss of limb control.

Do not move the victim.

Rib fractures can also be very serious. If the ribs have punctured the lungs, the victim will be severely shocked, cough up red, frothy phlegm, and have breathing difficulties. If the ribs have penetrated the skin surface, there will be an open, "sucking" wound.

Treat bleeding only if it is severe enough to endanger life (*see* p.516).

Action

Treat any "sucking" chest wounds immediately with an airtight dressing.

If the victim stops breathing, give artificial resuscitation. *See* **Breathing stoppage: the kiss of life,** p.518.

Summon medical aid as soon as possible.

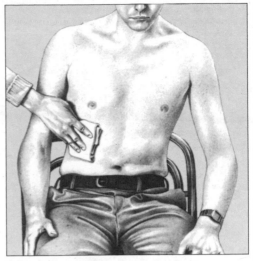

2a

If the victim has rib fractures, and there is no open chest wound or lung damage, place the victim in a sitting position and put bandages round the chest.

If the ribs have penetrated the skin, put an airtight dressing over the wound immediately.

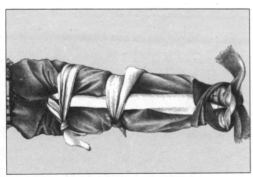

1

If medical assistance is available, **do not** move a victim with spinal fractures.

If medical assistance is not available, prepare the victim for transportation.

Using the utmost care, slide a wide board (a door will do) under the victim. Place padding between the thighs, knees, and ankles. Tie broad bandages around the thighs and knees, and a narrow bandage around the feet.

If the victim is unconscious, **do not** use the recovery position because this may cause further damage.

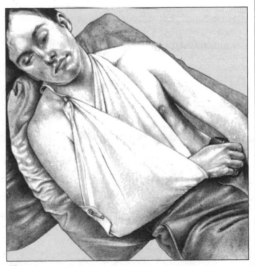

2b

Keep the airtight dressing in place and support the arm on the injured side in a triangular sling. Lay the victim down on the injured side.

If the ribs have punctured the lungs, keep the victim's head and shoulders raised. **Do not** bandage the ribs.

Head and facial injuries

Head injuries are potentially dangerous because brain damage may result. Indications of brain damage include coma, headache, convulsions, drowsiness, vomiting for no apparent reason, and loss of memory of the injury. There may be unequal pupil size and paralysis on the side of the body opposite the injury. *See* **Unconsciousness,** p.573.

Do not move the victim if there is a suspected fracture of the neck or spine. *See* **Fractures: the spine or ribs,** p.551.

If the victim has a fractured or dislocated jaw, there will be difficulty in talking, increased salivation, and the teeth may be out of alignment.

Action

If the victim has stopped breathing, apply artificial respiration. *See* **Breathing stoppage: the Holger Nielsen method,** p.520.

Treat any serious bleeding immediately.

Do not press too heavily if the bleeding is over a fracture site. *See* **Bleeding,** p.516.

An unconscious victim should be placed in the recovery position, with the wound uppermost. *See* **Fainting,** p.544.

Do not give the victim food or drink, in case a general anaesthetic is needed later.

Do not try to set a dislocated jaw.

Do not remove impaled objects from a wound; stabilize them and protect them from further movement.

Bleeding from the ear without any obvious cause may indicate a fractured skull.

Do not try to remove objects from the ear.

Blood trickling from the nose together with other head injuries may indicate a fractured skull. Treat as a skull fracture.

A broken nose will be swollen and painful. Tell the victim to breathe through the mouth, and treat the injury as a nosebleed. *See* **Nosebleeds,** p.590.

If there are corrosive chemicals in the victim's eye, *see* **Poisoning and dangerous chemicals,** p.562.

Summon medical assistance.

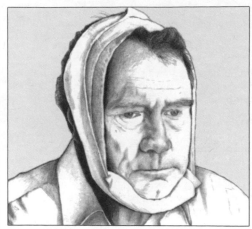

1

Jaw fractures: If unconscious, place the victim in the recovery position and ensure there is a clear air passage. Remove any dentures and carefully support the jaw using a pad secured with a bandage.

If conscious, place the victim in a sitting position with the head well forward. Remove any dentures and maintain a clear airway. Support the jaw as described above.

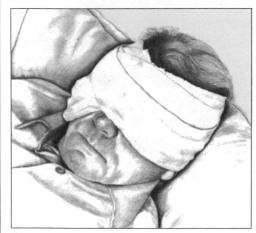

4a

Eye injuries: Do not try to remove any object that is impaled in the eye, that is on the pupil, or that is not readily visible.

Instruct the victim to close both eyes and to remain immobile. Place a dressing over the eye in such a way that it does not touch the eye or the eyelids and secure it with a broad bandage that covers both eyes. Lay the victim down and summon medical aid.

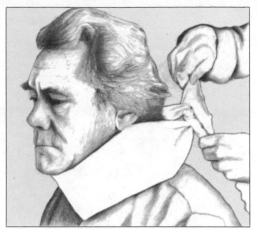

2

Neck injuries: Do not move a victim with a suspected neck fracture. *See* **Fractures: the spine or ribs,** p.551.

If it is certain that the neck is not fractured, the neck should be supported with a collar. A collar can be made from a folded towel or newspaper. Cover this with a bandage, place it around the victim's neck, and tie the ends.

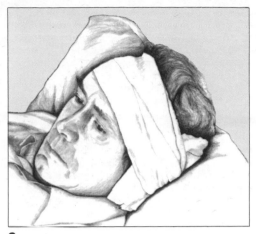

3

Ear injuries: Do not put anything into the ear canal.

Treat bleeding from a wound by pressure over the wound. Place a clean dressing over the ear and secure it with a broad bandage. Lay the victim down, with head and shoulders raised and the head tilted towards the injured side.

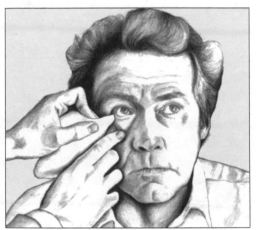

4b

If there are loose fragments in the eye, they should be removed. If the fragments are visible, place the victim in a sitting position facing a light.

Pull down the lower eyelid with a forefinger.

Instruct the victim to look upwards and remove the fragments with the corner of a clean handkerchief.

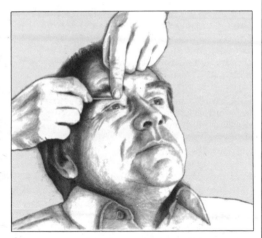

4c

If there is a fragment under the upper lid, instruct the victim to tilt the head back.

Stand behind the victim; steady the hand.

Place a matchstick at the base of the upper lid and press gently backwards. Grasp the lashes and turn the lid over the match-stick. Remove the fragment with a clean handkerchief.

Heart attack 1

A heart attack is caused by reduced blood supply to the muscles of the heart, resulting from an obstruction of the coronary arteries. The result is that the heart muscle is damaged, either temporarily or permanently.

When the blood supply to an area of heart muscle is cut off, the tissue no longer receives oxygen and food which initially results in cramp of the muscle and finally in death of the affected area.

There are two degrees of heart attack. The milder form, called angina pectoris, is caused by partial obstruction of the coronary arteries. For the more serious, often fatal, form, *see* **Heart attack 2,** p.556.

Action

The victim feels a severe pain in the chest. It starts in the middle of the chest and may spread to the shoulders and the upper arms, particularly on the victim's left side; to the abdomen; and to the neck.

The victim should rest, immediately, in the position that is most comfortable. A sitting position is often best because it makes breathing easier and allows the best flow of blood to the heart. Loosen any tight clothing.

Call medical assistance immediately and allow the victim to rest until help arrives.

Do not leave the victim until medical aid arrives, unless the victim recovers from the pain within five minutes.

If the victim has suffered angina pectoris before, tablets may have been prescribed by the doctor and may be in the victim's pocket. Before giving any tablets to the victim, ask if they are the right ones.

Feel the victim's carotid pulse (in the neck) to make sure that the heart is still beating. If the victim is unconscious and the heart has stopped, *see* **Heart attack 2,** p.556.

Do not apply heart massage unless you are sure that the heart has stopped.

Keep calm and reassure the victim.

Observe the victim's pulse and breathing.

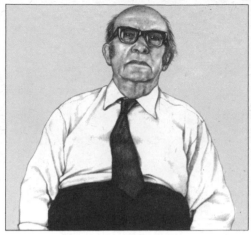

1
Angina pectoris may occur during or after physical exercise. The pain may be sudden and sharp, dull and continuous, mild or severe, but is always of short duration.

The pain usually starts in the centre of the chest and may spread to the left arm to give a tingling sensation in the fingers. The pain may also spread up the neck, across the chest, and to the right arm.

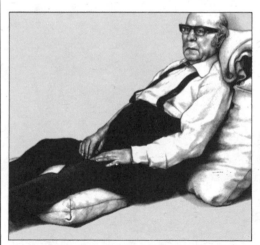

4
A victim with angina pectoris should rest in the most comfortable position possible until medical help arrives.

Usually the victim is most comfortable when sitting, with the back well supported.

The knees may also be supported; care must be taken to see this support does not interfere with blood circulation in the legs.

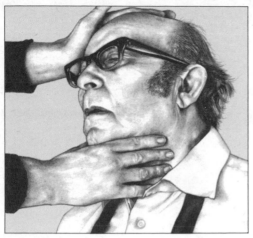

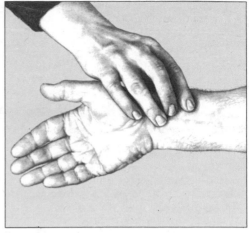

2

The strongest pulse is felt in the neck (the carotid pulse). This is caused by blood being pumped to the brain through the carotid artery.

To feel the carotid pulse, place your fingers alongside the windpipe near to the angle of the jaw. Do not press too hard. Check carefully for the carotid pulse. If no pulse is felt, *see* **Heart attack 2,** p.556.

3

The beating of the heart may be felt in the wrist (the radial pulse) as the blood is pumped down the arm to the hand.

Place your fingers in a line along the inside of the victim's arm, on the same side as the thumb, just above the wrist.

The radial pulse may be hard to detect if the heart is failing or the artery is small.

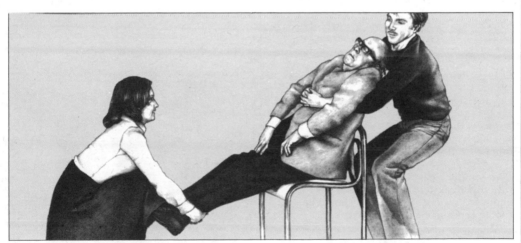

5

It may be necessary to move a victim with angina pectoris into a comfortable resting position.

To do this, one person should hold the victim's legs while another person holds the victim's shoulders.

You should try to move the victim as swiftly and as gently as possible.

If the heart has stopped, it is important to move the victim as fast as possible on to the floor, so that heart massage can be started.

Although the method illustrated is the most efficient way, almost any other method will suffice. The victim must lie face-up, so that heart massage can be started at once. *See* **Heart attack 2,** p.556.

Heart attack 2

A severe heart attack is caused by a blockage of a coronary artery. The heart may stop beating if blood fails to reach the heart muscle.

In such cases it is essential to start the heart beating as quickly as possible, or manually circulate the blood until the heart restarts. The best way to do this is to squeeze the heart in the chest until this mechanical stimulation starts the muscles pumping again.

Heart massage consists of pressing the chest wall over the heart so that the heart itself is pressed against the spine. In this way the pumping action of the heart is maintained artificially.

Action

The pain of angina pectoris follows a characteristic pattern. The victim must rest. *See* **Heart attack 1,** p.554.

The symptoms of a serious heart attack include severe and sudden chest pain; a grey colour to the victim's face; sweating; a rapid and feeble pulse; shallow, fast breathing; and loss of consciousness. The heart-beat and breathing may also stop.

Check the victim's pulse in the neck. If no pulse can be felt, start external cardiac compression at once.

Call for help immediately.

Lay the victim face-up on the floor.

Kneel at the victim's left shoulder. If no help is available, combine heart massage with mouth-to-mouth resuscitation.

Press on the victim's chest repeatedly at a rate slightly faster than once a second for about ten seconds (actual rate should be fifteen times in eleven seconds).

Move to the victim's mouth.

Breathe air into the victim's lungs twice so as to inflate them, and return to the chest.

Do not apply heart massage if the heart is still beating. *See* **Heart attack 1,** p.554.

Follow the instructions carefully. Keep calm so that your own breathing is regular and so that you do not get too tired.

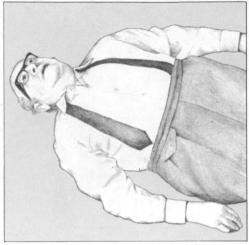

1a
The heart lies in the chest slightly to the left of centre. If the heart has stopped beating, rapid action to restart it is essential.

If the victim is wearing dentures, remove them as they may obstruct breathing.

The victim should be lying face-up on the floor, arms by the sides.

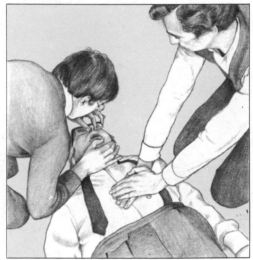

2a
To combine heart massage with mouth-to-mouth resuscitation, *see* p.518.

With two people, the one compressing the heart should kneel at the victim's shoulder. The other person, on the victim's other side, tilts the victim's head back, holds the victim's nose, and breathes into the lungs.

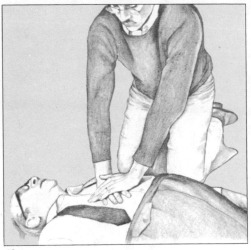

1b

To restart the heart you must press on the chest over the whole area of the heart.

Kneel at the victim's left shoulder and place your hands, one on top of the other, over the centre of the sternum (breastbone).

Press on the victim's sternum with the heel of your hand.

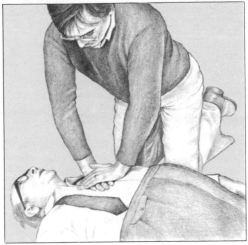

1c

Lean forward with the arms as straight as possible to compress the victim's heart within the chest.

Press at a rate of about 80 compressions a minute.

You should press firmly, but not hard enough to damage the rib-cage.

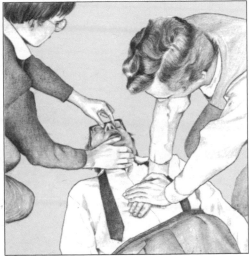

2b

The technique occupies a 15-second cycle.

The person applying cardiac compression presses 20 times during this period. At the same time, the person giving resuscitation ventilates the victim's lungs twice. It is necessary for both people applying aid to establish a steady working rhythm.

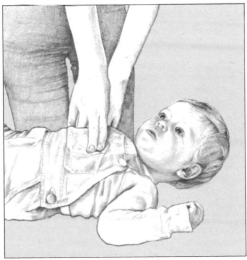

3

If the victim is a baby or a very small child, two fingers only should be used to press on the chest. A rate of about 100 presses a minute is required.

Particular care is essential when applying heart massage to small children because the chest and lungs are very delicate.

Hypothermia, exposure and frostbite

When a person is inadequately clothed for more than a short time, particularly in weather conditions that are also windy or wet, there is a danger that the body temperature will drop. Such a drop in body temperature affects the central nervous system, and causes the symptoms of slurred speech, loss of co-ordination, and confusion. In severe cases, hypothermia can lead to unconsciousness, coma, and death.

People who are hungry or tired, the elderly, people who are ill, children, and people who have drunk alcohol are particularly likely to suffer from hypothermia in cold conditions.

Hypothermia develops gradually. The greatest danger to a person in the early stages of the condition is that the confusion it causes may make the person careless. At the first signs of such carelessness, the person must find food, warmth, and shelter.

Action

It is important to recognize the symptoms of hypothermia so that the correct treatment can be given as quickly as possible.

The initial symptoms of hypothermia include sluggish physical and mental responses; slurred speech; muscle cramps and persistent shivering; and the tendency to miscalculate one's abilities, particularly with regard to strength.

First raise the temperature of the body as a whole, and keep a constant check on the temperature to prevent any further drop. Wrap the victim in dry blankets, or in a sleeping bag, with a warm person, if possible.

It may help to immerse the victim in a bath of water at normal body temperature (98.4°F; 37°C).

Give the victim warm, sweet liquids to drink.

Do not give alcohol to a person who is hypothermic, because alcohol causes the blood to circulate more freely in the cold extremities, such as the hands and feet, and so cools the body as a whole.

Warm the person gently but quickly so as to minimize the degree of damage to tissues.

In all cases, take the victim to a hospital as soon as possible. Be prepared to treat the victim for heart and breathing stoppage.

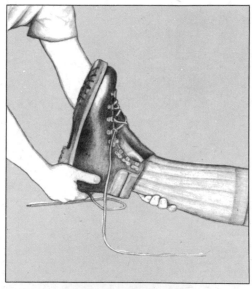

1
Find or build a shelter, if the victim is outdoors. It is important to prevent further exposure by protecting the victim from the cold and the wind as much as possible.

Give warm, sweet drinks, and food.

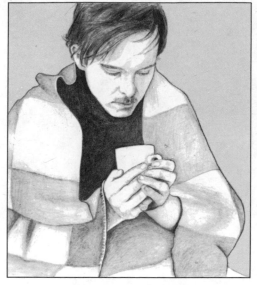

2
Loosen any clothing, such as boots or gloves, that constrict the blood circulation.

Replace wet clothing with dry clothes.

Keep the victim conscious and active.

Frostbite

Frostbite occurs when areas of tissue freeze in cold weather conditions. It is more likely to occur if the conditions are damp or windy. The underlying tissues, as well as the skin, may be affected. Frostbite may result in blistering and ulceration of the affected part. In severe frostbite, gangrene may occur.

The areas most commonly affected are the nose, ears, cheeks, fingers, and toes.

Frostbite usually occurs without pain. The frostbitten part becomes numb and stiff, and appears white. Because of the numbness, the symptoms may not be noticed. There may be an area of red, inflamed skin between the yellowish-white, frostbitten part and the normal tissues.

Stiff fingers or toes may be an indication that frostbite is occurring or has occurred.

Action

It is important to recognize the signs of frostbite so that first aid can be given at the earliest opportunity.

First of all, try to rewarm the affected part, but be careful about the way this is done.

Warm parts of the face by covering them with warm hands that are not frostbitten.

Warm frostbitten hands by placing them in the armpits, next to the skin.

Warm frostbitten feet by wrapping them in a blanket or by warming them against the abdomen of another person.

A person who has frostbite may also be suffering from hypothermia so protect the victim from further cold, and treat for hypothermia.

Do not apply direct heat to the frostbitten part. For example, do not warm the feet or hands in front of a fire.

Do not rub a frostbitten area, either directly with the hands, or with snow.

Do not exercise the frostbitten part, and do not try to walk on frostbitten feet.

Aspirin, paracetamol, or other painkilling drugs may be required to relieve the pain that occurs as frostbitten tissues gradually become warm again.

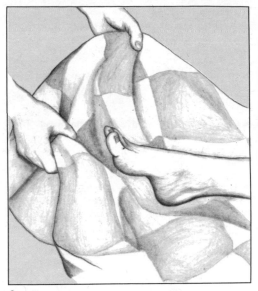

1

Gently warm the affected part. If the toes are frostbitten, wrap them in a dry blanket. Do not rub them, and make sure that their blood supply is not restricted. If part of the face is frostbitten, cover it with a warm, dry hand, until normal colour and sensation return.

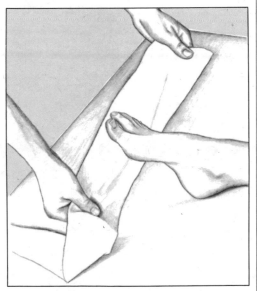

2

The injury caused by frostbite resembles a burn, and is vulnerable to infection.

Cover the frostbitten area with a sterile dressing. Take the victim to a hospital as soon as possible.

Miscellaneous serious injuries

Rupture (hernia)

A rupture is a protrusion of the abdominal organs, usually part of the intestine, through the wall of the abdomen under the skin.

Ruptures occur most commonly in the groin, but may also occur at the navel or through a surgical scar in the abdomen.

A rupture usually occurs gradually for no obvious reason, or as a result of straining the abdominal muscles when lifting a heavy object, exercising, or, rarely, coughing.

A rupture may produce a painless swelling which may remain or disappear, or there may be a sudden, painful swelling, which may be accompanied by vomiting.

Occasionally, the protruding part of the intestine may become twisted or trapped by the abdominal muscles; this is known as a strangulated hernia. It is an extremely serious condition, because the intestine may become obstructed and the blood supply may be cut off. If the blood supply is cut off, the intestine will develop gangrene. This can be fatal and requires an urgent surgical operation to restore an adequate blood supply and repair the rupture.

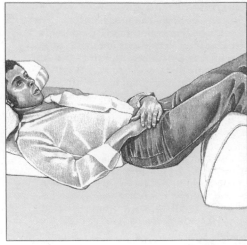

Painful rupture

For a painful rupture, summon emergency medical aid. Lay the victim down and support the head, shoulders, and knees.

Do not try to reduce the swelling.

If the victim vomits, turn him or her to the recovery position. *See* **Fainting,** p.544.

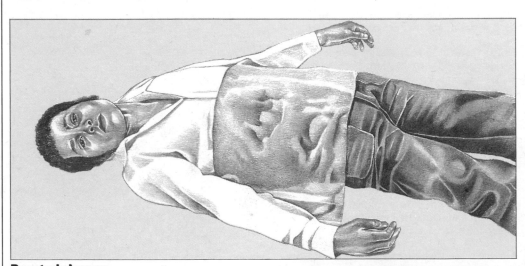

Burst abdomen

A burst abdomen is a rare injury but it is extremely serious because the exposed part of the intestine may become infected. In some cases, such an infection may be fatal.

A burst abdomen is commonly caused by the tearing of a wound following surgery, or, more rarely, the rupture of a surgical scar. It may also result from a deep knife wound.

Summon emergency medical aid.

Do not touch the exposed intestine.

Lay the victim down and cover the intestine with a clean towel or smooth cloth.

Do not give the victim anything to eat or drink.

Accidental amputation

Accidental amputation is the severance of a limb due to sudden trauma. It occurs most commonly as a result of road accidents, or of a limb being trapped in moving machinery.

The main danger of an accidental amputation is that the victim may bleed to death. This is most likely to occur if a limb has been severed.

Action

Summon emergency medical aid.

Try to stop bleeding by applying direct pressure over the end of the stump. If pressure alone does not stop the bleeding and another person is available, one person should continue to apply pressure over the stump while the other person tries to control the bleeding by pressing over an artery at a pressure point. Release the pressure over a pressure point every twenty minutes for a period of thirty seconds.

If possible, the severed limb should be kept. It may be possible for a surgeon to reattach it. Pack the limb in ice, and place it in a clean plastic bag.

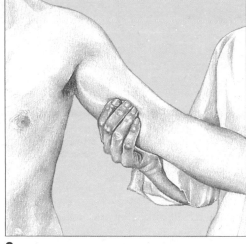

2

The arm pressure point is situated above the brachial artery, which runs along the inner side of each upper arm. The course of the artery is approximately indicated by the inner seam of a coat sleeve. To apply pressure to the brachial pressure point, put your fingers on the inner side of the victim's upper arm above the artery and press the artery against the underlying bone.

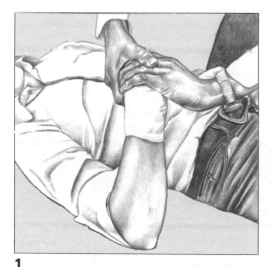

1

Lay the victim down and support the stump in a raised position. Cover the stump with a thick bandage or a clean towel. Apply continuous pressure over the bandage until the bleeding has stopped.

If the bleeding persists, apply more padding and maintain the pressure. **Do not** remove the original bandage.

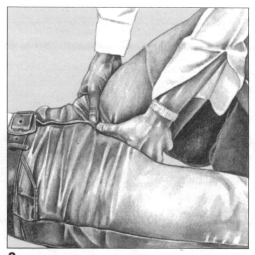

3

The leg pressure point is situated above the femoral artery where the artery passes into each leg at a point that corresponds to the centre of the fold of the groin. To apply pressure, grasp the victim's thigh with both hands and press directly downwards in the centre of the groin. Use both thumbs, one on top of the other, and press firmly against the edge of the pelvis.

Poisoning and dangerous chemicals 1

This section concerns substances which, when taken into the body, may damage the health or even kill.

There are four main methods by which poisoning may occur: breathing noxious fumes; swallowing poisons; absorbing chemicals through the skin; and by injection.

Most cases of poisoning through the lungs occur as a result of breathing traffic exhaust fumes. Poisonous fumes are also produced in some industrial processes, for example, carbon tetrachloride in the dry-cleaning industry.

Substances that are poisonous when swallowed affect the stomach or intestines, causing vomiting, pain, and diarrhoea.

If corrosives are swallowed, the lips, mouth, oesophagus, and stomach will be burned, causing intense pain, and serious damage.

Many household products, such as domestic bleach, are poisonous. Keep all household chemicals out of reach of children.

Some plants and mushrooms are poisonous. If the victim has eaten a poisonous plant, *see* **Dangerous plants,** p.530.

Some poisons may affect the nervous system, producing delirium, convulsions, and unconsciousness.

Poisoning by injection may result from intentional drug abuse. *See* **Drug overdose,** p.536. The bites of certain animals and insects may also "inject" poisons into the body. *See* **Bites and stings,** p.514.

Many pesticides and herbicides are poisonous if absorbed through the skin. These chemicals are also poisonous when swallowed, causing convulsions and unconsciousness. Be extremely careful when handling these sub-stances. Wear protective clothing. If any is spilled on the skin, wash it off immediately.

Action
Summon emergency medical aid.

If the victim is conscious, ask what happened.

If the victim is unconscious, check that the airway is clear. Place the victim in the recovery position (p.544). Check the victim's breathing and heart-beat at frequent intervals.

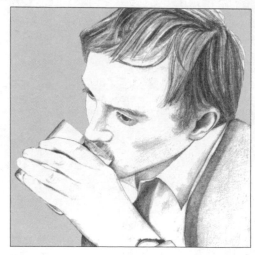

1
If the victim has swallowed a corrosive substance, the lips and the mouth will be burned.

If the victim is conscious, give large amounts of water or milk to drink. This will help to dilute the corrosive agent. **Do not** attempt to induce vomiting.

If the victim stops breathing, give artificial resuscitation. Use the Holger Nielsen method so that you are not affected by the poison. *See* **Breathing stoppage: the Holger Nielsen method,** p.520.

If the victim's heart stops, apply heart massage. *See* **Heart attack 2,** p.556.

Artificial resuscitation and heart massage may have to be continued until professional medical aid arrives because the victim's breathing mechanism may have been damaged or disturbed by the poison.

If the victim is having convulsions, *see* **Convulsions,** p.528.

If the victim's skin has been burned by a corrosive chemical, it should be thoroughly washed with water for about fifteen minutes and then treated as an ordinary burn. *See* **Burns and scalds,** p.524.

Keep any bottles, drugs, specimens of the poison, and samples of the victim's vomit. These may help a doctor identify the particular poison involved.

Benzene, toluene, and xylene

These substances are present in many commercial solvents and domestic paint removers.

Poisoning may occur after ingestion, or inhalation.

Burning sensation in the mouth leading to vomiting; chest pains; coughing; and dizziness. In later stages, lack of co-ordination; confusion; stupor; and coma. Death is usually from respiratory or heart failure.

Remove the victim from the source of poisoning.
Carefully remove the victim's clothing if contaminated.
Arrange for hospitalization of the victim.
If the victim is unconscious, put in the recovery position (p.544).
If the victim stops breathing, give artificial respiration using the Holger Nielsen method (p.520).
If the victim's heart stops, apply heart massage.

Carbon monoxide

The most common source of carbon monoxide is exhaust fumes.

Poisoning may occur following inhalation.

The victim may be overactive. There may also be mild headache; irritability; fatigue; vomiting; confusion; lack of co-ordination; transient fainting fits with convulsions; and incontinence. Death is usually from respiratory failure.

Remove the victim from the source of poisoning.
Arrange for hospitalization of the victim.
If the victim is unconscious, put in the recovery position (p.544).
If the victim stops breathing, give artificial respiration using the kiss of life method (p.518).

Carbon tetrachloride

Carbon tetrachloride is present in many solvents used for removing grease.

Poisoning may occur following inhalation or ingestion.

There may be vomiting; headache; dizziness; confusion; convulsions; difficulty breathing; and coma. Death is usually from respiratory or heart failure.

Remove the victim from the source of poisoning.
Carefully remove the victim's clothing if it is contaminated.
Arrange for hospitalization of the victim.
If the victim is unconscious, put in the recovery position (p.544).
If the victim stops breathing, give artificial respiration using the Holger Nielsen method.
If the victim's heart stops, apply heart massage.

Chlorate compounds

Chlorate compounds occur in some mouthwashes and weedkillers.

Poisoning may occur following ingestion.

There may be vomiting; diarrhoea; blood in the urine; jaundice; delirium; convulsions; and coma. Death is usually from kidney failure.

Arrange for hospitalization of the victim.
If the victim is conscious, give large drinks of water.
If the victim is unconscious, put in the recovery position (p.544).
If the victim stops breathing, give artificial respiration using the Holger Nielsen method.

Poisoning and dangerous chemicals 2

POISONS AND SOURCES	SYMPTOMS	TREATMENT

Corrosives

Strong acids, such as battery acid; strong alkalis, such as caustic soda; strong antiseptics; and tincture of iodine. Poisoning may occur following ingestion.	There may be burns around the lips and mouth; intense pain in the mouth, throat, and stomach; vomiting, sometimes with blood; shock; and difficulty breathing. Death is usually from respiratory failure.	Arrange for hospitalization of the victim. If the corrosive has been spilled on the skin, place the affected area under running water for at least ten minutes then treat the injury as an ordinary burn. If the victim is conscious, give small drinks of water. If the victim is unconscious, put in the recovery position (p.544). If the victim stops breathing, give artificial respiration using the Holger Nielsen method (p.520).

Metaldehyde

Metaldehyde is present in slug and snail poison. Poisoning may occur following ingestion.	There may be nausea; vomiting; exaggerated reflexes; convulsions; and difficulty breathing. Death is usually from circulatory failure.	Arrange for hospitalization of the victim. If the victim is conscious, induce vomiting. If the victim is unconscious, put in the recovery position (p.544). If the victim stops breathing, give artificial respiration using the Holger Nielsen method (p.520). If the victim's heart stops, apply heart massage.

Naphthalene

Napthalene is present in moth balls and air fresheners. Poisoning may occur following ingestion or contact.	There may be abdominal pain; vomiting; diarrhoea; difficulty breathing; delirium; convulsions; and coma. Death is usually from liver or kidney failure.	Arrange for hospitalization of the victim. If the victim is conscious, give sodium bicarbonate in water. If the victim is unconscious, put in the recovery position (p.544). If the victim stops breathing, give artificial respiration using the Holger Nielsen method (p.520).

Organophosphorus compounds

These substances are present in many insecticides. Poisoning may occur following ingestion, inhalation, or absorption through the skin.	There may be increased salivation; vomiting; abdominal pain; diarrhoea; pinpoint pupils; difficulty breathing; convulsions; and coma. Death is usually from respiratory failure.	Carefully remove all of the victim's contaminated clothing. Arrange for hospitalization of the victim. If the victim is conscious, induce vomiting. If the victim is unconscious, put in the recovery position (p.544). If the victim stops breathing, give artificial respiration using the Holger Nielsen method (p.520).

Oxalic acid

Oxalic acid is present in some bleaches,	There may be pain in the mouth; vomiting;	Arrange for hospitalization of the victim. If the victim is conscious, give Milk of

| --- | --- | --- |
| metal cleaners and stain removers.

Poisoning may occur following ingestion. | thirst; twitching; convulsions; and coma. Death is usually from heart failure. | Magnesia or ordinary milk to drink.
If the victim is unconscious, put in the recovery position (p.544).
If the victim's heart stops, apply heart massage. |

Paraffin and petroleum distillates

These substances are present in many domestic cleaning fluids, paint thinners, and polishes. Poisoning may occur following ingestion or inhalation.	Mild poisoning may produce a state similar to drunkenness. Severe poisoning may cause pain in the mouth, throat, and stomach; vomiting; diarrhoea; headache; blurred vision; agitation; lack of co-ordination; delirium; convulsions; and coma. Death is usually from respiratory failure.	Remove the victim from the source of poisoning. Carefully remove all of the victim's contaminated clothing. Arrange for hospitalization of the victim. If the victim is unconscious, put in the recovery position (p.544). If the victim stops breathing, give artificial respiration using the Holger Nielsen method (p.520).

Phenol and cresol

These substances are present in many strong antiseptics. Poisoning may occur following ingestion, inhalation, or absorption through the skin.	If inhaled or absorbed there may be difficulty breathing, and unconsciousness. If ingested there may also be burning of the mouth and throat, and vomiting. Death is usually from respiratory failure.	Remove the victim from the source of poisoning. Carefully remove all of the victim's contaminated clothing. Arrange for hospitalization of the victim. If the victim is unconscious, put in the recovery position (p.544). If the victim stops breathing, give artificial respiration using the Holger Nielsen method (p.520).

Phosphorus

Phosphorus is present in some rat poisons. Poisoning may occur following ingestion.	There may be burning of the mouth; a smell of garlic on the breath; vomiting; diarrhoea; delirium; and coma.	Arrange for hospitalization of the victim. If the victim is unconscious, put in the recovery position (p.544). If the victim stops breathing, give artificial respiration using the Holger Nielsen method (p.520).

Sodium hypochlorite

Sodium hypochlorite is present in domestic bleach. Poisoning may occur following ingestion.	There may be vomiting; pain and inflammation of the mouth and throat; difficulty breathing; delirium; and coma.	Arrange for hospitalization of the victim. If the victim is unconscious, put in the recovery position (p.544). If the victim stops breathing, give artificial respiration using the Holger Nielsen method (p.520).

Shock and heatstroke

Shock is caused by a sudden decrease in the blood supply, which adversely affects all the functions of the body.

Shock often accompanies severe injuries; haemorrhage; burns; heart attack; infection; poisoning; stoppage of breathing and heart-beat; a severe illness; an overdose of insulin in diabetics; vomiting; and fear.

The severity of shock varies depending on the gravity of the cause and individual reactions to it, and may vary from a feeling of weakness to total collapse.

The signs of shock include: pallor; cold, clammy skin; sweating; nausea; vomiting; low body temperature; weak, rapid pulse; and irregular breathing.

Action

Do not move the victim unnecessarily, especially if there may be a serious injury.

Do not give the victim any food or drink if there may be an injury to the head or abdomen; if the victim is unconscious, vomiting, or convulsing; or if expert help will arrive within one hour.

If the victim complains of thirst, moisten the lips with water.

Do not leave the victim alone. Ask somebody else to summon emergency medical aid.

Keep a close check on the victim's breathing and heart-beat at all times.

If the victim has stopped breathing, give artificial respiration. *See* **Breathing stoppage: the kiss of life,** p.518.

If the victim's heart has stopped, apply heart massage. *See* **Heart attack 2,** p.556.

If the shock has been caused by a burn, *see* **Burns and scalds,** p.524.

If the shock has been caused by an insulin overdose and the victim is conscious, give any food or drink that contains sugar. Artificial sweeteners will not help.

If the victim is unconscious or likely to vomit, place the victim in the recovery position, if injuries permit. *See* **Fainting,** p.544.

Treat any bleeding or serious injuries. *See* **Bleeding,** p.516.

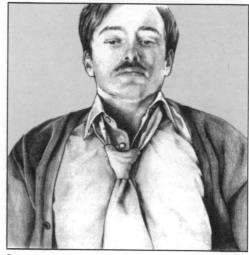

1

Loosen the victim's clothing at the neck, chest and waist.

Keep the victim warm by maintaining the body heat. Cover the victim with blankets or a coat.

Do not warm the victim artificially, because this may be harmful.

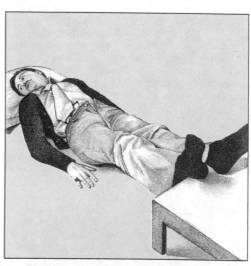

2

If the victim is conscious, lay him or her face upwards with the legs raised.

If there is any injury to the victim's head, chest, or abdomen, the victim's shoulders should be raised slightly and supported.

Turn the victim's head to one side.

Heatstroke

Heat exhaustion must not be confused with heatstroke. The victim of heat exhaustion is pale with cool, moist skin. He or she collapses, sweating profusely. The treatment is simple, and recovery quick.

By contrast, a victim of heatstroke looks flushed and has hot, dry skin. The condition results from a combination of high temperature and high humidity. It is caused by a breakdown in the sweating mechanism. Other symptoms of heatstroke include mental confusion; delirium; headaches; and dizziness. Shock and unconsciousness follow.

Action

Heatstroke is a major medical emergency requiring prompt action. Treatment is aimed at reducing the body temperature as quickly as possible.

The most effective method of cooling the victim is by immersion in a cold bath of water.

The victim's temperature must be brought down below 39°C (102°F). If this is not done immediately the victim could suffer shock, coma, and irreparable brain damage.

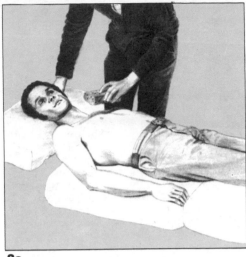

2a
If the victim is suffering from heatstroke, the body temperature must be reduced as quickly as possible.

Take the victim to a cool, shady environment immediately.

Sponge the victim down with plenty of cold water.

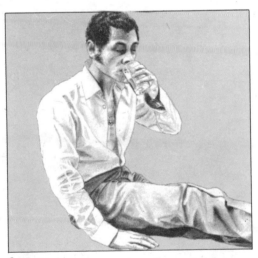

1
If the victim is suffering from heat exhaustion, place in a cool, shady environment. Give the victim cold water containing one teaspoonful of salt per pint to drink.

If the victim is unconscious, place in the recovery position. *See* **Fainting,** p.544.

Heat exhaustion may lead to heatstroke.

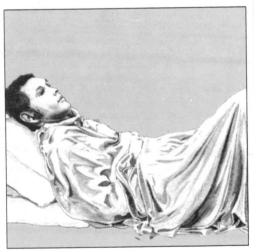

2b
Wrap the victim in a cold, wet sheet.

Lay the victim down in a fairly strong current of cold air.

If the victim is unconscious, place in the recovery position. *See* **Fainting,** p.544.

Summon emergency medical aid.

567

Transporting an injured person 1

Do not move the victim if medical help is available. If the victim's life is endangered by hazards, such as fire, the priority is to move the victim away. Remember that transportation may aggravate the victim's condition.

If there is no hazard, attempt to transport the victim, but first carry out a systematic examination to establish the extent of the injuries; any injuries should be treated before moving the victim.

The priorities of action are emergency rescue, if necessary, followed by treatment of breathing difficulties, bleeding, poisoning, and unconsciousness. Any injured limb should be supported and, if the extent of injury is in doubt, treated as a fracture and splinted before moving the victim.

The victim should be made comfortable and the most practical method of transportation ascertained.

The method of transportation chosen depends upon the nature and severity of the injury, the number of people available, the distance to be travelled, and the terrain to be traversed.

During the journey, keep a careful watch on the victim's condition, ensuring that the air passage is clear at all times, that there is no further bleeding, that the victim does not become unconscious, and that fractures remain immobilized. The journey itself should be as smooth and as safe as possible.

Transportation on a stretcher is the least tiring method, and should be used wherever possible.

Always transport an unconscious victim on a stretcher.

Head and facial injuries
If conscious, the victim should be moved in a sitting position with the head tilted forwards.

With a single first-aider and a lightweight victim, the cradle lift may be used. If the victim can walk, the human crutch method may be used. Standing at the victim's side, place one arm around the victim's waist and the victim's arm around your neck. If another assistant is available, the four-handed seat or the chair lift may be used.

If unconscious, the victim should be transported face upwards on a stretcher.

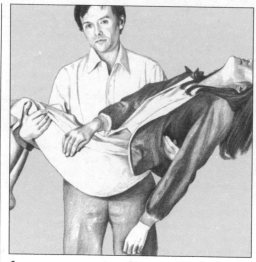

1
To do the cradle lift, place one arm behind the victim's knees and the other around the waist.

This lift is suitable only if the victim is lightweight, and for transportation over short distances.

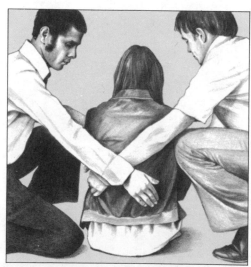

3a
The two-handed lift is useful when the victim's arms are disabled.

Two first-aiders stand facing each other and bend down, one on each side of the victim. Each first-aider places the arm nearest the victim behind the victim's back, just below the shoulders.

568

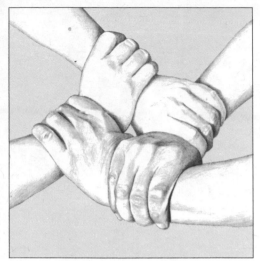

2a

For the four-handed lift, two first-aiders stand facing each other behind the victim.

Each grasps the top of his or her own left wrist with the right hand.

Each first-aider then grasps the other's right wrist with his or her own left hand.

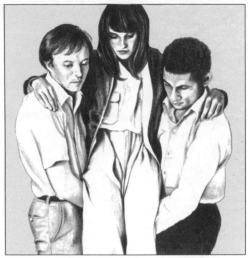

2b

The two first-aiders bend down and grasp each other's wrists.

The victim places an arm around the neck of each first-aider and sits on their interlocked hands.

This lift is tiring and so is suitable only for short distances.

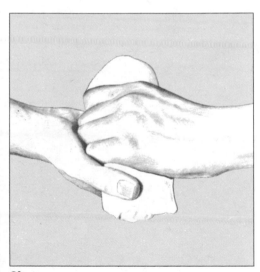

3b

The first-aiders raise the victim's back and pass their other arms underneath the victim's thighs, and clasp their hands in a hook grip. The first-aider on the victim's left side has the palm upwards and holds a handkerchief to prevent being hurt by the other's fingernails. The first-aider on the victim's right side has the palm downwards.

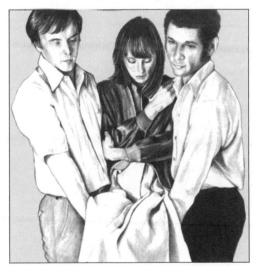

3c

The first-aiders rise at the same time and step off with their outside feet.

The first-aiders should walk forwards with a crossover step, not with sideways paces.

Transporting an injured person 2

Chest injuries

Chest injuries can be serious and may be accompanied by other injuries.

If the victim is unconscious or there are signs of internal injury (breathing is impaired, or there is an open chest wound), transport the victim in a semi-recumbent position on a stretcher.

If the victim is conscious and there are no obvious signs of internal injury, transport as a walking or sitting case.

When there is only one first-aider, a victim who can walk may be assisted using the human crutch method (see previous pages).

When other assistance is at hand, either the chair lift or the two-handed lift (see previous pages) may be used.

Arm injuries

Arm injuries may be associated with chest injuries. In the case of such an injury, the victim should be transported using one of the methods for chest injuries.

When there is only one first-aider and the victim has injured only one arm, the human crutch (see previous pages) may be used, the support being given on the uninjured side.

If the victim has injured both arms, the cradle lift (see previous pages) may be used.

If help is available, either the two-handed lift or the chair lift may be used.

Hip, pelvic, and abdominal injuries

These injuries often involve damage to internal organs. The victim should be transported face upwards on a stretcher.

Leg injuries

Where possible, a person with leg injuries should be transported on a stretcher; this is essential for serious leg injuries.

When there is only one first-aider and the victim has a minor leg injury, the pick-a-back method may be used. The first-aider bends down, back to the victim, whose arms are then placed around the first-aider's neck. On bending further, the first-aider lifts the victim and grasps behind the victim's knees. If other assistance is at hand the chair lift or the four-handed lift (see previous pages) may be used.

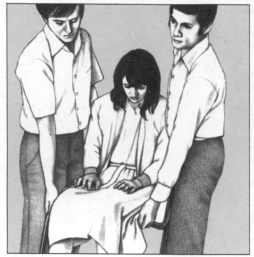

1
This method should be used only if the victim is conscious and not seriously injured.

Sit the victim on a straight-backed chair. Two first-aiders stand, one on each side of the chair, each holding one front leg and one rear leg. The chair is then tilted slightly backwards and lifted.

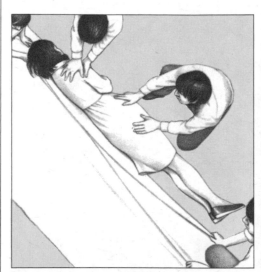

3a
Roll a blanket lengthways for half of its width.

One first-aider supports the victim's head and neck, another the victim's feet. Two other first-aiders roll the victim gently towards them. The rolled edge of the blanket is then placed alongside the victim's back.

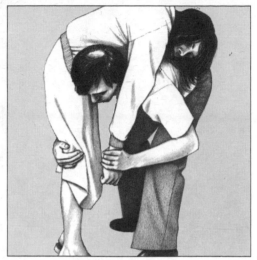

2a

Do not use this lift unless it is necessary to carry the victim a short distance. An inexperienced first-aider may suffer a strain from lifting such a heavy weight.

Help the victim to rise to an upright position. Grasp the victim's right wrist with your left hand. Bend down with your head under the victim's extended right arm.

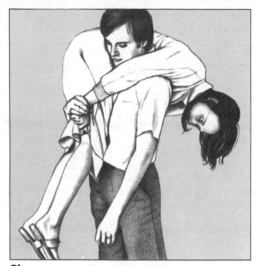

2b

Place your right arm around the victim's legs.

Take the victim's weight on your right shoulder and rise to an upright position. Pull the victim across both shoulders and transfer the victim's right wrist to your right hand.

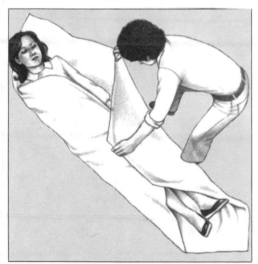

3b

Turn the victim on to the back over the roll of the blanket and then on to the victim's other side. Unroll the blanket and turn the victim on to the back.

Finally, roll the edges of the blanket to form hand grips.

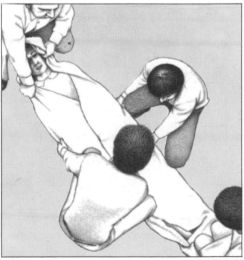

3c

One first-aider grasps the blanket by the side of the victim's neck, another grasps the blanket around the victim's feet. Two other first-aiders stand each side of the victim and grasp the rolls of blanket to support the victim's back and thighs. The first-aiders then rise together and lift the victim onto a stretcher.

Transporting an injured person 3

Neck and spinal injuries
Do not move the victim unless it is vital to do so; incorrect handling may cause paralysis. If it is essential to transport the victim, a stretcher must be used and the victim moved in a face-up position.

Before moving the victim, stiffen the stretcher by placing boards across it; a door would be suitable. Use extreme care when moving the victim on to the stretcher. The victim's body should be moved as a rigid whole. This requires six people, one supporting the head and neck, another supporting the feet, and two on each side of the victim supporting the body and legs.

The journey itself should be as smooth as possible.

Multiple and internal injuries
Do not transport the victim unless it is essential to do so.

If it is necessary to move the victim, a stretcher must be used, and the victim transported in the recovery position.

Do not give the victim food or drink during the journey.

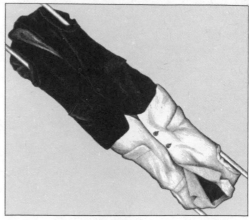

1b
Thread the poles through the sleeves.

Lash a strip of wood between the poles at each end to ensure that the poles stay apart and that the stretcher is taut.

Always test an improvised stretcher before using it to transport the victim.

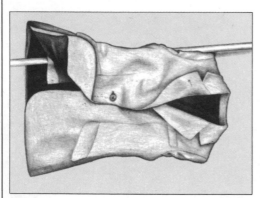

1a
A stretcher can be improvised using anything which provides a firm, flat surface and is large enough to accommodate the victim, for example, a door, a broad plank, or an ironing board. A layer of padding should be placed on it and covered with a blanket.

One form of stretcher can be made using two jackets and two strong poles.

Turn the jacket sleeves inside out. Lay the jackets down with the bottom hems touching and button the jackets.

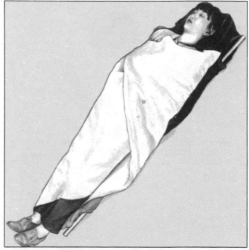

1c
Carefully move the victim on to the stretcher using the blanket lift (*see* p.571).

During the journey the victim should be kept warm and comfortable, but do not overheat the victim; one blanket should be sufficient for most conditions.

Unconsciousness

Unconsciousness occurs when normal brain activity is interrupted. It may progress rapidly from a state of drowsiness to a coma.

Any person who has been unconscious should consult a doctor, because unconsciousness may be a symptom of an underlying illness or a head injury that is not immediately obvious.

Do not give an unconscious person food or drink.

Do not leave an unconscious person alone.

Action

Remove the victim from any harmful gases. If the victim has stopped breathing, give artificial respiration. *See* **Breathing stoppage: the kiss of life,** p.518.

If the victim's heart has stopped, give heart massage. *See* **Heart attack 2,** p.556.

Control any bleeding. *See* **Bleeding,** p.516. If the victim is having an epileptic seizure, *see* **Convulsions,** p.528.

Treat any other injuries.

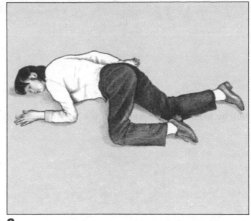

2
Place the victim in the recovery position, and elevate the feet.

If the victim has difficulty in breathing, the head should be pressed backwards and the lower jaw pushed forwards so that the chin juts out.

Check the victim's breathing and pulse at regular intervals.

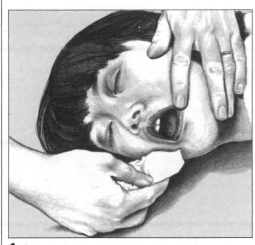

1
Ensure that the victim has a clear airway.

If the airway is blocked, remove any loose dentures and clear the mouth of mucus, blood, or vomit, using a handkerchief if necessary.

Ensure that there is plenty of fresh air.

Loosen clothing around the neck and waist.

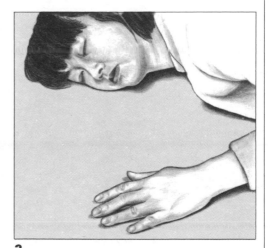

3
If the victim has no obvious injuries, look for clues as to why unconsicousness occurred. An emergency medical information tag or a syringe may indicate that unconsciousness was caused by an excess of insulin; a steroid card indicates that the victim is having cortisone treatment and may collapse in moments of stress. An empty pill bottle may indicate a drug overdose. Save the bottle and any pills; these will help the doctor.

Treating minor injuries and disorders

Section contents

If there is any doubt whether an injury or disorder is major or minor, *first see* the **Index of Emergencies,** p.504.

Introduction

This section discusses common wounds and conditions that are not life-threatening, but which require attention and treatment. **If there is any doubt whether an injury or disorder is minor or major, first see the Index of Emergencies,** on p.504.

All the injuries and disorders in this section can be treated at home and without professional aid. However, if the treatment is ineffective, or if there are indications of a more serious ailment, consult a doctor immediately.

Many minor injuries and disorders can be prevented if adequate safety precautions are taken. For advice concerning these, see the section entitled **Family safety,** beginning on p.604, and particularly the information given about Safety in the home (pp.606-609).

A store of basic first-aid supplies for the care of these minor injuries and disorders should be kept in the house. For advice about what a home medical chest and a first-aid kit should contain, see the section entitled **What you should have on hand,** beginning on p.630. The supplies most commonly used in the treatment of these ailments are bandages, gauze pads, and dressings, and simple pain-killing drugs such as aspirin or paracetamol. Treatment of minor wounds usually consists of taking elementary measures to clean the injured area and prevent infection. Painful conditions in the muscles and joints, such as cramp and strains, usually respond to rest and gradually disappear without further treatment, although over-the-counter pain-killing drugs may be used to relieve severe pain.

The people who are especially prone to minor injuries are the very young and the very old. Both these age groups are less capable than others of looking after themselves, and may not notice the dangers involved before performing some task.

Parents of young children together with those who care for the elderly therefore have a special responsibility to protect their charges from potentially dangerous situations.

Young children left in cots or push-chairs should be secured with a harness to prevent them from falling out. They should be dressed in clothes that are comfortable and appropriate to the climate, and should be shielded from direct sunlight. Sharp or jagged objects that are nearby and could cause cuts should be removed. Small objects that a child might swallow are especially dangerous. All medicines, cleaning fluids, and other household liquids should be kept out of the reach of children. Many of these may be poisonous. Furniture with sharp edges, stairs, and hard, slippery, or wooden floors may all be a cause of injury. Special care is needed with stoves and cookers in the kitchen, and with all electrical equipment and power-driven machinery. Plastic bags should be disposed of or locked away; they can easily cause suffocation if placed over the head. Such safety precautions cannot entirely eliminate all the dangers that young children expose themselves to, but they can prevent many accidents.

Elderly people are especially prone to falls, which often result in fractured bones. Slippery surfaces, loose carpets and rugs, and objects left lying on the floor are all possible hazards. Adequate lighting and handrails on staircases and in the bathroom are a sensible safety precaution.

Nosebleeds resulting from arteriosclerosis are also common among old people.

Children and old people with any of the minor injuries and disorders in this section usually require simple treatment that can be administered by another person. When treating an injured person it is always necessary to give reassurance and comfort, however minor the injury. The shock and anxiety experienced by the injured person can be greatly reduced by calm and efficient treatment.

When treating minor wounds, such as cuts and bruises, make sure that the victim is comfortably seated. Before washing the victim's wound, first wash and dry your own hands. If the wound is bleeding and there is nothing stuck in it, immediately apply a pad or dressing and hold it gently but firmly in place until the bleeding stops. If possible, wash the area around the wound. It may be necessary to use damp pieces of gauze to wash the wound itself. Apply these gently to the wound, working from the centre out-wards, and dispose of them immediately after use. The wound should then be dried, again using pieces of gauze if necessary. If there is any dirt or soil embedded in the wound, consult a doctor about its removal; antibiotics or an antitetanus injection may also be necessary.

Most minor wounds heal naturally, and do not need to be covered with ointments or lotions. A simple adhesive dressing is sufficient for most small cuts; for larger wounds, apply a pad of sterile gauze and secure it with an adhesive bandage. When applying any dressing, handle it carefully by the corners only; do not touch the part that is to cover the wound itself. If a dressing needs to be replaced, remove the old dressing with care and try not to touch the wound. If there is some discharge from the wound, it should be washed again. If the wound appears not to be healing, consult a doctor. All used dressings should be disposed of immediately.

The victim may often be reassured if the person dressing the wound explains what is happening, and why it is necessary. Many people become worried or frightened at the sight of their own blood, so any bloodstained tissues or towels should, if possible, be kept out of the victim's sight. None of the injuries or disorders in this section should cause any real anxiety; moreover, all can be effectively treated by the majority of people. If you suspect that an injury or disorder may be more serious than it appears, however, do not hesitate to consult a doctor.

Blisters

A blister is a collection of fluid beneath the skin.

The fluid is usually reabsorbed quickly into the underlying tissues. New skin then forms under the blister.

Blisters may be caused by a variety of injuries, such as friction from ill-fitting shoes; burns; scalds; exposure to certain chemicals; and contact with irritant plants.

Many diseases, such as chickenpox, eczema, impetigo, and herpes simplex also produce blisters.

Consult a doctor if you suspect that a blister is caused by a disease.

Action

If a blister is caused by a burn or a scald, *see* **Burns and scalds,** p.524.

If a blister is caused by contact with an irritant plant, *see* **Dangerous plants,** p.530.

If a blister is caused by contact with a chemical, *see* **Poisoning and dangerous chemicals,** p.562.

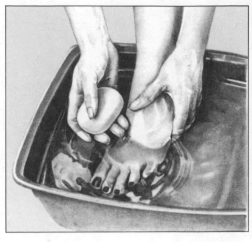

1b

Wash the affected area gently with soap and water.

Take care not to puncture a blister.

If a blister is punctured, it leaves a moist area that is extremely painful and exposed to infection.

Do not apply any lotions or ointments.

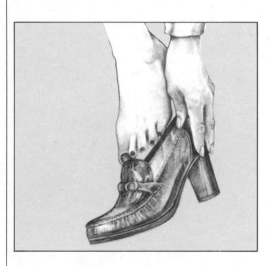

1a

If a blister is caused by friction, as with ill-fitting shoes, remove the cause of the friction as soon as possible.

If the cause cannot be removed immediately, place padding between the blister and the cause of friction. A handkerchief is suitable. This may ease the pain, and prevent further damage to the skin.

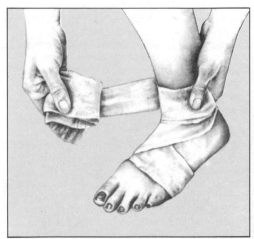

1c

Apply a light gauze dressing over the blister. A cushion can be made by cutting a hole in some folded gauze or sponge rubber, and bandaging it in place.

If the blister persists, or if there is increased redness and pain or other symptoms of infection after the apparent cause has been removed, consult a doctor.

Boils

A boil is caused by a bacterial infection deep in a hair follicle, usually in the actual root of the hair.

A person suffering from recurrent boils should consult a doctor. The boils may be a symptom of diabetes. A simple urine test can eliminate this possibility.

Boils on the nose or in the ear should be examined by a doctor. A large boil, or one that does not come to a head, also needs medical attention, and may have to be lanced.

If red streaks appear radiating from the site of the boil, or if a nearby gland becomes large and tender, seek medical advice urgently. This may indicate a dangerous spread of the infection.

Dressings impregnated with antiseptic cream cut down the risk of the infection spreading to neighbouring follicles.

Action

Boils generally heal themselves, and nothing can be done to speed up the process. Hot poultices, sometimes recommended, actually encourage the infection to spread.

Clean the skin carefully with an antiseptic.

Stretch an adhesive bandage over the area of skin to reduce skin tension.

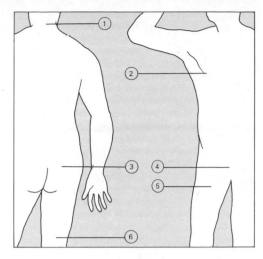

1
Boils occur more frequently in areas where the skin is constantly rubbed: (1) at the back of the neck; (2) under the arms; (3) on the buttocks; (4) around the groin; (5) at the top of the thigh; and (6) behind the knees. Boils on or in the nose, or in the outer ear, are extremely painful as they develop, because the tissues do not stretch easily, and the pressure is localized and intense.

Boils often complicate an existing skin disease, for example, acne. For this reason, they often occur at the onset of puberty.

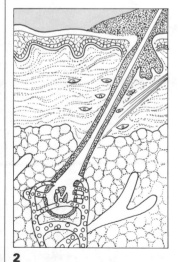

2
A red swelling forms deep in the hair follicle. The skin around the hair itches.

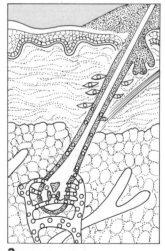

3
The skin around the hair forms a tight, red lump. The developing boil is extremely painful.

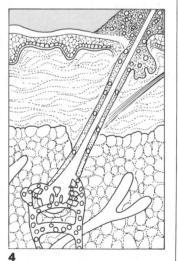

4
Within a few days, a yellow head forms. The boil bursts to discharge pus. The pain subsides.

Bruises

Bruising is a minor form of internal bleeding. It is commonly caused by a sharp blow or knock that is painful when it happens, but can also occur after a blow that at the time went unnoticed. Bruising is also common around the sites of other injuries. Before treating bruising, check for other injuries such as fractures.

Bruising that occurs apparently spontaneously can be a sign of several different conditions. Consult a doctor.

Most bruises are not serious; if the victim is in good health generally, there should be no need for alarm. The bruise will eventually disappear of its own accord. All bruises are different: there is no set healing time, although the process of healing can be gauged, to some extent, by the colour.

Usually, bruises are red at first, before turning blue, then finally yellow, as the blood is gradually reabsorbed. But bruises may not proceed through the whole sequence: they may start at the half-way stage, especially around the face. Blood blisters are another form of bruising. They display the same sequence of coloration, generally more vividly.

Bruising that occurs some days after an injury near a bone may indicate a fracture. A doctor should be consulted if this is a possibility. If a broken bone is left untreated, it may cause complications in the future.

Bruising in the abdominal region may be a sign of internal injury.

A black eye is another form of a severe bruise. Usually, it is the result of a blow just above the eye or between the eyes. But a black eye following an injury to the eye itself should always be seen by a doctor, because it may be a sign that there is some damage to the structure of the eye. A black eye following an apparently unrelated head injury is a possible indication of a fractured skull.
See **Head and facial injuries,** p.552.

People with blood disorders such as haemophilia bruise easily, sometimes without any apparent cause.

Bruising in people taking anticoagulant drugs may be a sign that the dosage needs adjustment, and should be regulated lower by the prescribing doctor.

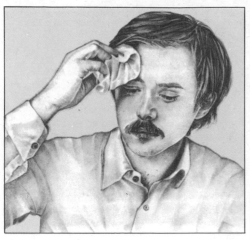

1a

Rest a bruise as much as possible. This may be difficult on the face, for example, or at a joint. But immobility allows for more rapid clotting of the blood, which in turn prevents further bleeding beneath the skin.

To discourage swelling, an ice pack or a cold compress should be applied to the bruised area, and held there.

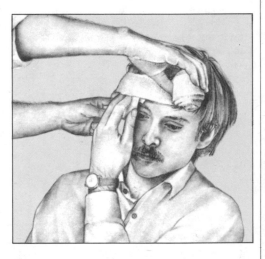

1b

When the bruised area has already swollen, a bandage should be applied to hold an ice pack or a cold compress on to the bruise.

The ice pack or cold compress should be replaced as often as necessary. The cold also helps to numb the pain.

Corns and bunions

A corn is a painful thickening of the outer layer of the skin of the toes. Corns are usually caused by the pressure of tight shoes. Inside a "hard" corn, usually a hard growth on the upper surface of a toe, is a cone-shaped core that extends downwards and presses on a nerve, causing pain. "Soft" corns are usually found between two toes; they remain soft because of warmth and moisture. Hard corns can also appear on top of the foot and even on the sole: anywhere that friction with the shoe occurs.

A bunion is a painful swelling at the base of the big toe. The tissue next to the big toe becomes inflamed, and forms a bursa which bends the toe inwards toward the other toes. Bunions are almost always caused by ill-fitting shoes.

Action

Anybody with either corns or a bunion should in the first instance ensure that they wear properly fitting shoes.

Do not attempt to lance or pare a corn (or bunion) with a sharp blade. This is dangerous and can cause serious infection.

To treat corns, soak the feet in hot water and then rub the corn gently with an emery board or pumice stone. This should painlessly remove the superficial hard skin.

A variety of corn remedies are available; many contain salicylic acid, which softens hard skin and may provide temporary relief. But it is advisable also to consult a chiropodist, who can remove corns and give advice as to preventing their recurrence.

With a bunion, do not put padding between the bunion and the shoe. This only causes extra pressure on the toes. Padding between the big toe and the second toe may, however, relieve pain.

The only complete and final cure for bunions is surgical removal of the bunion and part of any overgrown bone beneath it.

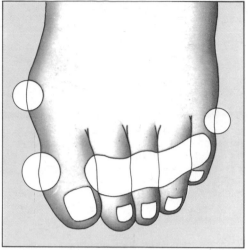

1

Corns are caused by friction in shoes that are too tight. The hard and painful thickening of the skin that results is formed where the inside of the shoe rubs the foot or toe. The most common site is the upper surface of the joint of a toe that is habitually bent in order to get inside the shoe. When toes are pressed together by tight shoes, soft corns may form between them.

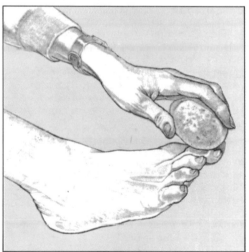

2

The best treatment for a corn is to wear wider and longer shoes. Shoes that come to a point, or that have high heels, are common culprits for producing corns. Soaking a corn in hot water softens the top layers of the hardened skin. An emery board or a pumice stone can then be used to file away the hardened skin.

Cramp and spasms

A spasm is a sudden, involuntary muscular contraction, either of a single muscle, or of a group of muscles. A convulsion is a general spasm that affects the whole body.

Spasms may be caused by various factors, such as muscular fatigue or emotional stress. Asthma is caused by a spasm of the bronchial tubes in the lungs.

Cramps are strong, painful spasms. Some forms of cramp, such as writer's cramp, may be caused by performing a repetitive task. Excessive salt loss may also cause cramp.

Night cramp usually affects the legs and feet. It occurs mainly in the elderly, and the cause is not known.

Some women suffer from abdominal cramp during menstruation.

Action

Certain chemicals and drugs may cause cramp if ingested in excessive quantities. If cramp or spasms are caused by a drug overdose, *see* **Drug overdose,** p.536.

If the victim is having convulsions, *see* **Convulsions,** p.528.

If an asthmatic attack lasts for more than 15 minutes and is getting worse despite the use of inhalers or other drugs, summon medical help.

If cramp is caused by excessive salt loss, replace the lost salt by drinking a glass of water to which half a teaspoon of salt has been added. Rest the affected part until the cramp stops.

Cramp may occur during vigorous exercise even in healthy people, particularly if exercise is taken after eating or drinking. This can be dangerous if cramp occurs while swimming.

Do not take exercise immediately after eating or after drinking alcohol.

Laryngeal spasms sometimes occur in children, usually at night. The child has difficulty in breathing and may even stop breathing for a short period. Although such laryngeal spasms are alarming, they are not usually serious medical emergencies.

If cramp or spasms persist or recur frequently, consult a doctor because there may be a more serious underlying cause.

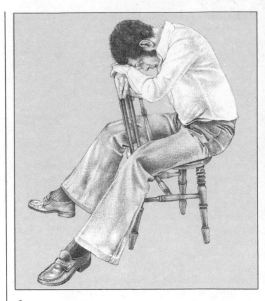

1
During an asthmatic attack, let the victim sit, with the arms at chest height.

Do not lie the victim down because this makes breathing more difficult. Allow the victim to use any prescribed medication.

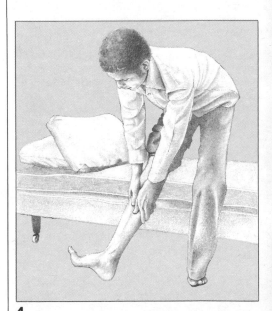

4
If the victim has night cramp in the legs or the feet, move the feet so as to stretch the affected muscles.

Night cramp in the legs or feet may also be relieved by massaging the affected part.

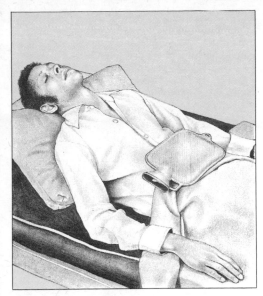

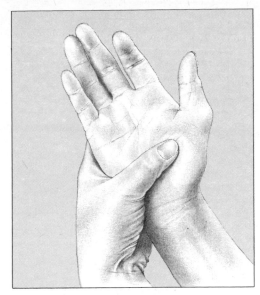

2
If the victim is having intestinal spasms, lay the victim down. Keep the victim warm and comfortable, possibly with a hot water bottle.

If the spasms are severe, or if the victim is vomiting, summon emergency medical aid.

3
If cramp is caused by excessive activity, such as swimming, running, or rowing, immediately stop the activity that has caused the cramp.

Rest and massage the affected part.

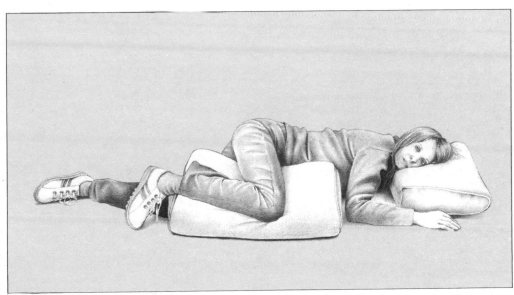

5
Menstrual cramp usually lasts for about three minutes, with an interval of about fifteen minutes between attacks.

If the victim has menstrual cramp, it may help to perform light exercise.

If exercise is ineffective, the victim should rest in bed.

Gentle heat applied to the victim's abdomen or middle of the back may relieve the pain. If it does not, give the victim pain-killers.

Cuts

A cut is a break in the skin which permits the escape of blood and may lead to infection.

Incised cuts, for example, made with a sharp blade usually bleed profusely. Lacerated cuts involving torn tissues bleed less than incised cuts but heal with more difficulty. Punctured cuts may have relatively small openings but may be deep, causing serious injury to the underlying tissues.

Most cuts are minor injuries and do not require expert medical attention.

If the victim has a deep and dirty punctured cut, a doctor should be consulted, because antitetanus injections may be necessary. Any large cut should be examined by a doctor, because stitches may be necessary.

Action

The first action is to control bleeding (*see* p.516). If there is suspicion of damage to internal parts of the body, summon emergency medical aid.

Control heavy bleeding by applying firm pressure over the wound.

Do not attempt to remove minor debris; such action may cause more bleeding.

If the cut is deep or there is an object impaled in the wound, **do not** interfere with the wound. However, it is imperative that bleeding is controlled. Summon emergency medical aid.

If the victim has a small puncture wound, wash it with soap and water, and dry.

Cover the wound with a clean, dry dressing.

If a fish hook is deeply impaled or is embedded in a part of the face, **do not** attempt to remove it.

If the fish hook is in any other part of the body, push the shank through the skin until the barb appears.

Cut off the barb with clippers or pliers and remove the shank from the wound.

Wash the wound and cover it with a clean dressing. Consult a doctor immediately.

If the wound is discharging pus when the dressing is changed, if it becomes inflamed and painful, or if there are other symptoms of infection, consult a doctor.

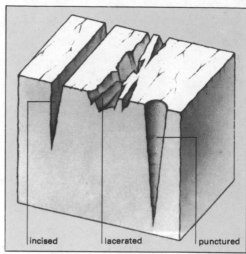

incised   lacerated   punctured

Types of cut

An incised cut is a clean cut made with a sharp edge.

A lacerated cut has irregular, torn edges.

A punctured cut is a wound that penetrates deeply into the skin.

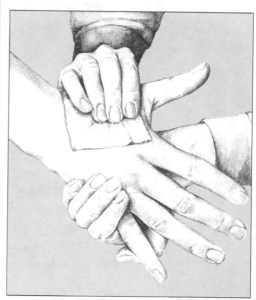

2
If the cut is deep, control any bleeding by pressing clean gauze directly over the wound with the palm of the hand. *See* **Bleeding,** p.516.

Do not wash or interfere with the wound.

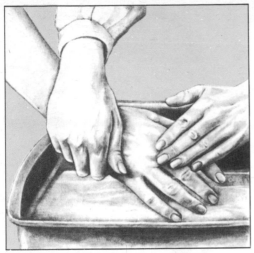

1a
If the cut is small, wash the wound with soap and water, rinse it thoroughly, and dry.

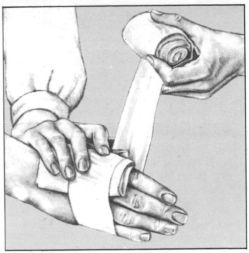

1b
Apply a clean dressing over the cut.

Do not touch the part of the dressing that will be applied to the wound.

Do not apply any salves or ointments.

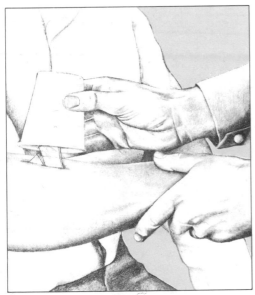

3a
Do not remove the impaled object that caused the wound if it is still embedded in the skin.

Carefully cut away any clothing from around the wound.

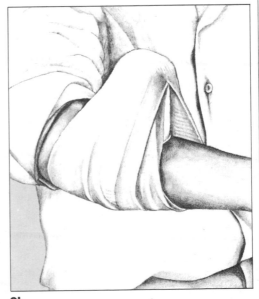

3b
Cover the impaled object with anything that will prevent it from being moved, such as a cup.

Bandage the protective cover in place.

Fever

Fever is a state in which the body temperature is above normal and is a symptom of a wide variety of illnesses.

Although there are individual differences, the accepted normal body temperature, measured orally, is 37°C (98.6°F). The underarm temperature is usually 0.5°C (1°F) lower than the mouth temperature. The rectal temperature is about 0.5°C (1°F) higher than the mouth temperature.

Young children and elderly people often have a temperature slightly above 37°C (98.6°F). A temperature of 40°C (104°F) is more common in infants and children than in adults and carries a different medical significance.

Fever may be accompanied by shivering, sweating, headache, restlessness, loss of appetite, weakness, confusion, and delusions.

Action

Take the patient's temperature. If it is 38.8°C (102°F) or higher on two occasions, four hours apart, call your doctor.

Try to establish the cause of the fever. There may be other complaints. If there does not seem to be a simple cause, or if the patient has a rash, a sore throat, or an earache, consult a doctor.

Put the patient to bed in a cool, quiet room.

If there is a moderate or high fever, undress the patient and sponge with lukewarm water.

Continue the sponging until the temperature has decreased. Between spongings, keep the patient lightly covered with a sheet.

Do not be alarmed if the patient has no appetite. Encourage the patient to drink plenty of fluids, especially fruit juices. **Do not** give alcohol.

Aspirin or paracetamol may be given to help reduce the temperature. The maximum adult dosage is two tablets every six hours for twenty-four hours. Children's aspirin should be used for children.

If the fever has not gone within forty-eight hours, consult a doctor.

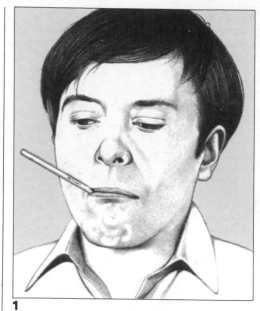

1
Before taking a temperature, make sure that the mercury has been shaken down. Place the bulb of the thermometer beneath the tongue. After one minute, remove the thermometer and note the mercury level.

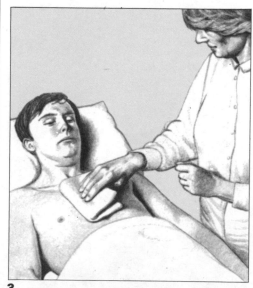

3
If the fever is over 40°C (104°F), place the patient on a waterproof sheet and sponge the body down with lukewarm, not cold, water. Check the patient's temperature every ten minutes.

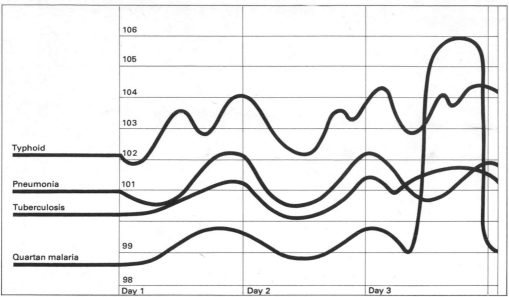

		Day 1	Day 2	Day 3

Typhoid
Pneumonia
Tuberculosis
Quartan malaria

106
105
104
103
102
101
99
98

2

It is thought that fever helps the body in its fight against disease, although the process is not yet fully understood. One possible reason may be that some microorganisms cannot live in temperatures over 0.5°C (1°F) above "normal" body temperature.

Fever patterns are an important diagnostic aid. Some diseases reflect the life cycle of the invading organism. For example, malarial protozoa break out from the red blood cells every seventy-two hours, causing a rapid rise in temperature.

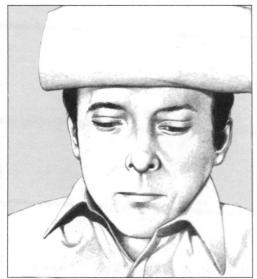

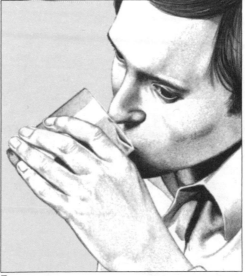

4

If the patient is obviously uncomfortable, put some crushed ice in a sealed plastic bag, and wrap the bag in a dry cloth. Place the bag on the patient's forehead, refilling when necessary.

5

Give the patient frequent drinks. The patient should eat a high protein diet, because the body can lose as much weight as a pound a day during a fever. If the patient cannot eat, the weight must be regained during convalescence.

Haemorrhoids

Haemorrhoids, also called piles, are painful swellings resulting from the formation of varicose veins in the anus and rectum.

Internal haemorrhoids occur at the junction of the anus and rectum and are covered with mucous membrane.

External haemorrhoids occur just outside the anus and are covered with skin.

Haemorrhoids can occur at any age, often without any obvious cause. But common causes include constipation or diarrhoea; pregnancy; liver disorders; rectal tumours; and the repeated use of laxatives.

Haemorrhoids cause itching and burning, and may bleed during a bowel movement.

Action

Anybody suffering from haemorrhoids should consult a doctor because self-medication provides only temporary relief, and because there may be a serious underlying cause.

Depending on the severity of the haemor-rhoids, a doctor may treat them with injections to shrink them, or may recommend their surgical removal (haemorrhoidectomy). Surgical removal provides a permanent cure.

Sometimes the blood in a haemorrhoid clots (thromboses), forming a firm nodule which can be very painful. The pain may be relieved by applying an ice pack to the affected area, and by taking pain-killing drugs.

A warm bath and scrupulous cleanliness may also provide some relief.

Avoid constipation by keeping to a high fibre diet. Do not use laxatives.

Haemorrhoids do not cause cancer, nor do they become cancerous. But bleeding from the rectum may be a sign of cancer, so any bleeding should be investigated by a doctor to exclude the possibility of cancer.

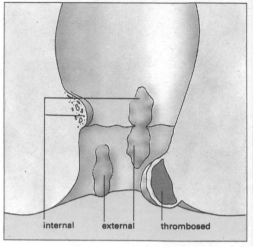

internal external thrombosed

1
Haemorrhoids occur in the lining of the rectum and the anus. They are swellings caused by collections of dilated (varicosed) veins. Swellings that occur inside the rectum (internal haemorrhoids) are covered by mucous membrane. Swellings in the lining of the anus (external haemorrhoids) are covered by anal skin. If the veins inside a haemorrhoid rupture, a blood clot forms.

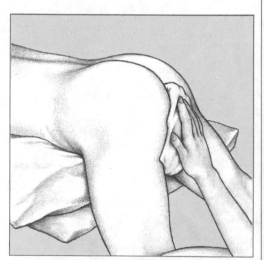

2
To relieve the pain caused by thrombosed haemorrhoids, apply an ice pack to the anal region. The patient should lie on the side or back with the legs open while another person presses the ice pack on to the affected area. At best, however, this method provides only temporary relief, and a doctor must be consulted for more permanent treatment.

Hiccups

Hiccups are usually not serious and may be caused by overeating; minor stomach disorders; excessive drinking; or emotional stress.

Persistent hiccups for hours or days may be a symptom of a more serious disorder, such as a brain lesion; a tumour in the chest cavity; various intestinal diseases; kidney or liver disease; or uraemia. These causes are all comparatively rare and in such cases there are usually other symptoms.

If hiccups are persistent or occur frequently, the patient should consult a doctor who may prescribe a tranquillizing drug; very rarely, it may be necessary to anaesthetize the nerve that serves the diaphragm.

Action

Most of the treatments for occasional bouts of hiccups are based on the principle of stretching the diaphragm.

When due to minor causes, hiccups usually respond to one or another of the following remedies, or may disappear spontaneously.

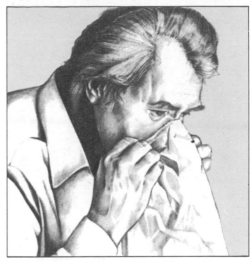

2a
Breathe into a paper bag for several minutes. **Do not** use a plastic bag.

If that is ineffective, take a deep breath and hold it for as long as possible.

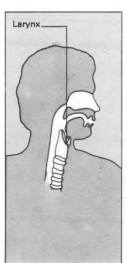
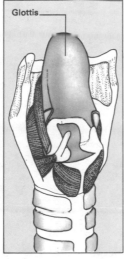

1
Hiccups are a succession of gasping sounds caused by spasmodic contractions of the diaphragm.

This causes a sharp intake of breath with the result that the glottis closes spasmodically, thereby producing the characteristic "hick" sound.

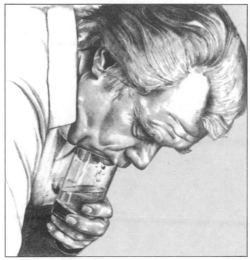

2b
Other remedies that may help include: Drinking cold water from the wrong side of the glass, as shown above.

Pulling the tongue forward with force.

A sharp blow on the back of the chest.

Miscellaneous minor injuries

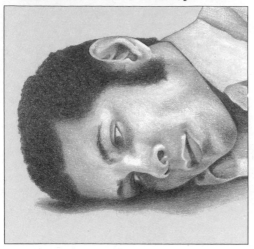

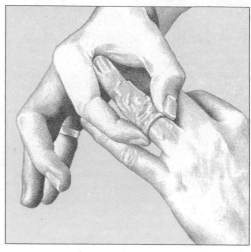

Foreign body in the ear

Do not attempt to remove any object from the ear.

Lay the victim down with the affected ear uppermost and calm the victim.

On no account attempt to remove the object. Obtain professional medical attention as quickly as possible.

Ring stuck on a finger

Place the finger in ice, then cover it with grease and try to slip the ring off.

If this method is ineffective, place a strong strip of thin plastic under the ring and over the knuckle. Gently try to pull the ring off. If both these methods fail and the blood circulation is constricted, urgently seek medical attention.

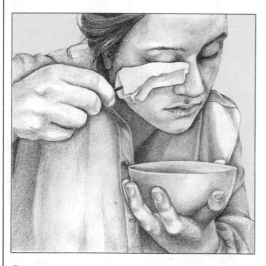

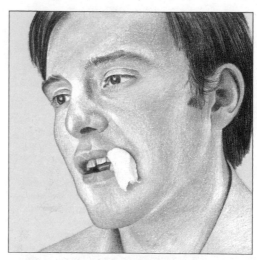

Stye

A stye is a pus-filled inflammation around an eyelash.

Treatment for a stye involves the application of a hot compress. Use water as hot as you can stand, on a cloth pad wound round a smooth object with a handle – like a spoon. Apply for ten minutes every two hours; if this is ineffective, consult a doctor.

Broken tooth

Try to avoid touching the tooth with the tongue. Place a piece of gauze over the jagged tooth.

Put another piece of gauze inside the cheek. This will prevent the tooth from damaging the inside of the cheek.

Consult a dentist as soon as possible.

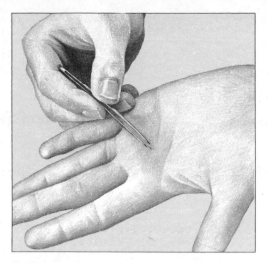

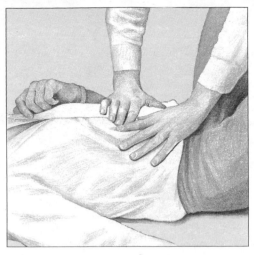

Splinter

Do not attempt to remove a large splinter or one that is not protruding from the skin. Consult a doctor.

If the splinter is small and is protruding from the skin, grasp the end of the splinter with a pair of tweezers. Carefully pull out the splinter in the opposite direction to which it entered the skin. Apply antiseptic.

Stitch

A stitch is a cramp-like pain in the abdomen that is caused by a spasm of the diaphragm. It occurs most commonly during exercise, particularly in those who are not fit.

Lay the victim down and gently rub the affected part of the abdomen. **Do not** start to exercise again for at least fifteen minutes after pain has gone.

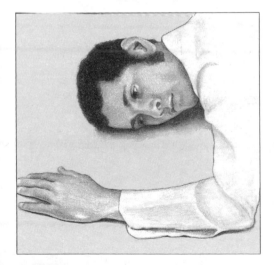

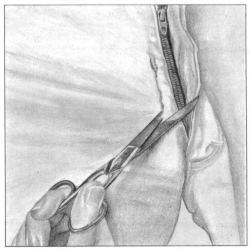

Winding

Winding results from a violent blow to the upper part of the abdomen. The victim may gasp for air or may even lose consciousness.

Place the victim in the recovery position.

Loosen the victim's clothing around the neck, chest, and waist. If the pain and adverse symptoms persist, seek medical advice.

Zip injuries

Loose skin may become trapped in the teeth of a zip, causing a painful but rarely serious injury. **Do not** attempt to force open the teeth. Using blunt-ended scissors, cut across the closed end of the zip at a point well below the site of injury, then pull open the teeth. If this fails, remove the end-stop of the zip in order to open the teeth. Apply a cold compress to the wound.

589

Nosebleeds

Nosebleeds in adults are usually the result of a direct injury to the nose that causes small blood vessels to rupture and bleed. Nosebleeds may occur without obvious cause.

A minor nosebleed may follow vigorous nose blowing or sneezing.

Nosebleeds may have more serious underlying causes, such as infection; allergy; tumours in the nose; high blood pressure; arteriosclerosis; various blood disorders; fever; or even possibly a skull fracture.

Nosebleeds may also occur in those taking anticoagulant drugs. This is an indication that the dosage needs adjustment.

Action

A trickle of blood from the nose may be a sign of a fractured skull. *See* **Head and facial injuries,** p.552.

A doctor should be consulted if nosebleeds occur without obvious cause; if the victim is taking anticoagulant drugs; if a broken nose is suspected; or if nosebleeds recur frequently when there is no known tendency that might explain them.

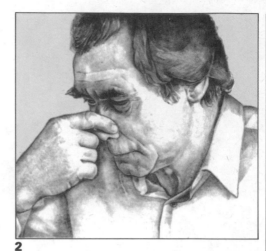

2

Firmly pinch the soft part of the nostril just below the bone for about ten minutes even if the bleeding has stopped.

Instruct the victim not to blow the nose for forty-eight hours.

If bleeding has not stopped within thirty minutes, telephone your doctor. Loss of blood may become serious.

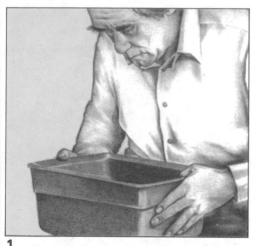

1

Place the victim in a sitting position with the head tilted forwards over a bowl.

Place a gauze pad in each nostril.

Instruct the victim to breathe through the mouth and to avoid swallowing.

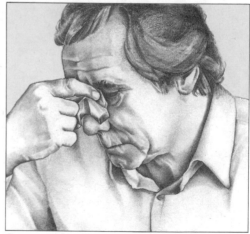

3

An ice pack can be applied to the bridge of the nose that is bleeding.

If the victim is injured but still conscious, elderly, or in shock, lay the victim down with the head and shoulders raised on a pillow.

Summon emergency medical aid.

Scrapes and abrasions

Scrapes and abrasions are superficial injuries to the skin and mucous membranes. Extensive abrasions are often sustained following motorcycle and bicycle accidents, for example.

Although scrapes and abrasions are relatively minor injuries, they may be painful and can easily become infected.

As with any open wound, there is the danger of tetanus. A doctor should be consulted about antitetanus injections.

If dust and grit are left in the wound, there may be permanent marks on the skin. Any such foreign matter should be removed before the wound has healed.

Action

Examine the victim for other injuries.

If the victim has extensive abrasions, summon emergency medical aid.

Do not remove any scabs that may form over the injury. They will fall off when the wound has healed. If scabs are removed before the wound has fully healed, the abrasion may begin to bleed again.

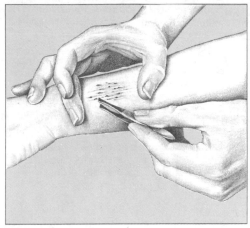

2a

Any pieces of grit lying loose in the wound can be removed with a pair of sterilized tweezers. **Do not** dig deeply into the wound.

If there is a lot of grit in the wound, or if the grit is too deeply embedded to be removed easily, dress and bandage the wound and seek medical attention.

Do not apply any lotions or ointments.

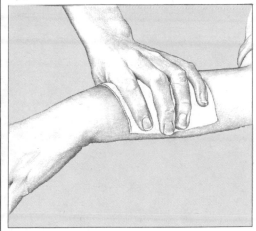

1

If the wound is bleeding, place a clean dressing over the wound.

Apply firm pressure over the dressing until the bleeding stops. Remove the dressing carefully once the bleeding has stopped.

If the bleeding is severe, control it and make sure medical aid has been summoned. *See* **Bleeding,** p.516.

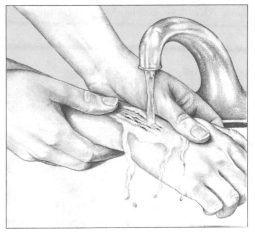

2b

Wash the wound with soap and water, rinse it thoroughly, and dry the area.

Do not cover the wound unless it is bleeding or is in a place where the victim's clothing will rub. Minor wounds heal better if left exposed to the air.

If the wound becomes inflamed and painful, or exudes pus, consult a doctor.

Sprains and strains

A sprain is an injury to the ligaments that surround a joint. The ligaments hold the joint in position, but may be stretched or torn.

A strain is an injury to a muscle in which the muscle fibres are torn or stretched. It is a less serious injury than a sprain.

Sprains most often occur in the ankle, knee, wrist, shoulder, or spine.

The area most often affected by strain is the lower back. This injury is usually caused by lifting heavy objects incorrectly.

Action

With a severe sprain, the joint usually swells rapidly. Several hours after the initial injury bruising may appear.

The major symptom of a strain is a sharp pain at the time of injury. The muscle may feel stiff and the pain may become worse.

The symptoms of both sprains and strains resemble those of a fracture. If in any doubt, treat the injury as a fracture and seek medical advice.

With any sprain or strain the injured part should be moved as little as possible.

Do not allow the victim to walk if there is any injury to any part of the leg.

A severe sprain may need expert splinting and bandaging.

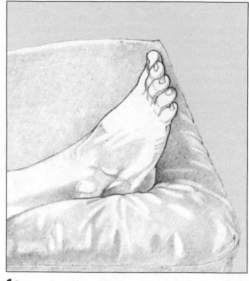

1a
If the victim has a sprain, elevate and support the joint with pillows in the most comfortable position.

Carefully remove the clothing around the joint.

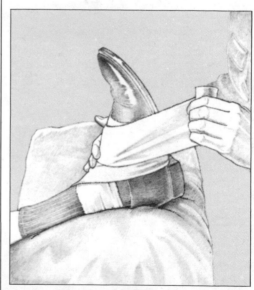

2
If an ankle is sprained out of doors, **do not** remove the victim's shoe.

Give additional support by applying a figure-of-eight bandage over the shoe.

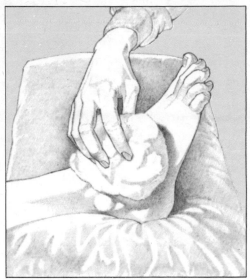

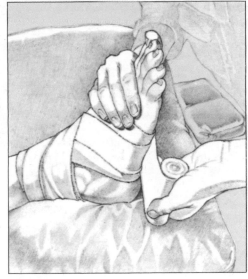

1b
Apply an ice pack to the affected joint for several minutes every hour. This eases the pain and minimizes the swelling. A cold, wet cloth may be used instead of an ice pack.

Do not immerse the joint in iced water.

1c
Immobilize the joint by surrounding it with a layer of cotton-wool, keeping it in place with a bandage.

If the joint begins to swell, loosen the bandage.

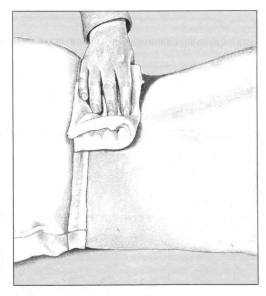

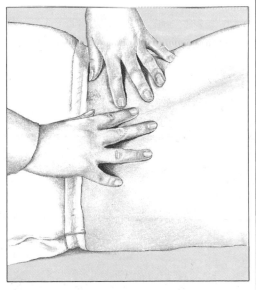

3a
If the victim has strained a muscle, apply heat to the injured area, unless a fracture is suspected.

A heat lamp or heating pad is a suitable way of relieving the pain. A hot bath also helps.

3b
Gentle massage of the strained muscle may help to relieve the pain.

Any strain that causes severe pain should be examined by a doctor.

Sunburn

Sunburn is an inflammation of the skin caused by excessive exposure to ultraviolet rays. In mild cases of sunburn, the radiation causes the skin to become red, but with severe sunburn, blisters may form. Later the burned skin flakes off in scales.

A person suffering from sunburn may suffer from headaches, dizziness, fever, vomiting, and mild shock.

Sunburn can be avoided by not exposing the skin to the sun for long periods, and by using sun filter creams.

Action

Get the victim into the shade immediately.

Cool the burned area with cold water or an ice pack. Immersion in a tub of cool water is soothing.

The first-aid treatment for sunburn is the same as that for other burns. *See* **Burns and scalds,** p.524.

If the burn is severe or extensive, or the victim experiences a strong reaction to exposure, treat the victim for shock. *See* **Shock,** p.566.

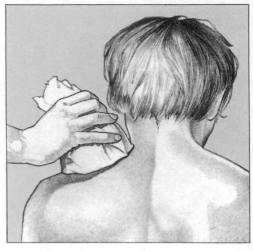

1b
The burned areas should be washed with lightly running cold water. If the burn is deep, and it is possible to leave it to soak in a basin or tub of water, then this will help to relieve the pain. The pain from burns on the shoulders and upper regions can be relieved with a cold compress, such as one made from crushed ice in a plastic bag.

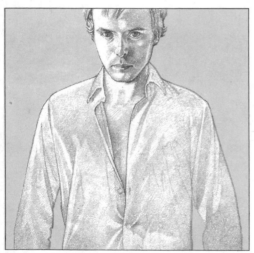

1a
To prevent further burning cover the exposed area with a loosely fastened shirt, or drape a towel over the exposed area. Remove the victim to deep shade, such as inside a house; the shade provided by trees is inadequate. If the victim remains exposed to the rays, deep burning is likely to occur, and may cause permanent damage to the skin. Heatstroke may accompany excessive sunburn.

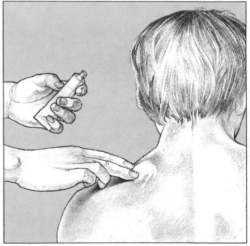

1c
A further soothing effect can be obtained from the use of sunburn lotion rubbed gently over the burned area. Plain, unperfumed moisturizers also have a cooling effect over the area of inflammation. Never use creams or moisturizers until after the skin has been cooled with ice or water. Do not cover the area, but leave exposed to the air. Let blisters heal naturally.

Toothache and gumboil

Toothache is a symptom of many dental disorders, but usually of tooth decay. The outer layers of the tooth are destroyed, and the nerve is exposed.

A filling which is too close to the pulp of a tooth may also cause toothache, especially after eating or drinking hot, cold, or sweet substances.

Occasionally, toothache may be caused by a disorder in another part of the body, such as an ear infection.

A gumboil is an abscess caused by infection adjacent to the root of a tooth. Pus forms in the abscess, causing swelling and extreme pain in the affected tooth.

There are several ways of reducing the likelihood of dental decay:
reducing the amount of sugar in the diet; taking fluoride tablets; regular brushing and use of dental floss; and regular visits to a dentist.

Toothache is common in infants who are cutting teeth. In addition to the pain, the gums may be inflamed; the infants may lose their appetite; and they may be irritable. Toothache caused by teething is normal.

Action

For treatment of toothache or gumboil, consult a dentist as soon as possible.

Pain may subside for a time, but it returns and is a sign that expert treatment is required.

If toothache is caused by a gumboil, there may be a discharge of pus.

Pain-killers such as aspirin or paracetamol may help. **Do not** exceed the recommended dose, no matter how painful the toothache is.

Do not eat or drink any hot, cold, or sweet substances.

Gently clean out a cavity with mouthwashes.

Do not put a pain-relieving tablet directly on an affected tooth. The position of the tablet cannot lessen the toothache and the drug may be harmful to the gum. Oil of cloves applied directly on to the aching tooth may give temporary relief.

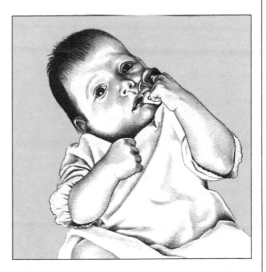

1
In some cases of toothache, cold may help to relieve the pain. Hold an ice pack against the cheek.

Alternatively, apply oil of cloves directly on the affected tooth.

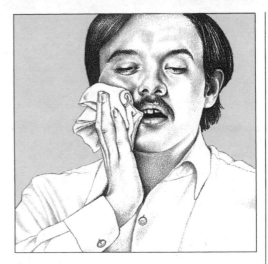

2
Toothache caused by teething in infants does not usually require expert medical attention. Give the infant a teething biscuit or a teething ring to chew. This helps the cutting process.

Do not use any medicines without expert medical advice.

595

Travel disorders

Precautions should be taken before extensive travel to ensure that problems of ill health do not arise or, if they do, they are prevented from becoming serious.

Pack clothing appropriate to the area and the type of holiday. Find out as much about the region to be visited as possible. Organize adequate health insurance for each person. Ensure that all protective immunization is up to date. If you suffer from any permanent or recurrent medical problem, consult your doctor before departure. Specialist advice should also be obtained before visiting the tropics. Some tropical diseases have long incubation periods, so it is important to inform your doctor at once if you become ill shortly after returning home. If you are recovering from a cold, you should consult your doctor before flying.

Drugs to travel with should include aspirin; antihistamine tablets; mild sleeping pills; antinauseant tablets; antidiarrhoeal mixture; insect repellents; antiseptic cream; and water sterilizing tablets.

Motion sickness

Motion sickness is nausea and vomiting that is caused by violent or repeated movement of the body, which affects the organ of balance within the ear. Motion sickness may be preceded by sweating, headache, and fatigue. It is most common in children, and may occur with any form of transportation.

If you suffer from motion sickness, you should take antinauseant drugs the night before the journey, and again on the morning of the journey. Antinauseant drugs may cause drowsiness and should not be taken if you intend to drive a car. If you are taking regular medication for other disorders, consult your doctor before the journey because these drugs may interact with some antinauseants.

A light meal should be eaten about half an hour before the journey, because an empty stomach may increase the feeling of nausea. During the journey, you should lie down with the head slightly raised. You should lie in a part of the vehicle with the least movement, such as the centre of a boat, or near the wings of an aircraft. If this is not possible, it sometimes helps to look at a level horizon or a point within the vehicle. Small amounts of food and drink should be taken at regular intervals. Alcohol should be avoided.

Altitude sickness

Altitude sickness occurs as a result of a lack of oxygen at high levels. It affects people who are not acclimatized to high altitudes. Individual susceptibility varies greatly, being most severe in the elderly and in those with heart or chest problems.

Symptoms of altitude sickness include mild confusion; increase in the rate and depth of breathing; dizziness; fatigue; headache; vomiting; nosebleed; and problems with seeing or hearing.

In time the body gradually adjusts to the lower oxygen concentration. But until you have become fully acclimatized, you should avoid physical exertion. For severe symptoms, breathing oxygen and immediate return to a lower altitude gives relief.

Food poisoning

Serious diseases can be contracted from infected food and water. You should avoid unwashed fruit, precooked foods, and unsterilized water. Bottled drinking water can be bought in many countries. If in any doubt about the water, use sterilizing tablets or boil the water first. Personal hygiene is vital when travelling. You should always wash your hands before handling food.

The symptoms of food poisoning include diarrhoea, vomiting, headache, and fever. If any of these symptoms persist for more than twelve hours, consult a doctor.

Jet lag

Jet lag is caused by a disturbance of the body's biological rhythms and is a common problem after long flights. It causes fatigue and slight disorientation during the period that the body readjusts to new sleeping and eating times. The symptoms of jet lag are often made worse by overeating during the flight, and a high alcohol consumption that results in slight dehydration.

Plenty of fluids should be taken during the flight, and small amounts of food should be eaten every few hours. A mild sedative, prescribed by your doctor, may help to ensure proper sleep after arrival.

Traveller's diarrhoea

Traveller's diarrhoea is an intestinal disorder that may be caused by several factors. The usual causes include a change in diet, which disturbs the microorganisms in the intestine; excessive intake of fruit; large quantities of alcohol; or true intestinal infections. The symptoms include severe stomach cramp, vomiting, and diarrhoea.

Plenty of fluids should be drunk to prevent dehydration. A bland diet and antidiarrhoeal drugs usually control the symptoms until there is a natural improvement. Consult a doctor if the symptoms persist for more than twelve hours, if the diarrhoea is blood-stained, or if there is a high fever.

Vomiting

Vomiting is the forceful ejection of the stomach contents through the mouth. The diaphragm presses downwards; the abdominal wall is drawn inwards; the wave of stomach contractions moves in reverse; the sphincter leading from the stomach into the small intestine closes; and the stomach muscles contract to expel the contents back up the oesophagus.

Vomiting may be caused by overeating; excessive drinking; swallowing an irritating substance; travel sickness; allergic reactions; shock; pregnancy; head injury; peptic ulcer; intestinal infections; and migraine.

If vomiting persists, or if there is blood in the vomit, a serious underlying cause, such as a bleeding ulcer or internal injury, is indicated.

Action

A conscious victim should lie down in a quiet room with a basin at the bedside.

Do not attempt to suppress vomiting.

Do not give the victim any food or drink.

Do not give the victim any medicines.

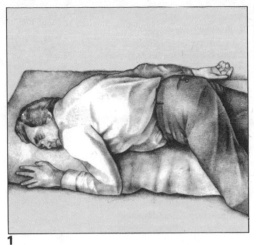

1

An unconscious or semiconscious victim should be placed in the recovery position, to prevent the inhalation of vomit. Check frequently that the victim's airway is clear.

If the victim has inhaled vomit and is choking, clear the airway. *See* **Choking and coughing, p.526.**

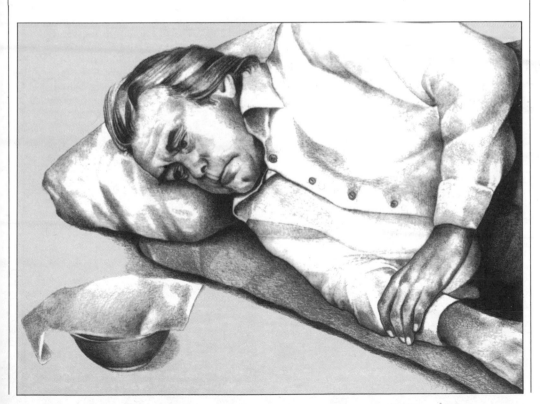

What could be wrong?

Assessment index

What could be wrong?

Somehow, it is only in the face of a minor domestic injury or disorder that people may think of applying first aid to themselves. And yet very often, at the outset of a serious illness or when an injury has been sustained but not assessed or treated, there are signs and symptoms that can be recognized, and a first aid procedure started to counteract possible further pain, complications, and discomfort.

This section examines all the most significant medical conditions that are common symptoms of disorders or injuries. The section is an index for the reader to use in assessing what the onset of one or more of these symptoms may require in terms of self-administered first aid. The relevant disorders and injuries are listed, with page-references to specific parts of the first aid section. A second list of other causes of each symptom is also given.

Most importantly, in addition, there are recommendations included concerning when (or whether) to consult a doctor.

The section should not be regarded as providing a conclusive assessment, much less a diagnosis, of all possible ailments. In all cases of doubt about health, it is essential that a doctor or a specialist should be consulted for an accurate diagnosis.

What could be wrong? is therefore an unusual section for a first aid manual in that it does not contain instructions aimed at a first aider surveying a victim. Instead, when you, the reader, are aware that something may be going wrong within your own body, the section may be referred to and action may be taken – by yourself.

Confused state

consult a doctor immediately

Dangerous plants	530-531
Drug overdose	534-537
Exposure	558-559
Faintness	544-545
Fracture	546-553
Frostbite	558-559
Head injury	552-553
Heart attack	554-557
Poisoning	562-565
Shock	566
Vomiting	597

Other possible causes of a confused state:
Allergy
Concussion
Dementia
Epilepsy
Fever
Hyperglycaemia
Neurological disorder
Stroke

Fever

consult a doctor

Burn	524-525
Drug overdose	534-537
Fever	584-585
Poisoning	562-565
Scald	524-525
Shock	566
Sting	514-515

Note: Any fever can cause delirium, especially in a child or elderly person.

Other possible causes of fever:

(1) *with a rash*
Chickenpox
German measles
Measles
Rheumatic fever
Roseola
Typhoid fever
Typhus

(2) *lasting for more than a week*
Brucellosis
Cancer
Endocarditis
Glandular fever
Hepatitis
Pneumonia
Pyelonephritis
Rheumatic fever
Tuberculosis

Haemorrhage

Abortion	540-543
Accidental amputation	561
Bite	514-515
Bleeding	516-517
Burn	524-525
Cut	584-585
Emergency childbirth	540-543
Fracture	548-553
Haemorrhoids	587
Nosebleed	591
Scrapes and abrasions	592

consult a doctor or seek emergency medical aid

Other possible causes of bleeding:

(1) *from the mouth*
Bitten cheek
Bitten tongue
Bleeding tooth socket
Bronchitis
Gingivitis
Infection
Injury
Laryngitis
Lung cancer
Nosebleed
Pneumonia
Tonsillitis
Tracheitis

(2) *from the stomach or anus*
Anal fissure
Anal fistula
Cancer
Diverticulitis
Gastritis
Growth in rectum
Haemorrhoids
Injury
Intestinal obstruction
Peptic ulcer
Sharp foreign body
Vomiting

(3) *in the urine*
Bladder disorder
Kidney disorder
Urethral disorder

(4) *from the genitals*
from the vagina
Blood disorder
Cervical cancer
Menorrhagia
Menstrual problem
Venereal disease

from the penis
Blood disorder
Cancer
Urological disorder
Venereal disease

Eye and vision problems

Note: Some of these symptoms may be serious. Where indicated, **consult a doctor immediately.**

See also the articles on Blindness and Eye disorders in the A-Z section.

Other possible causes of eye and vision problems:

1 Disturbances of the eye

Painful eye (usually red)

Common causes:		**Consult doctor immediately**	
	Conjunctivitis	Other causes:	Glaucoma
	Corneal ulcers and abrasions		Iritis or choroiditis
	Foreign body in eye		Tension headache
	Migraine		Trigeminal neuralgia
	Sinusitis		

Red eye

Common causes:			
	Common cold	Other causes:	Allergies
	Conjunctivitis		Corneal ulcers and abrasions
	Insomnia		Drugs or alcohol
	Sinusitis		Foreign body in eye
	Smoking		Glaucoma
	Subconjunctival haemorrhage		Hay fever
			Iritis or choroiditis
			Seborrhoea

Sensitivity to bright light (photophobia)

Common causes:			
	High fevers (especially children)	Other causes:	Brain disorders
	Migraine		Encephalitis
			Meningitis
			Snow blindness

Watering eye

Common causes:			
	Conjunctivitis	Other causes:	Allergies
	Emotional causes		Blocked drainage duct
			Common cold
			Foreign body

2 Disturbances of the eyelid

Irritation of the eyelid

Common causes:			
	Conjunctivitis	Other causes:	Allergies
			Blepharitis
			Seborrhoea

Swollen eyelid

Common causes:			
	Stye	Other causes:	Black eye
			Blepharitis
			Chalazion

3 Disturbances of vision

Blurred vision

Common causes:	Astigmatism (long or short sight) Cataract	Other causes:	Conjunctivitis Damage to retina Glaucoma Haemorrhage Iritis Migraine Neuritis of optic nerve Night blindness Poisoning Retinitis Stroke Thrombosis of eye artery or vein

"Dots" or "specks" in front of eyes

Common cause:	Fatigue	Other causes:	Conjunctivitis Iritis Low blood pressure or standing up too quickly Migraine Retinitis

Double vision

Consult doctor immediately

Common causes:	Alcohol (causing lack of co-ordination of eye movements) Concussion Fatigue Migraine	Other causes:	Encephalitis Hyperthyroidism Meningitis Myasthenia gravis Paralysis of nerve to eye muscle

"Floaters" ("black threads" in vision)

Causes:	Minor degeneration within eye Remains of artery and veins to lens "collapsed" at birth

Halos around lights

Consult doctor immediately

Common cause:	Cataract	Other cause:	Glaucoma

Lack of or disturbance of colour vision

Common cause:	Congenital colour blindness	Other causes:	Drugs Excessive sunlight Smoking

Momentary loss of vision

Consult doctor immediately

Common causes:	Low blood pressure Migraine	Other causes:	Emboli High blood pressure

"Zigzags" in front of eyes

Common cause:	Migraine	Other cause:	High blood pressure

Pain

Angina pectoris	554-555	Drug overdose	534-537	With any pain that has no
Bite	514-515	Electric shock	538-539	evident cause, or that lasts
Bleeding	516-517	Emergency childbirth	540-543	for an unexpected time,
Blister	576	Fever	584-585	**consult a doctor immediately**
Boil	577	Haemorrhoids	586	
Bruise	578	Head injury	552-553	
Bunion	579	Heart attack	554-557	
Burn	524-525	Poisoning	562-565	
Corns	579	Scrape	591	
Cramp	580-581	Sprains and strains	592-593	
Cut	582-583	Toothache	595	
Dangerous plants	530-531	Travel disorder	596	

Other possible causes of pain:

(1) *in the head*
Abscess on nose
Boil
Common cold
Diphtheria
Earache
Encephalitis
Gastroenteritis
Glandular fever
Headache
Influenza
Meningitis
Migraine
Mumps
Pharyngitis
Sinusitis
Sore throat
Stroke
Subarachnoid
 haemorrhage

(2) *in the limbs and joints*
Arthritis
Ankylosing spondylitis
Bursitis
Capsulitis
Dengue
Fever
Fibrositis
Frozen shoulder
Gout
Joint disorder
Osteoarthritis
Polyarthritis
Polyneuritis
Psoriasis
Reiter's disease
Rheumatic disorder
Rheumatoid arthritis
Still's disease

(3) *in the back*
Ankylosing spondylitis
Arthritis
Cancer
Dysmenorrhoea
Fibrositis
Gynaecological disorder
Kidney disorder
Muscle disorder
Myeloma
Nephrolithiasis
Neuritis
Osteoarthritis
Osteoporosis
Pancreatitis
Peptic ulcer
Pyelitis
Rheumatic disorder
Salpingitis
Scoliosis
Slipped disc
Spinal disorder
Spondylolisthesis
Strain

(4) *in the chest*
Abscess
Bornholm disease
Broken rib
Cardiac disorder
Heartburn
Heart failure
Hiatus hernia
Indigestion
Lung disorder
Pericarditis
Pleurisy
Pneumothorax
Tietze's syndrome

(5) *in the shoulder*
Ankylosing spondylitis
Arthritis
Frozen shoulder
Inflammation
Pulled muscle

(6) *in the stomach*
Anxiety
Appendicitis
Bornholm disease
Cancer
Coeliac disease
Colitis
Constipation
Digestive disorder
Diverticulitis
Dysmenorrhoea
Gall bladder disorder
Gastritis
Gastroenteritis
Hiatus hernia
Intestinal obstruction
Kidney disorders
Jaundice
Peptic ulcer
Peritonitis
Poisoning
Pregnancy
Pyloric stenosis
Pylorospasm

Breathlessness

Breathlessness without any obvious cause – with or without pain – is serious: **consult a doctor**

Bite or sting	514-515	Other possible causes of breathlessness:
Burn or scald	524-525	Anaemia
Choking	526-527	Asthma
Cramp	580-581	Blockage of airway
Dangerous plants	530-531	Breath-holding
Drug overdose	534-537	Bronchitis
Electric shock	538-539	Collapsed lung
Fainting	544-545	Croup
Heart attack	554-557	Emphysema
Heatstroke	567	Heart disorder
Hiccups	587	Kidney disorder
Poisoning	562-565	Pneumonia
Shock	566	Pleurisy

Faintness

Bite or sting	514-515	Other possible causes of faintness:
Bleeding	516-517	Brain abscess
Burn or scald	524-525	Brain tumour
Dangerous plants	530-531	Concussion
Drug overdose	534-537	Diabetes mellitus
Electric shock	538-539	Encephalitis
Fracture	546-553	Epilepsy
Head injury	552-553	Exhaustion
Heart attack	554-557	Meningitis
Heatstroke	567	Pneumonia
Poisoning	562-565	Stroke
Pregnancy	540-543	Temperature extremes
Shock	566	Uraemia
Sunburn	594	

Vomiting

Choking or coughing	526-527	Heatstroke	567	Vomiting with no obvious
Dangerous plants	530-531	Poisoning	562-565	cause, or persistent vomiting,
Drowning	532-533	Shock	566	is serious: **consult a doctor**
Drug overdose	534-537	Sunburn	594	
Fever	584-585			

Other possible causes of vomiting:

(1) *continuously or repeatedly*	(2) *with stomach-ache*	(3) *intermittently*
Brain tumour	Appendicitis	Alcoholism
Diabetes mellitus	Brain tumour	Anorexia nervosa
Encephalitis	Calculus	Brain tumour
Fever	Diabetes mellitus	Diabetes mellitus
Gastric flu	Fever	Encephalitis
Gastritis	Gastritis	Gastritis
Hyperemesis gravidarum	Intestinal obstruction	Hepatitis
Intestinal obstruction	Kidney failure	Hiatus hernia
Kidney failure	Otitis media	Intestinal obstruction
Labyrinthitis	Peptic ulcer	Kidney failure
Meningitis	Peritonitis	Motion sickness
Migraine	Pyelitis	Peptic ulcer
Motion sickness		Pregnancy
Pregnancy		Pyloric stenosis
Volvulus		Stomach disorder

Family safety

Section contents

Introduction

Although the information given in this section is practical and has a strong medical bias, much of the content of this section is intended as precautionary material to be read before an emergency occurs. Instead of providing information for reference in times of stress, or for instruction, this section is meant to be read for general information at the reader's convenience.

The emphasis in this section remains on health and the avoidance of injury. **Safety in the home** shows what kinds of accidents are most likely to occur in the living room, the bedroom, the bathroom, the kitchen, the garage, and the garden; it also suggests precautionary measures that may be taken to avoid these accidents. Because the home environment is so familiar, possible hazards often go unnoticed. However, the annual statistics compiled by the Royal Society for the Prevention of Accidents show that the number of deaths caused by accidents in homes and residential institutions is nearly as many as those caused by road accidents. The home is therefore one of the most dangerous places to be. The majority of children who die in home accidents are under five years of age, and the largest single cause of child fatalities is choking and suffocation. Parents of young children therefore have a special responsibility to take safety precautions and to supervise their children at all times. The comfortable familiarity of the home environment must not be allowed to result in carelessness and negligence.

The following section, **Fire prevention and control,** suggests further safety precautions to be taken in the home, and also deals with fire prevention out of doors. Specific advice is given concerning fireworks and electrical and gas appliances. The procedure to be followed if a fire does break out is outlined, together with information about fire-fighting equipment and methods.

The section **Car and motoring safety** is concerned with the health and safety of drivers and other road users, and no information is given about the servicing and maintainance of vehicles. Practical advice is given concerning clothing, equipment, and ways to avoid fatigue, which is a contributory cause of many road accidents. Fatigue can lead to carelessness, impatience, and lack of concentration. To allow this to happen while driving a vehicle is dangerously irresponsible. A high degree of mental alertness is essential for all road users, and no one should attempt to drive a car or ride a motorcycle or bicycle while tired, under stress, or under the influence of alcohol or drugs.

It must be emphasized that the advice given in this section applies to pedestrians as well as motorists. Everyone who uses roads is at risk, especially children. Child pedestrian casualties represent nearly half of all pedestrian casualties, and the great majority of road accidents involving children occur in built-up areas. Parents should teach their children how to cross roads safely at an early age, and should not allow their children to cross roads unsupervised until they have learned and fully understood the kerb drill or the Green Cross Code.

The next section provides advice about **Camping and caravanning safety.** As the cost of hotel accommodation rises, these types of holiday are becoming increasingly popular. Advice is given about hygiene and equipment. On crowded camp sites and caravan sites, where cooking often has to be done in cramped conditions and normal toilet facilities may be unavailable, personal hygiene is even more important than it is at home. This applies particularly to families with young children, who are more vulnerable to infection, and to those who take their holidays abroad, where the food may be unfamiliar and the water may contain harmful bacteria. Camping and caravanning holidays need careful planning with regard to food, warmth, and shelter. When packing, remember to include supplies of tinned food in case of emergencies, plenty of clothes suitable for all possible weather conditions, and, of course, a first-aid kit.

The section on **Hiking safety** also deals with an activity that is becoming increasingly popular. The benefits of extended exercise in the open air are substantial, but many city-dwellers imagine that they can set off for hikes in the countryside without any special preparation, and so expose themselves to unnecessary danger. The importance of suitable clothing and equipment is emphasised, and a procedure for obtaining help in case of accident is explained. The sections on **Sports safety** offer similar advice related to particular winter sports and water sports. Skill in most winter sports, especially skiing, cannot be acquired immediately: it is the result of good training, hard work, and long experience. Most accidents involving beginners occur because they are too impatient and ambitious, and attempt feats that are beyond their capabilities. With water sports, it is essential that anyone who participates must be able to swim. Children should be taught to swim at an early age, although not before they feel safe in the water. They should always swim with an adult trained in life-saving techniques while they are learning, and not be allowed to swim without adult supervision until they have become confident and experienced swimmers.

Throughout this section, emphasis is placed on the need to be aware of potential hazards and to take precautionary measures to prevent accidents before they can occur. Even the non-human causes of accidents – which include adverse weather conditions, mechanical defects, and environmental factors – can often be prepared for and guarded against. For the human causes – which include negligence, carelessness, impatience, and lack of supervision of children – there can be no excuse, and no amount of regret or self-reproach can undo an accident once it has occurred.

In all the activities discussed, children and the elderly are the people most vulnerable to accidents. Children are often led by their natural inquisitiveness and sense of adventure into situations whose dangers they cannot appreciate. Old people are vulnerable because of the natural process of ageing, which involves the gradual deterioration of the faculties of sight, hearing, mobility, and memory.

Safety in the home 1

The living room

Some television sets get very hot and are potential fire hazards. They must stand on a firm base to prevent them from being knocked over. Always turn the set off before leaving the room.

All fireplaces must be protected by a firescreen that covers the entire opening. Make the area above the fireplace as uninteresting as possible to discourage people from reaching over the opening, or standing too close to it. Do not place combustible furnishings near the fireplace opening.

Make sure the bottom shelf of a set of shelves is high enough to prevent a small child using them as a ladder. Keep sewing and knitting materials out of the reach of children. Cigarettes must also be kept out of a child's reach; a small child can be poisoned by eating one cigarette. Remove tablecloths and mats from the table; a child may pull the contents of the table on top of himself or herself.

Inspect all toys carefully for small detachable parts, like glass eyes, or for sharp edges. Be careful that a younger child does not get hold of a toy designed for an older child, for example, a marble, or a piece of a construction set small enough to choke on.

The bedroom and nursery

The cot in the nursery must be stable and high-sided. Make sure that between the sides and the mattress there is no gap in which a child could get trapped. A child under the age of one does not need a pillow; it is dangerous to provide one because an infant may roll over onto the pillow and accidentally suffocate. If older children sleep in bunk beds, the top bed must have a guard rail.

You can warm the baby's cot with a hot water bottle, but remove it before putting the baby to bed. Use a hot water bottle with a thick cover and button-down flap over the metal stopper.

Pyjamas are safer for children than nightdresses; they are less likely to catch in a fire or heater. Make sure that all nightclothes are made of flame-resistant fabric. Central heating in the bedroom and nursery should be set at a temperature low enough to prevent a burn if the radiator is accidentally touched. Never dim a lamp by covering it with anything. Instead, use a low-wattage bulb. Do not hang clothes over a heater to dry, or place a heater near curtains.

Never smoke in bed, but if a person insists on smoking, provide an ashtray. Do not use an electric overblanket under

How people died in domestic accidents in 1977

Type of accident	Age group (in years)						Total for all ages
	0-4	5-14	15-44	45-64	65-74	75 and over	
Falls	30	8	100	313	538	2725	3714
Fires	69	53	87	132	140	289	770
Poisoning	16	11	286	259	77	64	713
Suffocation and choking	148	20	136	153	85	70	612
Other causes	47	15	77	90	73	153	455
Total	310	107	686	947	913	3301	6264

you, or an underblanket over you. Always turn the blanket off before getting into bed, unless the blanket is a low-power kind designed to be left on all night. Check the blanket is serviced regularly and discard it when electrical parts become worn or broken.

Cover all plugs with safety covers when not in use. If a child remains fascinated by a plug, move a heavy piece of furniture in front of it. Keep all cosmetics, aerosol containers, and medicines that must be kept in the bedroom in a locked drawer or on a high shelf out of the reach of children.

Make sure that carpets or other floor coverings are in good repair; a loose or worn carpet or rug may cause a dangerous fall. Loose rugs on top of a polished floor are particularly hazardous.

The bathroom

Touching an ordinary switch with wet hands can give you a severe electric shock. Do not handle electrical appliances, such as an electric shaver, unless your hands are dry.

All medicines, razor blades, scissors, and disinfectants must be kept in a childproof cabinet. Make sure the cabinet is high enough to be out of reach of children.

Check basin and bathtub overflows regularly to make sure they are not blocked. If water overflows, it can make the floor dangerously slippery. Wipe up spills immediately.

Keep the bathroom well ventilated. If the room needs extra heat, have a heater installed by an electrician. It must be high on the wall or ceiling, away from the bathtub or basin, with a cord-pull switch. Never bring a portable heater into a room. Heated towel rails must be cool enough not to burn the skin if touched accidentally. Install a handrail by the bath to provide a safe handgrip when getting into and out of the bath.

At bath time, run cold water into the bath first. This way, if a child steps into the bath without the temperature having been tested with a hand, he or she will not get scalded. Use a non-slip strip or mat in the bath; a child or old person can easily slip when stepping into the bath.

Never leave a small child in the bath alone; a child can drown in less than 5cm (2 inches) of water. If the doorbell or telephone rings, take the child with you, or ignore the call. Never leave a small child in the bath with an older child.

Preventive measures against accidents in the home

Falls
1 Provide adequate lighting for all areas of the house.
2 Install handrails on stairways and in the bathroom.
3 Secure firmly all loose carpets and rugs.
4 Do not leave toys or other small objects lying around on the floor.
5 If there are children in the house, install safety bars at the top of stairways.
6 Do not allow young children to remain alone near open windows.

Burns and scalds
1 Place firescreens around all open fires.
2 Check regularly that all electrical appliances, sockets, plugs, and leads are in good repair.
3 Switch off all electrical appliances when they are not being used.
4 Keep all inflammable liquids out of the reach of children.
5 Do not hang clothes or towels over cookers or heaters to dry.
6 Buy children's clothes, especially night clothes, made of flame-resistant fabric.
7 When cooking, do not let the pan handles hang over the edge of the cooker.

Poisoning
1 Keep all medicines and other potentially dangerous substances and liquids in locked cabinets.
2 Keep all medicines and tablets in their original containers, clearly labelled.
3 Check the correct dosage for all medicines and tablets before taking them.
4 Destroy or return to the chemist all unused medicines and tablets.
5 Check regularly that all gas appliances are in good repair, and make sure that there is good ventilation when using them.

Suffocation
1 Keep all plastic bags inaccessible to children.
2 Check that all blankets in a baby's crib are secure, and cannot be pulled over the baby's face. Do not allow a young baby to sleep on a soft pillow.
3 Watch over a baby when he or she is feeding, and take appropriate action in case of choking.

Safety in the home 2

The kitchen

Keep a fire extinguisher in an accessible place. Make sure all the adult family members know how to use it. Install childproof locks on the fridge. Keep the kitchen well ventilated.

Make sure the kitchen cooker is well maintained and is working correctly. Turn it off when not in use. Turn pan handles away from the front of the cooker so that they are out of the reach of children but not over another burner. Use dry oven gloves to take hot pans and dishes from the oven; a dishcloth is both too thin and dangerous. If you spill something on the floor, wipe it up immediately to prevent the floor from becoming slippery.

Keep knives and sharp cooking utensils in a drawer. Install a childproof lock. Wrap dangerous refuse, like razor blades, in thick newspaper before throwing away.

Keep bleaches, disinfectants, and scouring powders in a high cupboard. Never store them next to fruit drink bottles where even an adult could make a mistake. Store china, glass, and plastic bags in a high cabinet or cupboard. Keep pots and pans and other unbreakables in the lower cupboards. If the highest shelves are difficult for an adult to reach, keep a sturdy kitchen stool available.

With small children in the house, it is essential to keep a play area physically separate from the kitchen, but within view. This eliminates the risk of tripping over a small child or a litter of toys while you are carrying a hot pan.

The garage

Keep the garage well ventilated. Never run a car engine inside the garage: poisonous gases may build up. To inspect the underside of a vehicle, a ramp is safer than a jack. Make sure the handbrake is firmly applied and put chocks behind the wheels. Always clean up after each job; wood shavings and oily rags are a fire hazard. Never smoke in the garage. A fire extinguisher should be kept within easy reach, and every member of the family old enough should be taught how to use it. Whenever you leave the garage, always lock the doors.

The garage should have its own electric socket and not rely on extension cords from the house. Special care should be taken in a garage to ensure that the electrical system is isolated from any place where water, petrol, or any other liquid is stored or used. The electric socket should have its own fuse and be of sufficient voltage to power an electric light plus other garage appliances.

Lock the car door whenever you leave it. A small child could climb in and release the handbrake, start the engine, or get a hand trapped in the door. Take extreme care when backing out of the garage. A small child may be standing behind the car below the level of visibility from the rear-view mirror.

Inside the garage, there should be shelves and hooks on which to store potentially dangerous items out of the reach of children. All bottles and cans of chemicals must be carefully labelled and have tightly fitting lids.There is a legal limit of one gallon of petrol that can be stored. It should be kept in cans specially designed for this purpose. Ladders and sharp tools should be secured to prevent them from falling.

The garden

Outside steps must be kept clean. They must also be adequately lit, and repaired when broken or cracked. Check fences regularly for holes and gaps, so that animals cannot get in and young children cannot get out, especially if the home is situated near a busy street. Fences should be high enough to prevent small children from climbing over. All gates must have childproof locks and be kept closed when not being used.

For safety, place swings, climbing frames, and slides on grass. If the grass beneath wears down to dirt, move the position of the equipment. Never let children play unattended in a swimming pool. The entire family should learn to swim; non-swimmers are a danger to others as well as to themselves.

Keep all garden tools and machinery away from children, preferably in a locked shed. Insecticides and other poisons must be locked in a cabinet, or at least placed on a high shelf. A light switch should be near the house door.

Keep ornamental paths in good repair, and sweep them regularly. Remove any uneven stepping stones and relevel the underlying sand before replacing them.

As early as possible, children should be taught never to taste any plant or fruit without first asking. Children should also never slam shut or kick open gates or doors: there may be somebody on the other side.

If you burn waste or have a barbecue in the garden, make sure that the fire or barbecue is situated in a place to prevent sparks from flying. Also make sure that the area around the fire is clear of inflammable objects. Keep children and pets at a safe distance. Keep a bucket of water or a hosepipe nearby. Never leave the fire unattended. When you have finished, make sure the fire is extinguished by dousing it with water. Do not leave a fire to burn out.

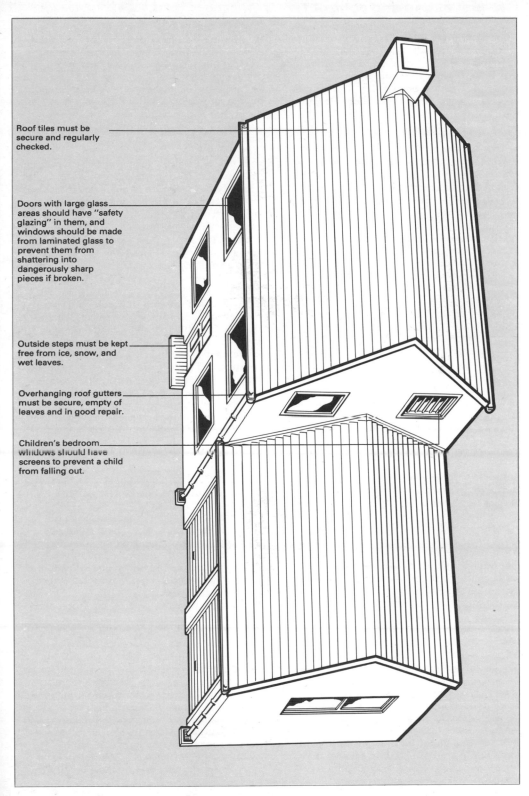

Roof tiles must be secure and regularly checked.

Doors with large glass areas should have "safety glazing" in them, and windows should be made from laminated glass to prevent them from shattering into dangerously sharp pieces if broken.

Outside steps must be kept free from ice, snow, and wet leaves.

Overhanging roof gutters must be secure, empty of leaves and in good repair.

Children's bedroom windows should have screens to prevent a child from falling out.

609

Fire prevention and control 1

The cost of accidental fires in terms of both money and human life is often out of all proportion to the accident or oversight that caused the fire. A number of precautions that may help to prevent the outbreak of accidental fires is listed on this page. These precautions should be remembered and incorporated into the daily routine of every safety-conscious family.

In the home

All open fires should be protected with fire guards and fire screens, especially when there are children or elderly people in the house. Never use petrol or paraffin to help light a fire, or use newspaper to make it draw. Chimneys should be swept regularly, at least once every year. Keep the area directly above the fireplace free of decorations such as mirrors or ornaments; these could tempt an interested person to step too close to the fire.

Never carry any portable heater when it is alight. When refilling oil or paraffin heaters, take care not to spill any of the fuel on the floor or on clothes. No heater should be placed near curtains, clothes, or any other inflammable materials. The most suitable type of heater for children's rooms, bathrooms and garages is a wall-mounted heater, which cannot be accidentally touched or knocked over.

If you want a dimmed light in a bedroom, buy a low-wattage bulb: never attempt to dim a light by covering it with a cloth or other material. Pyjamas and other night clothes should be made of flame-resistant fabric. Remember that it is extremely dangerous to smoke in bed, especially when feeling tired.

In the kitchen, do not hang clothes or towels over the cooker in order to dry them. When cooking, turn all pan handles inwards (but not over another burner) so that the pans cannot be knocked over. Chip-pans should never be filled over half-full with oil, and should never be left unattended while cooking.

In the garage, clearly label all bottles and cans containing inflammable liquids, and keep them out of the reach of children. Keep all aerosol containers away from heat, and never burn them or puncture them even when they are empty. Sweep up all wood shavings as soon as you have finished work. Do not smoke in the garage, and do not use naked lights or flames.

Before you go to bed at night, close all the doors in the house; this could prevent the flames and smoke from spreading if a fire does start during the night.

Out of doors

In hot, dry weather there is an ever-present risk of forest fires. These fires may spread rapidly and fiercely, especially when fanned by even a slight wind.

In these conditions, even a single lighted match may cause a sudden conflagration. All cigarettes and matches must be carefully extinguished before being disposed of, and should never be thrown from the window of a travelling vehicle.

If you are using a gas burner or charcoal grill to cook food in the open air, place it securely on level ground and away from trees or bushes. If you are making an open fire, never use petrol or paraffin to help to light it. It is sensible to position any fire near a running stream or other source of water, and in a sheltered place where the sparks cannot be blown far by the wind.

Fireworks

Fireworks are exciting to watch but dangerous to handle. Each year in Britain over 500 people are injured in accidents involving fireworks during the period around November 5th, and are taken to hospital for treatment. The majority of those injured are children under the age of sixteen. Most of these injuries could be prevented if a series of simple precautions are taken.

All firework displays should be supervised by an adult. If many children are present, screen them away from the firing area with a low fence, and keep the boxes inside the fence. Keep buckets of water close by to dowse any fireworks that get out of control. Make sure that the box is closed after a firework is taken out.

Sort through all the boxes and take out all the hand-held fireworks. These should be kept separate, and handed out individually.

A strict code of rules must be followed when lighting the fireworks, and all children present must understand these rules before the procedure begins.

Light the firework with a long taper, and move away immediately.

If the firework does not light immediately, dowse it with water before approaching. Although it may not appear to be alight, it could explode unexpectedly as you approach.

Never try to rescue a firework that has fallen over. Leave it to burn out on the ground.

Follow the manufacturer's instructions about placing and securing the firework.

Carry a torch with you. Never try to read the instructions by the light of a match.

Carry only one firework at a time. Never carry fireworks around in the pocket of a coat or trousers.

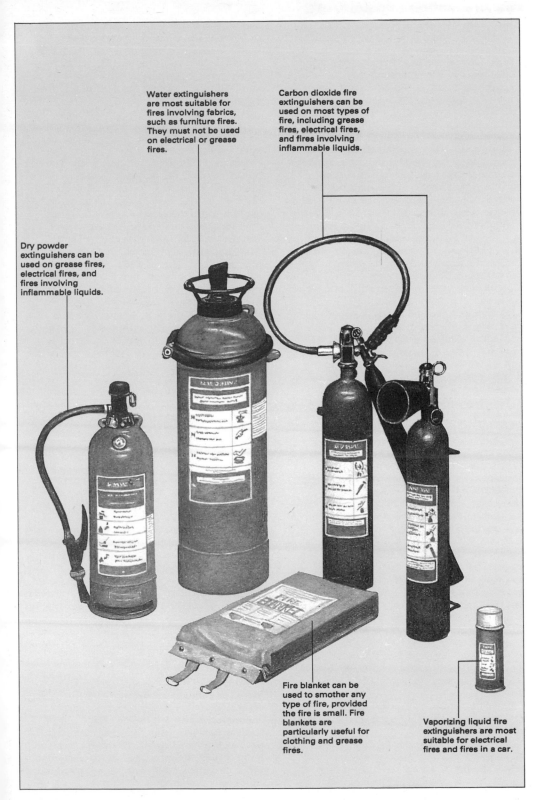

Water extinguishers
are most suitable for
fires involving fabrics,
such as furniture fires.
They must not be used
on electrical or grease
fires.

Carbon dioxide fire
extinguishers can be
used on most types of
fire, including grease
fires, electrical fires,
and fires involving
inflammable liquids.

Dry powder
extinguishers can be
used on grease fires,
electrical fires, and
fires involving
inflammable liquids.

Fire blanket can be
used to smother any
type of fire, provided
the fire is small. Fire
blankets are
particularly useful for
clothing and grease
fires.

Vaporizing liquid fire
extinguishers are most
suitable for electrical
fires and fires in a car.

Fire prevention and control 2

Electrical equipment

Your house should be fitted with a sufficient number of three-pin sockets for all your needs. Do not overload the electrical points by using multi-way adaptors: this can result in overheating and a serious risk of fire. There should be one socket for every appliance that you use, and all sockets should have childproof covers. Do not plug an iron or other appliance into a light socket.

All circuits and plugs should be correctly fused; keep a supply of spare fuses. So that you can change a plug safely, learn the correct wiring colours: green and yellow stripes for earth (E), brown for live (L), and blue for neutral (N).

Do not trail long flexes around a room, and replace all flexes when they become worn or frayed. Be especially careful with the flex of an electric kettle in the kitchen. Do not place flexes under carpets or rugs, as they may become worn or frayed without anybody noticing.

Before going to bed at night, switch off the electricity at the sockets.

Electric blankets need special care. They must never be folded or creased while on or still warm. They should not be used to dry damp bedding, not put on a child's or elderly person's bed if bed-wetting is likely.

When buying new electrical appliances, check that they conform to the appropriate standards of the British Standards Institution.

Gas equipment

A mixture of air and gas is potentially explosive. Never check any suspected leak of gas with a naked flame. A safe method of checking for a leak is to brush soapy water on the suspect part of the pipe or connection, and watch to see if bubbles appear.

Before lighting a gas water-heater or cooker, be fully ready to light it. Check that all pilot lights are lit. If the gas supply is controlled by a coin-operated meter and the gas runs out, turn off all gas taps before inserting more coins.

Gas cylinders and other containers should be kept away from heat, and should be changed in the open air.

All gas heaters should be protected with a metal guard, and should be situated away from curtains and other inflammable furnishings.

Gas taps should be fitted with removable keys, which should not be left in place after use.

In case of fire

When staying in a hotel or working in a school, office, or other public building, read and learn the fire drill for that building. This should tell you what to do if you discover a fire or hear the fire alarm sound. All public buildings must conform to strict safety regulations governing their design, construction, and facilities, and must have a fire drill on public display.

If you discover a fire in a building, the first duty is to bring everyone to the ground floor and evacuate them from the building. You must then call the fire brigade, using the emergency telephone number (999). The last person to leave the building must close all doors and windows as he or she leaves; this reduces draughts, which can fan a fire and cause it to spread rapidly.

If the fire is small or in its early stages, and you are confident that you can tackle it without danger to yourself, use any available equipment to fight the fire. If you use a fire extinguisher, however, make sure that it is suitable to the type of fire, and be careful not to scatter burning material with the jet.

If you are trapped in a room by a fire immediately outside, you should close the door and any other means of access and block all cracks with any available material. This is to prevent smoke from filling the room.

Then go to a window and try to attract attention. If smoke fills the room, lean out of the window. If this is impossible, lie on the floor where the air is clearer.

If you have to escape before help arrives, make a rope by knotting together sheets or upholstery materials and tie the end to a heavy object or fixed point. If there is no material available, throw cushions, mattresses, or other soft material from the window; then lower yourself from the window and drop onto these materials, which should break your fall. Lower yourself (or a child or other person) to the full extent of your arms before dropping.

If you are in a room above the first floor, you should drop to the ground only if there is no other possible means of escaping from the building.

If your clothes catch fire, you should roll on the ground to extinguish the flames. Wrap yourself in blankets or rugs if available.

Chimney fires

Whether you use smokeless or non-smokeless fuel, you should have your chimney swept at least once every year. If the wall becomes very hot, or if the chimney catches fire, you should call the fire brigade immediately. Remove the hearth rug and all other inflammable objects from around the fireplace, and dampen the fire.

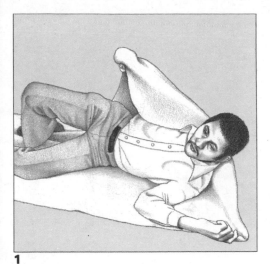

1
If your clothing catches fire, the most important thing to do is to lie on the ground immediately. This slows the flames spreading up the body towards your face. Once on the ground, roll across the floor to extinguish the flames. If there is a rug or blanket close at hand, wrap yourself in it, but do not delay lying down in order to reach for these things. Roll on the flames to smother them.

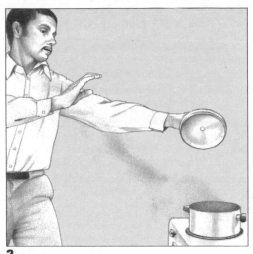

2
If a pan of grease is smoking, then it is too hot and likely to catch fire. If this happens, turn off the heat, and put the fire out with a fire extinguisher, or quickly slide a lid or some other rigid cover over the pan. It is vital to use the correct type of extinguisher. Dry powder extinguishers or fire blankets are suitable for use on grease fires. Never use water on a grease fire.

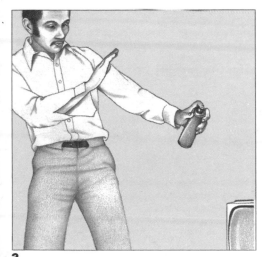

3
All electric circuits and plugs should be correctly fused, and all electrical appliances should be unplugged when not being used. If an electrical appliance or a socket does catch fire, it is essential to use the correct type of extinguisher. Under no circumstances should an electrical fire be fought with water unless the electrical equipment has first been unplugged from the electrical source.

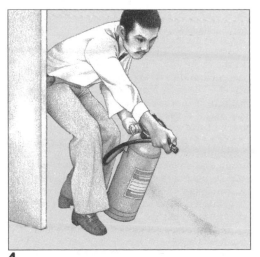

4
It is wise to keep a fire extinguisher near fire hazards. In the event of a fire, position yourself near a clear exit. Stay at a safe distance from the blaze. Direct the jet at the base of the fire, and sweep the jet left and right. Never use water to try to extinguish grease or electrical fires. The best general extinguisher for all fires contains carbon dioxide.

Car and motoring safety 1

Equipment

Motor vehicle accidents are the leading cause of accidental deaths, and the number of road accident fatalities rises steadily. Anyone who drives a car or other vehicle on a road is exposing himself or herself to unavoidable dangers, but it is important to realize that many accidents can be prevented by taking simple safety precautions.

When choosing a car, consider carefully the number of safety factors incorporated into the car's design. Safety regulations now demand that cars are designed in accordance with certain specifications, but above these minimum legal requirements there are wide variations in design.

If you already own a car, there are a number of items of equipment that can improve its safety and for which you, as the owner or driver, are responsible. Some of the items are illustrated on these pages. They are not just attractive accessories: they might actually save your own life and the lives of other road users. Children are especially at risk: each year approximately 22,000 children aged seven years or under are killed or injured in road accidents in Britain.

Of course, it is important not just to equip your car with these accessories, but to use them every time you drive. You should wear your safety belt for every journey, no matter how short. Every time you travel with young children, make sure that they are placed securely in their child seats or harnesses in the back seat. This not only protects children in the event of an accident, but also prevents them from distracting the driver or reaching for the controls. Make sure that the doors are locked. If there is a dog or other animal in the car, it should travel behind a grid in the back of the car.

As well as a first-aid kit and a fire extinguisher, you should carry in your car a torch and a reflective triangle. This triangle can be placed on the road and used as a warning sign in the event of an accident or a breakdown. Also carry a tool box, a tyre pressure gauge, and a jack.

Your mirrors should be aligned to allow the best possible vision of the traffic behind. A simple wide driving mirror is safer than a convex-shaped one, which distorts distances and so makes judgement of speeds more difficult. You should have your car regularly serviced, and you yourself should be able to check the condition of the tyres, shock absorbers, brakes, windscreen wipers, and lights. By caring for the running condition of your car as you care for your own health, you minimize the dangers of accident or breakdown.

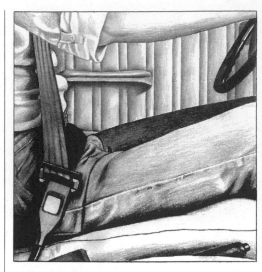

Safety belts

Safety belts with shoulder and lap straps should be worn by the driver and front-seat passengers for every journey, no matter how short. Rear-seat passengers should wear their lap belts. They reduce the danger if an accident occurs. Check that they are fitted securely, and that they are easily accessible for passenger use.

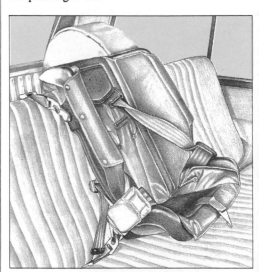

Child seat

Children under the age of five should travel in a crash-tested child safety seat. The seat should be secured to its own car fittings, or by the existing adult lap belt. If the seat is equipped with a top tether strap it must be properly anchored to the car. The back centre seat position is the safest location in the car.

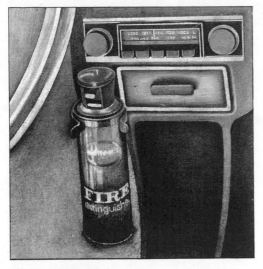

Fire extinguisher

A fire extinguisher should be fitted securely to the interior of the car. It can be of the dry powder, liquid, or gas-filled type, and must be capable of extinguishing fuel and electrical fires. Check the pressure regularly. If a fire does start in the car, get all the passengers out of the vehicle, and well away from it, before returning to fight the fire.

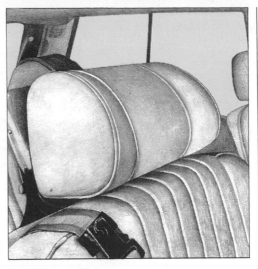

Head restraint

Head restraints prevent whiplash injury to the neck in the event of a collision from behind. They should be an integral part of the seat or anchored securely to it, but should not obstruct the driver's rear vision. Head restraints that clip on to the seat merely provide a head rest, and do not give enough protection to prevent whiplash injury.

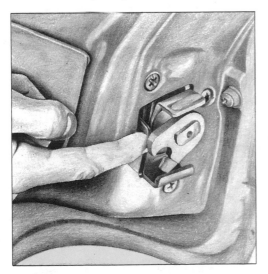

Childproof locks

Any car in which children travel regularly should be fitted with childproof locks. These make it impossible for a child to open the door accidentally. Similar locking devices can be fitted to the windows, to prevent a child from opening the window beyond a certain level. Children should always travel in the back seat of a car, not the front.

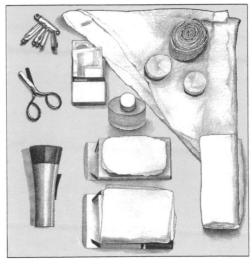

First-aid kit

A first-aid kit should be carried in the car at all times. It should contain at least bandages, adhesive tape, gauze pads, antiseptic, aspirin, scissors, and a first-aid handbook. The box must be closed with a childproof catch, but not locked. Check its supplies before setting off on a long journey. It is also useful to keep tissues in the car.

Car and motoring safety 2
Emergencies

A responsible driver is aware that at any time he or she may be expected to deal with emergencies. The lives of passengers and others may depend on the driver's knowledge and skill, and the driver should take all possible precautions to minimize the risks of accident or breakdown.

Planning ahead

Firstly, before starting any journey, the driver should ensure that the car is in good condition. Check the engine oil level, the tyre pressures (including the spare tyre), the brakes, the headlights, the water level in the cooling system, and the petrol. Take a plastic bottle or can in which to carry an emergency supply of water in case you run out. Check over the car's equipment, make sure that the jack and the tool box are in the car, and that all movable objects in the boot are secure.

For longer journeys, work out your intended route carefully before setting out, and take maps with you. If possible, find out the weather forecasts for the areas you intend travelling through. Tell a reliable person details of the route to be taken, and your estimated time of arrival.

Check the supplies in your first-aid box, which should be carried in the car at all times. For long journeys, you should also take emergency supplies of energy-giving food. Chocolate, nuts, raisins, and glucose or dextrose tablets are especially nourishing.

In snow, take some means of warmth, light, and shelter. If waterproof sleeping bags are not available, take plenty of woollen blankets for every person. For warmth, take a small solid fuel burner. Candles and matches can also be useful, and a torch and flares should be carried in the car.

If your car breaks down in a remote area, you may need to attract rescuers by using some kind of signalling device. This can be done by using, for example, flashing lights, fires, a whistle, or the car's horn. The letters SOS are an internationally recognized distress signal. In the International Morse code these letters are represented by three dots, three dashes, and three dots (··· ––– ···), and this pattern can be formed by flashes of light, blasts on a whistle or the car's horn, or by sticks or strips of light-coloured clothing placed on the ground. Another international distress symbol is a triangular pattern of three fires.

Careful planning of a journey can minimize fatigue, which reduces a driver's concentration and judgement and so increases the chances of an accident. There should be no long, uninterrupted periods of motoring, and it is often sensible to share the driving with a person you are travelling with. Plan your journey to avoid rush hours in big cities, and stop the car at least once every two hours for physical exercise or light refreshment.

In case of accident

If you are involved in a road accident, or arrive at the scene of one, you must act promptly and efficiently to help any injured people and to protect them from further danger. The following actions should be carried out:

(1) To prevent further collisions, warn oncoming traffic by displaying warning signs at least 50 metres (or yards) from the accident (at least 150 metres at night). Use reflective triangles, if these are available, or ask another person to give the warning and wave the traffic past. If your car is fitted with hazard warning lights, switch them on.

(2) To prevent a petrol explosion or any other form of fire, instruct all drivers present to switch off the ignition in their cars. Spread earth or sand on any petrol that may have spilled on the road. Do not let anyone smoke. If a fire does start, use an extinguisher, a blanket, or a coat to put it out.

(3) Make sure that an ambulance and the police are summoned immediately. Use the emergency telephone number (999), and give the exact location of the accident and the number of people injured.

(4) Examine all injured people and look for any who may have been thrown clear of the accident. Do not move the victims unless they are in immediate danger. Undo safety belts and remove any safety helmets. If a victim's heart has stopped, give immediate heart massage (see p.556). Then give first aid to all injured people in order of priority (see p.508). If an injury is bleeding, apply firm but gentle pressure to the wound with some clean material, and fasten a pad over it with a bandage or strip of cloth. If a limb is not broken, it may be raised to lessen bleeding.

(5) Stay with the victims until an ambulance and the police arrive. Reassure them about their condition, and keep them warm. Do not give them anything to drink or eat.

If the accident involves a vehicle containing inflammable or dangerous chemicals or other goods, inform the fire department and police immediately, giving the code number on the back of the vehicle.

Make sure that others present are aware of the danger, and keep them away from the vehicle.

Escape from a sinking car

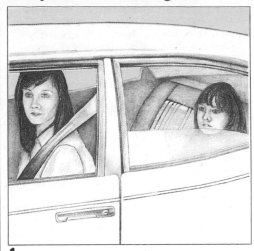

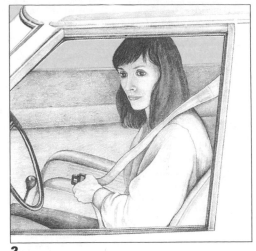

1

If the car floats for a short time, try to escape immediately. If the car starts to sink quickly, close the windows to prevent the water from gushing in. The water enters the car through the many holes in the floor; for example, around the handbrake cables and pedals.

It is not possible to open the doors until the inside and outside pressures are equal.

2

Shut off the car's engine, but keep the lights on to aid rescuers.

As the water rises, release the seat belts. Make sure that all the passengers are free from restraints. Check that the doors are not locked. Keep a hand on the door handle.

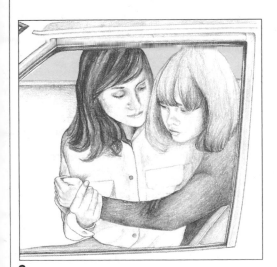

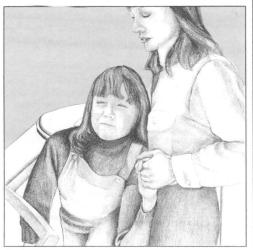

3

Make sure that the heads of all passengers, particularly children, or injured people, are above the water level as it rises.

Wait until the water has reached chin level and try to open the doors. They may need several hard pushes.

Do not panic.

4

The moment the doors are open, the car begins to sink rapidly.

With non-swimmers, form a human chain by holding tightly onto the other passengers.

Still holding tightly onto the other passengers, swim strongly and swiftly to the surface.

Car and motoring safety 3

Fitness to drive

The degree of concentration demanded by driving is greater than that demanded by almost any other routine activity. The driver must be able to deal capably and confidently with the changing traffic conditions, and must be prepared at all times for unexpected dangers. In an emergency situation, the lives of the driver and the passengers may depend on the speed of the driver's reactions.

To sustain this degree of concentration, the driver must be mentally alert and physically fit. The most common threat to a driver's mental alertness is fatigue, especially on long journeys. To avoid fatigue, the following measures can be taken:

(1) The driver should be seated comfortably, be able to see everything around and be able to reach all the controls without difficulty.
(2) The car should be well ventilated, with a continuous current of fresh air.
(3) If there is a radio or tape player in the car, the driver must take care that his or her alertness is not dulled by music that is too loud or too soothing.
(4) The driver should avoid eating heavy meals or drinking alcohol either before or during a journey.
(5) On long journeys, the driver should stop the car at least once every two hours in order to exercise the muscles by walking around or by doing physical exercises, such as those suggested on this page.

The harmful effects of alcohol on a driver's concentration and judgement are well known, but still need to be emphasized. The particular danger of alcohol is that it may increase the driver's subjective feeling of self-confidence, while at the same time decreasing the actual powers of judgement. Drugs also may have similar effects, and a driver who has been prescribed drugs, or who is taking any medicines regularly, should consult the doctor about the possible effects on driving.

A less obvious factor that may affect a driver's concentration is nervous tension and stress. One cause of tension may be worries about the car itself. These can be reduced by ensuring that the car is regularly serviced and in good condition, and by repairing or replacing faulty parts as soon as the fault becomes apparent. A driver can also suffer from nervous tension if he or she is un-necessarily distracted by other passengers in the car. Children especially become bored and restless on long journeys, and another adult in the car can help the driver by keeping them amused with games of observation. Such games are preferable to reading, which not only is difficult to do in a moving car, but also may induce sickness.

It is impossible to eliminate all stress from driving, but careful planning before every journey to allow enough time for different road conditions does produce a more relaxed, and therefore a more alert driver. If at any time during a journey you feel yourself becoming sleepy, draw to the side of the road, and take a short walk.

Travel sickness

Travel sickness is more likely to affect children than adults. It is often preceded by yawning and a general loss of interest; sweating, with a cold and shivery feeling; and pallor of the face. If any of these signs is present, stop the car and let the victim walk around for a while. Give the victim a sip of water, and when getting back into the car let the victim sit in front.

Attacks of travel sickness may be prevented by driving smoothly, with gentle cornering and braking, and by maintaining a flow of fresh air through the car. Make sure that all people in the car are seated comfortably and that seat belts are worn. Any dangling object, such as a soft toy, should be taken down. Make frequent stops for a little exercise and perhaps some light refreshment, such as a picnic lunch.

There are a number of commercial preparations available for the prevention of travel sickness. Drivers should not take travel sickness pills without first checking with a doctor that it is safe to do so, because most of these preparations cause drowsiness.

Body exercises

Here are a few simple exercises that a driver can do during stops to relieve body tension.
Neck. Relax the shoulders and lean the head back as far as possible for two seconds. Let the head fall forward so that the chin rests on the chest. Relax and repeat.
Shoulders. Rotate the shoulders in a forward motion, one at a time then both together, with the arms dangling loose. Relax and repeat.
Arms and hands. Clench the fists, bring them to the shoulders, and flex the biceps. Relax and repeat. Alternatively clasp the hands together with the fingers interlocked, and try to separate the hands without breaking their grip. Count to ten and relax.
Stomach. Take a deep breath and brace the stomach muscles. Hold to a slow count of ten and breathe out slowly. Repeat several times.
Legs. Squeeze the thighs together and press the hands against the outside of the legs near the knees. Maintain hand pressure and separate the legs. Count to ten and relax.

618

Kerb drill

Crossing a road is dangerous, especially for children. Before children are allowed to cross a road alone, parents should make sure that they understand and can apply the following rules:

Look for a suitable place to cross, such as a footbridge, a pedestrian crossing, or traffic lights. If you cannot find any suitable place like these, find a safe place from where you can see clearly along the road in both directions. Look and listen in both directions for approaching traffic. If you see traffic coming, let it pass. When the road is clear, walk straight across to the other side. Do not cross the road diagonally and never run.

At night, it is often difficult for drivers to see pedestrians until they are very close. For their own safety, pedestrians at night should wear light-coloured or reflective clothing, or carry a torch. Fluorescent material is conspicuous in daylight, but of little use at night. Where there is no pavement, walk on the left-hand side of the road, towards the oncoming traffic. Walk single file and keep to the side of the road. At all times, keep children under close control, and never allow them to run into or along the road.

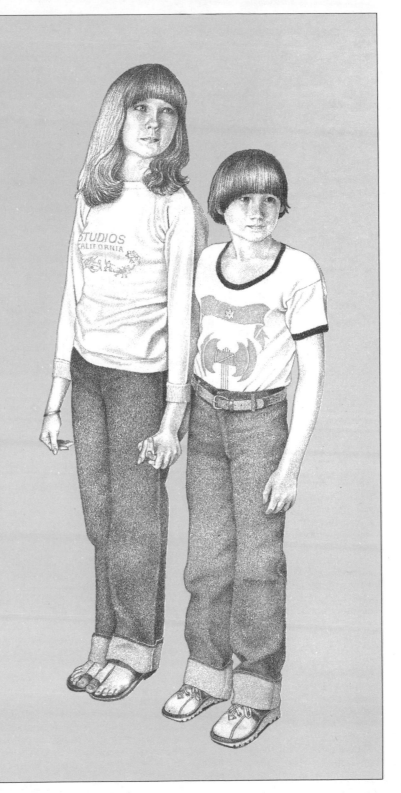

Car and motoring safety 4

Safety on two wheels

Cyclists and motorcyclists are more vulnerable than car drivers: their vehicles are less visible to other road users, and give them less protection in the event of an accident. Car drivers often do not notice motorcyclists and cyclists until they are very close, and allow them little space when overtaking. For this reason, all motorcyclists and cyclists should take special care of their equipment, and should wear clothing that is both protective and conspicuous.

Motorcyclists

If you are buying your first motorcycle, safety should be a more important consideration than speed. Choose a machine of reasonable size and power, one that you will be able to ride with confidence. Inspect the motorcycle carefully before committing yourself to buy it, especially if you are buying it second-hand. Get an expert to advise you, and to help you check the condition of the tyres, the brakes, the wheel and steering bearings, the chain, the exhaust, the suspension, the lights, and the engine. For the sake of your own safety, you should learn how a motorcycle works and how to maintain all the parts in good running condition.

You should choose your clothing carefully. The helmet is especially important. Whichever type you buy – fibreglass or polycarbonate, full-face or open-face – make sure that it bears the kite-mark of approval by the British Standards Institution. It is important that the helmet fits correctly. Try on a helmet and fasten the straps; if you can wriggle out of it, it is the wrong size. If a visor is fitted to the helmet, remember it is dangerous to ride with the visor open, because this exposes you to eye damage from particles in the air, and also it can lift the helmet. Replace the visor when it becomes scratched. Wash your helmet in water only, and never allow it to come into contact with petrol, grease, or other organic solvents. Also, do not paint your helmet or stick tape or transfers on it: this can damage the shell structure, and the helmet may then shatter at only a slight impact. Check the straps regularly to see that they do not become worn or frayed. Never use a helmet for longer than three years, and throw it away if it has been involved in an accident or even if you have dropped it, because many helmets are designed to absorb a single impact only. All other clothing should provide long-term protection against the weather.

Having taken all necessary precautions concerning equipment and clothing, motorcyclists can further increase their safety by practising correct riding techniques at all times. Give clear, positive hand signals before turning left or right in busy traffic. Never assume that because you can see other drivers, they can see you. Use your headlights and sound your horn to make sure other road users are aware of your presence.

Many techniques can be learned only by experience, and should be practised on quiet roads before they are attempted on main roads or in heavy traffic. These techniques include controlled, progressive braking on wet or slippery roads, leaning into the bend combined with the correct use of gears and brakes when rounding a corner, and allowing for slipstreams when overtaking.

Cyclists

Much of the information given above to motorcyclists also applies to bicyclists. Because of the simplicity of a bicycle it is tempting to assume that it demands less care and attention: your personal safety, however, remains equally important.

As with motorcycles, choose a bicycle that you will be able to ride with comfort and confidence. When you are seated on the saddle, the toes of both feet must be able to touch the ground without tilting the bicycle. The thigh, leg, and heel of the foot on a pedal at its lowest should form a straight line as you ride along. The saddle should be almost parallel to the ground. Except on a high-riser, the handlebars should be almost level with the saddle.

Keep the bicycle clean and well oiled, and make sure that there are no loose parts. Pay special attention to the brakes, tyres, and lights. Check regularly the tightness and alignment of the wheels, handlebars, pedals, and chain.

Bicyclists are even less visible to car drivers than motorcyclists, so it is even more important for them to wear safe and conspicuous clothing. Bright-coloured vests or belts can be worn over your normal clothing. Do not wear wide-bottomed trousers, flapping skirts, trailing scarves, or any other loose clothing that may catch in the spokes or on the chain. The bottoms of trousers should be tucked into socks or secured with bicycle clips. Shoes should have low heels. For riding at night, reflective material can be sewn into clothing or stuck onto the bicycle.

At all times, cyclists must give clear and positive hand signals when turning. Do not weave in and out of traffic, or ride close to moving vehicles. Special care is needed at pedestrian crossings, near parked cars, and on uneven road surfaces.

The motorcyclist's clothing should be protective, conspicuous, and durable. The most important item is the helmet. These are usually made of polycarbonate or fibreglass. Full-face helmets offer more general protection, but require the use of a visor. Open-face helmets can be used with either a visor or goggles, and allow better vision. Whichever type you choose, the helmet must be kept in good condition, and replaced at least every three years.

For jackets and boots, leather is probably the most popular material. When buying a suit, check that the areas round the knees, hips, and elbows are padded, and that the clothing is comfortable in the riding position. However, leather can never be entirely waterproof, even when coated with special oil. Alternative materials include nylon, waxed cotton, and PVC. Whichever you choose, pay careful attention to the stitching, the zip fasteners, and the neck, which are the weak points of a suit.

Other essential items of clothing are overboots, which should be at least calf-high, and gloves. For comfort and warmth, leather is the most suitable material. Overgloves of nylon or waxed cotton offer good waterproof protection.

Bright-coloured clothing increases your safety by making you more conspicuous to other road users. You can also wear a reflective vest or belt, or put reflective tape on your clothing (not the helmet).

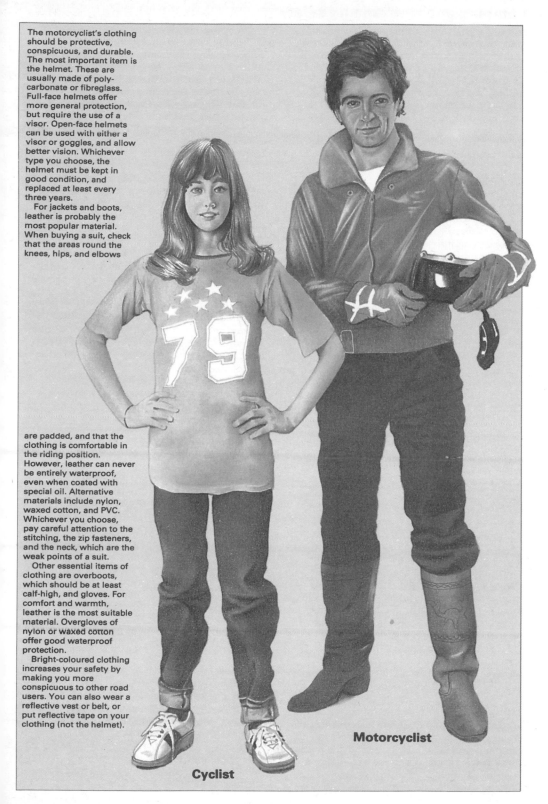

Cyclist

Motorcyclist

Camping and caravanning safety

Camping and caravanning holidays have many advantages, especially for families with children: they allow flexibility and freedom of movement, and provide city-dwellers with a rare opportunity to spend an extended holiday in the countryside without having to pay the prohibitive costs of hotel accommodation. Anyone planning such a holiday, however, must be aware of the special responsibilities involved if the holiday is to be successful.

Hygiene

Hygiene and cleanliness are especially important during holidays with young children. Normal standards of hygiene should not be allowed to deteriorate because of cramped conditions and lack of facilities. Badly organised camp sites and caravan sites can become breeding grounds for harmful bacteria; children are especially vulnerable to infection, and if only one member of a family or group becomes ill, the holiday can be ruined for everyone else.

Normal rules concerning personal hygiene must be strictly applied. Hands must be washed carefully before preparing food, especially food for babies. Cups and plates must be washed after every meal and kept covered until they are used again. Refuse should be disposed of quickly and hygienically: waste food and empty containers should be wrapped in paper and placed in covered bins. Empty tins and broken glass that are left lying around can cause severe injuries.

Water taken from streams, as well as local water on many camp sites and caravan sites, may contain harmful bacteria: it should therefore be boiled and then cooled before it is drunk. Alternatively, sterilising tablets may be used. All fresh fruit should be washed thoroughly before being eaten.

All fresh meat and fish that are bought during the course of a holiday should be eaten on the day of purchase if possible. If there is no refrigerator available, it should be sealed against insects and stored in a cool place until eaten.

Finally, all toilet facilities need special care. If a private toilet compartment or portable lavatory is used, it must be emptied and disinfected at least once every day.

Equipment

Well-chosen equipment and accessories can greatly increase the material comfort of any camping or caravanning holiday. Many motor caravans and trailer caravans are equipped to luxurious standards: the fittings may include carpets, curtains, convertible beds, insulated walls, central heating, gas cookers with ovens and grills, a refrigerator, a shower compartment, a flushing toilet, and a water storage tank with electric pump and pressure switch. On the other hand, it is of course possible to have an enjoyable camping holiday with only a tent, a groundsheet, a sleeping bag, and a minimum of cooking equipment. Remember that accessories such as cooking stoves and insulated food storage containers are available for hire.

It is essential to take safety precautions with all cooking and heating equipment. Gas cylinders should be stored securely in their special cupboards if appropriate; they should be kept away from all naked flames, and from electrical wiring and appliances. When camping, always cook in the open air, never inside the tent. Set up the cooker or charcoal grill firmly on level ground and away from trees and bushes. Wear an apron and gloves when cooking, and use long-handled cooking utensils. It is possible to increase the safety of all cookers by fixing a steel or brass rod around the top of the cooker so that the pans cannot slide off. When using an open fire, never attempt to light it by pouring paraffin or petrol over the fire.

Electrical installations in caravans need special care. The caravan battery must be firmly secured and, if located inside the caravan, must be placed in a separate compartment with a lid that gives an air-tight seal and also permits easy access. The inside of the compartment must be acid-resistant. 12 volt wiring and mains wiring must be installed as separate systems, and the caravan must be uncoupled from the towing vehicle before any mains connection is made. All wiring must be fused; if the supply is drawn from the towing vehicle, the fuse in the caravan should be kept as close to the source as possible. When touring abroad, remember that foreign electrical systems and wiring practices may differ from those in Britain, and mains connections need special attention.

Safety precautions to protect against fire are also essential. All heating and cooking appliances should be kept clean and in good repair. When changing gas cylinders, check that the hose connections have not deteriorated. Never look for a gas leak with a match or other naked flame. Do not place clothes, towels, or other inflammable materials above cookers and heaters. Never use portable gas or paraffin heaters inside a tent or caravan. Always keep a fire extinguisher or fire blanket easily accessible, but remember that liquid-type fire extinguishers should not be used for fat or electrical fires.

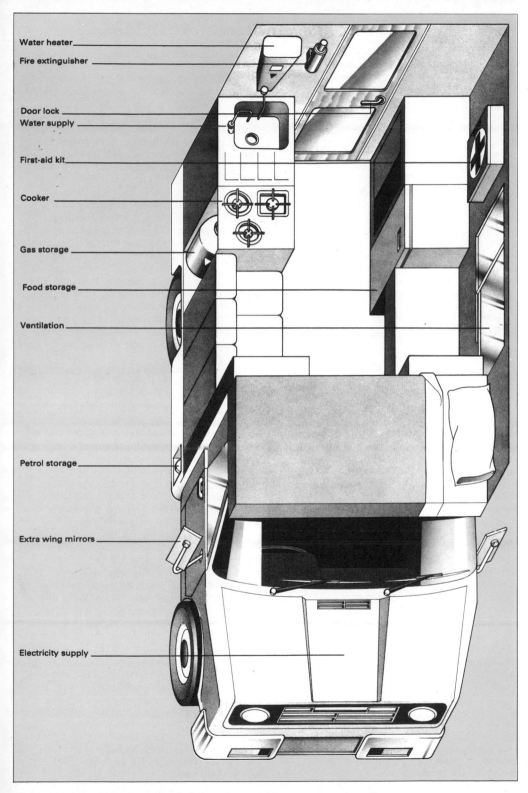

Water heater

Fire extinguisher

Door lock

Water supply

First-aid kit

Cooker

Gas storage

Food storage

Ventilation

Petrol storage

Extra wing mirrors

Electricity supply

Hiking safety

Preparing for a hike

Never set out on a hike alone: on day trips travel with at least one companion. If the planned hike takes the party more than five hours away from habitation on any part of the route, travel with three companions. Plan the route carefully from maps and guide books. A responsible person must be given a copy of the intended route, and the estimated time the party hopes to arrive at a given point. Do not stray from the plan, and let the same person know when the party is back safely. Make a note of mountain rescue posts and of any telephone boxes that are accessible should an emergency arise. The itinerary should be within the capabilities of the slowest and least experienced of the party: do not plan anything that puts an inexperienced walker at risk. Check the weather forecast before leaving. On the route, check weather forecasts for individual mountains. Weather conditions at the top of a mountain are often displayed on notice boards at the beginning of well-used routes. Make sure that the walk can be completed within daylight hours.

The rucksack

Make sure that the rucksacks for the hike are completely waterproof. Check that the frame sits easily on the back of the person carrying it, and is adjusted accordingly. A well-adjusted rucksack makes load-carrying easy, but when packing the sack, put in the essentials before planning the luxuries. Next to the sack frame carry enough spare, dry clothing for any weather condition. A survival kit must be carried by each member of the party. It should be lightweight and compact and each item should satisfy the basic needs of fire, shelter, signals and first aid. The kit should contain: a map and compass; signalling devices (a whistle or metal mirror); matches or fire-starting materials; a nylon rope; a first aid kit. This should contain: at least one elastic bandage; a triangular bandage; safety pins; antiseptic ointment; soap; a three-day supply of antibiotic and antidiarrhoea medicines; lip salve; aspirins; commercial antihistamine tablets; and water-sterilising tablets. Each member of the party must carry plasters in an easy-to-reach part of the pack, to deal with minor cuts and blisters. Each person must carry enough water for the trip. There should be at least one torch, spare battery, and bulb carried by the party. Emergency food should include chocolate, biscuits, glucose (dextrose), and salt. A bag of nuts, raisins, and boiled sweets can provide nourishing snacks during the walk.

During the hike

The party must match the rate of walking to the pace of the slowest member of the party. If one member begins to lag behind, let that person take the lead. Rather than one large meal halfway through the day, it is advisable to take a few small meals and to drink small amounts frequently. An overfull stomach slows walking down. Walk rhythmically to conserve energy. If one member of the party has to stop for any reason, do not walk on, expecting that person to catch up because he or she may get into difficulty and may need help.

General accident procedure

Should a member of a party of four or more have an accident that prevents further travel, two people should go in search of help. One person must stay with the injured person, marking the site of the accident carefully. If possible, the victim should be moved to a sheltered spot. If this is not possible, erect a bivouac around the victim. This can be made from branches, a pile of rucksacks, or a bank of snow. Place plastic waterproof clothing under the victim to protect him or her from the cold ground. Try to keep the victim's morale high until help arrives.

Hypothermia

Hypothermia is the medical term for an abnormally low body temperature. It is the most dangerous condition a hiker is likely to face, and can occur under the most unexpected circumstances. Hypothermia is caused by a combination of things: cold; wind; humidity; fatigue; and hunger. The most dangerous aspect of the condition is that the hypothermia victim is not aware of the danger and that until the signs are obvious no one else may realise. The victim begins to act strangely, as if drunk. He or she may suddenly lose all regard for personal comfort or safety, walk through deep puddles instead of around them, try to sit down or sleep on the ground, or start swearing and complaining about the walk. Hikers should be on the lookout for such signs.

The treatment for hypothermia is to try to warm the whole body of the person affected. Layers of clothing should be wrapped around, and a warm drink administered. No alcohol should be given; alcohol lowers the blood temperature and only maintains the condition. If there is a warm bath available within a short distance, that would also help.

Hypothermia can be prevented by adequate preparation for cold, wet, and windy conditions.

Wearing correct clothing is one of the most important safety measures a hiker can take. Natural fibres are very efficient at controlling heat loss, even when wet.

Wear a hat or head cover of some kind, preferably made of oiled wool.

Under the wool, crew-necked sweater, wear two or three layers of light, easy-to-remove shirts. These can be tucked into the rucksack or tied round the waist when the weather gets hot.

A brightly-coloured, windproof and waterproof parka or anorak is essential. It must have a waterproof hood, a protected zip fastener, and tie-strings around the hood, waist, and base seam. The cuffs must be tight-fitting. Carry waterproof over-trousers in the pack at all times.

The rucksack should be made of a non-absorbent, waterproof material. The integral frame must be adjusted to fit the back comfortably when the rucksack is refilled. A hip strap distributes the weight of the pack over the spine, and keeps the rucksack from moving. When packing the rucksack, put the heaviest part of the load at the top of the pack. When the rucksack is adjusted correctly, the weight is above the pelvis when standing normally. If heavy things are packed at the base of the sack, the weight pulls away from the pelvis. Pack spare clothing next to the sack frame. This protects the back against sharp objects in the rest of the pack.

Mittens are warmer than gloves. Waterproof over-gloves are also useful.

Wear woollen walking trousers, preferably breeches. Never wear jeans. Cotton does not retain the heat efficiently.

The boots should be made of leather, have enough support for the ankles, and be soled either with cleated rubber or nailed leather. Never set out on a long trip wearing a pair of boots that have not been broken in for a total of at least eight walking hours. The laces should be made of natural fibre: synthetic fibre tends to slip. Carry a spare pair of laces in the rucksack.

One pair of long socks should be covered by one or two pairs of short woollen socks. Gaiters stop grit, small pebbles, twigs, and snow from falling into the top of the boot.

Sports safety – winter sports

Safety on the ice

Safe ice is usually found on slow-flowing streams, small areas of water, such as ponds, or on small lakes. Ice is thinner at the edges of pools, under overhanging trees or bushes, and under bridges. Areas that should be avoided altogether are tidal water, and where fast-flowing water has iced on the surface. Although ice there may be thick, it is constantly submitted to strain, and may break up under the weight of a person. Ice of this kind should not be used if the water beneath is over one metre (3 or 4 feet) deep. In fact, such ice tends to be rough and uneven.

During the first freeze of winter, "black" ice forms. It is completely transparent, and is usually tough and elastic. Once it has frozen to a depth of at least 12 or 15 centimetres (5 or 6 inches), it is probably safe to use for walking, skating, and skiing.

At the end of the winter, the sun and wind begin to melt the ice. Although the ice may look safe, and may be several inches deep, it may become waterlogged, and break up at a slight increase of weight on the surface.

Ice accidents tend to happen in two different ways. The ice user may break directly through the ice, and struggle to reach hold of the edge of the ice. The body jack-knifes, the ice breaks away, and the victim is drawn under the surface. The following procedure prevents this.
(1) Do not attempt to climb out immediately.
(2) Kick the feet to the surface behind.
(3) Extend hands and arms onto surrounding ice.
(4) Adopt a horizontal swimming position.
(5) Work carefully forward in this position until firm ice is reached.

The other form of accident occurs when the ice splits, and the ice user trips over the raised edge of ice. The automatic response is to get to the feet. But this increases the pressure on a small area of already fractured ice, and the victim falls through. To prevent this happening, the ice user must intentionally sprawl forward during the fall, then wriggle or roll away from the danger area where the ice is weak.

Rescue from the ice

If a person falls through the ice, speed is essential for a rescue. The longer a person is in icy water, the greater the chance that he or she will panic and either attempt to struggle onto the ice, breaking more away from the edge, or become exhausted and slip under the surface. The other great danger is cold.

It is essential that rescuers do not rush forward to help. The area around the hole in the ice is cracked and extremely dangerous.

The rescue must be conducted from firm ice a few metres (yards) away, or as far away as necessary. It is important that any person approaching the victim across the ice distributes the body weight evenly by wriggling at full stretch over the ice and has at least one helper to pull him or her back to safety if the ice gives way for a second time.

If a victim fails to catch hold of the edge of the ice, and disappears beneath it, the decision to attempt a rescue must be carefully considered to avoid a double tragedy. Some experts feel that the risk is never justifiable. Once beneath the ice it is almost impossible to find the hole again, because visibility is poor. The only circumstances that can justify an attempt is if a very powerful swimmer goes down attached to a strong line. The rescuers must pull the swimmer up after a very short time.

All skaters should learn how to fall on ice properly and safely. A fall on ice is far less serious than a fall on solid ground, because the body tends to slide along the ice, and much of the impact is absorbed. A skater must not be afraid of falling on the ice. The automatic response to loss of balance is a struggle to regain it, but a skater is safer if he or she relaxes and lets the fall take a natural course. A skater should lean forward at the beginning of a fall. An outstretched hand slides on the ice, and the elbow can bend to absorb the jolt. Wearing gloves, a skater is unlikely to come to any harm.

Skiing safety

It is essential that all skiers, whatever their standard, should be properly clothed and equipped (see the illustration on the opposite page).

The probability of suffering from fatigue, which can greatly increase the chances of an accident, can be reduced if the skier has done some pre-season exercises. Flexibility and endurance exercises to strengthen legs and ankles are traditionally recommended for skiers. It is also wise to do quick warm-up exercises without skis before the first run.

It is unwise to continue to ski if snow conditions deteriorate, and no skier should continue if visibility is reduced by fog or by snowfall. Skiers should also beware of sunburn, particularly from rays reflected off the snow, and of intense cold, which can lead to frostbite.

Beginners should stay within their class, and not be tempted to follow the more experienced skiers in their party. If a skier falls, he or she should flatten down any dents made in the snow that might be dangerous for following skiers.

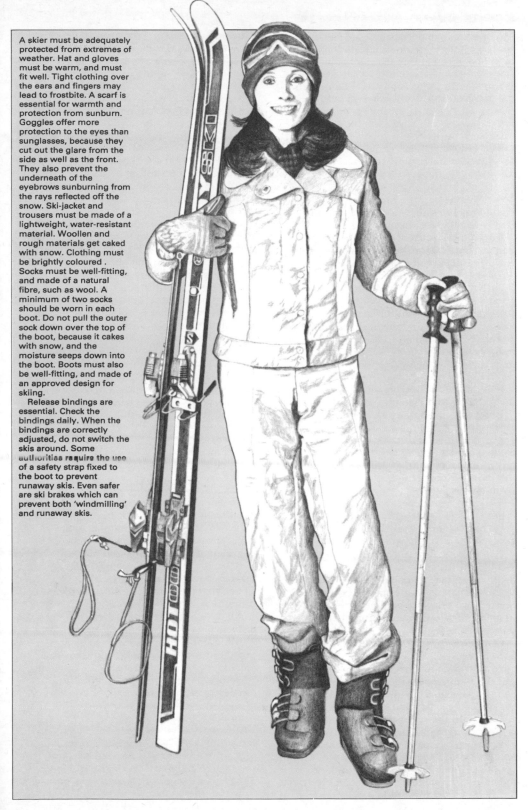

A skier must be adequately protected from extremes of weather. Hat and gloves must be warm, and must fit well. Tight clothing over the ears and fingers may lead to frostbite. A scarf is essential for warmth and protection from sunburn. Goggles offer more protection to the eyes than sunglasses, because they cut out the glare from the side as well as the front. They also prevent the underneath of the eyebrows sunburning from the rays reflected off the snow. Ski-jacket and trousers must be made of a lightweight, water-resistant material. Woollen and rough materials get caked with snow. Clothing must be brightly coloured . Socks must be well-fitting, and made of a natural fibre, such as wool. A minimum of two socks should be worn in each boot. Do not pull the outer sock down over the top of the boot, because it cakes with snow, and the moisture seeps down into the boot. Boots must also be well-fitting, and made of an approved design for skiing.

Release bindings are essential. Check the bindings daily. When the bindings are correctly adjusted, do not switch the skis around. Some authorities require the use of a safety strap fixed to the boot to prevent runaway skis. Even safer are ski brakes which can prevent both 'windmilling' and runaway skis.

627

Sports safety – water sports

There are two important rules for all water sports, whether you are interested in sailing or skin diving. (1) Buy the right equipment. There is seldom a safe way to cut costs. Generally the more you pay for equipment, the more reliable it will prove to be. In the same way, (2) the more you spend on expert instruction, the safer you will be, and therefore, the more fun you will have.

The following points should act as a safety checklist for water sportsmen and women, however experienced they are.

Swimming

Swimming is a skill every member of the family should learn from an early age.

The sun can seem misleadingly cool when you are in the water, and it is possible not to realize until later that you have been badly burned across the shoulders and back.

There are certain times when, however good a swimmer you are, you must not go in the water. Never swim within half an hour of eating a large meal; it might cause muscle cramp. Never swim after drinking alcohol; it reduces your awareness of the cold, and you may begin to vomit and choke. Never swim when feeling tired or cold.

It is dangerous to swim on your own, or at night. Swim with a partner of equal ability.

Before beginning a swim, pay careful attention to notices and warning signs concerning tides and strong undercurrents. Never sunbathe on an inflatable air mattress in the ocean. You could drift a long way from the shore without realising, and be unable to swim back.

Children must never swim unsupervised. It is not enough to have an adult nearby. The adult must stand at the edge of the water and keep constant watch over the children.

Waterskiing

Waterskiing safety depends as much on the skiboat driver as on the skier. For this reason, two people should be in the boat, one to navigate safely, the other to pass on the skier's handsignals.

Operate clear of swimmers and other water users. Keep well away from rocks and buoys.

Always wear a lifejacket. Clothing should suit the weather conditions. One can suffer bad sunburn on a day that seems overcast, or get chilled on a day that seems mild.

Wait until the ski tips are up and the rope is taut before signalling to the boat to start.

Watch the water ahead all the time. If you feel yourself falling, curl up into a ball to stop yourself falling forward. Let go of the rope the moment you feel yourself going. Retrieve the skis as soon as possible.

Canoeing

You must be a competent swimmer before taking up canoeing as a sport. Always wear a lifejacket and clothing appropriate to the weather conditions.

Always canoe with a companion. Canoe with at least two other boats when on fast rivers or in the ocean.

Before setting out on a trip, tell a responsible person where you are going and how long you expect to be away. Check the weather forecast for that area, and make sure you know what conditions you are likely to encounter.

Learn how to deal with a capsize. In calm water it is safer to hold on to a floating overturned canoe than to try to right it. In fast, white water, get away from the boat.

A canoe must be equipped with bow and stern toggles, deck lines, paddle parks, towing cleat, adequate buoyancy bags, and a spare split paddle secured to the stern deck.

Never carry more people than the canoe is designed to take. In a canoe, never change places with another person while afloat.

Keep clear of other boats. Remember that large boats are less manoeuvrable than you are, and that a canoe can use shallower water than other craft. Keep away from weirs.

Keep clear of rowing boats. It is often difficult for rowers to see a canoe.

Sailing

Every member of a sailing crew must be a competent swimmer and wear a personal lifejacket.

Familiarise yourself thoroughly with the boat. The safest way to learn about the boat's equipment and handling is to join a class with a local boating club. Failing this, sail with an experienced colleague until he or she is confident that you can go out alone.

A dinghy must have enough inbuilt buoyancy to keep afloat after a capsize. Check that the boat has a standby means of propulsion, such as oars.

All sizes of boats should carry the right distress flares.

All motor boats must carry fire extinguishers. Every member of the crew must know how to operate the equipment.

Before setting out, get the latest weather forecast. Let someone on shore know where you are going and how long you are likely to be out. Report your return.

Never overload the boat. If you have to carry fuel, keep it in an approved container.

If a fire breaks out, head the boat into the wind and use the fire extinguisher. However, if there is a danger of an explosion, get away from the boat as quickly as possible.

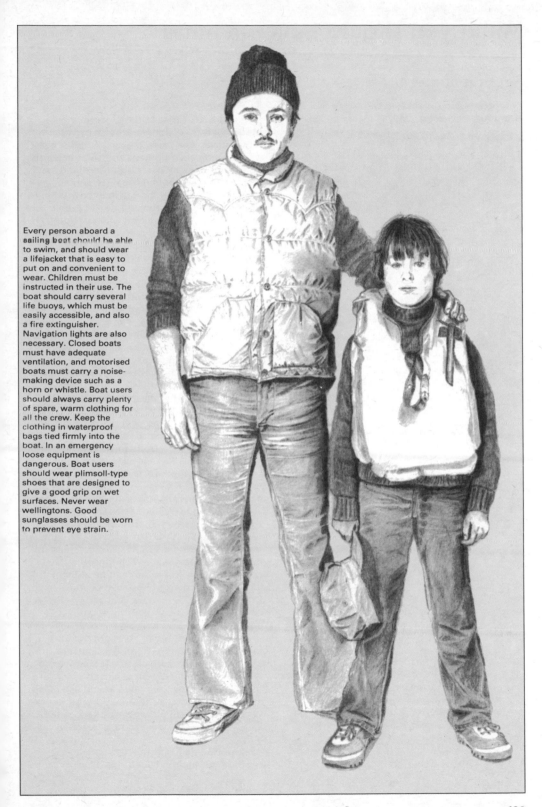

Every person aboard a
sailing boat should be able
to swim, and should wear
a lifejacket that is easy to
put on and convenient to
wear. Children must be
instructed in their use. The
boat should carry several
life buoys, which must be
easily accessible, and also
a fire extinguisher.
Navigation lights are also
necessary. Closed boats
must have adequate
ventilation, and motorised
boats must carry a noise-
making device such as a
horn or whistle. Boat users
should always carry plenty
of spare, warm clothing for
all the crew. Keep the
clothing in waterproof
bags tied firmly into the
boat. In an emergency
loose equipment is
dangerous. Boat users
should wear plimsoll-type
shoes that are designed to
give a good grip on wet
surfaces. Never wear
wellingtons. Good
sunglasses should be worn
to prevent eye strain.

What you should have on hand

Section contents

Introduction

The purpose of this section is to provide a visual checklist first of the emergency medical kit that should accompany you on any journey in a private vehicle, and second of the medical equipment and treatments that you should keep – carefully stored and safely out of the reach of children – at home.

A first aid box in the car may be vitally important not only to you or your family, but perhaps also to the victims of an accident that you may witness or arrive at. The kit should therefore be kept in an easily accessible spot within the car, and not in the boot. It should be marked with a red cross and should be visible also from outside the vehicle, in case a stranger has to locate and use it in a hurry.

Useful items associated with a first aid kit in a car are: a notebook, for recording the details of any accident actually witnessed; a torch; a battery-operated beacon, preferably a flashing red light; and a blanket.

The home medical chest is often located in an upstairs bathroom. The most common accident site in the house – the kitchen – is quite a distance away, perhaps with a flight of stairs in between. The obvious place for a medical chest, therefore, if there is room, is the kitchen or a centrally located position. The kitchen has the added advantage in most houses of leading directly to the garden – which is the next most common site for accidents, generally minor ones to children.

It cannot be stressed too much or too often that it is dangerous to position the home medical chest within the reach of the younger members of the family. Many medicines still do not come in so-called childproof containers, and therefore can be a danger. The home medicine chest also contains such things as lotions, scissors, and safety pins. All of these things are dangerous to young children.

In both the kit for the car and the home medical chest, it is extremely important to keep any medicines well stocked and up to date, and the equipment replaced as it is used. Items of ordinary household use (such as scissors or torch) should never be "borrowed" from either car or home medical kits. Bandages once used by children in their games should also never be rewound and put back in the medical kits. New bandages should be bought instead.

Emergency first aid kit

A large number of accidents happen on the roads every year, so a first aid box should always be carried in a visible, accessible place in your car.

Being prepared for an emergency is no substitute for preventing accidents. *See* **Car and motoring safety**, p.614.

A first aid kit for the car can be bought already prepared, or you can equip one yourself.

In addition to the equipment illustrated below, other useful items to carry are a rug or blanket; plastic bags for vomit and used dressings.

Check the equipment regularly and replace any items that have been used.

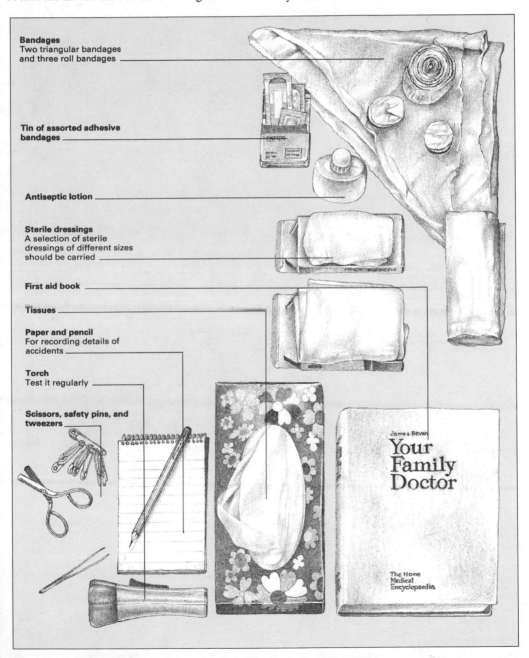

Bandages
Two triangular bandages and three roll bandages

Tin of assorted adhesive bandages

Antiseptic lotion

Sterile dressings
A selection of sterile dressings of different sizes should be carried

First aid book

Tissues

Paper and pencil
For recording details of accidents

Torch
Test it regularly

Scissors, safety pins, and tweezers

James Bevan
Your Family Doctor

The Home Medical Encyclopaedia

Home medical chest 1

First aid equipment, for the emergency treatment of injuries, should be kept in the home. The site in the house where accidents most commonly occur is the kitchen. Most kitchens also have direct access to the garden, where accidents to children are also common. The kitchen is in many ways, therefore, the most advisable place in which to keep the home medical chest.

A first aid kit is a potential danger to small children. Keep all equipment in a box or cupboard with a childproof lock. Keep the first aid box out of reach of children.

Label the first aid box clearly and put it in a place where it can easily be found.

Replace equipment once used.

Do not hoard prescribed medicines. Flush outdated medicines down the toilet. Label all medicines with an expiry date and check them regularly. Keep only basic medicines.

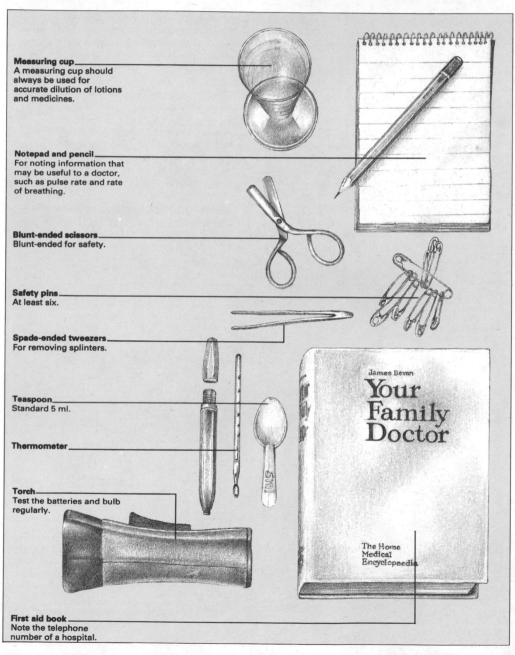

Measuring cup
A measuring cup should always be used for accurate dilution of lotions and medicines.

Notepad and pencil
For noting information that may be useful to a doctor, such as pulse rate and rate of breathing.

Blunt-ended scissors
Blunt-ended for safety.

Safety pins
At least six.

Spade-ended tweezers
For removing splinters.

Teaspoon
Standard 5 ml.

Thermometer

Torch
Test the batteries and bulb regularly.

First aid book
Note the telephone number of a hospital.

James Bevan
Your Family Doctor

The Home Medical Encyclopaedia

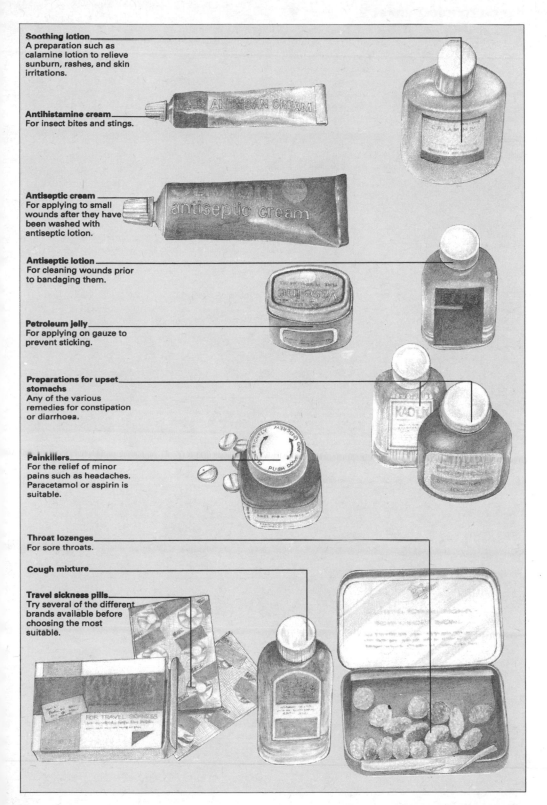

Soothing lotion
A preparation such as calamine lotion to relieve sunburn, rashes, and skin irritations.

Antihistamine cream
For insect bites and stings.

Antiseptic cream
For applying to small wounds after they have been washed with antiseptic lotion.

Antiseptic lotion
For cleaning wounds prior to bandaging them.

Petroleum jelly
For applying on gauze to prevent sticking.

Preparations for upset stomachs
Any of the various remedies for constipation or diarrhoea.

Painkillers
For the relief of minor pains such as headaches. Paracetamol or aspirin is suitable.

Throat lozenges
For sore throats.

Cough mixture

Travel sickness pills
Try several of the different brands available before choosing the most suitable.

Home medical chest 2

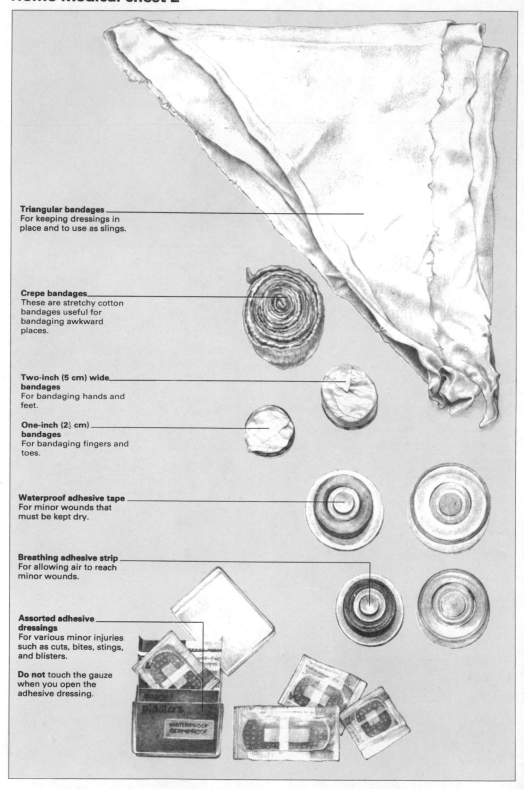

Triangular bandages
For keeping dressings in
place and to use as slings.

Crepe bandages
These are stretchy cotton
bandages useful for
bandaging awkward
places.

**Two-inch (5 cm) wide
bandages**
For bandaging hands and
feet.

**One-inch (2½ cm)
bandages**
For bandaging fingers and
toes.

Waterproof adhesive tape
For minor wounds that
must be kept dry.

Breathing adhesive strip
For allowing air to reach
minor wounds.

**Assorted adhesive
dressings**
For various minor injuries
such as cuts, bites, stings,
and blisters.

Do not touch the gauze
when you open the
adhesive dressing.

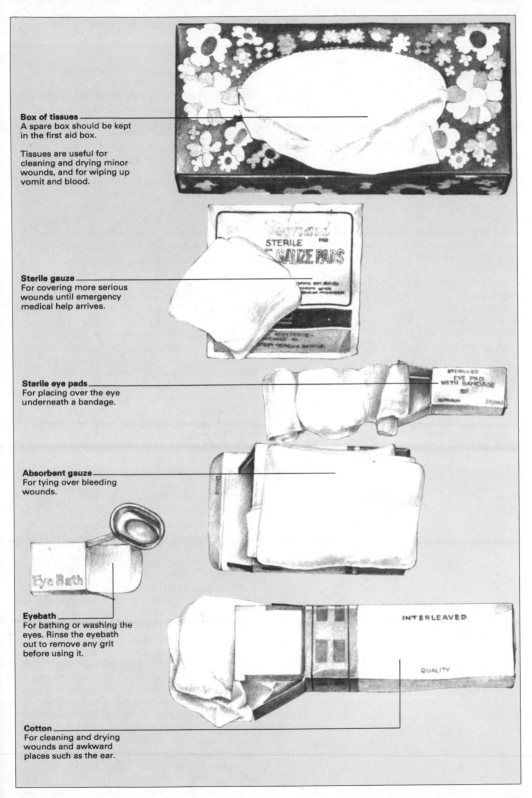

Box of tissues
A spare box should be kept in the first aid box.

Tissues are useful for cleaning and drying minor wounds, and for wiping up vomit and blood.

Sterile gauze
For covering more serious wounds until emergency medical help arrives.

Sterile eye pads
For placing over the eye underneath a bandage.

Absorbent gauze
For tying over bleeding wounds.

Eyebath
For bathing or washing the eyes. Rinse the eyebath out to remove any grit before using it.

Cotton
For cleaning and drying wounds and awkward places such as the ear.

635

Care of the sick at home

Section contents

Introduction

The aim of this section is to explain how to look after a patient in a well-organized and caring way, at home, and in such a way that family life is not disrupted too much.

Nursing skills take time to acquire. But with the step-by-step illustrations of basic nursing techniques presented here, even an inexperienced person can soon learn essential routines. What may be lacking in professionalism, however, can be compensated for with good will, thorough organization, and affection. The spirit in which the task is approached can make all the difference between drudgery and the satisfaction that comes from doing a worthwhile job.

The task of home nursing must often be combined with family and career commitments. Some families share the caring, however, which lightens the burden for everyone and can also make life more interesting for the patient. It also has the advantage of teaching compassion to the younger members of the family.

With planning, much trudging up and down stairs can be eliminated. Good organization means saving time and energy. For this reason there are some pointers on how to choose the room most suitable for use as a sick room.

A number of factors are taken into account. Is the position of the room convenient for the family? Is the room near the toilet? Is it well-heated and ventilated? Is it the most practical room for the season of the year? But at the same time, of course, the patient should not be isolated from the rest of the family just because the room has all the other advantages.

Furnishing the room also requires careful thought. For example, the bed should be high enough so that it is convenient for the patient to get in and out of, yet not inconvenient for the family and visitors who have to bend over the patient. Other qualifications for various items of furniture are discussed, taking into account how they are to be used by patient, nurse and visitors.

Safety is another important factor when planning living space for someone who is ill or physically disabled. An ordinary bathroom can present many potential hazards; instructions are given for making the bathroom both safe and easy for the patient to use.

Doctors agree that boosting the patient's morale is an important part of nursing. The bored patient has time to linger on unhappy thoughts which may lead to depression or to excessive demands on the family. Some advice is given on how to keep the patient cheerfully occupied by encouraging an interest in family matters, personal appearance, and hobbies.

Just as the patient needs to be kept cheerful, so do those in attendance need to be refreshed from time to time by a change of surroundings. Relatives and friends could be called upon to substitute.

Many parents have experienced how exhausting it can be to nurse a child who is bedridden with some common complaint. But there is always the comfort of knowing that the illness will run a known course and that recovery is assured within a certain time.

The problems are much more complex with patients who are chronically ill. It can often be very discouraging to care for such a patient, often an elderly parent suffering from increasing immobility.

The seemingly never-ending chores of bed-making, washing and feeding, offering the bedpan, administering medicines, turning the patient to prevent bedsores, and so many other necessary actions, become less burdensome when carried out in as professional a way as possible. The illustrations in this section show how to accomplish these tasks skillfully.

One common problem in nursing the chronically ill is ensuring that enough nourishment is taken. Loss of appetite is usual during illness and the patient may have to be encouraged to eat. In these pages you will find set out the basic requirements of a well-balanced diet and a suggested dietary timetable. Special diets for the sick are discussed, using foods that are especially nutritious and easily digested.

Prolonged periods in bed can lead to poor muscle tone, and to blood clotting in the legs (thrombosis). To help a patient overcome these conditions, the home nurse can encourage participation in the gentle exercises illustrated in this section.

Making the patient as independent as possible of physical help should be a prime aim. Accordingly, ideas are included here for devising simple aids to walking or general mobility, with the emphasis on safety. Other useful aids are also mentioned to help the chronically ill person cope with daily life.

The patient needing perhaps the most loving care is the one who is either mentally confused or retarded. The senility of old age, the more common forms of mental illness, and the problems arising in the care of a retarded child, are discussed. There may come a time when the care of such a person is beyond the capabilities or endurance of the family. The general practitioner may then recommend special care in hospital or a place that can provide professional attention. The family should not regard this as defeat but make every effort to continue to maintain links with the patient by frequent visiting.

Finally, there is a sympathetic discussion of the care of the dying and the testing of family ties when death overtakes a loved one. Practical advice is offered concerning the handling of funeral arrangements, death certificate, and other legal matters.

The sick room: summer and winter

The choice of any one room as a sick room requires some consideration. Many factors should be taken into account, and it may not be enough just to put the sick person in what is usually a bedroom. A room that best fills all needs should become the sick room.

The room should of course be pleasant for the sick person, but should also be in a position of maximum convenience for the rest of the family. In a house of two or more stories, the ground floor is usually by far the most practical for a sick room, especially if there is a downstairs toilet. For the patient it may be preferable also because no stairs

intervene between the sick room and the centre of family life. And not having to go up and down stairs is convenient for the family when carrying trays and other articles to and from the patient.

On the other hand, if the only toilet is upstairs, the most suitable place for the sick room may also be upstairs, depending on the individual patient. Another consideration is that a room upstairs may provide more peaceful, less stressful, and more therapeutic surroundings. It is also generally easier to arrange for a more pleasing view through a window from an upstairs room.

The bedroom
The room that is to be home to a bedridden patient should contain all the necessary furniture and equipment without appearing to be overfilled.

The bed should have a firm mattress. It must be of the right height: low enough to make getting in and out of the bed easy, yet high enough not to cause difficulty to a member of the family bending over the patient. Generally, the most practical position for a bed is such that a person can approach from either side. But when the patient is senile or in a confused state, it is sometimes better to have one side of the bed against a wall; this does tend to make bed-making difficult, however.

There should be two chairs fairly close to the bed. One should be specially comfortable, for the patient's use when allowed, or able, to get out of bed. The other chair is for visitors, and for use in holding bedclothes and pillows when stripping and remaking the bed.

A commode can be useful if the patient is able to move to it.

There should also be a chest of drawers or a cupboard of about waist height in which to store essential equipment, such as spare linen. The top can be used as a working surface by members of the family, and by the doctor.

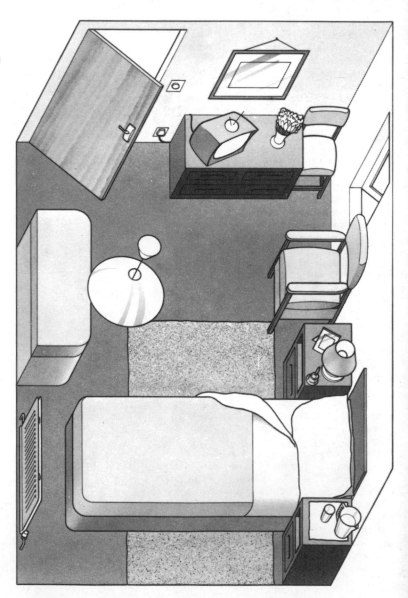

Ventilation of the sick room is of great importance: sick people need fresh air, although they should not be bothered by it. A small window, or part of a large one, can be kept open at all times, as long as the patient is not in a draught. In summer, the room should be kept cool; an electric fan may be necessary in extreme heat. In winter, the room temperature should be maintained at a comfortable and constant warmth by reliable and strategically placed heaters. Any additional open flame or red-hot element should be guarded and away from articles such as bedclothes.

A small bowl of cold water placed in front of a heater helps to maintain a reasonable humidity.

The sick room should be made to seem homely to the patient. There should be favourite pictures, furniture, and other articles. Some form of entertainment should be provided, such as radio or television, that can be switched on and off from the bed.

In cases where the patient has difficulty in moving, aids such as rails and extra flat surfaces are extremely useful in the sick room, although the room in which they are most needed is the bathroom, as illustrated.

The bathroom

Of all the rooms in a house, the bathroom is the one in which most ingenuity and care has to be exercised to make it safe for a patient. There are many simple improvements that can be made or bought.

The light switch by the door should be on a cord at an adjusted height.

The bathtub itself should have a mixer tap, so that neither hot nor cold water is flowing into the bathtub at any one time, but water of the required temperature. There should be rails on each side of the bathtub, and on the wall slightly above. A rubber mat with suction-cups beneath provides a secure footing. A seat above the bath makes getting in and out much easier. A short plank from a nearby chair may help a patient to reach the bath seat.

The toilet should have a lever or a push-bar, rather than a suspended chain. If necessary, the height of the seat can be altered by adding specially-shaped pieces of wood. A rail alongside helps the patient to sit down and to get up. Here too, a rubber mat provides a non-slip surface for the feet.

It is more practical for the washbasin to have a flat surface surrounding it.

The door should never be locked when an unsteady person is taking a bath, and make sure some responsible person knows when the patient is in the bathroom.

Some audible non-electrical means of alarm can be useful, for example a handbell.

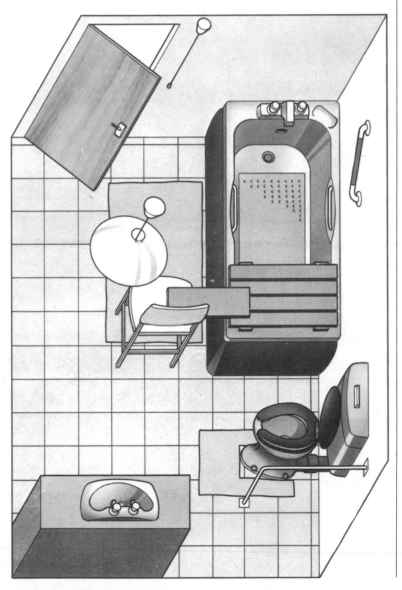

The sick room: what you should have

The sick room should contain not only the means for maintaining the patient's physical comfort, but also enough aids and items to keep the patient cheerful and occupied.

The room should be well provided with light, and it should be possible for at least one lamp in the room to be dimmed, or shaded from the patient, at night.

Because a bedridden patient tends to collect many things to have within reach at all times, it is generally more practical to place a bedside table or a locker on each side of the bed. These can hold the usual bedside lamp; radio; tray, with jug and glass; bowl of fruit or sweets; clock; and a favourite photograph or picture.

A bedside lamp is of great importance: most patients spend much of their time reading. A lamp that is easily adjusted to the desired height and direction is the most suitable. The lamp should be within easy reach of the patient and should be heavy enough at its base not to be easily toppled.

For patients who for one reason or another are less able to concentrate, it is advisable also to have an alarm bell, an intercom system, or some other audible means of summoning help in emergencies.

Beside the bed
Somewhere close to the bed, space must be found for the means by which a patient can take pride in his or her own appearance and wellbeing. It is also important to have the articles and materials used for bodily hygiene near to the patient. Even if patients cannot attend to their own hygiene, they are then convenient for those who assist the patient.

If they are physically able, patients generally prefer to wash themselves, and keep themselves tidy. For this purpose, at least two flannels or sponges are required, with soap, talcum powder, and deodorant. For drying, there should be two or three bathtowels for the body, and a soft towel for the face. To keep teeth clean and encourage mouth freshness, a toothbrush, toothpaste, and a small mug or bowl, should be provided, with denture brush and denture bath if necessary. For hair care, there should be a hairbrush, a comb, and a mirror.

To ensure adequate fluid intake, supply a jug of water (or fruit juice) with a glass, on a tray for easy carrying.

Medical equipment that should be kept on hand includes: a clinical thermometer; a medicine glass and one or two 5 ml. teaspoons; a clock or watch that records seconds (for use in taking the pulse); and a small napkin.

It is also useful to have a container for dirty clothing, a box of tissues, and a wastepaper basket.

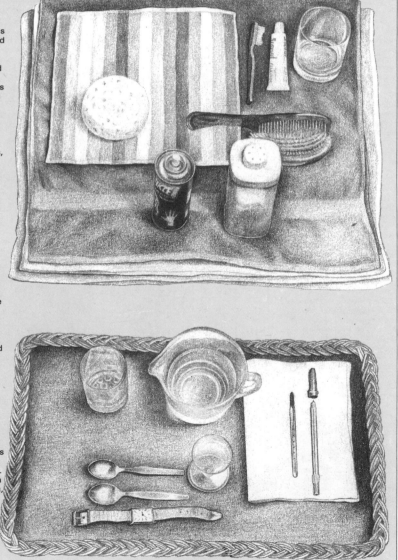

There should be an adequate supply of bedclothes for the bed: not just blankets for warmth, but enough sheets and pillowcases in case of an accident in bed, from incontinence to an upset breakfast tray. Where incontinence is to be expected, drawsheets and at least one waterproof sheet are also necessary. For more details on a well-made bed, *see* **Bed-making**, p.642.

Much of the equipment now used in sick rooms is disposable. But other items, made of glass, metal, or ceramics, should be thoroughly washed after use. And if the patient has an infectious illness such equipment should be washed, placed in water that is brought to the boil, and boiled for at least five minutes.

The patient's attitude to his or her surroundings can affect his or her wellbeing. If possible, there should be something either in the room or visible through a window that is of great interest to the patient, or perhaps new and unexpected. The patient's interest should also be encouraged in the rest of the family and its daily life, in order to avoid becoming self-centred. An occasional change of scenery within the room, such as flowers or a plant, is suggested.

Hygiene

People who are confined to bed still need to wash frequently, and a good wash and brushing of teeth can do much to improve a patient's morale.

If there is no built-in wash-basin in the sick room, some attempt must be made to provide hot and cold water. The most convenient way to maintain a hot water supply is to use a vacuum flask, although pouring may be difficult in bed. An alternative is a large enamel jug. Both containers may be refilled when necessary. Cold water can be provided in a light, plastic bucket or jug, preferably with a lip or spout and a handle. All such vessels should stand on a flat surface no higher than the patient's mattress.

The patient should be provided with a large inflexible plastic bowl to wash in. It should be at least 15cm (6 inches) deep, to stop water from splashing out.

A smaller bowl is also useful, either as a vomit bowl or for holding the patient's dentures.

Urination and defecation can be both difficult and embarrassing for a bedridden patient. The family should respect the patient's need for privacy to carry out such bodily functions. Bedpans and, for men, urinals should generally be kept and carried under cloths. The toilet paper should be kept out of the sight of visitors. Frequent washing and sterilization are essential for all equipment of this kind.

Space may also be needed in the sickroom for medical equipment such as bandages and dressings.

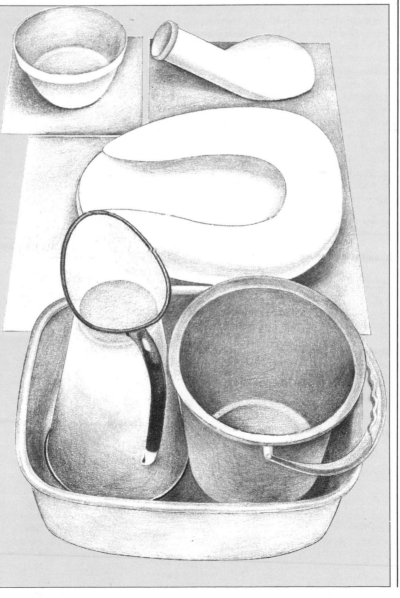

Bed-making

The most important piece of furniture in the sick room is, of course, the bed. It is essential that the bed is firm to lie on: a sagging bed provides only poor support for the back and tires the patient in time. To make a sagging bed firm, simply place a board between the bedsprings and the mattress. Make sure, too, that the mattress is firm and well-sprung. Patients who suffer from back problems will always need a firm bed. A doctor can give advice about this.

Choose bedclothes with care. Nylon sheets are easy to launder but tend to slip off the bed and are not as absorbent as sheets made from cotton or linen. Flannelette sheets have a slightly raised nap and so they are warmer than sheets made from other materials. It is advisable to always have an adequate supply of bed linen available. Woollen blankets are warm but the patient may find them to be too heavy. Cellular blankets of cotton or Dacron are lighter than woollen ones and are also easier to wash. The patient may require three or four blankets on the bed. Patients who suffer from painful joints or poor circulation may prefer the lightness of a duvet to the weight of blankets. It is advisable to have no fewer than four pillows available for a sickbed. Additional pillows may be needed to support the patient and prevent fatigue at various places, such as the elbows and arms, or under the heels.

To make up the bed, the mattress should first be protected with a waterproof sheet, such as polythene. Place a blanket over this to provide a soft and warm surface for the patient. Place the sheets on the bed and keep the right (nap) side of each sheet innermost. (A waterproof sheet and a drawsheet placed over the bottom sheet save unnecessary changing of linen if the patient is likely to dirty the bed frequently.) Place the blankets on the bed and cover them with a light eiderdown and an attractive, cheerful-looking bedspread. When the bed has been made up, give the bedclothes a slight upward tug over the area of the patient's feet to allow plenty of freedom for movement. Remember that elderly patients feel the cold easily, and may prefer to keep a shawl or light blanket between them and the sheets.

When sitting up in bed, the patient will need a minimum of four pillows for support (see right). It is possible to buy a ready-made triangular pillow that provides the shape of the first three pillows in the armchair position, so that only a soft head pillow has to be placed on top. However, the triangular pillow is harder than ordinary pillows, and the patient may not find it quite as comfortable.

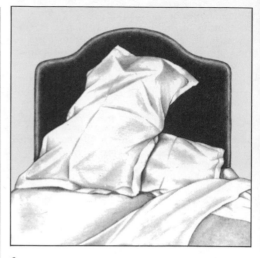

1

The armchair position provides the most comfortable and popular arrangement of pillows for those who like to sit upright in bed. At least four pillows will be needed altogether. Place a fairly solid pillow horizontally at the head of the bed. Position another pillow vertically on top of this and to one side, followed by another propping it up from the other side.

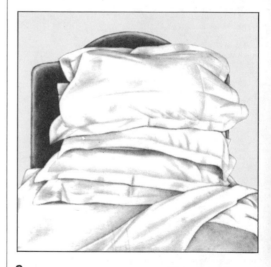

3

Alternatively, you can arrange the pillows in the upright position. Stack at least four pillows on top of each other; the number of pillows once again depends on how tall the patient is. As many as six or seven pillows may have to be used for complete comfort. The firmest pillow is placed at the bottom of the pile and the softest one at the top to support the head.

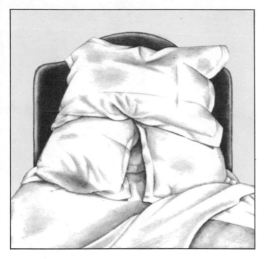

2

On top of this triangular shape place the final
soft pillow for the head. Taller people may
need extra pillows to make up for their
height. The two upright pillows provide good
support for the small of the back and make
an especially comfortable arrangement for
the patient who has trouble breathing
because it helps to keep the shoulders back
and the lungs unconstricted.

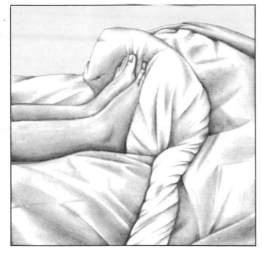

4

Frail or elderly people have a tendency to
slip down the bed and may need a foot-rest.
Take as hard a pillow as you can find. Roll it
up in a sheet, twisting the ends firmly around
it. Place the pillow hard up against the
patient's feet and tuck the ends in each side
of the bed. Alternatively, raise the foot of the
bed a few inches on to a pile of books.
Telephone directories are ideal for this.

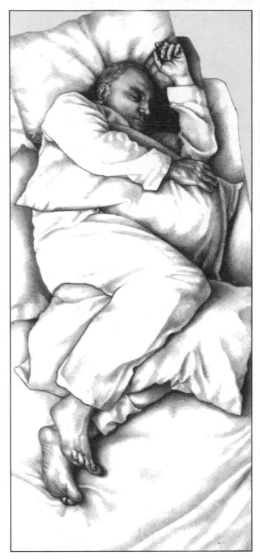

5

A patient who is unable to sit up in bed may
like to lie on one side with just two pillows to
support the head. This position is a good
alternative to lying on the back and may be a
necessity for the victim of a stroke who has
become paralysed down one side of the body.
Extra pillows can be arranged to make this a
most comfortable position. Place one pillow
in the small of the patient's back to provide
support and to prevent the patient from
rolling backwards. Now place a pillow
between the patient's legs for general
comfort as well as to prevent any soreness
developing from the knees rubbing together.
Finally, place a third pillow under the
patient's free arm.

Bed-changing

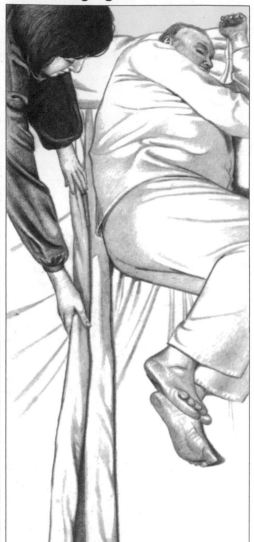

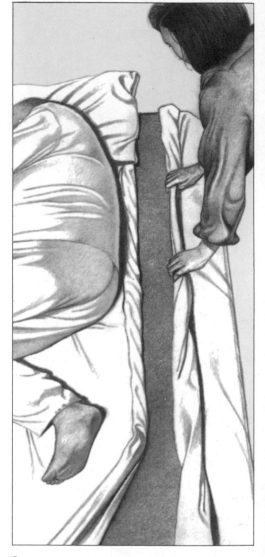

1
It is easy to change the bottom sheet without having to move the patient from the bed. Tell your patient what you are going to do. If it is not uncomfortable for the patient, remove all but one of the pillows. Remove the top bedding but keep the patient covered with a blanket (not shown in illustration). Take a clean sheet and roll it up lengthwise to the middle crease and place on one side over a bedside chair. Roll the patient over to one side of the bed. Untuck the dirty sheet and roll it up lengthwise (in as small a roll as possible) to the middle of the bed up to the patient's back. Take the clean sheet and place it on the bed so that the two rolls meet. Tuck in the clean sheet.

2
Turn the patient back the other way again over the two rolls of bedding on to the clean sheet, which is now in position. The smaller the rolls of sheeting have been made, the more comfortable it will be for the patient to be turned from one side to the other. Move the pillow if necessary so that the patient has support for the head and is comfortable. The dirty sheet can now be removed and put on one side to be washed. Keep talking to your patient. It is reassuring for the patient to know exactly what you are doing and how you are going to do it. It is important, especially with elderly or senile people, that the patient should not be worried unnecessarily by your movements or actions.

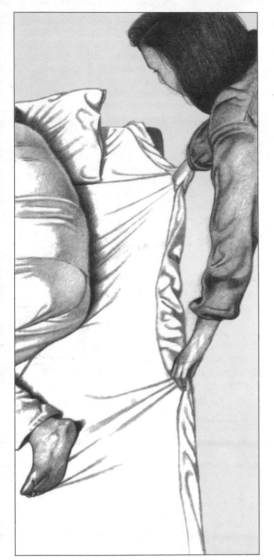

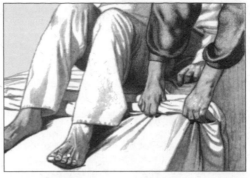

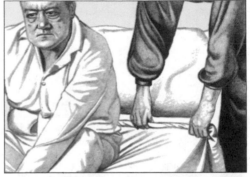

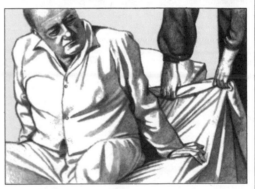

3

After you have removed the dirty sheet, unroll the clean sheet to the other side of the bed. Draw it taut, smoothing out any uncomfortable creases, and tuck in all around. Changing the bottom sheet can be a fast and easy operation if there are two people to do it, but one person should be able to manage adequately. Make up the bed with a clean top sheet, pillowcases, and bedspread, if these need changing. Finally, reposition the pillows according to whether the patient wants to sit up in bed or to lie down. The best time to change the bottom sheet is probably just after the patient has had a bed bath. In this way, two routines can be combined into one.

4

Occasionally, you may have to change the bottom sheet from a different direction, working from the bottom to the top of the bed as opposed to across it. This may be necessary when dealing with a heart patient, or any person who finds that lying flat causes a feeling of breathlessness. Place the two rolls of sheeting together underneath the patient's knees. Lift the patient up by placing one hand under the thighs. The patient can help by pushing down with the hands on to the clean sheet in front. Meanwhile, swiftly take the dirty sheet back and draw the clean sheet up into place. Of the two methods, this one in particular is far easier when done by two people working together.

Pressure points

One of the most important aspects of nursing the patient at home is, without doubt, the prevention of bedsores. This is even more essential when caring for a patient confined to bed for any length of time.

The first warning sign that the skin is under stress is a slight local reddening of the skin. At this stage good nursing care can prevent a bedsore from developing. The importance of changing the position of the patient every two hours cannot be emphasized enough. If this procedure is not carried out, the skin is more likely to break, leaving the underlying tissue exposed and open to infection. A doctor should be consulted immediately, so that appropriate treatment can be given without delay.

Protective heel-pads or elbow-pads may be useful. To make one, take a piece of foam rubber about 2.5 centimetres (1 inch) thick and cut out two strips, each 25 by 10 centimetres (10 inches by 4 inches), long enough to reach around the patient's ankle or heel. Attach Velcro or tapes to the ends to act as a fastening. Other methods include the use of sheepskins and foam rubber rings. (*See* **Comfort in bed,** p.648.)

When turning a patient apply gentle massage to the area which has been subjected to pressure. Careful rubbing with the palm of the hand helps to stimulate the blood supply to the skin. Sprinkle on some talcum powder at the same time. This will be a pleasant freshener for the patient, as well as reducing the friction of your hands against the skin. Alternatively, there are a number of lotions, any of which could be used. A simple and cheap lotion can be easily made using equal parts of surgical spirit and glycerin (glycerol).

Apply a little lotion to the palm of the hand. Massage should be firm but gentle so as to move the top layers of tissue over those underneath. This helps to get the blood moving again. Too heavy and grinding a pressure will break the skin.

Every day, when the patient has a blanket bath, pay particular attention to the pressure areas. Rub these areas twice a day to prevent any soreness occurring.

When coping with an incontinent patient, it is extremely important that you wash all urine off the skin. Any urine remaining may cause irritation, making the formation of bedsores more likely and encouraging infection. A barrier cream helps to give adequate protection.

A little silicone cream (not as greasy as petroleum jelly) is particularly good for dealing with drier areas of skin, such as the elbows or heels.

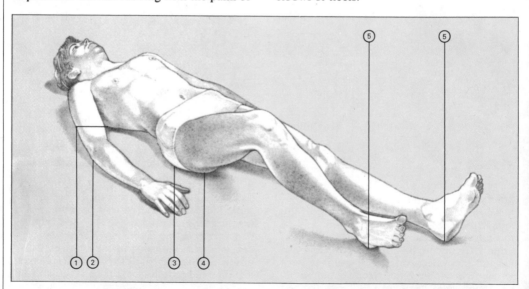

Primary pressure points
The parts of the body most liable to pressure sores are the shoulder blades (1), the elbows (2), the sacrum (3), the buttocks (4), and the heels (5). Pressure sores form because the weight of the bedridden patient's body causes sustained pressure on the skin, depriving it of normal blood circulation. Deprived of blood, the skin tissues start to break down. The sores accordingly appear most commonly on the bodies of people who have difficulty in changing position in bed. Old people are particularly susceptible because their skin is less supple and an elderly person stays in one position for longer than a young person.

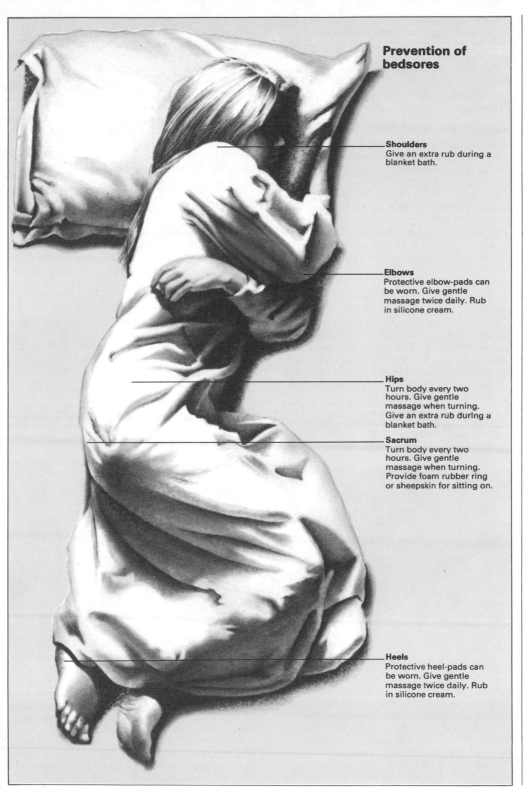

Prevention of bedsores

Shoulders
Give an extra rub during a blanket bath.

Elbows
Protective elbow-pads can be worn. Give gentle massage twice daily. Rub in silicone cream.

Hips
Turn body every two hours. Give gentle massage when turning. Give an extra rub during a blanket bath.

Sacrum
Turn body every two hours. Give gentle massage when turning. Provide foam rubber ring or sheepskin for sitting on.

Heels
Protective heel-pads can be worn. Give gentle massage twice daily. Rub in silicone cream.

Comfort in bed

There are a number of devices available on the market that have been designed specifically with the comfort of the bedridden patient in mind.

Bedsores are one of the main causes of discomfort for anyone who has to spend a great length of time confined to bed (*see* **Pressure points,** p.646). The discomfort is likely to be increased if the patient is overweight or seriously underweight. A sheepskin placed beneath the patient's body can help prevent the formation of bedsores. Placed with the fleecy side up, a sheepskin provides a soft springy surface for the patient to lie on. The wool of a sheepskin allows circulation of air, which evaporates any excess moisture.

Natural sheepskins are available but very expensive. The acrylic type are much more practical since they are easier to wash and also to dry. They are sold in full- and half-length sizes. For a patient who is bedridden for a long time it is advisable to have two: one in use, one in the wash.

Some patients may prefer to use either an air mattress or a water bed. One air mattress that is especially effective in preventing bedsores is the Ripple Bed, which has an electrical device that constantly changes the pressure of air in the mattress. The changes in air pressure within the bands of the mattress cause a gentle rippling beneath the patient's body and a continual shifting of the area of the patient's weight.

Patients who are able to sit up in bed may prefer to sit on a foam rubber ring or a ring-shaped air cushion, either of which removes pressure from the sacral area. To make your own foam rubber ring, use a piece of foam rubber about 7 to 10 centimetres (3 to 4 inches) thick and cut a hole out of it to suit the size of the patient. Then cover it with a pillowcase. An air cushion can be inflated or deflated in size according to individual preference, but is seldom as comfortable as a foam rubber ring.

A free-standing adjustable bed table can be of great benefit to patients who are able to sit up in bed. The bed table is designed so that its foot can be slipped under the side of the bed and the table's top placed directly in front of the patient. The table's top can be raised or lowered and its angle altered from the horizontal to the perpendicular, if required. Patients can use the table not only at meal-times, but also for doing jigsaw puzzles, for reading books, or for drawing or painting. All of these activities can make a long-term confinement to bed more tolerable.

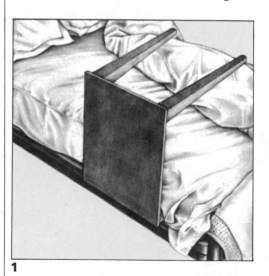

1

A frame for carrying the weight of bedclothes provides relief for a patient's feet or legs. Patients who suffer from varicose ulcers or a sprained ankle will find such a frame of particular value. You can use a stiff cardboard carton or a coffee table turned onto its side and slipped under the mattress at the side of the bed. The other two legs will carry the weight of the bedclothes.

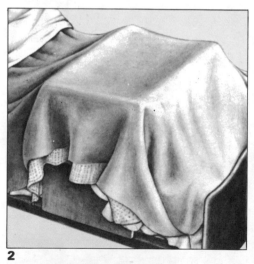

2

Lift the bedclothes up and over the top of the frame, and tuck them in if possible. Elderly patients feel the cold easily and may like the extra warmth and comfort of a light blanket over their feet when the bedclothes are placed over a frame. The most usual position for the frame is over the feet. However, if the patient has pain in the legs you can move the frame farther up the bed as necessary.

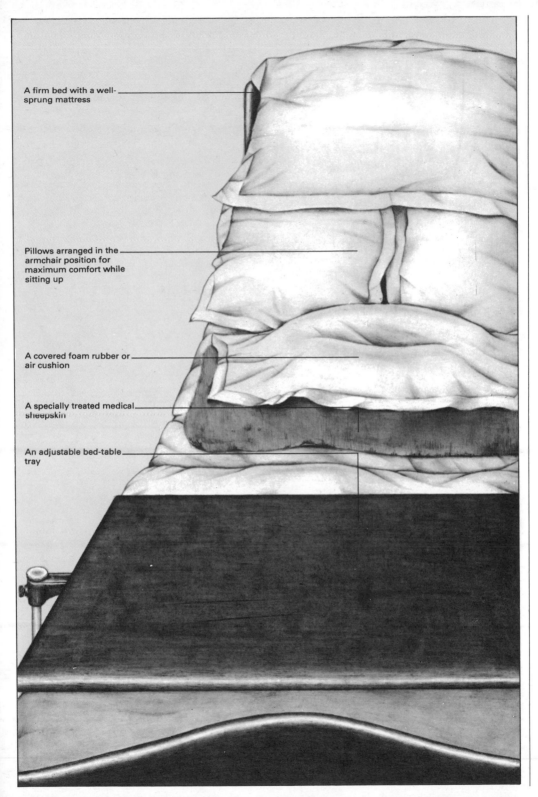

A firm bed with a well-sprung mattress

Pillows arranged in the armchair position for maximum comfort while sitting up

A covered foam rubber or air cushion

A specially treated medical sheepskin

An adjustable bed-table tray

649

Turning a patient

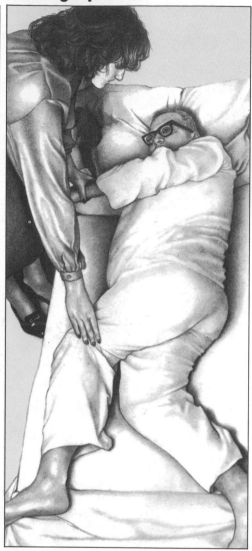

1

A bedridden patient should be turned at least
every two hours. This can be carried out by
one person alone, or by two, depending on
just how much help the patient needs. Gain
the patient's co-operation by explaining how
the turning is to be done. Remove the top
bedding and all the pillows but one. To turn a
patient from the lying position to the right
side, provide enough room for safety and
gently ease the head, shoulders, and hips to
the left side of the bed, supporting the
patient under his body with your hands and
forearms, on a drawsheet. Turn the patient's
head to the right. Bring the patient's left arm
across to the right arm and the left leg across
the right leg.

2

Still standing on the same side of the bed,
place one hand on the patient's left shoulder
blade and the other on the buttocks. Firmly,
but gently, pull the patient up and over onto
the side of the body. Use pillows to position
the patient. Any movements the patient is
able to make alone and unaided should be
encouraged whenever possible. Praise will
boost the patient's morale enormously and
this in itself can help to speed up the process
of improvement and recovery. Move the
pillow across the bed to support the patient's
head. Take this opportunity to talk to the
patient who may have new information to
give you regarding his or her concerns and
state of health.

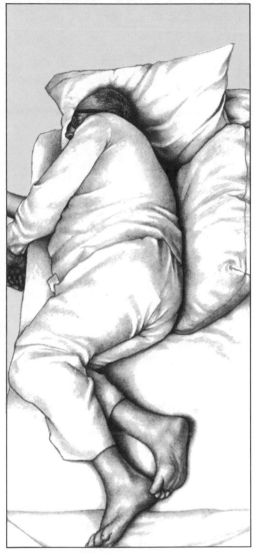

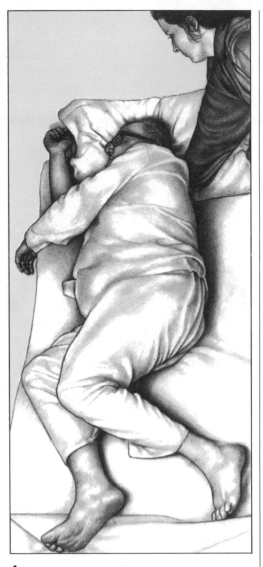

3

Having got the patient into the sideways
position, place a pillow in the small of the
back to prevent the body from rolling
backwards again. A patient who is strong
enough can help at this point by holding on
to the side of the bed while you move round
to the other side. Some elderly people,
however, might be afraid of falling off the
bed while you are moving around to the
other side, and gentle reassurance or bedrails
would make the patient feel more secure. If
there are two of you working together, you
can stand on opposite sides of the bed.
Furthermore, two of you will complete the
task much more quickly and so cause less of a
disturbance to the patient.

4

Standing at the other of the bed, you should
gently push the top of the patient's left
shoulder and the left hip forwards. Gently
pull the right shoulder back from underneath
being careful to prevent excessive friction.
The patient's lower leg should be bent
slightly and extended to a comfortable
position. The upper leg should be bent more
forwards and upwards so as to prevent the
trunk from rolling over. Position the pillow
under the patient's body to make the patient
as comfortable as possible (*see* **Bed-making,**
p.642). To turn the patient to the left, follow
the above directions substituting left for
right. The patient must be kept warm, so heat
up the room beforehand if necessary.

Lifting a patient

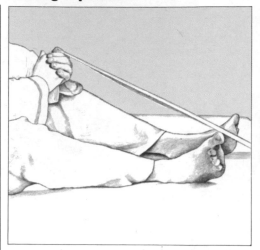

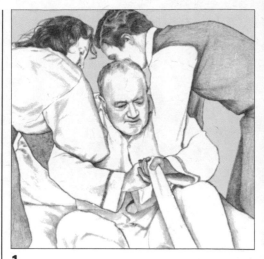

1

Elderly or infirm people may appreciate some means by which to pull themselves up in bed. A pull strap secured around the foot of the bed and long enough to reach the patient's hands will enable the patient to do this. You can make a pull strap with webbing, a scarf, or crepe bandage, or any material that is soft on the patient's hands, but strong enough to take the strain.

A patient should always be encouraged to do whatever possible alone and unaided by anyone else. This is good for the patient's morale and gives the bedridden patient a welcome sense of independence.

Using the pull strap described above, the patient can sit up without your help. This leaves your two hands free for washing the patient's back or brushing the hair. The pull strap also enables a patient to move more freely within the bed than might otherwise be possible. If the patient has a physical disability however, a pull strap is unlikely to be of use; indeed it may require two people to lift a helpless patient up or down in the bed.

One person, working alone, can easily help a patient out of bed. When not in bed, the patient should wear night clothes, a dressing gown, socks and slippers. You should prepare an armchair for the patient by placing a blanket across it and a pillow for the patient's head. Wrap a blanket around the patient's body, and provide a footstool to keep the feet off the floor and away from draughts. If you should decide to use a heater in the room, make sure that the patient is not placed too close. Ensure too that everything that the patient might need is within reach. If it is the patient's first time out of bed, do not leave the patient up for too long.

Two people are needed to lift a helpless patient. Tell the patient what you are going to do. Stand each side of the patient facing the head of the bed. Next, you should each slip one hand under the patient's arms, and use your other hand to support the patient's back, and help the patient into a sitting position. If the patient can assist by pulling up on the pull strap, so much the better.

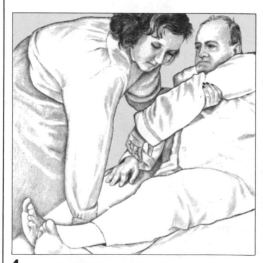

4

A patient may wish to use a commode, but may need help to get out of bed. One person can easily give this help. Bring the commode up next to the bed. One hand is used to lift the legs round to the edge of the bed to get the patient into the sitting position. Your other hand and arm can pass around the patient's upper arm and provide a support for the patient to hold on to.

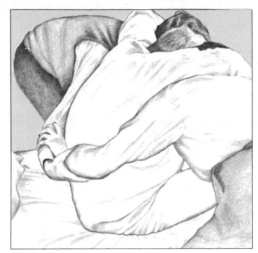

2
You can now move the patient backwards (or forwards, according to what is wanted). You should each stand on either side of the patient, facing each other. Bend your knees in preparation for lifting the patient. Now, each of you should put the arm that is nearer to the foot of the bed under the patient's thighs and grasp hold of the other's elbow, so that your forearms are locked together.

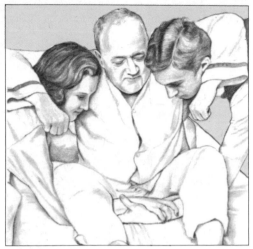

3
Put your other arm as low down the patient's back towards the buttocks as it will go. The lower the arm is, the easier it is to lift the patient. Once again lock forearms with the person who is helping you, by gripping one another's elbows. Count one, two, three, and lift the patient backwards. The patient can help by pushing down into the bed with the heels.

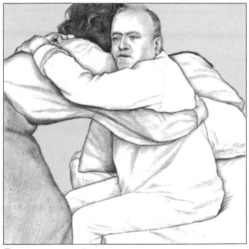

5
Bend your knees and place them securely on each side of the patient's knees. Your knees should always be bent when doing any sort of lifting to prevent backstrain. Ask the patient to clasp hands around your neck or around the top of your back. Meanwhile, nestle your head into the patient's shoulder and clasp your hands around the patient's back, holding the patient tightly to you.

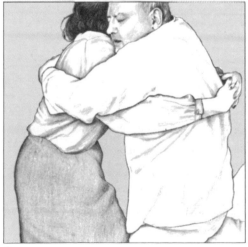

6
With a gentle rocking motion, backward and forward, count one, two, three. On the count of four, come up, with each of you holding on to the other, and round on to the commode. Keep your knees bent while doing this so as to take the weight of the patient's body more easily. To get the patient back into bed again, repeat the process in reverse order, keeping your knees bent when you lift the patient.

Blanket bath

A patient who is lying in bed all day needs to wash just as often as an active, healthy person. For a bedridden patient, a blanket bath can be extremely refreshing. Ideally, a blanket bath should be given every day. But if this is not possible, the patient should be bathed at least every other day.

Remember that the patient may feel that he or she is putting you to a great deal of unnecessary trouble, or may feel embarrassed at being bathed by someone else. Your calm and efficient manner can do much to reassure the patient that this is not so, and the patient may come to enjoy the routine.

Equipment needed includes a jug of hot water; a fairly large bowl; a bucket; soap; two flannels, one for the face and one for the body; talcum powder; a small soft towel for the face; and plenty of larger towels, for drying the patient and for placing under each part of the body as it is being washed.

Shut all the windows and make sure that the room is warm. It may be better if the patient is first accompanied to the toilet or is given a bedpan, to avoid interrupting the blanket bath.

Undress the patient and remove the top bedclothes. Place an old towel or blanket on the bed underneath the patient and a blanket on top to keep the patient warm. If the patient is comfortable lying flat, arrange two pillows for the head. If not, wash the patient in the sitting position.

Expose only one part of the patient's body at a time, as it is being washed. Change the washing water half-way through the routine, after washing the legs and before starting on the back.

A blanket bath is a good opportunity to massage any potentially sore areas of the body, such as the shoulder blades, base of the spine, and hips. While soaping, give these areas a few extra gentle rubs. If the patient's elbows and heels are dry, rub them with a non-greasy cream.

Always dry the patient's body carefully before putting the night clothes back on. Pay particular attention to any crevices or cracks, because these can get sore if left moist. For a female patient, do not forget the areas underneath the breasts, and in fat people the groin area at the top of the legs. When the patient is completely dry, dust on some talcum powder.

Brush the patient's teeth, and brush and comb the hair. Perhaps the patient would like to use a deodorant, and a woman might want to apply lipstick or a dab of perfume. All these will contribute towards the patient's general sense of wellbeing. Finally remake the bed, with clean sheets if necessary.

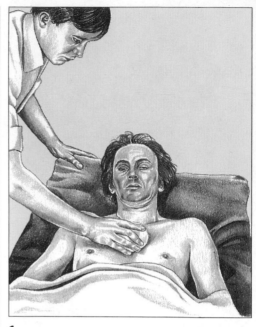

1
Start with the face, neck, and ears. The patient may be well enough to do this unaided. Pat the skin dry with a soft towel.

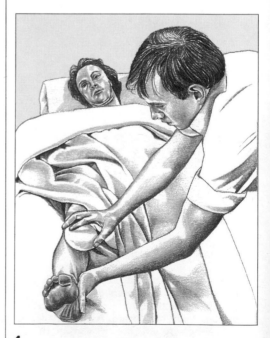

4
Wash the legs, one at a time, paying particular attention to the area between the toes. Cut the toenails if they need it.

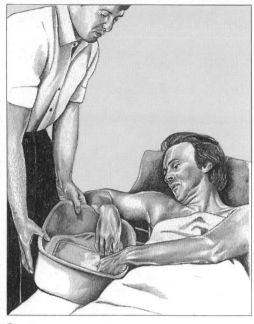

2
Wash and dry the chest and arms. Let the patient dip the hands in the bowl of water to rinse off any soap.

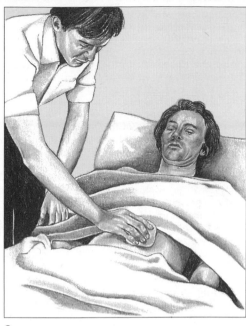

3
Keep the chest and lower parts of the body covered while you wash the patient's abdomen. Do not forget the navel.

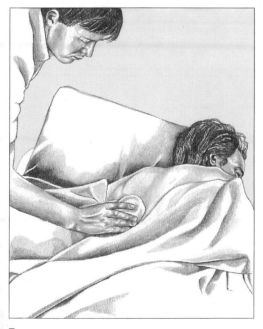

5
Turn the patient on to one side, then the other, to do the upper half of the back. Alternatively, get the patient to sit up.

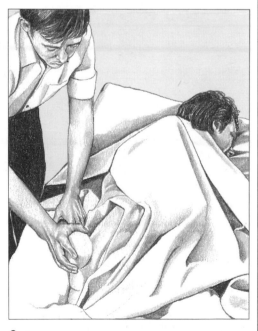

6
Lastly, wash the lower part of the back. Most patients prefer to wash their genital area themselves.

Helping a patient into the bath

The first bath after a long illness can greatly help a patient's morale. The fact that it is being attempted at all is a good sign that the patient is recovering.

Prepare the bathroom beforehand. Close the windows to keep out any draughts, and half fill the bath with warm water. The temperature should not be hotter than normal body temperature (37°C, or 98.6°F). Test the temperature of the water with your hand; the water should feel comfortably warm.

Equipment needed includes soap; two flannels (one for the face and one for the body); a face towel; and two body towels.

If the patient has difficulty getting into the bath, place an upright chair of about the bath's height alongside the bath. Hang one towel over the back of the chair and one on the seat.

Patients who are unable to lie down may miss the pleasant sensation of warm water splashing around the shoulders. Do this for them by splashing water on the shoulders using cupped hands.

Make sure the patient is dried thoroughly before accompanying him or her to the bedroom. Keep the patient covered and warm at all times.

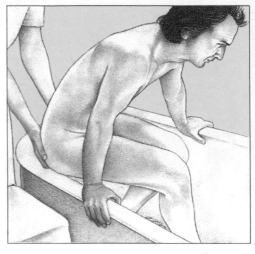

2

Some patients, especially the elderly, may have difficulty in lowering themselves into a sitting position. They can be helped by placing one hand just below the buttocks. A bath seat in the bottom of the bath is also a great aid. You can improvise by using a low stool or a wooden block.

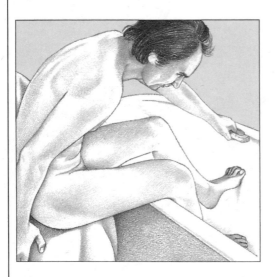

1

Help the patient to get into the bath by lifting the legs together up and over the side. The patient should be well enough to be able to pull himself or herself forward on the bathrail, placing the free hand on the edge of the bath for support. A non-slip mat in the bottom of the bath may give confidence to a person who is afraid of a fall.

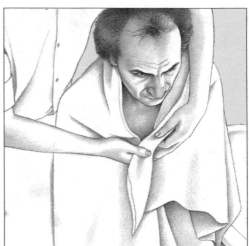

3

Help the patient out of the bath by guiding him or her on to the chair beside the bath, which should already have towels draped over it. Wrap the towel from the back of the chair around the patient's body and shoulders, leaving the other one for sitting on. It is pleasant for the patient if the towels have been warmed beforehand.

Hairwashing in bed

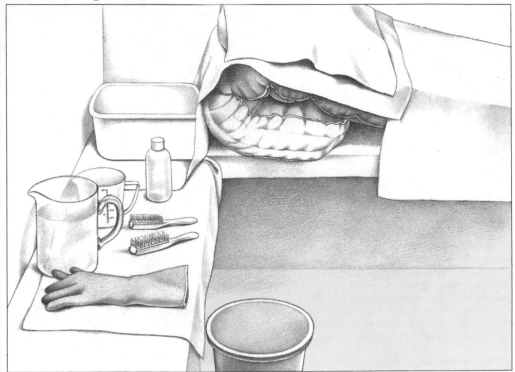

Care of a bedridden patient's hair is important. The hair should be combed or brushed at least twice a day. If necessary, use a dry shampoo to prevent grease. But washing the hair with water and liquid shampoo is not difficult, and can boost the patient's morale.

Ensure that the top of the bed is near an electric socket into which the hairdrier can be plugged. Ask the patient to move towards the foot of the bed, giving help if needed. Sit the patient upright and roll the top of the mattress under itself.

Place one or two pillows on top of the mattress, so that the top of the patient's back is well supported.

Put rubber sheeting over the springs of the bed to protect them, and cover the bedclothes with polythene sheeting and a towel. Put a plastic cape and a towel around the patient's shoulders, and get the patient to lie back so that the head can hang down over a bowl placed underneath it.

Other equipment needed includes two jugs, a large one containing a supply of warm water, and a small one to work with; a bucket, in which to pour used water; shampoo; a brush and comb; towels; and a hairdrier. A female patient may also need rollers and pins to set her hair.

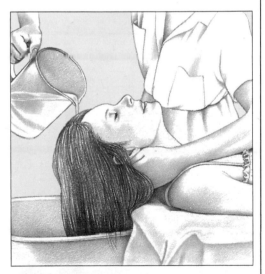

Washing the hair
Support the patient's neck with one hand, and wash the patient's hair with the other. Use water from the small jug to wet the hair. Pour on the shampoo and rub it gently into the hair.

Rinse and repeat. After the final rinse, dry the hair with a warm towel. Finish off using an electric hairdrier.

657

Feeding in bed

To prepare a patient for a meal, make sure
the pillows are comfortable and support the
back when the patient is in the sitting
position. If there is a bed table, place it in
front of the patient. Adjust it to the
appropriate height and angle for the patient
to eat off comfortably.

A bedridden patient may have a poor
appetite. Careful presentation of food can
help to overcome this. Make use of attractive
table linen and tableware. The simplest foods
can be brightened up considerably with a
sprig of parsley or a slice of lemon to add
colour and decoration. A bunch of flowers,
or even a single bloom, picked from the
garden and placed in a vase, provides a
delightful finishing touch.

Serve only small helpings of food. Too
large a helping heaped on to a plate may take
away the appetite of the sick or elderly. If the
patient is still hungry after the meal, a further
portion can always be given. The patient may
enjoy helping to plan the menu and may
welcome the opportunity to be useful.

The food must be fresh and served at the
right temperature. Preparing food at home
does not mean you can ignore the strictest
rules of a good restaurant: hot food should
always be served hot, and cold food served
cold.

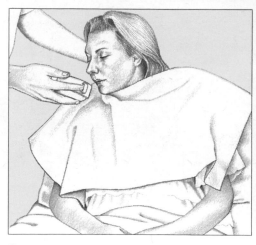

2

If possible, prop the patient up in a sitting
position. Lay a napkin over the patient's
night clothes in case of spillage. Check the
temperature of the liquid. It should be
neither too hot, nor too tepid. Support the
patient's neck with one hand, tilt the cup with
your other hand, and gently pour into the
patient's mouth. As well as tea, and coffee,
you may give the patient nutritious
soups.

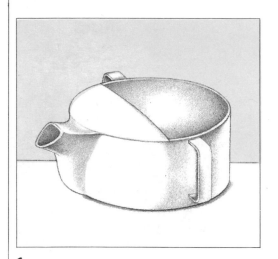

1

The feeding cup is a useful utensil for the
patient who is unable to cope alone with
feeding. It is easier to use than an ordinary
cup because it is light, and has a spout-like
opening. This allows a greater control over
the flow of liquid. The handles on each side
of the cup allow the patient to hold the cup if
able to do so. The handles also make it easier
for you to pour.

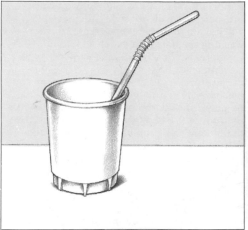

3

Often, a feeding cup is not available just
when you need it most. One practical
alternative is to let the patient drink through
a flexible straw. Ordinary drinking straws are
not satisfactory unless the patient can incline
the head towards the straw.

Flexible straws can be used again and
again, and are best used with a slim cup or
flask to stop the straw from falling out.

Food
Serve only small portions
of food at a time.

Position of patient
A minimum of four pillows
arranged in the armchair
position gives the best
support for sitting the
patient up in bed.

Presentation
An attractive plate and
napkin, and some sweet-
smelling flowers add an
extra-special touch.

Adjustable table

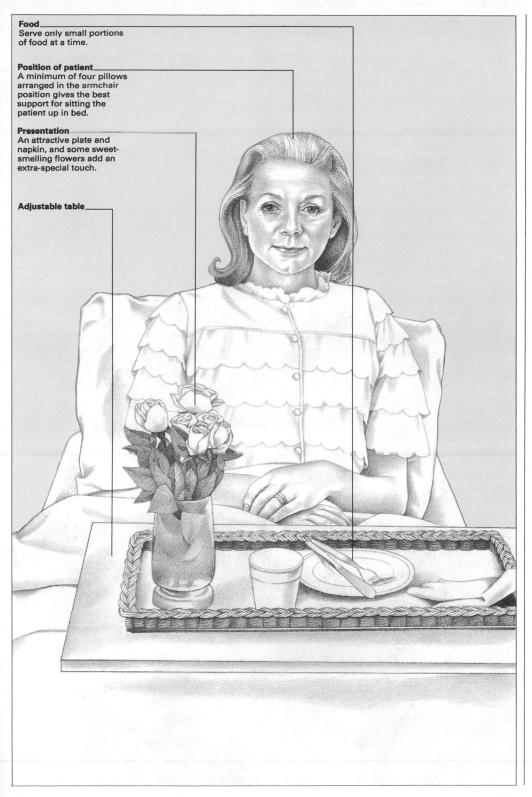

Taking temperatures and pulse

The average human body temperature in health, taken under the tongue, registers 37°C or 98.6°F on the thermometer.

The average adult pulse rate varies from 68 to 84 beats per minute at rest. In men the normal pulse rate is 68 to 76 beats a minute; in women, 70 to 84; in infants and children, still higher, 100 to 120. A baby's pulse rate is much higher, about 120 to 140 beats per minute at rest. The pulse of a twelve-year-old is about 80 beats per minute at rest.

Having taken the patient's pulse, you should keep hold of the wrist, and observe the patient's respiration rate. Do not let the patient know what you are counting. The patient's awareness could cause a subconscious reaction that would change the rate of breathing. One respiration consists of one complete inhalation and exhalation. Count the respirations for a full minute. For a healthy adult, the total is 16 to 22 respirations per minute; for a baby it is 30 to 50. A twelve-year-old's respiratory rate is the same as an adult's.

It is important that you write down the daily readings of the patient's temperature, pulse rate and respiration rate. A temperature chart can be bought from the chemist to help you to do this more efficiently. The doctor may want you to keep a record of other bodily functions, such as how often the patient moves the bowels, or the patient's fluid intake and output. When the patient's illness has passed and a thermometer is no longer needed, swab it in disinfectant before finally putting it away.

Taking the temperature under the tongue gives the most accurate reading. However, this method is not suitable for babies or for senile or confused patients. A reading taken under the arm (axillary) is a suitable method for the elderly and senile. Alternatively, a reading can be taken by placing the thermometer in the patient's rectum. This may be necessary when a patient is unable to have the thermometer placed under the tongue (sublingually) because of, say, inflammation of the mouth. A rectal temperature reading is usually taken in children under four years.

Never use a long-tipped mercury thermometer for taking a rectal temperature: use only the short-tipped stubby type of thermometer with a bulb the same diameter as the stem. Lubricate the thermometer bulb with petroleum jelly before inserting it about 2-3cm (1 inch) into the rectum. Hold the thermometer in place for one minute. Remove the thermometer and record the reading. A rectal temperature is about 0.5°C (1°F) higher than a sublingual temperature.

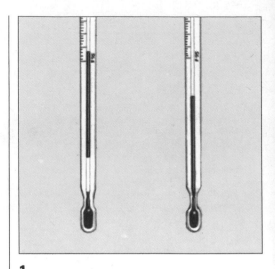

1
Before taking the patient's temperature you must ensure that the mercury ribbon in the thermometer is well below the "normal" mark of 37°C (98.6°F). To do this, you hold the thermometer at the opposite end to the bulb firmly between the finger and thumb. Give the thermometer two or three sharp flicks of the wrist. Check the new reading, repeating the flicking action if necessary.

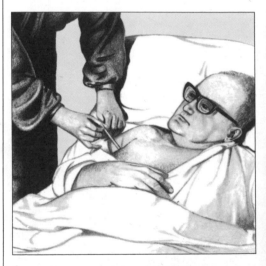

4
Lift up the patient's arm, and slip the thermometer under it so that the bulb rests in the armpit. Bring the patient's arm across the chest to ensure that the thermometer stays securely in place. Leave the thermometer in position for at least three minutes. Remove it and record the reading. An axillary temperature is about 0.5°C (1°F) lower than a sublingual temperature.

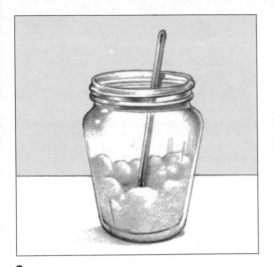

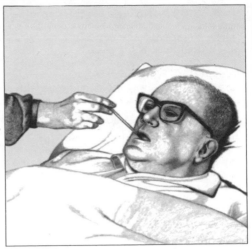

2

During the time when you are using a clinical thermometer, keep it in a jar with a wad of absorbent cotton at the bottom.

After you have used the thermometer, rinse it thoroughly under cold running water to wash away any germs, dry it, and replace it in the jar. Never rinse the thermometer under hot water. The mercury may expand too much and break the bulb.

3

Check that the patient has not had a hot or cold drink, or a smoke, within the last half hour. Place the bulb of the thermometer under the patient's tongue. Ask the patient to close the lips (but not the teeth) gently around the stem of the thermometer. Leave the thermometer in place at least one minute. Remove the thermometer and record the reading.

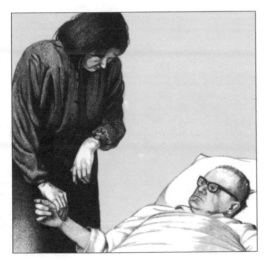

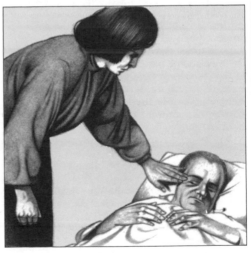

5

You can feel a pulse wherever an artery lies across a bone. The usual place to take a patient's pulse is at the wrist. Place the first and second fingers of your hand gently on the patient's wrist at the base of the thumb. After a few moments you should feel the beats of the pulse. Count the number of beats during one full minute by watching the second hand of a clock or wrist-watch.

6

If the patient is asleep, or whenever the wrist is not readily accessible, simply place two fingers lightly on the patient's temples, and take the pulse reading. The most accurate reading is obtained by counting the beats over a full minute. You should avoid taking the pulse for a shorter time and multiplying the number of beats by a factor to get the result.

Medicines, inhalants, and eye drops

Wash your hands before administering any medicines. Always check the instructions and dosage on the container before use, whether pills or liquids are being given.

If the medicine is liquid, thoroughly shake the container. When pouring liquid from a medicine bottle, always hold the bottle with the label uppermost to prevent the label from becoming damaged and therefore illegible as a result of spillage. Fill the standard 5 ml. teaspoon right to the top as often as the prescribed dose requires. Large doses may be given in a graduated medicine glass.

If the medicine is in tablet form, give the patient a glass of water to drink, to make swallowing the tablets easier. Children in particular, and some elderly people, may find a tablet difficult to swallow even with a drink of water. In these circumstances, crush the tablet between two spoons, and if necessary disguise the powder by mixing it in a little jam before giving to the patient. Wash the medicine glass or spoon after use.

Be sure always to follow accurately the instructions given on the medicine container. For example, when specifically directed to give tablets only before meals, do not give them at any other time. If a medicine has to be given four-hourly or six-hourly, keep to the times as closely as possible, without unnecessarily disturbing natural sleep patterns. If the medicine has to be given three times a day, breakfast, lunch and supper times provide an easy timetable.

Once such a pattern has been established, make it a routine and keep to it. A routine encourages calm acceptance by the patient. Such a timetable also ensures that a balanced concentration of the drug is maintained in the bloodstream.

Always make sure, personally, that the patient takes the medicine. Do not assume, for example, that it will be taken after you have left the room.

All medicines should be kept outside the sick room, preferably in a locked and childproof cupboard.

Dealing with styes

Styes may often be helped by some form of heat treatment.

A simple and effective way of applying heat is to take a wooden kitchen spoon and wrap the rounded part in cotton wool or a handkerchief. Keep the cotton in place with loosely wound bandages. Dip the spoon into boiling water and then hold it up close, but not too close, to the stye.

The steam rising from the spoon has a soothing effect that can provide great relief.

Ear drops

Unless the instructions on the container state otherwise, warm the ear drops by placing the container in a bowl of warm water. Drops containing an antibiotic should not be heated. The patient should lie with the head flat and the affected ear uppermost. Take hold of the earlobe and carefully pull it back so as to create as large an opening as possible. Draw up the liquid into the dropper. Rest the end of the dropper over the ear opening and allow the prescribed number of drops to trickle gently into the ear. Leave for a few moments before placing a small plug of cotton in the outer ear to prevent the liquid from leaking out. The patient should continue to lie in this position for about five minutes.

Nose drops

Place two pillows under the patient's shoulders so that the head is tilted backwards. The further back the head rests, the more effective is the treatment. Insert the end of the dropper into one nostril and release the prescribed number of drops. Instruct the patient to sniff gently. Repeat with the other nostril. The patient should stay with the head back for about one minute. Wipe away excess fluid with cotton wool.

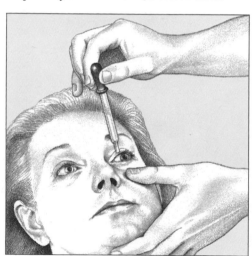

1 Eye drops

Ask the patient to look upwards, with the head resting on a pillow. Gently ease down the lower lid with one hand. Apply the eye drops with the other. Try to place the drops towards the inner corner of the eye. Ask the patient to shut the eye for a few seconds immediately after; this ensures that the liquid is distributed evenly. Gently swab away excess liquid with a piece of cotton wool.

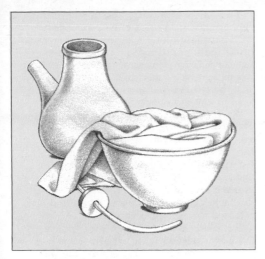

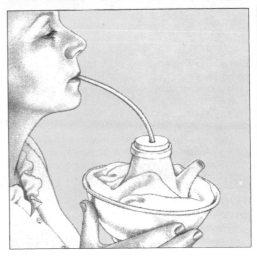

2 Closed inhalation

The Nelson's Inhaler is used to loosen sticky mucus from the lower lungs, a common symptom of bronchitis or pneumonia. Fill the inhaler with boiling water to just below the spout. Add half a teaspoon of Friar's balsam, if desired. Wrap a towel around the inhaler, leaving the spout clear. Attach the cork stopper and glass mouthpiece. If the glass is too hot, wrap a piece of gauze around it.

3

Place the inhaler in a bowl or on a table in front of the patient, ensuring that the spout is facing away from the body. Ask the patient to breathe in deeply through the mouth and out through the nose for about ten minutes. Hold the bowl steady if necessary. The treatment can be repeated every three to four hours. The patient must be kept warm for at least half an hour after the inhalation.

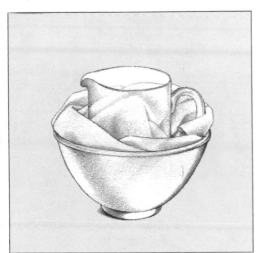

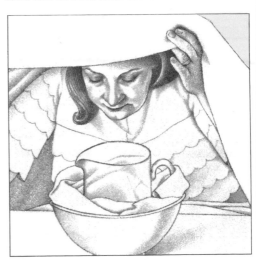

4 Open inhalation

Open inhalation is effective in the treatment of head colds or blocked sinuses.

Fill a two-pint enamel or glass jug up to five centimetres (two inches) from the top with boiling water. Add one 5 ml. teaspoon of Friar's balsam or, alternatively, one small crystal of menthol (the size of a large pin's head). Wrap a towel around the jug and stand it upright in a bowl.

5

Drape a towel over the patient's shoulders. Bring the towel over the patient's head so that it also covers both the jug and bowl. It is important that the towel completely covers the bowl as well as the patient's head so that no steam is lost. Ask the patient to breathe in and out through the nose for about ten minutes. Make sure the patient is kept warm for half an hour afterwards.

Use of bedpans and drawsheets

When giving a bedpan or urinal, allow the patient as much privacy as possible. Most people will prefer to be left on their own.

The bedpan or urinal should be carried to and from the patient covered with a clean towel. A urinal should be placed in position for a helpless or confused patient.

A bedpan should be warm and dry. Warm it with running water from a hot tap, and dry it thoroughly. Raise the patient's buttocks with one hand, while gently slipping the bedpan underneath with the other. Two people are needed to give a bedpan to a helpless patient. Take care not to graze the patient's skin. Provide a supply of soft toilet paper, and give assistance only if specifically requested.

Remove the bedpan or urinal and cover it immediately with a towel. Give the patient a bowl of water, some soap, and a towel with which to wash the hands.

Observe the contents of the bedpan or urinal before emptying it down the toilet. Rinse the bedpan thoroughly under running water, and clean under the rim with a mop, which should be kept for this purpose in a jug of disinfectant.

The doctor may prescribe glycerin suppositories or an enema for a patient who is having bowel difficulties.

To insert a suppository use a pair of thin rubber gloves. Lubricate the suppository with petroleum jelly. Use the first finger to insert the suppository into the rectum as far as it will go. This may be embarrassing to the patient, so remain calm and be efficient. Tell the patient that the longer it is kept in, the more effective it will be.

An enema comes in the form of a plastic sachet with a nozzle attached. Immerse the sachet in a bowl of hot water for ten minutes to warm the contents. Lubricate the nozzle with petroleum jelly and insert it slowly about 8 cm (3 inches) into the rectum while gently squeezing out the sachet's contents. The enema should be retained for as long as possible.

Retention is made easier if the foot of the bed is raised slightly. It also helps if the patient can be distracted in some way. Let the patient lie on the back while listening to the radio or reading a book.

When retention is no longer possible, help the patient out onto a commode or give a bedpan. Provide toilet paper, followed by a bowl of water and soap for washing.

The patient should then be left in peace and quiet. Having an enema can be exhausting, particularly for an elderly person.

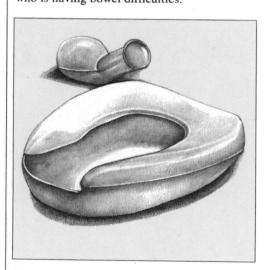

1

For some patients it is necessary to keep a record of the intake and output of fluids. Keep two separate measuring jugs, one to measure the intake of fluids as the patient drinks them, the other for measuring the output of urine. Some urinals have a measuring scale down one side. The liquid from a bedpan, however, has to be separated out.

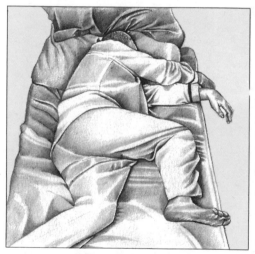

2

Enemas and suppositories should be given to a patient lying, if possible, on the left side. This position provides easy access to the rectal area. Encourage the patient to empty the bladder first. Place an old towel under the buttocks, and keep the patient warm with a blanket, leaving a minimum of skin exposed. Ask the patient to take shallow breaths.

Elderly people suffering from incontinence often feel distressed and de-
graded by it. Getting annoyed with them
only aggravates the problem. The home
nurse should make the situation as easy
and comfortable as possible for the patient.
Often incontinence can be prevented
altogether by giving the patient a bedpan
regularly every two hours.

An incontinent patient should always
have a protective waterproof sheet placed
over the mattress of the bed. Disposable
incontinence pads can be obtained, with your
doctor's help, from the local health authority,
or from a chemist.

The patient should use night clothes that
are easy to wash and dry. Female patients
should wear nightdresses that open down the
back. The lower part can then be arranged so
that it does not become wet.

Urine is a skin irritant, and so should
not be left in contact with it for any length
of time. Change the patient's bedclothes
and wash and dry the skin as soon as
possible, applying a barrier cream.

To avoid frequently changing bed
linen, make up the bed with a drawsheet.
This is a long narrow sheet placed across
the bed under the area of the patient's
buttocks.

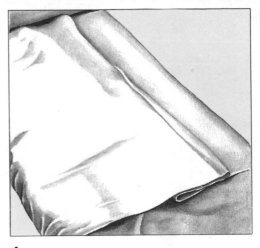

4

If the drawsheet becomes damp, or if the
patient feels hot and wants to lie on a
cooler piece of sheet, the large fold can be
untucked and some of it moved across the
bed as necessary. When the required
amount has been moved across, tuck what
remains of the large fold back underneath
the mattress for future use. (A dirty sheet,
however, will have to be removed.)

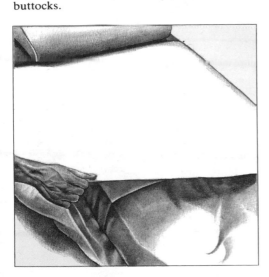

3

First place a polythene sheet across the bed
over the bottom sheet, and tuck in.
Take the drawsheet (an old sheet torn in
half is ideal for this) and tuck in under the
mattress at one side of the bed. Take the
other end of the sheet to the other side of
the bed, and tuck in only the end so that a
fold hangs down. Tuck in the whole of the
remaining length of fold.

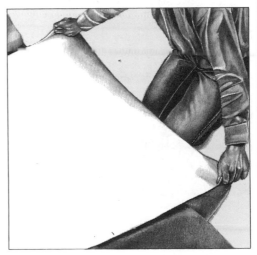

5

From the other side of the bed pull the
new piece of sheet taut, smoothing out
any creases. Tuck the used piece of sheet
underneath the mattress on this side of the
bed. If the slack in the drawsheet is always
moved in the same direction across the
bed, it is possible to get about four clean
pieces of sheet. If it has not got dirty, it
can be moved back in the other direction.

Exercises in bed 1

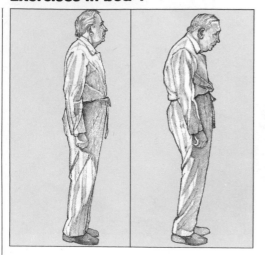

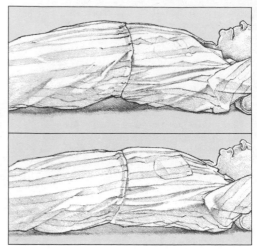

Good posture (*above left, this column*) depends on the correct tilt of the pelvis – the body's centre of gravity is located there. The buttocks should be tucked in so as to flatten the lower back. This movement automatically rolls the pelvis upwards and tightens the stomach muscles. The shoulder blades are pulled together to straighten the upper back, and the shoulders allowed to relax downwards. The neck should be stretched up comfortably from the top of the back so that the head is pulled up, and the chin is kept parallel with the floor. The knees are kept straight, not bent, and the weight of the body is distributed evenly on both feet.

Bad posture (*above right, this column*) results from not following these actions. The pelvis tilts forward so that the stomach and buttocks are sticking out. The shoulders are slouched and the head hangs down. The knees are slightly bent and do not provide a strong support for the body. Bad posture can strain ligaments because the body's weight is not distributed correctly.

After spending a long time in bed, a patient's muscles become weak. This is particularly true of the postural muscles. Other, stronger muscles may then pull the body down into positions that lead to bad posture. To avoid this happening, the patient while still in bed should perform exercises that strengthen the postural muscles. The patient's doctor should be consulted before any exercises are undertaken.

Lack of exercise leads to poor muscle tone, a loss of strength, and a sense of fatigue. Regular gentle exercise not only produces strong muscles and a sense of wellbeing, but also prevents the slow movement of blood in the legs and reduces the likelihood of clots.

The patient performs the first exercises while still lying in bed. Later, exercises are done at the edge of the bed, and finally on the floor. As well as strengthening muscles in preparation for standing and walking again, these exercises are also good for the patient's morale. As each new exercise is mastered, it gives the patient a feeling of progress on the road to recovery.

Each bed exercise should be practised three to five times in the morning, afternoon and evening. The number can be increased, with the doctor's consent, as the patient gets stronger. Progress from one exercise to the next as the muscles strengthen. During exercise, get the patient to breathe in when contracting the muscles, and breathe out when relaxing them.

The following exercises are given as direct instructions to the patient. However, it is more satisfactory to have someone to assist and supervise in order that the exercises are done correctly.

Start the exercises by practising the pelvic tilt (*above, this column*). Lie flat and straight on the bed with one small pillow under the head. Squeeze the buttock muscles together and feel the lower back flatten on to the bed. This action will roll the pelvis upwards at the front and so flatten the stomach muscles.

Having mastered the pelvic tilt, combine this with work on the leg muscles. "Roll" the pelvis upwards. Push both knees downwards and tighten the thigh muscles. Pull the feet upwards to make a right angle at the ankles. Feel the pull down the back of the legs.

Finally, combine the exercises to involve the head and shoulders as well. Relax the shoulders down and tighten the muscles between the shoulder blades. Stretch the neck gently behind the ears. Keep the chin parallel with the pulled up feet.

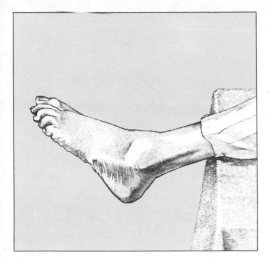

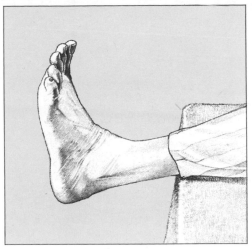

1

Lie flat on the back with the arms relaxed by the side of the body.

Extend the feet and ankles over the end of the bed to allow greater freedom of movement during the exercises.

Starting with either the right or the left foot, point the toes and feel the stretch down the sides of the leg and around the ankle.

2

Draw up the toes so that they are pointing towards the ceiling, and push forward with the heel as far as it will go.

Feel the stretch of the muscles up the back of the leg and around the ankle joints, and in the muscles of the thigh.

Continue this up and down movement with one foot before repeating with the other foot.

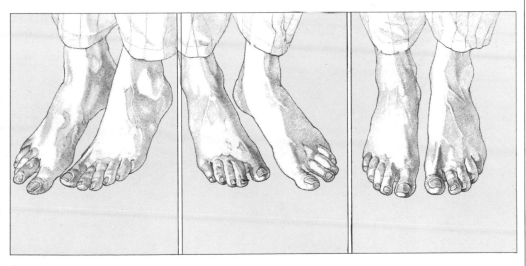

3

Rest both feet together over the edge of the bed, and relax before the next exercise.

Rotate the ankles, pointing the feet round to the right as far as they will go.

Continue the circular movement. Point the toes down to the floor and up again to the left until they have returned to their original position, with toes pointing upwards.

Repeat the exercise, but this time rotate the feet in the opposite direction.

As the feet point to the side, feel the pull on the ankle muscles.

The downward movement stretches the muscles at the front of the leg. As the feet move upwards, the stretch returns to the back of the leg again.

Exercises in bed 2

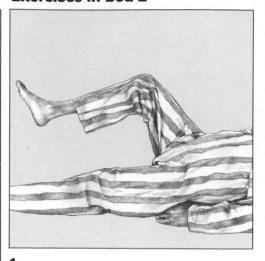

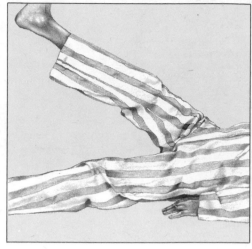

1
Lie flat on the back with the arms relaxed by the sides of the body. Straighten the left leg and try to get the back of the knee flat on the surface of the bed. Keep this leg flat throughout the exercise. Bend the right knee as far as is possible while still keeping the left foot on the bed.

Stretch the right knee out, keeping the foot at right angles to the leg. Feel the stretch of the muscles down the back of the leg, and the tightening of the muscles around the knee joint. Keeping the leg straight, let it down slowly on to the bed. Repeat with the left leg.

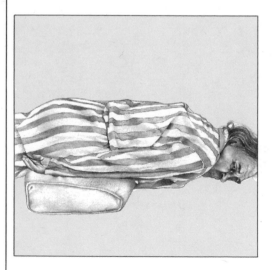

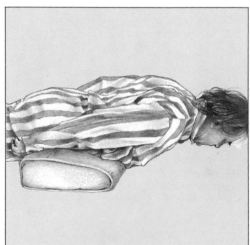

3
Lie flat on the stomach with a pillow placed underneath the abdomen so as to avoid arching the lower spine. Keep the arms relaxed by the sides of the body, and rest the head on one side. The breathing should be regular. Experience the feeling of relaxation before starting the exercise.

Breathe in, and raise the head and shoulders as far upwards as possible. Feel the muscles of the back working to hold the chest and shoulders off the bed. Be careful not to overstrain the muscles. Slowly let the upper trunk down on to the bed again. Breathe out with the downward movement of the trunk.

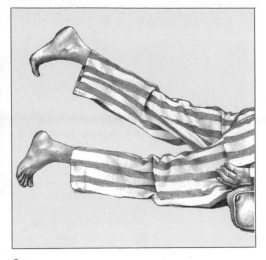

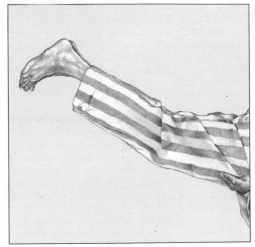

2
Lie flat on the stomach with a pillow placed underneath so as to prevent too great a hollowing of the lower back. Raise one leg at a time, keeping the foot at right angles to the leg. Push the heel as far back as it will go and feel the stretch down the back of the leg.

Lift both legs together, as high as you can without straining. Stretch the legs by pushing from the heel as hard as possible. Keep the pelvis flat on the pillow throughout the whole of this exercise. Concentrate on the muscles of the legs, on the buttocks, and around the hips.

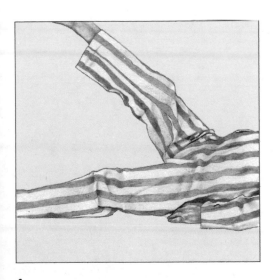

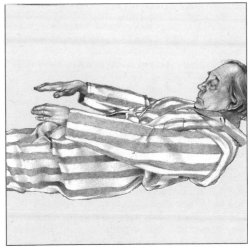

4
Lie flat on the back, with the arms relaxed by the sides of the body. Straighten the left leg and try to get the back of the knee flat on the bed. Raise the right leg with the foot pulled well up. Keep the knee straight and feel the stretch of the muscles at the back of the leg and in the buttock. Lower the leg.

Stretch the arms forward. Raise the head and tuck in the chin. Bring the body up and across to the right-hand side. Touch the right knee with the left hand, without bending the knee. Come back slowly, keeping the chin tucked in, and repeat the whole exercise on the left-hand side of the body.

Exercises on the edge of the bed 1

After toning up the muscles while lying in the bed, the next stage is to get the patient to exercise while sitting on the edge of the bed. This involves slightly more strenuous activity, and includes exercises for the upper part of the body as well as for the lower part. The following exercises, on these two pages and the next two, are designed particularly to strengthen the postural muscles of the trunk, shoulders, and legs. It is advisable, however, to get a doctor's advice on whether the patient is ready for such exercise.

Encourage the patient to think about the way that muscles and joints inside the body work. Apart from making the exercises more interesting, it will also help the patient to do them better.

Get the patient to stretch and extend the body as far as is comfortable, but be careful not to overstrain the muscles. Movements are more helpful and easier to carry out if breathing fits in with the actions. The patient should breathe in as muscles are being tightened, and breathe out again as the muscles are relaxed.

Always keep the patient's comfort in mind. On no account let the patient get cold. Before exercise begins, make sure that the room is warm enough.

It has already been mentioned that lack of exercise reduces both the tone and strength of muscles. Lack of exercise also slows the circulation of the blood. The heart, which is a muscle, becomes less responsive to increased exercise so that the pulse rate increases and shortness of breath occurs.

A patient who has been lying in bed for a long time has less need of a full range of thoracic movement. The lungs are not fully expanded and so air does not enter the lower regions of the lungs. Normal drainage may not take place, and this may lead to infection of the lung, for example, pneumonia. The lungs are situated inside the rib-cage. Pressure on the ribs encourages the lungs to expand. If a towel or something similar is placed around the ribs and pulled inwards, the lungs are made aware of the pressure on them. They tend to move outwards against any resistance, and so squeezing the rib-cage stimulates them into activity.

Patients who are going to have to use crutches or a similar walking aid may find it useful to exercise the arms. Strong arms are necessary because they will have to carry most of the body's weight. To strengthen the arm muscles, sit on the bed and place the hands in a fist shape on each side of the body, with the thumbs facing forward. Keep the arms straight and press them downwards on to the bed to raise and lower the trunk.

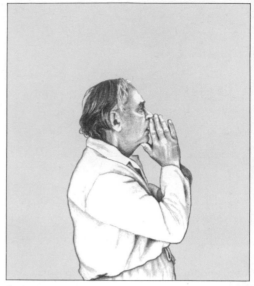

1
Sit on the edge of the bed with the legs and feet together, and with a straight back. Put the hands together. Breathe in. With the thumbs, touch the chin, the nose, and the forehead. This ensures that the shoulder muscles are stretched gradually.

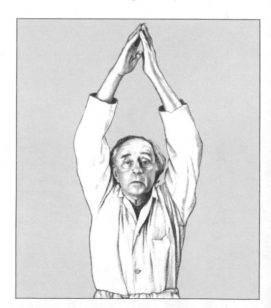

4
Breathe in and return to the vertical position. Stretch upwards, keeping the head, arms, and trunk in a straight line, and the chin parallel with the floor. Check that the back is still straight. Feel the stretch in the rib-cage as well as in the shoulder muscles.

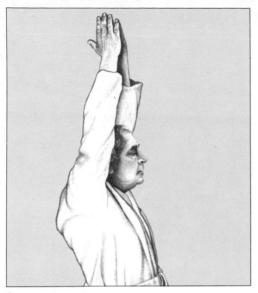

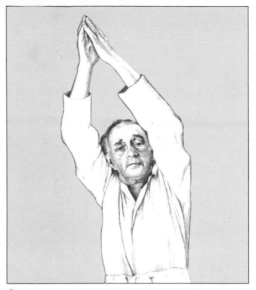

2
Continue the movement upwards, with the hands still touching one another. Stretch the arms up above the head until they are positioned behind the ears, and in as straight a line as possible with the body. Remember to keep the chin parallel with the floor.

3
From this position, breathe out and tilt the trunk over to one side. Keep the arms well stretched up above the head and behind the ears. Keep them as straight as possible; this will increase the stretch down the side of the waist and the rib-cage.

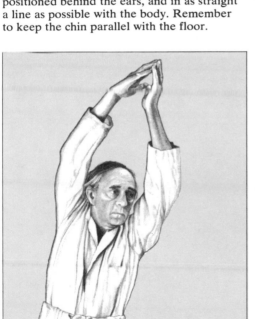

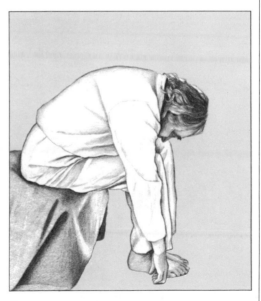

5
Breathe out and tilt the trunk over to the other side of the body. Keep the arms as straight as possible up above the head. Tilt the body only as far as is comfortable. Feel again the stretch along the side of the body. Return to the upright position.

6
Finally, relax slowly and "roll" the body forwards. Concentrate on controlled relaxation downwards, until the arms are hanging loosely by the side of the body. Do the whole exercise once or twice to start with, and then gradually increase the number.

Exercises on the edge of the bed 2

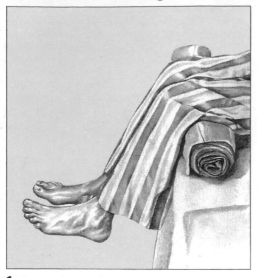

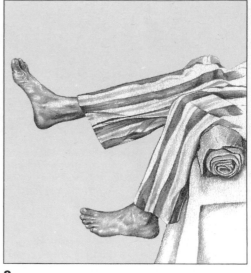

1

Sit on the edge of the bed. Place a rolled-up towel under the thighs (just above the knees) so that the feet are no longer resting on the floor, and the legs feel relaxed. Support the shoulders by placing both hands on the bed behind the body.

2

Straighten one knee until the knee joint is locked and the leg as straight as possible. Pull the foot upward and feel the muscles and tendons stretch up the back of the leg. Drop the foot, lower the leg, and relax. Repeat with each leg ten times.

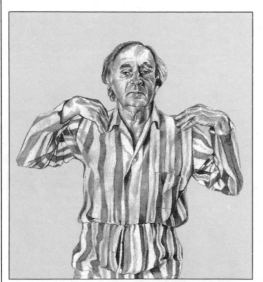

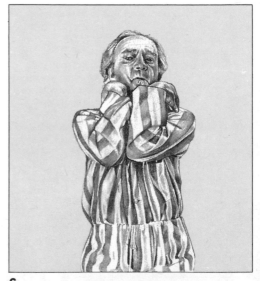

5

Sit upright on the edge of the bed with the back straight, the shoulders down, and the feet and legs together. Keep the head steady and the chin parallel to the floor. Bend the arms and place the fingertips of the hands at the front of each shoulder.

6

Keep the fingertips in position, and slowly raise the elbows up from the side of the body, and bring them forward. Try to make them touch at the front if possible. You should feel the pull and stretch this action causes between the shoulder blades.

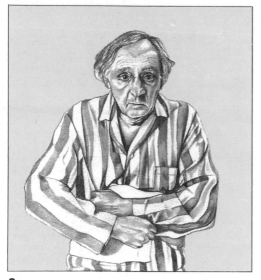

3
Take a towel and fold it lengthways to a width of about 15cm (6 inches). Sit upright on the edge of the bed. Put the towel around the lower rib-cage and hold the ends firmly with the hands. Breathe out, slowly pulling the towel to help expel air from the lungs.

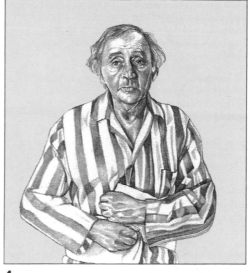

4
Hold the towel tightly and breathe in slowly. Feel the pressure of the ribs against the towel as the lower lungs expand. Keep the upper chest relaxed, and the shoulders down. Repeat the exercise only two or three times at first, gradually building up to more.

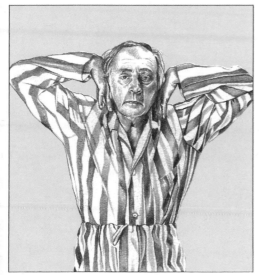

7
Continue the upwards movement, and raise the elbows as high as they can go. The bigger the circles you can describe with your elbows, the more effective the exercise. Keep the shoulders down. Concentrate on the movement at the shoulder joints.

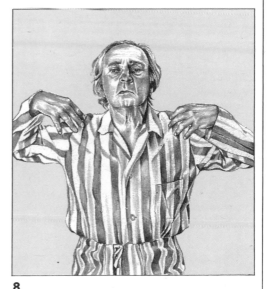

8
Swing the elbows downwards and as far back as you can. Bring the elbows round until the circle has been completed. Do the full exercise five times to begin with, gradually building up to ten times. Never try to do more than you know you can cope with.

Exercises for heart patients

A damaged or weak heart cannot stand any sudden or violent strain. Patients who suffer from any form of heart disorder should cultivate a calm, detached outlook on life. Don't allow yourself to become tense, worried, or excited. Any emotional upset or excitement can have disturbing physical effects on your heart. A calm mental attitude will help you to take life at a relaxed pace, without hurrying or expending your energy in sudden bursts. Walk at a steady, regular pace, even when you are late.

However, it is equally necessary for patients to keep themselves as fit and healthy as possible. It is now recognized that the regular practising of planned exercises can strengthen a weak or damaged heart, and can help to restore it to its former condition. Practise the first three exercises to warm up the body before attempting the other ones. If there is a sudden increase in the rate at which your heart beats, do not attempt the complete series of exercises at one time.

Above all, you should consult a doctor before starting these or any exercises, and should practise them with caution. If you feel chest pain or get short of breath while performing these exercises, you should stop immediately and lie down.

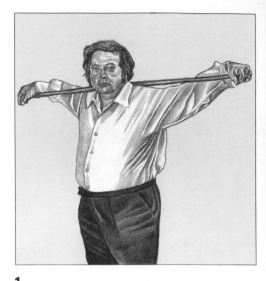

1
Stand with feet apart, and support the arms outstretched on a bar. The hips and legs should remain steady while the shoulders turn. Turn the head and shoulders as far as possible to the left, then to the right, in a steady movement. Repeat about ten times in each direction.

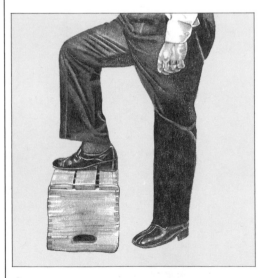

4
Stand facing a box that is about 46cm (18 inches) or 60cm (2 feet) above the floor. Step on to the box with the left foot first, then bring the right foot up before stepping down again with the left foot first. Repeat this sequence five times, then do the same again but leading with the right foot. Choose a stable box that won't tip over.

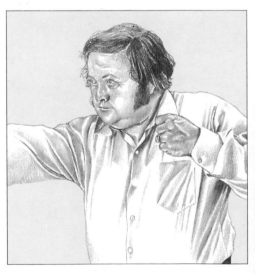

5
Stand with the feet apart and the fists clenched in front of the chest at about the level of the shoulders. Punch straight forward as far as possible from the shoulder, first with the left arm, then with the right. Keep the head and the legs still, but allow the torso to swing from the waist with each punch. Do about ten punches.

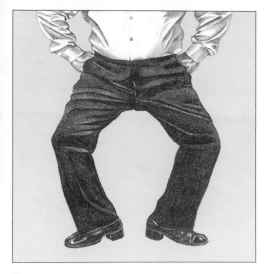

2
Stand with the heels about 60cm (2 feet) apart, and with the toes turned out. Bend the legs at the knees and squat as far as possible, keeping the heels on the ground and the back straight. If balance is difficult, hold the arms out sideways. Squat down and then stand up about ten times. Do not rush.

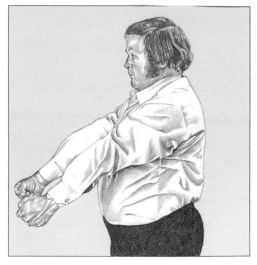

3
Stand with the feet apart, and the palms together in front of the body. Lift the arms forwards and upwards. When the arms are above the head, separate the hands. Then continue to rotate the arms backwards in as wide a sweep as possible, until they are in front of the body again. Repeat ten times.

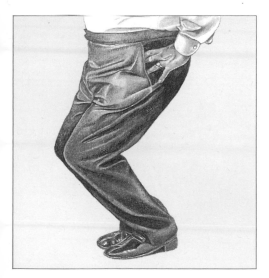

6
Stand upright with the legs and feet together and, once the exercise is known, the heels on a 5cm (2-inch) block. Squat down, bending the knees as much as possible. Keep the head up and the back straight. After squatting as long as possible, stand up again and drop the hands to the sides. Squat and stand up about ten times.

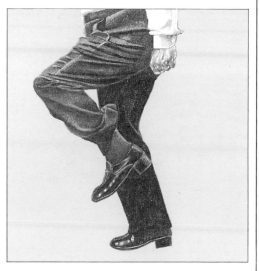

7
Other exercises that can benefit heart patients include running on the spot and skipping. Jogging is another useful exercise, but again requires caution at first. Heart patients who attend special clinics may also pursue a supervised course of exercise rehabilitation using cycling machines, rowing machines, and treadmills.

Remedial exercises

The patient has now reached the final stage of exercising in preparation for getting out of bed and resuming a normal active life.

By this stage, correct posture should have become a habit. This is especially important with the more difficult exercises as extra strain on muscles and joints is increased. Observe all postural areas, but particularly the pelvic tilt, the proper positioning of the shoulders, head and neck, and straight legs. There is always a tendency to bend the knees with correct tilting of the pelvis. But this should be overcome with practice.

Prepare the room beforehand, turning on the heating if necessary. Keep the room well aired, but free from draughts.

Each of the following exercises is designed to strengthen certain postural muscles. But whenever possible get the patient to stretch other muscles, even those that are not specifically being worked upon. The patient should consult the family doctor before attempting this group of exercises.

As with previous exercises, they should be practised as a set in the morning, afternoon, and evening. Each exercise should be done at least five times, eventually building up to ten times. As with all exercising, get the patient to breathe in as the muscles are tightened and out again as they are relaxed.

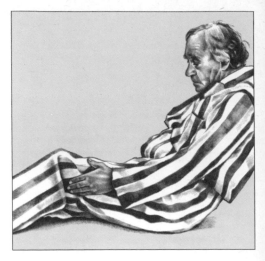

1
Lie flat on the back with the hands by the side of the body and the legs straight. Keep the knees tight, and the toes turned up. Roll the pelvis up towards the ribs and feel the stomach muscles shortening. Keep the chin tucked in so that it is parallel with the feet. Bend one knee up. At the same time slowly pull the trunk upwards and forwards, still with the chin tucked in.

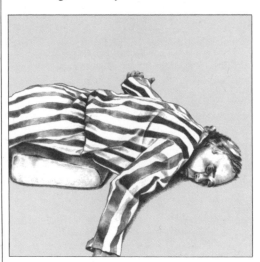

4
Place a pillow under the stomach. This flattens the back and prevents too great a hollow from forming at the bottom of the spine. Rest the head on one side. Stretch out the arms each side of the body at shoulder level. Extend the legs. Keep the knees straight and feel the stretch of the muscles. Extend the fingertips. Relax. Compare the two states of stretching and relaxing.

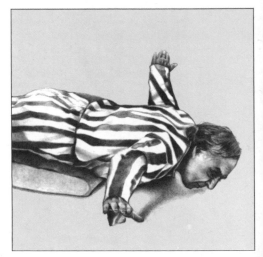

5
Breathe in. Raise the arms and the legs together as high as possible. Keep the chin tucked in to avoid neck strain. Feel the muscles of the lower back working to hold the trunk upwards. Draw the shoulder blades together to help in raising up the trunk. Keep the legs straight and feel the tightening in the muscles of the buttocks. Lower the limbs while breathing out, and relax.

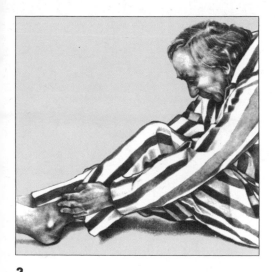

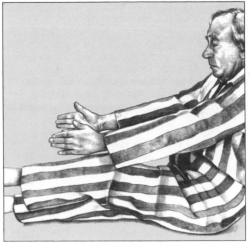

2
Continue to bring the head and shoulders forward. Bring the forehead down and make a serious attempt to touch the knee. It is important to move the head forward (rather than bringing the knee up to the head) to get the maximum exercise for the stomach muscles. If it is too difficult to raise the trunk, place two pillows lengthways under the back.

3
Stretch out the leg, keeping the body bent. Pull the leg straight to tighten the muscles at the knee. Keep the foot at right angles to the leg, so that the toes are pointing towards the ceiling. Make sure that the other leg is still straight, and try to keep the back of the knee flat on the floor. Slowly lean backwards into the lying position again, while breathing out. Repeat the exercise with the other leg.

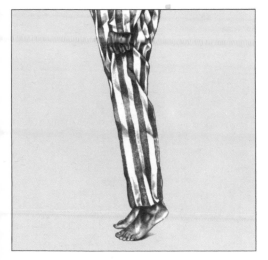

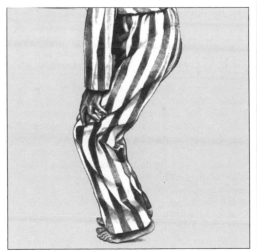

6
Stand up straight by rolling up the pelvis and drawing in the buttocks and the stomach. Pull the shoulder blades together and let the shoulders relax downward. Keep the chin parallel with the floor. Let the weight of the body rest evenly on both feet and keep the knees straight. From this position raise both heels, while still maintaining good posture and keeping the back flat.

7
Bend the knees and gradually move the body downwards. This is easier if the feet are kept slightly apart. Bend the knees as far as possible towards the ground. Keep the back straight and the chin parallel with the floor. Feel the muscles tighten down the front of the thighs and down the back of the legs. Come gradually back up again on to the toes. Lower the heels to the floor.

Aids and devices 1

Walking aids include sticks, walking frames, elbow crutches, and long crutches. It is important that walking aids are the right height for the patient who is using them. The use of any at the wrong height can lead to neck or shoulder tension. Long crutches should not be so high that they push upwards under the patient's armpits. Most of the body's weight should be supported by the hand grips attached to each crutch, and carried by the arms and hands.

A useful aid for moving from room to room is a chair trolley. This can be made by attaching small wheels to the legs of a kitchen chair. The upright back can then be used as a support while the patient walks and pushes the chair along. The seat can be used as a tray or trolley on which to carry things.

Rails and handles fixed at strategic places around the home can be an enormous help for those who have difficulty in walking and moving independently. Whenever possible, a handrail should be placed on both sides of the stairs. Grab rails should be secured wherever a person has to get up or sit down.

A wheelchair should be chosen with great care. When in the sitting position, the patient should be able to relax the arms comfortably on the armrests. The armrests may also be used to lever the body up into the standing position. The back should be well supported, and the feet placed flat on the footrest. Sitting down for long periods of time can lead to discomfort in the pelvic area. To help to prevent this, an effective cushion can be made by cutting a circular hole in a piece of foam rubber.

Moving about the home in a wheelchair is made considerably easier if steps are replaced by slopes or ramps. A short slope can be made by placing triangular wooden blocks against a step. Ramps can be bought or improvised. They consist of two tracks for the wheels of the wheelchair to run along. The ramp is placed between the upper and lower levels of a step, thus allowing the patient to move up the step by his or her own efforts.

For chronically ill patients, local authorities provide financial help for necessary structural changes in the house, and hospitals or local health authorities may supply essential equipment.

Make sure that the home has no potential hazards for the patient. Loose furniture fittings can be extremely dangerous; they should be securely attached. Check also that carpets are well tacked down. Keep a fireguard in front of an open fire, and do not position seats close to radiators. A torch kept at the patient's bedside may be useful at night or during a power failure.

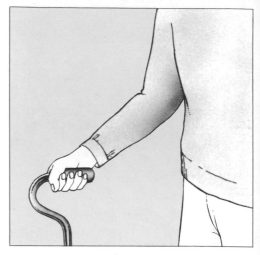

1
To calculate the correct height for a stick, the patient should hold his or her arm by the side of the body, with the arm loosely bent at an angle of about 160°. Measure the distance from the palm of the hand to the floor. This measurement should allow for the rubber grip (ferrule) at the bottom of the stick. Wooden sticks can be cut to the right length. Most metal sticks are adjustable.

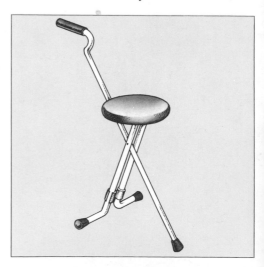

4
The seat stick is a combination of a stick and a hinged seat. The actual seat must be strong enough to be both secure and comfortable for the patient, and yet the whole device can be folded up. It is lightweight, so that it can be carried and used like an ordinary stick. The seat stick encourages a patient to be mobile, by allowing rest to be taken when required.

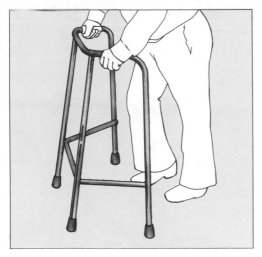

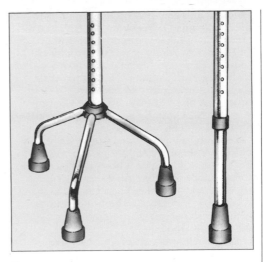

2
A walking frame of the right height can provide a great deal of stable support. But as with all walking aids, great care should be taken to ensure that it is the right height. If a walking frame is too high, it causes a hunching of the shoulders, which in turn leads to tension around the neck area. If it is too low, the patient is forced to stoop unnecessarily, putting strain on the muscles of the back.

3
All walking aids should have a large rubber ferrule at the end to prevent them from slipping. A ferrule can be purchased separately and is essential if the walking aid is to be used with any degree of confidence. This is important on a hard, resistant surface, such as linoleum or wood. A stick with three legs at its base provides greater stability and support than does an ordinary stick.

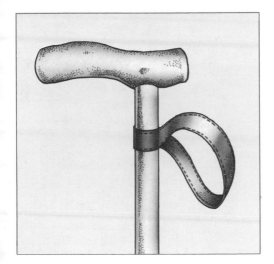

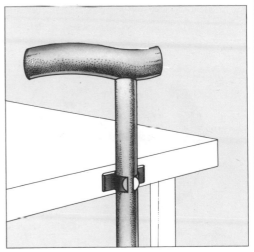

5
A loop around the top of a stick can be useful. Use a piece of tape, or any material that does not chafe the skin.

The loop can be slipped over the wrist, becoming a means of holding on to the stick when both hands are needed for some other purpose, especially when climbing stairs. The loop can also be used for hanging up the stick when it is not needed.

6
Clips to hold a stick can be attached to various pieces of furniture or wherever is convenient, for example, on the edge of a table or on a wall. Clips are most commonly required in the kitchen, next to a favourite armchair in the living room, next to the bed, and in the bathroom, one near the bath and another close to the toilet. A clip can also be attached to a wheelchair.

Aids and devices 2

Personal aids and devices give a physically disabled patient or an elderly person a new independence that is essential for morale. But recovery from a physical disability can sometimes be actually retarded by overuse of such aids. For in some cases, the patient should be encouraged to make an effort, in order that his or her condition may improve. Always check with a doctor, before providing a patient with an aid or device.

Dressing and undressing can be extremely difficult if there are many zips and buttons to deal with. A stick with a hook at the end is a simply made tool that can be used to pull a zip to which a loop has been attached. Alternatively, replace all zips and buttons with Velcro fastenings, preferably sewn into the front of clothing.

People who wear spectacles may like to keep them on a cord around the neck. This ensures that they remain at hand and are not mislaid.

A long mirror in the bedroom or bathroom is always useful for checking that clothes have been fastened correctly, and for practising correct posture. Attach the hand towel in the bathroom to a piece of loose elastic that can be hung over a hook. This enables the towel to be pulled and used, without it having to be unhooked and replaced.

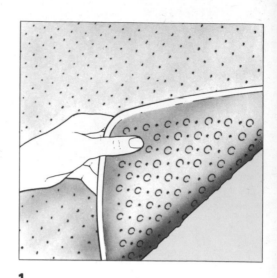

1
A rubber mat with safety suckers on its underside gives added security to unsure walkers. One can be placed wherever there is a chance of the feet slipping, especially in the bottom of the bath or in front of the toilet or a chair. Patients who are likely to be unsteady should always wear shoes that give firm support. Soft-soled shoes should be avoided, however comfortable.

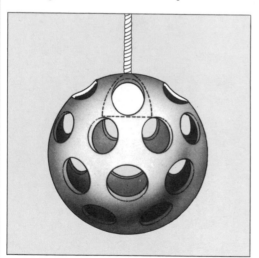

4
An electric light cord can be lengthened if the patient has difficulty reaching it. The end of the cord can be enlarged by attaching a hollow plastic ball.

Switches and power sockets throughout the home may have to be repositioned so that a physically disabled person can reach them without strain. The cost involved may be paid by the local authority.

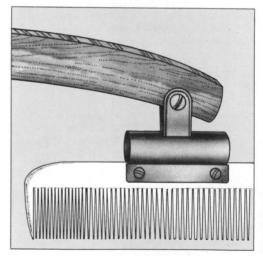

5
A long-handled comb can be simply made using an old wooden coat hanger. Remove the metal hook from the top. Screw a spring clip into one end of the hanger and attach the comb as shown in the illustration. Aids like this can give a patient an enormous feeling of independence. It can be demoralizing to ask other people to do such a simple and personal thing as to comb one's hair.

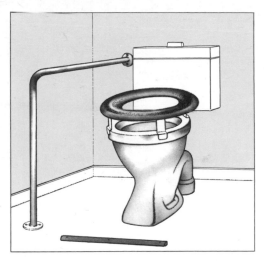

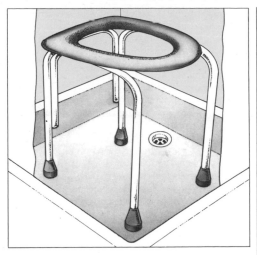

2

An elevated toilet seat can help a patient who has difficulty in rising from the sitting position. A strong rail secured by the side of the toilet can also be a great help. To prevent the feet slipping when standing up, put a safety mat in front of the toilet, or screw a wooden wedge into the floor. The door can be left unlocked, if help might be needed, and an "occupied" tag hung on the outside.

3

For patients who like to use a shower, a shower seat may be necessary. Ensure that this is the right height, so that the patient is able to stand up and sit down without difficulty. A magnetic soap clip or a piece of soap on a rope may be useful to prevent the soap from slipping out of reach. A nailbrush attached to a wall helps when cleaning the nails, and leaves the other hand free.

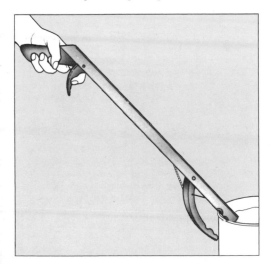

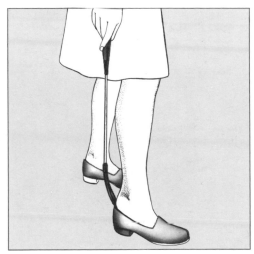

6

The device illustrated acts as an extended hand. It is particularly useful for people who have difficulty bending over, or reaching up; with it, they can pick things up off the floor, or take things down from shelves. But it should not be used to such an extent that a patient becomes unnecessarily lazy. Designs range from the simple to the sophisticated; some even have magnetic attachments.

7

A shoehorn with a long handle can help considerably in putting on a pair of shoes. Some shoehorns have a flexible spring attached near the end, so that the foot can be slipped into the shoe from practically any angle. Patients with laced shoes may also find it useful to have elastic shoelaces. This makes the shoe enlarge around the foot without having to untie and tie the laces.

Aids and devices 3

Life can be made easier for anyone with physical disabilities if the objects around the house, especially those used in daily chores, are adapted to suit that person's particular needs and capabilities.

Working surfaces should always be at the correct height, so that the patient's shoulders do not have to be hunched. If a seat is needed, its height should also be measured with care. In the kitchen, suction cups can be attached to tables or other surfaces in order to hold articles such as a bowl or plate, freeing at least one hand for other duties.

Another extremely useful item in the kitchen is a large funnel, which can be used when pouring liquids into containers. It is particularly useful when pouring out hot liquids.

An automatic electric kettle that switches itself off when the water is boiling is appreciated in any home. It will be especially useful to a person who has to move slowly. Such a device can prevent the kitchen from getting steamed up, and the kettle from boiling dry.

Finally, an apron with several pockets can be handy. It is one way of keeping various useful small items, and prevents having to move continually around the room searching for them.

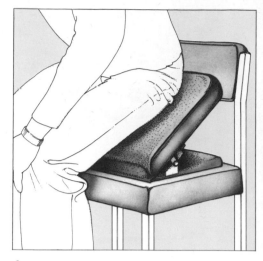

1
The tip-up chair can be a great help if a person has difficulty rising to the standing position. Springs attached to the seat raise it up at the back when the person sitting on it leans forwards in preparation for standing. The seat thus acts as a lever. It is also possible to obtain these chairs with armrests, which help a disabled person to sit down and stand up, as well as providing extra comfort.

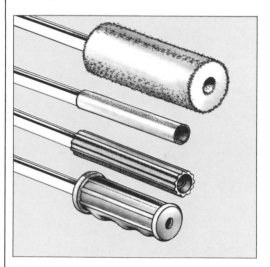

4
Handles can be enlarged according to requirements by using a variety of different materials. The illustration above shows, from top to bottom: a paint roll cover, aluminium tubing, a piece of garden hose, and a bicycle handle grip. To enlarge the handle of a telephone, wrap a piece of foam rubber around it and tie it securely in position with a bandage.

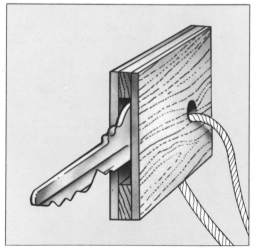

5
A key can be enlarged by enclosing its "head" in a piece of cork or wood. It is then readily found in a bag or pocket, and is easier to turn in the lock.

If a person has difficulty in selecting the right key from a number of similar ones, it may be helpful to attach the keys to strings of different colours. This enables a person to identify particular keys easily.

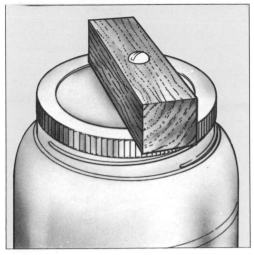

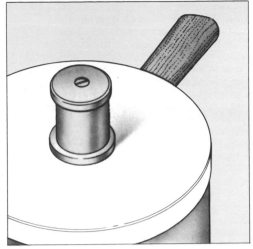

2

Unscrewing the lid of a jar can be a difficult task for a patient with arthritic hands. A block of wood screwed on to the top of the lid will provide something substantial to hold on to. Alternatively, screw two strips of serrated metal in a "V"-shape under the surface of a table or under a wall cupboard. Slide the lid between the two pieces of metal until tight against both and then turn.

3

Lids of pots and pans may be difficult to lift off if the knob is rather small. A knob can usually be unscrewed quite easily, and a cotton reel or larger block of wood put in its place. Buy only pots and pans with handles that do not conduct heat. When arranging a kitchen it may be preferable for the stove to be placed close to the sink so that dirty pans can be transferred easily.

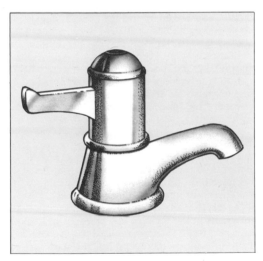

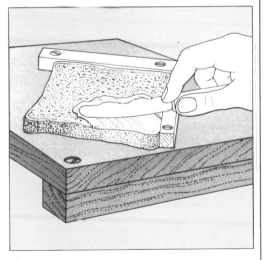

6

An elderly person, or someone suffering from arthritis of the hands, may be unable to operate a normal tap fitting. The rounded type of tap gives little to grasp, and can be almost impossible to move if it has been turned tightly. The lever-type tap solves these problems. It provides a handle, and is designed so that it cannot be turned too tightly. It can be fitted easily.

7

A wooden chopping-board can be held firmly in place if an extra piece of wood is fixed on to the underside of one end. This ensures that it will not slip forwards when being used. Two wedges of wood placed in a "V"-shape on the top of the board can also prevent anything on its surface from slipping. For example, a piece of bread can be pushed up against it while being spread with butter.

Special diets 1

Advice concerning well balanced diets for people in normal health is given in the section on **Nutrition,** beginning on p.960. The information given here concerns the special diets that are sometimes prescribed by doctors for patients suffering from or recovering from various disorders, or for children or adults who are in normal health but who have special nutritional requirements. It must be emphasized that no person, healthy or unhealthy, should make any radical or long-term change in his or her diet without first consulting a doctor.

The medical profession are generally less enthusiastic about diets than they were in the past. However, most doctors will recommend weight-reducing, diabetic, and, with increasing frequency, high-fibre diets. Doctors, like the rest of the population, tend to have fashions for new ideas which may change when later evidence alters their views.

Some diets, such as the low-sodium diet and the low-purine diet for patients with gout, are seldom recommended, as drug treatment is much more effective than special diets. Other diets are only prescribed when there is a serious underlying disorder, such as the low bulk diet for ulcerative colitis, as both the patient and the family find it difficult to maintain a special diet for any length of time unless there is a very good reason.

The diets in this section are an indication of the types of food that may or may not be eaten. More detailed information may be obtained from a dietician, or from a book on the subject recommended by your doctor.

Bland diet

A bland diet is often prescribed for patients who are confined to bed, including those who have a fever or who are convalescing. This diet is also suitable for patients suffering from gastritis, or for those with stomach or duodenal ulcers.

The main principle behind a bland diet is ease of digestion. Permissible foods include milk; cream; prepared cereals, such as cornflakes; soup; potatoes (without skins); white, long-grain rice; butter or margarine; white bread; eggs; strained, cooked vegetables and fruits; fruit juice (but not citrus fruit juices); lean, fresh meat; fresh fish; cottage cheese; custard; white sugar; tapioca; pudding rice; and plain cakes.

Foods to avoid include all fried and highly-seasoned foods; spices; strong tea and coffee; alcohol; whole-grain cereals and bread; pork; strong cheese; pies; pastries; rich sauces; nuts; olives; raisins; and raw vegetables and fruits.

The daily food intake should not contain more than about 2,000 calories. Meat and fish should be grilled or baked, not roasted or fried, and eggs should be poached or boiled.

All food should be served as attractively as possible, in order to stimulate the patient's appetite.

High-calorie diet

A high-calorie diet is usually recommended for patients who are underweight, or following a serious illness. The patient's normal diet is supplemented with high-energy foods such as milk and dairy products; sweets; cakes; puddings; and meat. There are also commercial food supplements available that may be included in this diet.

Bulky and low-carbohydrate vegetables and fruit should be avoided, and those containing a high proportion of carbohydrate used. A doctor may also recommend supplementary vitamins.

High-calorie, semi-solid diet

A high-calorie, semi-solid diet is usually recommended for patients who cannot tolerate a high-calorie normal diet. Small meals at frequent intervals should be given rather than three large meals a day.

Recommended foods include fruit juices; white bread; refined cereals; milk, cream, butter, and cream or cottage cheese; eggs; strained vegetables and fruit; thick, creamy soups; custard; tapioca; and sugar and jam. A doctor may also recommend supplementary vitamins.

Foods to avoid include whole-grain bread and cereals; raw fruit and vegetables; strong cheese; fried food; rich desserts; and fish and solid meats.

Soft diet

A soft diet is usually recommended for patients who cannot tolerate a normal diet because of poor teeth, general physical weakness, or intestinal disorders.

A soft diet should provide essential nutrients in the form of low-fibre, easily digested foods. Recommended foods include strained soups and vegetables; refined cereals, white bread; cooked fruit (without skin or seeds); fruit juices; potatoes (without skins); white rice; finely minced beef or chicken; milk; eggs; cream or cottage cheese; custard; ice-cream; tapioca; and plain cakes. A doctor may also prescribe vitamins.

Foods to avoid include raw vegetables and fruit; whole-grain cereals and bread; strong cheese; pork and veal; dried fruits, such as raisins; rich desserts; and all food that is fried, spiced, or seasoned.

Liquid diet

A liquid diet is usually prescribed for patients who cannot tolerate a soft or even a semi-solid diet. The patient may be given any food that can be served in strained or liquid form; custard; milky drinks; ice-cream; plain puddings; and very soft scrambled eggs. Commercial food supplements may also be given.

High-calcium diet

A diet rich in calcium is usually advised for pregnant and breast-feeding women. For the duration of a woman's pregnancy, and also while she is breast-feeding her baby, her food has to supply both her own needs and those of her baby. Her food should be rich in protein, calcium, iron, and vitamins. In particular, she needs more than twice the usual amount of calcium required by a normal healthy adult.

Milk, in quantities of up to two pints a day, is especially recommended. Other foods rich in calcium include cheese; fish, especially pilchards, sardines, sole, sprats, and whitebait; eggs; yoghurt; nuts, particularly almonds and brazil nuts; figs; gooseberries, dried peaches; vegetables, such as broccoli, parsley, peas, spinach, spring greens, and watercress; and certain sweet foods, such as milk chocolate, ice cream, and black treacle.

A high-calcium diet should be followed from the beginning of pregnancy. Symptoms of nausea and vomiting are often an indication that the amount of fat in the diet is too high, and constipation is usually an indication that the fluid intake is inadequate. A pregnant woman should be guided by her doctor in her choice of foods, and in the methods of preparing them. If there are signs that she is gaining too much weight, her diet will be adjusted so that the calorie content is reduced while the essential factors (protein, calcium, iron, and vitamins) remain adequate.

A high-calcium diet with plenty of milk is also suitable for adolescents, who require more than the normal amount of calcium to sustain the rapid physical development that takes place between the ages of twelve and fifteen.

Low-sodium diets

These diets are sometimes prescribed for patients suffering from disorders associated with retention of body fluid (oedema). Such disorders include kidney and liver diseases, high blood pressure, and congestive heart failure. A low-sodium diet may also be prescribed for patients taking coriscosteroid drugs.

There are three main low-sodium diets, classified according to the amount of sodium permitted: a mild sodium-restricted diet, a moderate sodium-restricted diet, and a severe sodium-restricted diet. The most suitable of these diets depends on the severity of the underlying disorder. During the acute stage of illness a moderate or strict sodium-restricted diet may be combined with a low-protein diet. When the patient begins to recover, the low-protein diet may be replaced by a high-protein diet, with plenty of eggs, cream or cottage cheese, and fresh meat and fish. The patient may also be allowed a mild sodium-restricted diet. A combined high protein/mild sodium-restricted diet may be advised as a long-term measure.

The main dietary source of sodium is salt (sodium chloride), but other sodium compounds are used in the preparation and preserving of foods. For example, baking soda and baking powder both contain sodium and are both used in the preparation of bread; tinned foods often have sodium benzoate or sodium glutamate added to improve their flavour and prolong their shelf-life.

The general rules when following any of the low-sodium diets are (1) avoid the use of salt in the preparation and serving of food; (2) avoid laxatives or other proprietary medicines that contain sodium compounds; (3) avoid drinking or cooking with water that has been treated with a water-softener because some of these devices add sodium to the water; and (4) avoid all foods with a high salt content.

Foods with a high sodium content include many cereals and cereal products, such as bread and crispbreads; cheese (except unsalted cream and cottage cheese); bacon, ham, sausage, and tongue; haddock and kippers; baked beans; chocolate; ice-cream; cakes and biscuits; and many tinned and preserved foods. Salted sauces, dressings, gravies, meat extracts, and other condiments also have a high sodium content.

Foods with a low sodium content include milk; lean beef, mutton, rabbit, and liver; most vegetables, provided they are cooked without salt; most fruits and nuts (unsalted); rice; pasta; sugar and preserves; and unsalted butter. It is also possible to buy bread, cereals, and other products that have been specially prepared for low-sodium diets.

A drastic reduction in the amount of dietary sodium may unintentionally result in a dangerous deficiency of other minerals. For this reason, low-sodium diets should be followed only on the advice of a doctor and

Special diets 2

the patient should be under medical supervision for the duration of the diet.

High-protein diet

A high-protein diet is usually recommended for patients suffering from protein depletion from any cause, as may occur with extensive burns or a serious illness. Such a diet may also be combined with other special diets as part of the treatment for a specific disorder. For example, a high-protein diet may be combined with a low-sodium diet in the treatment of congestive heart failure.

The general principles behind a high-protein diet are to ensure an adequate intake of calories, vitamins, minerals, and water; to increase the protein intake to twice or three times that of a normal diet; and to ensure that the foods included in the diet are easily digestible.

Milk and eggs form the basis of a high-protein diet. Some of the proprietary food supplements are also good sources of easily-digestible protein. Other easily-digestible, high-protein foods include digestive biscuits; bread; steamed fish; chicken; turkey; and veal. Some of the less fibrous vegetables, such as mashed potatoes and spinach, may also be included in a high-protein diet. Cheese is another good source of protein but some patients may find it hard to digest.

There are no specific foods to avoid when following a high-protein diet, but it may be advisable to restrict the intake of foods such as sugar and jam that contribute little to the diet apart from calories. It may also be necessary to omit some foods that the patient finds hard to digest.

Low-protein diet

A low-protein diet may be prescribed for patients suffering from chronic kidney failure. Such a diet may also be combined with other special diets as part of the treatment for a specific disorder. For example, a low-protein diet may be combined with a low-sodium diet in the initial stages of treatment for kidney failure.

A drastic reduction in the amount of protein in the diet may lead to malnutrition. Therefore, a low-protein diet should be followed only on the advice of a doctor, and the patient should be under medical supervision for the duration of the diet.

If a low-protein diet is necessary, a doctor will give specific instructions for each individual patient. Generally however, a low-protein diet involves omitting all meat, fish, cheese, and nuts. A small amount of protein may be allowed, usually in the form of one egg and six ounces of milk per day. The

doctor may also allow restricted amounts of foods with a very low protein content, such as apples, pears, pineapple, rhubarb, cucumber, lettuce, runner beans, carrots, marrow, butter, honey, and marmalade.

Diabetic diet

A strictly controlled diet is an important part of the treatment for patients suffering from diabetes mellitus, in which there is a disturbance of the normal carbohydrate metabolism resulting in a partial or complete inability of the body to use carbohydrates. Consequently, a diabetic patient's diet has to be adjusted according to the ability of the body to deal with carbohydrates.

The general principle behind a diabetic diet is a reduction in the amount of carbohydrate and an increase in the amount of protein. Food should be free of all sugar, but must contain adequate calories, vitamins, and other essential nutrients. The amount of calories and the proportions of carbohydrate, protein, and fat should remain constant for every meal and for every day. Most doctors restrict alcohol and advise diabetics to eat small amounts at regular and frequent intervals. Each patient will receive an individual diet sheet from his or her doctor.

The British Diabetic Association has developed a system of food exchanges which enables individual diabetic patients to choose a varied diet while remaining within the necessary restrictions. The food exchange system lists foods that are permissible for a diabetic patient, and gives the amount of each food that contains ten grams of carbohydrate. A list of some of the food exchanges is given opposite. Meat, fish, eggs, cheese, and butter do not appear on the list because they contain negligible amounts of carbohydrate and do not need to be restricted unless the patient needs to lose weight.

Low-fat diet

A low-fat diet is usually recommended for patients suffering from gall-bladder disease or from disorders in which food is inadequately absorbed in the intestine. A low animal-fat diet may also prevent the onset of arteriosclerosis and coronary heart disease.

All foods with a high fat content should be excluded from the diet. Fats to be omitted include butter, margarine, lard, and cooking fats. Foods with a high fat content include whole milk, milk products, such as cheese and cream; egg yolks; pastry; biscuits; cakes; nuts; chocolate; creamy sauces; and preserves. Meats to be omitted include duck; goose; ham; pork; sausage; tongue; and all

Food exchange list for diabetic patients

Amounts of various foods that contain about 10 grams of carbohydrate			
Food	**grams**	**Food**	**grams**
Cereal foods		**Nuts**	
Biscuits (plain or semi-sweet)	15	Almonds (shelled)	230
		Brazil nuts (shelled)	250
Bread (brown or white)	20	Chestnuts (shelled)	30
Cornflakes	10	Hazel nuts (shelled)	150
Cornflour (uncooked)	10	Peanuts (shelled)	120
Cornmeal	15	Walnuts (shelled)	200
Custard powder (uncooked)	10		
Flour	15	**Vegetables**	
Macaroni (uncooked)	15	Beans (baked, tinned)	95
Noodles (uncooked)	15	(broad, boiled)	140
Porridge (cooked in water)	120	(butter, boiled)	60
Rice (uncooked)	10	(haricot, boiled)	60
(boiled)	30	Beetroot (boiled)	100
Sago (uncooked)	10	Carrots (boiled)	230
Semolina (uncooked)	10	Corn on the cob	80
Spaghetti (uncooked)	15	Lentils (boiled)	60
Tapioca (uncooked)	10	Onions (fried)	100
		Parsnips (boiled)	80
Fruit		Peas (tinned, garden)	140
Apples (raw with skin)	100	(fresh, boiled)	130
(baked with skin)	120	(tinned, processed)	70
(stewed)	120	(frozen, boiled)	130
Apricots (fresh with stones, stewed)	190	Potatoes (boiled or jacket)	50
		(chips)	25
(fresh with stones, raw)	160	(crisps)	20
(dried, raw)	25	(mashed)	60
(dried, stewed)	60	(roast)	40
Bananas (ripe, peeled)	50	Sweet corn (tinned)	45
Cherries (raw with stones)	100	Sweet potatoes (boiled)	50
(stewed with stones)	120	Yams (boiled)	35
Currants (dried)	15		
Damsons (stewed with stones)	140	**Miscellaneous**	
Dates (with stones)	20	Honey	15
(without stones)	15	Jam	15
Figs (green, raw)	100	Jelly	15
(dried, raw)	20	Ice-cream (plain, non-dairy)	50
(dried, stewed)	35	Marmalade	15
Grapes (whole)	60	Oatcakes	15
Oranges (peeled)	120	Sausages	80
Peaches (fresh with stones)	130	Syrup	15
(dried, raw)	20	Treacle	15
(dried, stewed)	50	Yoghurt (plain)	150
Pears (raw with skin)	130		
(stewed)	125	**Drinks**	**millilitres**
Pineapple (fresh)	85	Grapefruit juice (tinned, unsweetened)	125
Plums (raw with stones)	110		
(stewed with stones)	210	Milk (fresh or sterilized)	200
Prunes (dry, raw with stones)	30	(condensed, sweetened)	20
(stewed with stones)	50	(evaporated, unsweetened)	80
Raisins (dried)	15	Orange juice (fresh or tinned, unsweetened)	110
Raspberries (raw)	180		
Strawberries (fresh)	160	Pineapple juice (tinned, unsweetened)	90
Sultanas (dried)	15		
Tangerines (peeled)	120	Tomato juice (tinned)	285

tinned meats, such as corned beef and luncheon meat. Fish to be omitted include bloaters; eels; herrings; kippers; mackerel; salmon; and all types of tinned fish, such as pilchards and sardines.

A low-fat diet should consist of foods that have a high carbohydrate and protein content and that are easily digestible. Low-fat foods include skimmed milk; egg whites; most types of fruits and vegetables; white fish; and certain meats, such as chicken, kidney, liver, turkey and veal.

The preparation and method of cooking food is important in keeping the fat content low. All visible fat should be trimmed from meat before cooking. Food should not be fried or roasted because these methods increase the fat content. Methods of cooking that do not increase the fat content include grilling, baking, and steaming.

High-fibre diet

A high-fibre diet is recommended for patients suffering from constipation or from diverticular disease of the colon. Additionally, recent research indicates that a high-fibre diet may help to prevent various diseases, such as certain types of intestinal cancer, diverticular disease, and heart disease.

The patient should eat plenty of bulky foods with a high fibre content, as this increases the bulk of the faeces and stimulates the movement through the intestine. The patient's normal diet should be supplemented with whole-grain bread and cereals (bran is a particularly good source of fibre); raw and stewed fruits; vegetables; and salads. It is also important to drink plenty of water.

Low-fibre diet

A low-fibre diet is sometimes recommended by doctors for patients suffering from a variety of intestinal disorders.

The patient should eat small amounts of easily digested food at regular and frequent intervals. Recommended foods include eggs; milk; cream or cottage cheese; refined, cooked cereals; white bread; lean meats, such as beef, lamb, and chicken; fresh fish; tender root vegetables that have been cooked and strained; creamed soups; stewed, strained fruits; plain cakes; and jelly.

Foods to avoid include whole-grain bread and cereals; raw fruit and vegetables; pork and veal; nuts; pastry; and excessive fat. It is also advisable to omit foods that are fried, spiced, or seasoned because these may irritate the intestine.

All food should be chewed thoroughly.

The patient should have plenty to drink but should avoid alcohol.

Low-purine diet

A low-purine diet is, rarely, recommended for patients with gout. Gout is caused by an excess of uric acid in the body, so foods with high amounts of this substance should be avoided.

Foods to avoid include liver, kidney, sweetbreads, anchovies, sardines, herrings, beans, lentils, spinach, meat extracts, and soups.

However, treatment of gout with modern drugs is much more effective than dietary treatment, and doctors seldom bother to recommend dietary restrictions.

Gluten-free diet

A gluten-free diet is prescribed for patients suffering from coeliac disease or non-tropical sprue, which are caused by sensitivity to the protein gluten. Gluten is found in wheat, barley, rye, and oats. Patients who are sensitive to gluten react adversely to even minute quantities of the protein. All traces of the gluten-containing cereals must therefore be eliminated from the diet.

Foods to avoid include beverages that contain gluten, such as malted milk, malted cocoa, and beer; all bread, cakes, and cereals that are made with wheat, barley, rye, or oat flour; pasta; sausages and other meat products that may contain bread or flour; and ice-cream. Patients should also ensure that desserts, sauces, gravies and sweets do not contain wheat, barley, rye, or oat products.

Foods that may usually be eaten include most fruits and vegetables, unless the patient is also sensitive to foods with a high sugar content; most meats and fish, provided that patients who cannot tolerate fat eat only the lean parts and avoid meats and fish with a high fat content (for example, herrings, trout, mackerel, salmon, and sardines); and carbohydrate foods, such as potatoes, rice, and sago, which are not associated with the forbidden cereals.

It is also possible to buy many gluten-free foods, such as gluten-free flour, for the preparation of food at home. Some manufacturers also provide special recipes for gluten-free dishes.

Vegetarian diets

Most people who follow a vegetarian diet in Western countries do so for moral reasons, not because of economic necessity. A vegetarian diet may be more healthy than a conventional diet, and research has shown that a vegetarian diet can significantly reduce the chances of heart disease.

A vegetarian diet can be as rich, varied, and nutritious as any diet that includes meat. The main vegetarian protein sources are soya; leguminous vegetables, such as kidney beans and broad beans; nuts; cheese; and eggs. Fats are provided by nuts, oil in salads, and vegetable fats used in cooking. Vitamins and minerals are provided by vegetables, which should be steamed or cooked in minimal amounts of water in order to retain these nutrients.

Roughage is provided by whole foods eaten raw, and by brown rice and wheat germ cereals, which should be eaten in preference to polished rice and products made from white flour. Dried skimmed milk mixed with water has a higher proportion of protein and calcium than fresh milk.

Vegans, who exclude from their diets all animal products including eggs and cheese, must supplement their diet with yeast extract or vitamin tablets to avoid vitamin B_{12} deficiency and other serious medical problems.

Macrobiotic diet

This diet is highly restricted and is not recommended because it is nutritionally unbalanced and scientifically unsound. Many nutritionists have criticized the macrobiotic diet because it is supposed to replace all medical treatment, and also because, as the stages of the diet progress, there is the danger of developing serious nutritional deficiencies of such essential nutrients as proteins, vitamins, and minerals. There have been many cases of deficiency diseases and even several deaths as a result of following this diet.

Weight-reducing diets

On p.960 there is a chart that shows a person's desirable weight range in relation to his or her height. A person who weighs up to 20 per cent more than his or her desirable weight is considered by most doctors to be overweight. A person who weighs 20 per cent or more than the desirable weight is considered to be obese.

The more overweight a person is, the greater the likelihood that he or she will suffer from various disorders, such as osteoarthritis and high blood pressure, and the lower is that person's life expectancy. Consequently, if you weigh more than is considered normal for your height and sex, then you should try to lose the excess weight and improve your physical fitness, thus reducing the probability of developing disorders associated with excess weight.

If you are overweight or obese, this is because the food you eat contains more calories than you use in physical activity. The aim of all reducing diets is, therefore, to reduce the amount of calories you take in, while retaining the necessary amounts of proteins, vitamins, minerals and other nutrients that are essential for good health. There is no easy or simple way to lose weight, and you should be cautious of diets you hear of or read about that claim to produce spectacular results within a short time. Be particularly careful of diets that allow you to eat as much as you like of certain categories of foods, and also of diets which claim that grapefruit, lemons, or other citrus fruits can speed up the conversion of fat to energy. There is no scientific evidence to support these claims. Although such diets may result in a short-term weight loss, they are not very effective for long-term weight control because as soon as you revert to your normal eating habits, you will gain weight again.

Fasting is not advisable unless it is done under medical supervision. This is because, in addition to fat, some of the essential tissues of the body, such as muscles, may be used as an energy source.

Fasting may result in deficiencies of essential nutrients, such as proteins, vitamins, and minerals, which the body needs all the time. It also shares the disadvantage of other faddish diets, namely that it is generally ineffective for long-term weight loss.

Commercial preparations that claim to aid you to slim may be misleading. Many of the products that claim to reduce appetite are ineffective, and even the tablets that may be prescribed by a doctor can sometimes have disturbing side-effects, notably restlessness and emotional tension. Artificial sweeteners that can be used to replace sugar in drinks and in cooking contain fewer calories than sugar, but they may also produce side-effects; for example, some people find that artificial sweeteners leave a metallic aftertaste. If is far more sensible to adjust your eating habits, and accustom yourself to unsweetened food and drinks. Substitute foods, low-calorie drinks, and foods that are specially prepared for dieters are expensive, and often have a less satisfactory taste than the natural products they claim to replace. Foods with special bulking agents that swell inside the stomach can make you feel so full that you actually eat less food, but these can lead to an unbalanced diet.

The weight-reducing diets that are most effective are of two types: the low-carbohydrate diet and the calorie-controlled diet. Both of these diets may be followed with complete safety, and they do not require artificial aids. However, they do require self-discipline and commitment. They are most effective, especially if you wish to improve your physical fitness, when combined with a programme of physical exercises.

Low-carbohydrate diet

With this diet, you eat only the most nutritious foods, and reduce or eliminate from your diet altogether the foods that have high fat and sugar contents. This will result in a reduction in the amount of calories in your diet without any reduction in essential nutrients.

The following lists of foods are intended as a guide to what you should and should not eat. The first category includes foods with high sugar or fat contents: you may remove these from your diet completely without losing any essential nutrients. The second category includes foods that contain some fat or sugar, but also contain essential nutrients: you should eat these foods only occasionally, and in small amounts. The third category includes foods that contain large amounts of essential nutrients, low amounts of fat and sugar, and relatively low amounts of calories: these foods should form the main part of your diet.

Foods to avoid:

Sugar, sweets, chocolate.
Cream, butter, margarine, oils and fats.
Cakes, pies, pastries, biscuits, puddings.
Honey, syrup, jam, marmalade.
Fruit tinned or bottled in syrup, dried fruit.
Fried potatoes, crisps, nuts.
Salad cream or mayonnaise.
Alcoholic drinks.
Most commercial soft drinks.

Foods to eat in restricted amounts only:

Fatty meats, such as salami, paté, bacon, and sausages.
Milk, eggs, cheese (except cottage cheese).
Breads and cereals (wholemeal varieties are preferable).
Potatoes, rice, pasta.
Oily fish, such as sardines, herrings, and anchovies.
Thick, creamy soups.
Pre-packed and tinned foods.

Foods that may be eaten in unrestricted amounts:

Liver, kidney, heart, brain.
Poultry (except duck), game.
White fish, seafood.
Green and root vegetables.
Salads.
Fresh fruit.
Skimmed milk.
Cottage cheese, natural yoghurt.
Clear soups, herbs, spices.
Water, low-calorie soft drinks.
Tea and coffee without milk.

If you follow this diet with self-discipline, you should lose weight at a rate of about one or two pounds (0·5-1kg) a week.

Calorie-controlled diet

The average adult male needs about 2,500 calories a day; the amount for women is slightly lower. However, the exact energy expenditure of an individual depends upon several factors, such as height, age, and occupation. A person who is on a calorie-controlled diet sets a target figure, usually about 1,000 calories a day less than the daily energy expenditure, and plans all meals so that the food eaten does not contain more than this number of calories. This target figure will vary according to your personal needs, for example, the target figure for a manual worker will probably be higher than that for an office worker because manual work involves a higher daily energy expenditure. Your doctor should be able to advise a suitable target figure with which to start the diet. The lower your target figure, the more rapid will be your weight loss, but a target figure of less than 1,000 calories a day can be dangerous.

To calculate the number of calories your food contains you will need a detailed calorie chart, giving the number of calories in stated amounts of specific foods. An abridged version of such a chart appears opposite; you may be able to obtain a more comprehensive chart from your doctor or at a bookshop. A calorie-controlled diet will probably consist mainly of the foods recommended in the low-carbohydrate diet. The number of calories varies according to the method of cooking, and you should therefore avoid all fried foods.

If your daily food intake contains 1,000 calories less than the amount you expend in physical activity, your average weight loss should be about two pounds a week. But, as with any weight-reducing diet, your weight loss during the first week or two will probably be more than this because of the loss of extra water. Also, your weight will probably not fall steadily and may even remain constant for some time. It is during such periods that most people abandon their diets, and it is therefore important to persevere if you wish to succeed.

Calorific value of selected foods

	Calories per 100g (3.5oz approx.)		Calories per 100g (3.5oz approx.)		Calories per 100g (3.5oz approx.)
Dairy produce		**Fish**		**Fruit**	
Butter	770	Cod (fried)	140	Apple (raw)	47
Cheese (Cheddar)	420	(steamed)	82	Apricot (raw)	28
(cottage)	83	Haddock (fried)	175	Banana (raw)	77
(cream)	800	(steamed)	100	Blackberries (raw)	30
(processed)	350	Halibut (steamed)	130	(stewed, no sugar)	13
Cream (double)	460	Herring (fried)	235	Blackcurrant (raw)	29
(single)	200	Kipper (baked)	200	(stewed, no sugar)	22
Eggs (fried)	239	Plaice (fried)	234	Cherries (raw)	47
(poached)	160	Salmon (steamed)	200	Dates (peeled)	248
Milk (whole)	66	(tinned)	137	Figs (dried)	214
(condensed)	320	Sardines (tinned)	294	(raw)	35
(dried)	500	Sole (fried)	274	Gooseberries (raw)	18
(skimmed)	35	(steamed)	84	Grapes (raw)	60
Yoghurt (natural)	54	Turbot (steamed)	100	Grapefruit (peeled)	22
		Whiting (fried)	193	Lemon (peeled)	17
Cereal foods				Mandarins (peeled)	33
Barley (boiled)	120	**Vegetables**		(tinned)	64
Biscuits (plain)	430	Asparagus (boiled)	18	Oranges (peeled)	35
Bran	311	Beans (baked)	90	Peach (raw)	37
Bread (white)	243	broad (boiled)	42	Pear (raw)	42
(wholemeal)	228	butter (boiled)	90	Pineapple (tinned)	63
Cornflakes	364	runner (boiled)	7	Plums (raw)	35
Cornflour	350	Broccoli (boiled)	14	(stewed, no sugar)	22
Custard powder	350	Brussels sprouts	17	Prunes (dried)	140
Flour (white)	349	(boiled)		(stewed, no sugar)	81
(wholemeal)	333	Cabbage (boiled)	10	Raisins (dried)	247
Macaroni (boiled)	112	Carrots (boiled)	17	Raspberries (raw)	25
Oatmeal porridge	45	Cauliflower (boiled)	10	Rhubarb (stewed, no	5
Rice (boiled)	122	Celery (raw)	6	sugar)	
Sago (raw)	355	Cucumber (raw)	10	Strawberries (raw)	26
Semolina (raw)	350	Leeks (boiled)	24	Tangerines (peeled)	34
Tapioca (raw)	357	Lentils (boiled)	96		
		Lettuce (raw)	10	**Nuts**	
Meat and poultry		Marrow (boiled)	7	Almonds (shelled)	598
Bacon, back (fried)	600	Mushrooms (fried)	217	Brazils (shelled)	644
streaky (fried)	530	Onions (fried)	355	Chestnuts (shelled)	172
Beef, corned	230	(raw)	23	Cobnuts (shelled)	398
sirloin (roast)	385	Parsley (raw)	21	Peanuts (shelled)	603
steak (grilled)	300	Parsnips (boiled)	56	Walnuts (shelled)	549
Chicken (boiled)	203	Peas (fresh, boiled)	49		
(roast)	190	(tinned)	84	**Alcohol**	
Duck (roast)	315	Potatoes (boiled)	80	Beer	28
Ham, lean (boiled)	210	(crisps)	560	Spirits	220
Kidney (fried)	210	(fried)	245	Wine	70
Liver (fried)	250	(roast)	123		
Mutton (roast)	280	Radishes (raw)	14	**Miscellaneous**	
(stewed)	315	Spinach (boiled)	24	Chocolate	590
Pork (roast)	455	Swedes (boiled)	17	Honey	280
Rabbit (stewed)	180	Tomato (raw)	14	Jam	260
Sausage, beef (fried)	280	Turnips (boiled)	14	Lard	910
pork (fried)	326	Watercress (raw)	12	Margarine	800
Sweetbreads (stewed)	180			Marmalade	260
Veal (roast)	232			Sugar	390
				Syrup	300

Care of the chronically ill

We are not all born nurses, and caring for the sick does not come easily to everyone. However, loving someone is the essential quality for the care and attention that you give your patient. Like love in all its forms, there are times of irritation and frustration, but these should not prevent you trying to put yourself in the patient's place.

Personal hygiene is important. It is essential to have clean hands, and short nails to prevent scratching. If you have long hair, tie it back to prevent it dropping across your face, and into the patient's eyes when moving him or her. Sharp rings, other jewellery, and watches should be removed from your hands and wrists. They not only scratch, but may become entangled in the bedclothing or soaked by water.

You may find it more comfortable to keep a special pair of old, rubber-soled, low-heeled shoes in the sickroom. Such shoes are less likely to slip and become damaged if the soles get wet or dirty.

Your doctor gives you instructions about medicines. It is important that you should know exactly when and how they should be given. If you do not understand, ask your doctor again. This is essential. Do not guess and give medicines because you think they are needed.

The best way of working out a routine of looking after a chronically ill patient is by discussions with your doctor and the visiting nurse, and adapting your other priorities, such as getting your family off to work and cooking meals. Prepare the sickroom. This has already been described. If the patient is incontinent, or likely to be so, the mattress must be protected with plastic sheeting, and covered with an easily removable drawsheet. Incontinence pads must be readily available. It is important to remember to offer the bedpan or commode every three or four hours as this may prevent further incontinence. Bed bathing, or washing, should be done in the morning as incontinence and perspiration during the night leaves the patient's skin moist and vulnerable to ulceration. If a patient is entirely confined to bed, the pressure areas on the buttocks, heels, and elbows should be thoroughly rubbed with surgical spirit and powder twice a day. Part of your daily routine must include care of your patient's hair, teeth – even false ones – and nails. A little make-up for a female patient helps her morale as well as yours.

Prepare food attractively, and serve in small portions. Fluids are essential and can be of different varieties, coffee, fruit juice, or milk. Used medicinally, alcohol is useful as a sedative at night, and may act as a stimulant to the appetite before a meal.

A patient who is inactive may have two additional problems. The first is constipation, and this may be helped by a high roughage diet, regular laxatives, or suppositories. The second problem can arise if your patient has a good appetite and gains weight. This can make nursing more difficult, but can be avoided by leaving carbohydrates, such as sugar, out of the patient's diet and increasing the bulk with fruit and vegetables, which also helps to prevent constipation.

Visitors not only help to share the care of the patient but also to boost his or her morale. They can talk about old times, the family, and future plans for grandchildren, as well as discussing friends at work. This acts as a stimulus, provided the visit does not last too long and leave the patient overtired. You need tact to end a visit before this point is reached. It is usually wise to warn the visitor that the doctor only allows visits to be a certain length of time. This gives you the chance to intrude without making the visitor feel that he or she is being sent away.

Unless the patient is completely bedridden, a wheelchair gives some degree of mobility and allows the patient to be moved from one room to another, out into the garden or, sometimes, for a drive in the car. This may tire the patient, but the stimulus is good for morale. The sickroom can be thoroughly cleaned while the patient is out, and the caring relative can have a rest.

Household pets, a favourite dog or cat, can give great pleasure to the chronically ill. Their companionship is undemanding and removes the feeling of loneliness that so often becomes a fear to someone who spends most of the time in one room.

The overall responsibility for the patient's care usually falls on a wife, daughter or daughter-in-law. The rest of the family can help in various ways. Someone can do the shopping, another may prepare food to be kept in the freezer, and another can take responsibility for exercising and looking after the dog. Even children in the house can help by carrying trays, fetching books, or helping with bedmaking. Involvement of the whole family makes everyone realize they are part of a team, and prevents the patient feeling too much of a burden to one person. It also gives the family a feeling of responsibility to each other, and to the patient.

Relatives and friends often share the work to give the wife, daughter, or daughter-in-law time off. Time to go to the hairdresser; time to walk and think; time to be alone; or to visit and talk to friends, away from the surroundings of her own home without the feeling of always being "on call"; time to rest and sleep if tired from disturbed nights.

If you are going out, it is useful to write down exactly what happens and when, so that a different person can become acquainted with the patient's routine. Even details about the way pillows are arranged in bed are important to the patient who may feel that this is essential for comfort and sleep.

Sometimes, when dealing with a long-term invalid, arrangements must be made for the carer to have a complete change and holiday. Another member of the family can take over, after a day or two in the house to see how things are done. If this is not possible, your doctor can make arrangements for a temporary stay in hospital for the patient. If this is going to happen it is essential to explain everything to the patient, who may momentarily feel frightened and deserted. He or she soon realizes the need for this change and can look forward to the return home. If the patient is being moved to hospital, a preliminary visit by a member of the family enables the nurse to discover any problems that may have to be faced, and the details of the routine that has been established at home. This helps the nursing staff to look after the patient in a way which he or she has become accustomed to. In addition the relative can tell the patient about the hospital and the staff. This acts as a preliminary introduction. If the change has been a success, further arrangements can be made from time to time, which give the family the feeling that outside help is available and acceptable when it is necessary.

As time goes by, the patient becomes used to the daily routine. Any changes that are made may prove to be distressing, so they should be explained before they occur. For example, lunch may be earlier than usual because of the expected visit of the doctor or a relative.

Smoking in the sickroom should be forbidden. The smell of stale cigarette smoke is unpleasant, unless the patient smokes. This is always a problem and a source of anxiety. A dropped cigarette may burn the bed-clothing, or patient, or start a fire. There is no easy answer to this as it may be one of the few pleasures for the patient. Luckily the number of cigarettes smoked often becomes less and, with tact, the packet and lighter can be put out of sight and reach.

Apart from the obvious hazards of smoking there are some other things that are dangerous. Never use a hot-water bottle. It may leak and cause burns, or a sedated patient may not feel the burning heat of a

bottle against his or her leg. A tray containing very hot fluids should not be balanced on the patient's legs because it may easily overturn. A light positioned above the patient's head must be securely fixed to the wall, or the patient may pull it down while feeling for the switch. If you cannot fix the light, change the position of the bed. A bed on casters may move if the patient tries to get out of bed. Instead of giving support, the bed could slide away, allowing the patient to fall, even if you are helping. Always be sure the bed is secure and that the carpet on the floor cannot slip.

The comfort of the patient is your main concern. Patients with heart and chest problems are usually helped by sitting upright on a rubber ring, with plenty of pillows arranged behind the back and head. Often, a small cushion or pillow behind the patient's head gives additional support to the neck and allows these muscles to relax. The patient may have a tendency to slide down the bed. You can prevent this by tucking a box, suitcase or pillow, rolled firmly in a sheet on the mattress at the foot of the bed. This allows the patient to push gently with the feet, maintaining a comfortable position and, at the same time, exercising the calf muscles, so preventing deep vein thrombosis. If necessary the end of the bed can be raised on wooden blocks or large books.

Many of the details of physical caring for the sick have already been described, but the patient's morale depends on your care and attention. If you are overtired you find yourself less able to help. It is for this reason that you need time away from the patient to rest and recover. Even a short time away refreshes you and helps you remain cheerful.

The patient gets great comfort from listening to your voice giving details about the family, the outside world, and neighbourhood news. It is not necessary for the patient to talk to you. Some families are more musical than others, and humming or singing old familiar songs gives the patient pleasure and brings back memories. A radio or a cassette recorder often gives greater comfort and entertainment to the patient than television. The fast moving pictures and rapid speaking voices often require a greater concentration. Flowers in the room and a favourite picture positioned so that it can easily be seen, are restful and give the patient enjoyment. Photographs of the family can be placed on a bedside table. All these things are simply and easily done and help to make the invalid's life cheerful and less monotonous.

Night-time is a particular problem for the chronically sick. The patient needs some kind of telephone or some other means of communication. Open doors may not be sufficient to hear what is happening in the sickroom. Last thing in the evening, make sure the patient's bladder has been emptied and the necessary medicines have been taken. Tidy the bed, and make the patient comfortable. Leave a shaded light in the room to stop the patient being confused in the night if he or she wakes up. The confusion could be due to the illness, the drugs, or the dark. It is greatly reduced if the patient recognizes familiar surroundings. Usually, however, an invalid feels sufficiently secure at home to have a reasonable night's sleep.

The rewards of nursing a chronically ill patient are often difficult to appreciate. The destruction of your family and personal life is a high price to pay. This is easier to sacrifice if the patient is someone you love, who returns this affection by showing his or her appreciation and thanks.

Providing care is much more difficult to do when the patient is confused, irritable, demanding or unable, or unwilling, to show any gratitude for your help. This is the most testing of all relationships, and you can only survive with sufficient outside help to allow you to escape occasionally.

Sometimes the burden is too much and you must be prepared to take outside advice from friends, family, and doctor if both you and your patient are suffering. There is no shame in admitting that you have undertaken an impossible task, because you have the justification that you have tried. Often, however, the care of a patient in your own home is an immensely satisfying, though tiring, job. You have shared in a human experience that gives you a deeper understanding of other people's problems, fears and troubles. You know that you have done a job well.

Depression and anxiety

These are two of the commonest problems of mental illness, and are often associated because depression leads to anxiety. Anxiety may be realistic, stemming from worries about a dying parent or an alcoholic wife. Sympathy and understanding from relatives and friends are a far better treatment than drugs, because they can help with the practical burdens of the problem.

Anxiety associated with depression may be unrealistic; the fears are due to the mood change. You can help by reassuring the person and finding a practical answer to the problems. Decision making is always difficult for someone who is depressed. Your

assistance may make life easier, even if it is only keeping the anxious patient company. If it is a neighbour who is depressed, frequent visits from you help.

Severe depression may lead to a state of complete hopelessness and suicidal despair. Suicidal talk is a serious symptom, and must not be ignored. You must either get in contact with a near relative of the patient, or a doctor. The doctor can recommend treatment with antidepressant drugs or, occasionally, hospitalization. Your role is one of friendship and understanding toward the patient. Unfortunately the depressed patient may feel that he or she has failed and let you down, and this sense of inadequacy is increased. It is important that you let the patient feel that your friendship outweighs any of the burdens that are being placed upon you. This human warmth is a lifeline that gives the patient hope of recovery.

Hysteria

Hysterics are an escape from an unpleasant reality. The symptoms can take many physical forms. For example, pain in the neck, head, or stomach; uncontrollable laughing or crying; choking sensations; dimness of vision; inability to urinate; or even dizziness and fainting. Your firmness and support are necessary. It is important not to give way and let the person "escape" from the reality. If you can help him or her to face and cope with the situation, then the patient can build up confidence and increase the ability to cope with the next problem.

Occasionally you can get control of the patient only by giving him or her a sudden shock, like a slap on the face or the traditional bucket of cold water. However, holding the patient's arms firmly in your hands and talking slowly, quietly, and with emphasis usually controls the symptoms and produces calmness. It is a matter of imposing the strength of your personality on the patient's emotions.

Mental instability

Instability is difficult to define. Even doctors disagree on the range of normal human behaviour. Some specialists accept behaviour that others would consider to be definitely abnormal. Instability may be considered to be a disorder of the patient's normal thought processes so that conclusions are reached that do not fit in with the facts of the situation and the reactions of the individual do not follow any apparent logical pattern.

Some patients have fixed delusions. In this form of instability, the patient is convinced that some underlying force is working against him or her, for example, that men in grey over-coats are agents of a secret enemy and must be avoided. These beliefs modify the patient's behaviour so that the particular "enemy" is avoided but behaviour is normal in all other respects. This is a form of paranoia.

The patient with more serious paranoia may hear unexplained voices, receive messages and instructions, and see visions of things that the rest of us cannot see. In the elderly patient this can usually be ignored, but in a younger person great care must be taken. The paranoia may be a symptom of schizophrenia, or drug addiction. You must avoid conflict with the patient's views; to him or her, they are very real. You should talk to the relatives about the problem or, if it is a member of your own family, discuss it with a doctor. It is important to try and get the patient to accept medical help. Sometimes the patient is aware of this mental confusion, and this makes it easier for you to persuade him or her to seek help. Often the problem is more difficult. A direct confrontation may produce a physical reaction and violence. You must be careful, and ensure that help is at hand. If you disagree with the patient you may be treated with suspicion, so you have to be subtle in your approach. If you fail, do not try again unless you feel the patient is a danger to himself or herself or to others. If you feel this is the case then you must get help from a doctor or, if necessary, the police. The patient may be so ill that admission to hospital is necessary. This decision is not taken by you, and depends on psychiatric and medical advice.

Mania is another form of mental illness. This occurs when an overactive mind overflows with enthusiasm, and ideas replace one another so quickly that there is often no time to carry them out. The patient is convinced he or she can change the world. The excessive enthusiasm ultimately leads to physical fatigue and confusion, but the patient cannot tolerate any frustrations, or attempts to prevent what he or she desires to achieve. The patient may react violently if you try to hinder these intentions. It is safer to gently deflect the patient from the ideas while apparently agreeing with his or her intentions. This gives the ideas a chance to spontaneously change, and a new course of action to start. It is important not to become personally involved in these schemes. In an extreme form the patient's loss of judgement, physical exhaustion, and confusion need to be treated by hospitalization and sedation. Only the doctor can help.

When you are dealing with a mentally disturbed patient it is important not to get hurt. Try to ensure that you are not alone, and that the patient is not between you and the door. Be prepared to leave quickly and, if necessary, move a chair between yourself and the patient as you escape from the room. There is no point in being brave and getting hurt. It is more sensible to admit that you cannot help any further and leave the problem to experts.

Confusion

Confusion, like mental instability, is difficult to define. It is not the same as dementia, which is a mental deterioration due to age and gradual changes in the brain tissue. Confusion and dementia may occur together. Confusion is usually of recent and fairly rapid onset. The patient loses sense of time and place, feels agitated and sometimes has hallucinations, hears voices, or feels that he or she does not really exist.

If the patient is confused, the presence of a friend or relative will prevent him or her coming to any harm. Sit the patient down, preferably in familiar surroundings, and talk quietly about familiar things. Reassure the patient in a calm voice that everything is all right and that you can help. Ask someone else to contact a doctor or make arrangements to take the patient to the doctor.

Confusion can be a symptom of physical illness, such as the onset of diabetes, pneumonia, or heart failure, which reduces the oxygen content of the blood reaching the brain. It may be caused by alcohol, drugs, concussion from an accident, or from a stroke. A doctor must make a diagnosis before treatment of the cause of the confusion can begin.

Elderly people may become confused at night only, through a combined effect of sleeping pills, slight anaemia, and a heart failure.

A permanently confused patient is probably suffering from dementia.

Dementia

This is a major problem in old age. The patient can still lead an independent life even if absent-minded and forgetful. But in a serious form of permanent confusion, the patient loses all sense of time, feels there is no need for meals, cannot remember how to dress or wash, is occasionally incontinent, and fails to recognize relatives or friends.

The family often has great difficulty persuading the patient that the time has come to join them in their own home or to move into a home for the aged. Although the patient's confusion is increased by a move, it has to be made. Your doctor is an ally to the family, and a friend to the demented relative.

A demented patient at home alone is constantly at risk. He or she could fall and break a bone; fall into a fire; get burned while lighting a cigarette or cooking; become undernourished from failing to eat; get skin problems from failing to keep clean; feel constantly persecuted from the imagined voices and persons that populate a disorganized mind.

The problems you and your family must deal with are to keep the patient safe, nourished and clean, as well as to control any agitation and disturbance in the patient's mind.

Set a room aside with a guarded fire, hidden light cords, carpets that do not slip, and a bed that is against a wall to prevent the patient from falling out on one side. A chair can be pushed firmly against the open side of the bed after the patient has gone to bed. A comfortable armchair is essential and a bed table can be placed across the chair to prevent the patient getting out without help. The furniture in the room should be simple, preferably containing some of the things from the patient's own home, with his or her favourite pictures on the wall. If the room is upstairs it is advisable to have a gate on the staircase. Make sure that the lock on the lavatory door can be opened from the outside. If not, remove the lock altogether.

Although the progress of the dementia cannot be prevented, a normal, healthy diet with plenty of fresh fruit and additional vitamins helps to maintain the patient's general health and well-being. The doctor may prescribe a tranquillizer to be taken last thing at night to ensure a good sleep for the patient and the family.

A strict routine helps the patient to achieve a comfortable rhythm to his or her life. Meals, washing, and visits to the lavatory should be at regular times. However irritated you may feel, talk to the patient in a calm voice. It produces better results than shouting. Even when you are in the room tidying or bedmaking use a gentle voice to tell the patient about neighbours, visits by the children, and other potential disturbances. This form of communication still penetrates the demented mind, and the topics keep the patient in touch with normal life.

Care of the demented person is likely to be long-term, so you will need your own time off. Relatives and friends may help, but, occasionally, you need a holiday. Ideally, someone should take over your work in the home as the patient is almost always made worse by the move to hospital with a change of routine, then worse again on the return home. However, if it is not possible to arrange for someone to come in, you must accept the patient's increased confusion on your return in order to get your holiday.

Eventually the elderly demented patient is unable to get out of bed, get dressed or go to the lavatory. Occasional incontinence becomes constant. The patient's skin may ulcerate and form bedsores, and the problems of home-nursing a chronically ill patient are aggravated by the dementia. You may feel you cannot cope any longer, because of exhaustion, the destruction of family life and, most of all, the physical inability to move and help your relative. You need to talk to your doctor, who will make arrangements for the patient to be hospitalized.

Mental retardation

The mentally retarded child is likely to have physical disabilities as well, for example, epilepsy, or cerebral palsy; the hydrocephalic child may suffer from spina bifida; the child with Down's syndrome may have a congenital heart disease; the child of a mother who had rubella in early pregnancy may be deaf or blind. The physical handicaps may increase the child's likelihood of dying before adult life.

However, if the child is physically normal, a mental disability may not be obvious in the first few weeks. It is only as the child fails to develop normally in many fields that the parents become suspicious. By the time the child reaches a year old, the suspicion is a certainty. Most parents blame themselves for their child's mental state. They must realize that mental handicap can afflict any family.

Most parents decide to look after the mentally backward child themselves. The problems they have to face are many. The child's learning ability is poor. Sitting, crawling, and walking develop late, and bladder and bowel control may not occur until the age of four or five.

The mentally retarded child can learn, but the process is slow. The parents have to persevere patiently, and praise the child's slightest success. The progress of a retarded child, however limited, is as rewarding to watch as the progress of a normal child. The child slowly learns to handle a spoon and cup; to get washed and dressed; and to remain continent. Only the most severely retarded children fail to learn these skills eventually.

It is difficult for parents with a handicapped child to spend enough time with other children in the family. Often they are too young to understand what is happening, and feel that one child is a "favourite". This may cause resentment toward the handicapped child, who already has enough problems. The skill with which this is handled depends on the awareness of the parents to the problem.

Normal children are often frustrated and annoyed by a disciplined upbringing, but a mentally handicapped child settles well into the security of a regular routine.

Depending on the severity of the handicap, the parents must decide whether the child should go to a special school. Many retarded children benefit from the company of normal children, but if your doctor advises you to choose a special school, it is wise to accept this advice. The mentally handicapped child often feels less conspicuous with other handicapped children, and realizes that he or she is not unique.

Parents of mentally retarded children need the help and advice of their paediatrician, and the support of special organizations. Grandparents, relatives, and friends help by giving the parents a well-earned rest. As the child grows up, he or she can go to special holiday camps that have specially-trained staff who can cope with the problems.

The parents of a mentally handicapped child have to cope with the problems all parents have to cope with. But when the child reaches puberty, the problems may become magnified; for example, the mentally subnormal boy can become highly aggressive. If you feel the time has come for the child to leave home, for instance, if the rest of the family is suffering, you must not feel guilty. The child can still be treated as one of the family, even though living away from home. The important thing is that the child began life at home, and that is an advantage that remains for the rest of life.

Many mentally retarded persons learn to do simple jobs and support themselves independently. They can work with other handicapped people, and feel secure in a comfortable working routine.

As parents, your responsibility to a handicapped child is to prepare him or her for as independent a life as possible, and to give the child the opportunity to develop to his or her fullest capacity. Remember that the role you play in caring for a handicapped child will determine largely the extent to which he or she realizes his or her potential capabilities in life. Any decision must be based on the effect of the handicapped child on the rest of the family, and the advice from your doctor and other experts.

What is meant by "retarded"

IQ is short for Intelligence Quotient. Parents may worry that an IQ test will prevent their mentally retarded child from going to a normal school. Children are not assessed on an IQ test alone. The test reveals one facet of the child's make-up, but the complete diagnosis does not depend on it. A child with an IQ of less than 70 is termed "mentally subnormal" and is in need of special schooling. A child with an IQ of between 50 and 70 is termed "educationally subnormal (mild)", and a child with an IQ of less than 50 is termed "mentally subnormal (severe)". At each level of handicap, the child is able to have some kind of education.

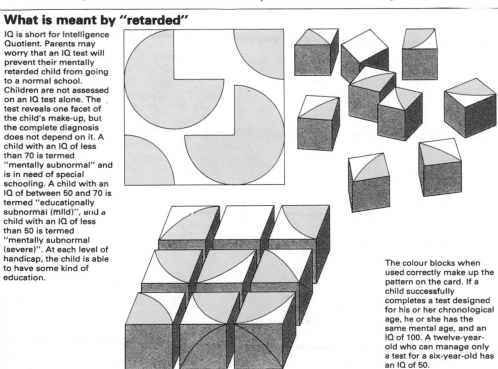

The colour blocks when used correctly make up the pattern on the card. If a child successfully completes a test designed for his or her chronological age, he or she has the same mental age, and an IQ of 100. A twelve-year-old who can manage only a test for a six-year-old has an IQ of 50.

Care of the dying

The sadness and inevitability of death bring problems and difficulties that few people have the knowledge or experience to cope with alone. Most people would like to die at home close to family and familiar possessions. Every help must be given to the patient who wishes to die at home and not in hospital. The expense of private nursing homes is often prohibitive, and this is an additional psychological as well as financial burden for the patient and family.

Some people have more experience of helping with the dying than others. The doctor knows about the patient's physical needs, and has the skill to prevent or relieve pain. He or she becomes a leader, and supports the family during the weeks ahead. A member of the clergy can give a spiritual support that may not have been needed by the patient or the family for many years.

At the onset of a fatal illness, the doctor and family are faced with the decision of what to tell the patient. If the course of the illness is rapid, the decision may not have to be made. The problem usually arises when an inoperable cancer is present; when there is an incurable muscular disorder; or when a cardiac condition begins to rapidly deteriorate. Often the patient's mental state remains unaffected and alert.

Every family doctor must be free to tell the patient what is necessary and appropriate. The problem is discussed with the patient's family. The doctor does not like to lie to the patient, because the patient will lose confidence in the doctor if the truth is ever discovered. Often, the dying patient never asks a direct question about his or her condition. This does not mean that the patient is not aware of what is happening, but that he or she prefers to help the family, the doctor, and himself or herself by maintaining the pretence that all will be well. The patient may not want to know how many months or years of life are left. It is enough for the patient to know that suffering will not occur.

Sometimes, however, the patient wants to know exactly what is the matter, what can be done about it, the likelihood of successful treatment, and eventually, the length of time the doctor expects him or her to live. Most doctors give truthful answers to direct questions such as these. This honesty may in itself help the patient through moments of mental anguish. It also gives the patient a chance to put his or her affairs in order. The patient may not want the family to know that he or she understands the predicament. This makes it easier for them all to maintain a façade of cheerfulness.

Sudden death

The violence of a car crash or the swift death caused by a heart attack gives the individual no time to know what is happening. Even death that occurs a day or two after an accident, operation, or acute illness is too entangled with the treatment of the condition for the patient to realize that he or she is dying. There is little time for the doctor to discuss the matter with the family, other than to warn them of the possibility. The patient rarely suffers, but the family is left unprepared and appalled by the disaster.

The family needs expert help from the doctor, the nurses, and the clergy. Medical help can soften the initial grief. The doctor can prescribe tranquillizing drugs and sedatives. The children and relatives can help each other. The very fact that they are being constructive produces an unexpected strength to cope with funeral arrangements, lawyers, and the hospital. Friends and neighbours can help the bereaved family in a practical way by helping with the shopping and other domestic chores.

Adjusting to life after the sudden death of a loved one is difficult. The surviving relative needs a chance to talk over the death. The bereaved person may suffer from a feeling of guilt, and needs encouragement and support. Grief sometimes takes the form of anger directed at the outside causes of death. The bereaved person is looking for someone to blame for the disaster. This feeling passes as the bereaved person's normal perspective on life returns, but it can be alarming to the family and friends who are trying to help.

Acute and despairing grief is understandable and common after a sudden death. As grief lessens, the support and care of the family and friends can gradually be softened. The relative or friend can come to terms with the situation as he or she would have been able to do had the death been gradual and anticipated.

Gradual death

The period of normal life must be maintained for as long as possible. At first, it is difficult for someone to accept that a relative has a fatal illness. One day the relative is complaining of a variety of symptoms, some of which might be severe, and the next day the doctor gives the family the information that they fear most of all. They could be told after the relative has had an operation, or after some minor investigation.

Usually, there is some form of treatment that produces a temporary improvement in the patient's health. Although this gives a false hope to relatives, it helps the patient's morale. If the doctor recommends a short holiday for the patient, it is wise to accept the advice.

It is sensible to discuss the practicalities of the situation with the doctor. The family needs to know how the disease will progress, how to make the patient comfortable and happy, and how long the patient can expect to live. The doctor can advise them on the possibilities of caring for the patient at home in the later stages of the illness, and whether special arrangements need to be made.

The normal routine of life should be continued for as long as possible. It is important for the patient's morale, as well as for the financial situation, to work for as long as possible.

Weekends should be set aside for the patient's recuperation. There may be a loss of stamina and endurance, so additional rest is advisable. The doctor may suggest a mild sedative at night to ensure a good sleep for the patient, and to reduce any worry or anxiety.

Increasing weakness and onset of symptoms means that sooner or later the patient's period of normal life comes to an end. The patient often suffers from a gradual loss of vitality, and an increasing fatigue makes a full day's work impossible. A relatively minor illness, such as a feverish cold, can develop into bronchitis and rapidly reduce the patient's strength. Other symptoms become worse, or develop. The patient may suffer from weight loss, weakness, and a loss of appetite.

Other problems that frequently occur with the terminally ill are nausea at the sight of food; vomiting after a meal; and constipation. The patient's weakness and lethargy leads to a feeling of profound depression and misery. The patient's awareness of the developing situation is magnified by worry, and there is a fear of becoming a burden to the family.

The doctor can help in a positive manner. Antidepressant drugs can be prescribed to help the patient's mood; a change of treatment to improve the patient physically; and support for the patient's family.

Although the patient is weaker, he or she can remain independent, and continue getting up and going to bed, going to the lavatory, and getting dressed and undressed unaided. Short walks can still be enjoyed, or drives and visits to friends and neighbours. Such trips should be planned carefully to coincide with the patient's strongest time of day. Although the trips may be exhausting, the patient will enjoy them.

The family routine begins to change. Make household rearrangements small and gradual. The patient needs a chair that is easy to get into and out of. Organize a downstairs room with a day bed. The patient will then be able to be with the family for most of the day without having to use the stairs.

Encourage friends and colleagues from work to visit the patient.

Work out a sensible daily routine and encourage the patient to relax.

If the patient is not in pain at this stage, his or her anxiety is increased by the onset of vague discomforts and aches. Reassurance is needed from the doctor, who may prescribe mild painkillers, antidepressant drugs, or a sedative to be taken at night to ensure a good sleep for the patient.

If the patient talks about the future, the comments should not be ignored. The patient needs reassurance about what will happen to the family. It is important to remain cheerful about the future, whether or not the patient knows the truth.

The role of the friend is a very important one. Friends want to help the patient and the family. The friend may not know the details of the illness, but has probably guessed the outcome, and can give the family and patient both moral and practical support. Visits from the friend ought to be brief, but they offer the patient an opportunity to talk about cheerful subjects, such as family, work, or old times. It is wise to avoid talking at length about the illness at the early stage, unless the patient shows signs of wanting to.

The friend can show appreciation of the work being done by the family, and offer to stay with the patient if the family need a little time away from home.

If the patient shows signs of wanting to talk about his or her illness and future, the friend can listen quietly. The patient can discuss practical problems with the friend that may be difficult to say to the family, for example, who will care for and guide the family in the future. Do not ignore the questions by convincing the patient that all will be well in the end, when the patient obviously needs practical reassurance.

During the later stages of the patient's illness, the friend can help the family with chores such as shopping. Sometimes, the patient's courage and strength prevent him or her from showing real emotions to the family, but will reveal them to a friend. The patient may feel that the doctor does not have the time to listen, and the friend can be a sympathetic listener to whom the patient can pour out many worries and fears. Often, a sudden release of emotion can be of enormous value to the patient.

The bedridden patient accentuates the practical problems of dealing with a terminally ill patient. The routine of caring for a chronically sick person is by now well established. The family must realize that deterioration is going to continue. Although the patient's loss of weight makes some aspects of nursing easier, the skin is more likely to be damaged without the protection of fat and muscle. It may take two adults to move the patient on and off the bedpan. A visiting nurse can help with bedbathing, and can show the family how to carry out the more complicated procedures. The doctor may advise the family on the use of drugs, and how to insert suppositories to treat constipation or other symptoms.

Pain may become a permanent part of the patient's life. The doctor prescribes painkilling drugs in adequate amounts, and explains how to use them. Do not wait until the patient complains of pain before giving the drugs. It is easier and more effective to administer them at regular intervals.

Nausea and vomiting are often more distressing symptoms for the family and patient to deal with than pain. The symptoms may be combined with hiccupping, which exhausts the patient. The doctor can prescribe drugs to control this. These drugs can also have a sedative effect if taken with painkillers. Although they can produce confusion and drowsiness, the drowsiness often benefits the patient. The drugs may prevent the patient from feeling thirsty, so it is important to encourage him or her to drink. Assist the patient by offering frequent drinks of cool, sweetened fluid, such as fruit juice, iced water, or herbal teas that freshen the mouth but do not have strong flavours.

If the patient is suffering from a heart or lung disease, coughing may be one of the symptoms. This distresses and exhausts the patient. The family also finds it disturbing. It is most important to control the coughing at night and so allow the patient and family a peaceful sleep. Try changing the patient's position in bed. A steam inhalation last thing at night reduces the irritation, and helps to prevent an unproductive cough. Broken sleep is exhausting for the family and the patient. If sleeplessness continues, it is sensible to arrange alternative care every other night if this is possible.

Another symptom of heart or lung disease is shortness of breath. Coughing, or the smallest physical activity, can make the patient gasp for breath. This causes great distress. The doctor may prescribe oxygen that can be used effectively after a bad bout of coughing or rapid physical movement.

The patient's strength and personality may cope with pain in a surprising manner. However, incontinence of urine and faeces is a humiliation few can tolerate. The situation requires immense care and tact, as well as tolerance, from those nursing the patient, because they must cope with the physical and psychological misery that incontinence produces. It is important that, despite the unpleasantness, the family should not let the patient feel that he or she is an intolerable burden. Incontinence must be accepted with sympathy and understanding.

As the patient becomes physically weaker, the doctor administers more drugs. The mental state of the patient changes from an alert, realistic individual, to one who is often confused about time and place. This confusion varies, and periods of normal discussion fluctuate with moments of drowsiness and loss of reality. Often the patient is aware of this temporary confusion, and is apologetic for the trouble caused.

Visitors should come for only a short time. It is best if they know the patient well, and can remain peaceful and silent. If necessary, they can just hold the patient's hand. This physical contact is a form of communication that can produce peace and contentment.

During the patient's deterioration, the appetite is usually lost. Offer the patient small amounts of his or her favourite foods, jellies, or soups.

If at any time the family feels that they cannot cope with the situation any longer, discuss the problem with the doctor. It may be that the time has come for the patient to be hospitalized, and it is wise to accept the doctor's advice on this.

The time of death is sometimes difficult for the doctor to estimate beforehand. The patient may become unconscious some hours, even days, before death, or may remain alert and conscious to the end. Painkilling drugs sometimes produce a state of semicoma that can be misinterpreted by the family as a forerunner to death. The patient may develop an alarming breathing pattern called Cheyne-Stokes breathing, in which breaths increase in rapidity and volume until they reach a climax, then gradually subside and stop altogether. This period can last from five seconds to one minute before the process begins again. The syndrome is common in sick or elderly persons. Although it can be a forerunner to death, it is just as likely to last for several months, or even to disappear altogether.

Do not be alarmed if the patient's breathing makes a groaning or croaking sound. It does not mean he or she is in pain.

When a dying patient slips into a coma, the position of the neck and body produces the noise, which can be reduced by gently turning the patient's shoulders or body.

Another alarming noise the dying patient may make is known as the "death rattle". This happens because the unconscious patient is unable to cough up the secretions that accumulate in the back of the throat.

The attitude of the family and the patient alters at this stage. As the patient suffers from increased weakness, lethargy, discomfort, and pain, he or she begins to come to terms with dying. Death is no longer frightening. Often a person's last days are spent more happily in the knowledge that he or she is dying, than in a state of uncertainty and doubt. It is easier for the family and patient to talk about death in a way that may not have been possible earlier in the illness. It brings comfort to everyone, and often a closeness not experienced before.

The patient or family may need additional comfort from a member of the clergy or from a doctor. The length of life remaining to the patient no longer matters. The important thing is the quality of the patient's last days, or hours. The doctor is aware that the application of medical skill can sometimes prolong the patient's suffering and bring no real benefit. Although the doctor may prescribe large doses of painkilling drugs if necessary, it is unlikely that new treatment will be started.

The actual moment of death is difficult to define, and for the family, difficult to accept. Even when the patient has stopped breathing and a pulse cannot be felt, the heart gives feeble contractions for another minute or two. Even a doctor may find it difficult to give an exact time of death, but leave it to the nurse or doctor to decide.

If the family is present at the moment of death, it is comforting for everyone to stay quietly at the bedside without talking. Each member of the family needs a chance to touch or to kiss the dead relative, and such physical contact helps to bring home the reality of death.

Often no one is present when the patient dies, for he or she may have been left alone to sleep. Although death is expected, it is still a shock for the member of the family who first enters the room. It is sensible to tidy the bedclothes, and comb the patient's hair before telling the rest of the family. When they come in to see the body, it has an appearance of calm and peacefulness.

A child's reaction to death depends on many factors. A child's first experience of a death is often the death of a pet. A child under the age of eight cannot understand that death is irreversible, and may expect the mother or father to bring the pet back to life. After the age of eight or nine, the child's understanding is usually as rational as that of an adult.

However, it may still be difficult for the child to understand that someone in the family is dying, neither is it important that the child should understand. What is important is that the child sees that the family is united and involved in caring for the sick relative. The child can then become part of the team, and help in caring for the patient.

If the patient slips into a coma, or is confused by drugs or illness, it is wise to keep the child out of the sickroom. The child may be frightened to see the familiar and loved person in this state, and the child's presence does not help the patient.

When the patient is about to die, the family may decide to send the child away to a neighbour or relative. Although this sending away is well intentioned, the experience can be frightening for the child, who may feel that death is going to involve another member of the family while he or she is away. The parents need to give the child a careful explanation about everything that will happen during the child's absence. Often, however, the child can stay at home and continue to feel part of the family.

The parents may decide to let the child see the dead relative. If the child does want to, someone should take him or her into the room and only stay long enough for the child to see how peaceful the person looks in death. If the child does not want to see the body, the family must respect that decision.

The parents may explain carefully and simply to the child what happens between the death of the relative and the funeral. A young child cannot understand a funeral or cremation service, so it is probably wise to leave the child with a close friend during the service. An older child may want to take part in this important family occasion.

Parents may be confused by the child's reaction to bereavement. The child may seem indifferent or aggressive, or may seem grief-stricken or guilty. The parents must encourage the child to discuss his or her feelings. The child must be reassured that these feelings are not unusual, but that they become unreasonable if taken to extremes.

The child soon learns that the sadness is made easier by sharing the emotion with the family. As time passes, the grief becomes less acute, and the child gains a better understanding of the concept of death.

Death of a baby

The intrauterine death of an embryo ends in a miscarriage (inevitable abortion). Ten per cent of pregnancies end in this way, commonly between the sixth and the tenth weeks, and usually because of an abnormality in the embryo. If a foetus is rejected between twenty and thirty weeks, however, the cause may be more serious. But with care, subsequent pregnancies are usually successful.

Stillbirth is the term used to describe a foetal death occurring after the twenty-eighth week of pregnancy. The mother may become aware that the baby's movements have stopped, and an obstetrician can check for foetal movement.

If the foetus is dead, the mother and father must be told. Labour is induced with drugs if it has not begun within a few days. The mother is usually kept under sedation until the baby is born. It is important that the baby's father is with the mother for the delivery to give comfort. The parents find it easier to cope with the reality of death if they are able to see the baby immediately after the birth.

The parents need to know the chances of subsequent pregnancies ending in this way. They also need time to mourn the loss of the dead baby before embarking on another pregnancy.

Perinatal death refers to death occurring between the moment of birth to a week after birth. Because the majority of babies are now born in hospital, the number of perinatal deaths has dropped. However, if death does occur, the parents need the same help and support that parents of a stillborn child need.

Sudden infant death syndrome is commonly referred to as "cot death". Sometimes a perfectly healthy baby between the age of three weeks and seven months is found dead in the cot. There is seldom an adequate explanation. The parents are left shocked and grief-stricken. They feel desperately guilty and in some way responsible. All that is known definitely about cot death is that it is not caused by choking, smothering, or any of the other popular myths. Neither does it run in families.

Before the parents can recover from the shock, they need careful counselling. A psychiatrist, family social agency, guidance clinic, member of the clergy, or the Foundation for the Study of Infant Deaths may help.

Death of an older child or an adolescent

From the age of five years onward, a child begins to understand the concept of death and dying. The dying child feels protective toward his or her parents. Although the child desperately needs to talk about what is going to happen, he or she may never get close to the subject. The child may attach himself or herself to a nurse or doctor while still relying on the parents. By doing this the child is sharing out the emotional responsibility. The parents may find this difficult to accept, but must realize that someone else can give more unemotional help, and listen dispassionately to the child's fears and anxieties.

The child who seems to have no idea about what is happening is better left in ignorance, but the child who asks "Am I going to die?" may be happier knowing the truth. He or she can then talk more openly about the worries and uncertainties, and bring comfort to himself or herself as well as to the parents. The child may be comforted by knowing the religious beliefs that surround death. Often it is the moment of death that the child fears. He or she needs to know that dying is usually calm and peaceful.

An adolescent in the same situation has reached a more logical and dispassionate view of life, and may reject the comfort that religious beliefs can bring. An adolescent rightly feels that life is unjust and unfair. He or she has been striving to find independence only to become totally dependent on the family once again. It takes a wise doctor or friend to help in this situation.

Parents who lose a child of any age need help and sympathy after the death. The doctor's job is to help the bereaved parents. This help must be extended to brothers and sisters too, whose grief may go unnoticed by the overburdened parents.

Grief

Death in the Western world has become a private affair that is concealed as far as possible. Grief is therefore a socially difficult emotion. A bereaved family may find themselves isolated because friends and relatives feel afraid in case they are unable to cope with another person's grief.

At first, grief takes the form of shock and numbness; then great waves of emotion sweep over the person accompanied by uncontrollable tears; and finally the person becomes calm. This cycle of emotion can continue for some weeks, even months. The emotional, tearful phase should not be suppressed.

Grief is often accompanied by tremendous fatigue. There is a great deal for the family to organize. For the single bereaved person, the burden is even greater. He or she also has to deal with a quiet home and a loss of routine;

there are usually feelings of guilt; and gone is the feeling of being wanted and needed. The person needs company and others to talk to. It is a time for other members of the family to give support and help to prevent a deepening of the depression that follows a death.

Professional people offer a great deal of support to the bereaved. A doctor can make sure that the bereaved are in mental and physical health; a lawyer can handle the financial and legal future; and a member of the clergy can offer spiritual support.

Gradually the bereaved person adopts a more normal life, and becomes more outgoing. Grief remains, but with understanding and sympathy the bereaved can begin a new life.

Death and arrangements
Death is sometimes expected when it comes as the end of a long illness. But it can be sudden and unexpected, for example, as the result of an accident or heart attack. It may take place at home, in a hospital, or elsewhere. Death can be a test of a family's strength and can bring out the best or the worst aspects of the family and friends. It is a time when strength, understanding, and love are of paramount importance. It is neither a time for noisy protestations of grief nor for competition among family members. Perhaps the best guide to conducting oneself is to try to act in a manner that would have been approved by the deceased.

A death certificate is required for every death. It will be issued, and signed either by a doctor familiar with the deceased or by the doctor in attendance at the time of death. This certificate should be taken to the local Registrar's office, where the death should be registered within five days. Registration may be delayed for a further nine days, but only if the Registrar receives, in writing, all the relevant details concerning the death. The Registrar will need to know the date and place of death, the profession or occupation of the deceased and all names by which the deceased has ever been known. The information given must be endorsed with the signature of the next-of-kin.

In the event of an accidental or unexplained death, the death certificate will be issued by the coroner. A post-mortem examination may have to be carried out in order to discover the cause of death. If the coroner decides that there are reasonable grounds for suspecting that the death was due to unnatural causes, an inquest will be held.

If the death occurs in hospital, the death certificate will be issued by the hospital.

The services of a funeral director can ease the administrative burden of death arrangements. On notification by the family, he will obtain permission to remove the body to the funeral home and arrange for burial or cremation. He then consults with a responsible relative on details, such as the type of coffin and service required, hours of visiting so that people can pay their respects, and whether the head and shoulders are to be on view or the coffin closed. A downpayment is usually needed to cover initial expenses, such as having a grave prepared at the cemetery. The director can, and usually does, take care of announcements of the death in the newspaper.

Somebody must take charge of family affairs. Often, the eldest child of the deceased or a trusted friend, who may be executor of the estate, is given the task. It is better than the individual concerned be able to keep a clear head and take the burden off the most grieving survivor, usually the widow or widower, particularly in the details of the funeral. The cost of funerals can be high, and while most funeral directors are honest and sympathetic, there are authentic stories of unscrupulous directors who try to sell the higher-priced arrangements to grief-stricken relatives.

The telephone will be in frequent use in the first few hours and it makes sense for the person in charge of affairs to use a nearby phone, leaving the home phone clear for calls from friends and relatives.

The family lawyer, if any, should be contacted immediately to find out whether the deceased had left any special instructions. The family priest, minister, or rabbi should also be informed at the earliest opportunity.

Some people leave their kidneys for transplant surgery, and usually carry a card in their wallet to this effect in case they are killed in an accident. The local eye bank will send a technician immediately upon notification if the deceased has bequeathed his or her corneas for transplant or experimental use.

When somebody dies in hospital, there is often a request for an autopsy. It is as distasteful to the hospital staff as it is to the bereaved to have to face this decision at the most grievous time, but so much has been learned from autopsy studies that the request should never be resented.

Death is never convenient. We can each spare our loved ones a great deal of unnecessary anguish by thinking out clearly all the details mentioned above, writing them down and placing the instructions in a safe place known to all, while we are in good health.

The sick child

When you are caring for a sick child at home, you should follow the same general rules of diet and comfort that have already been described (see **The sick room,** p.638, and **Special diets,** p.684). However, extra skill is needed to encourage the young patient to take medicines, and to relieve a child's boredom. Many of the childhood illnesses, such as German measles and mumps, cannot be cured with drugs, so careful home nursing to relieve symptoms is even more important.

It is better to assume that your child is going to enjoy a medicine before you administer it. Approach the exercise in a relaxed manner. If you begin with a lengthy explanation and apology, your child expects not to like it. Nowadays most medicines for children have a pleasant taste.

If your child refuses to take the spoonful, mix it with a drink. Make sure the drink is an unfamiliar one, like apple juice or grape juice, because most children notice a change in the taste of familiar drinks.

Tablets can be crushed up in the first spoonful of a strong-tasting food, such as stewed fruit. Bitter pills are more acceptable given in a teaspoonful of jam, marmalade, or honey. If your child has to swallow a capsule, put it in soft food, such as chopped banana.

Eye drops and eye ointments can be carefully applied while the child sleeps.

Always remember to keep medicines out of reach of children, and throw them away once the illness is over.

A comforting eyewash can be made from half a litre (one pint) of tepid boiled water containing one teaspoonful of salt. This is particularly soothing for the child with crusted eyes, for example, in measles. Whenever you are bathing eyes, use a clean piece of cotton wool for each eye to prevent spreading a possible infection from one eye to the other.

A child troubled by itching spots, for instance in chickenpox, runs a risk of infecting the spots by scratching. Keep the fingernails short and wash your child's hands three times a day. The itching can be relieved by bathing the child in a solution of two cups of bicarbonate of soda to a large tubful of water. Dabbing spots with calamine lotion often helps as well.

With some childhood complaints, such as measles and mumps, the mouth can get sore and dry. Frequent mouthwashes are a relief. If your child has a blocked nose, a handkerchief scented with the parents' favourite perfume or aftershave is comforting to take to bed at night.

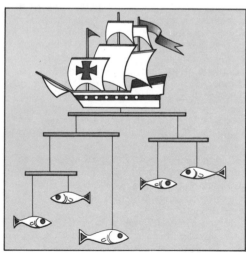

1
Mobiles are easy for a bedridden child to make and fun to watch when completed and hung over the bed. A child can paste pictures from magazines onto cardboard before cutting them out. Together you can make more complicated objects to hang on the mobile: cotton-reel animals, origami shapes, ribbon, cooking foil shapes, and wool pompoms.

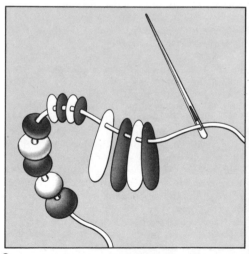

2
Bead stringing can amuse a convalescent child who does not feel over-energetic. Give the child a blunt darning needle and some thick cotton thread. Strings of beads can be made out of the dried pits of apples, oranges, lemons, and melons. Large seeds such as sunflower seeds and lentils can be used and even painted before stringing. Small coloured buttons also work well.

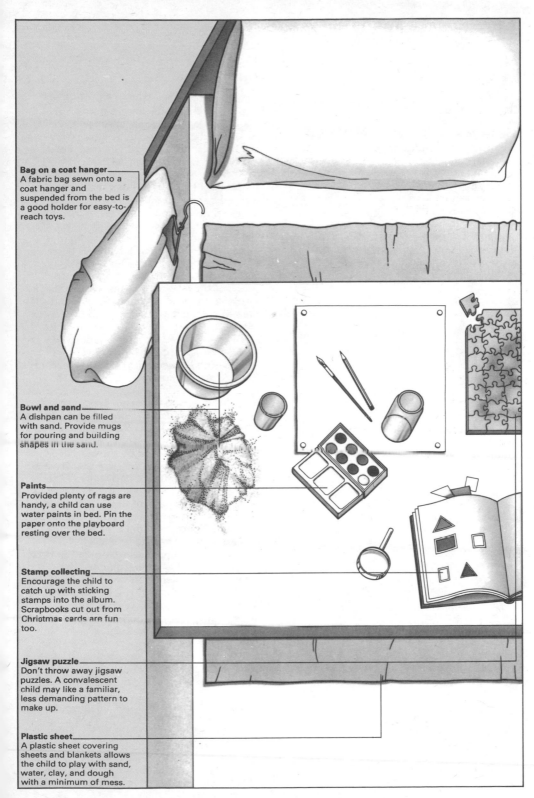

Bag on a coat hanger
A fabric bag sewn onto a coat hanger and suspended from the bed is a good holder for easy-to-reach toys.

Bowl and sand
A dishpan can be filled with sand. Provide mugs for pouring and building shapes in the sand.

Paints
Provided plenty of rags are handy, a child can use water paints in bed. Pin the paper onto the playboard resting over the bed.

Stamp collecting
Encourage the child to catch up with sticking stamps into the album. Scrapbooks cut out from Christmas cards are fun too.

Jigsaw puzzle
Don't throw away jigsaw puzzles. A convalescent child may like a familiar, less demanding pattern to make up.

Plastic sheet
A plastic sheet covering sheets and blankets allows the child to play with sand, water, clay, and dough with a minimum of mess.

Professional care for the sick

Section contents

Introduction

Every citizen of the United Kingdom is
entitled to free medical care through the
National Health Service, which was
established in 1948 with the aims of relieving
the financial problems of illness and of
improving access to medical care. The NHS
has become such an established part of the
pattern of life in Britain that many people
now take it for granted, and are not fully
aware of the vast scale of its resources and
the many different benefits it provides. **How
the NHS works** explains how the NHS is
administered and financed, and its basic
hierarchical structure is shown in a diagram.
Information is also given about private
practice, the alternative to NHS care that is
available to those who can afford it and who
are not completely satisfied with the NHS
services.

The patient and the GP includes a
discussion of the changing pattern of
relationship between the patient and his or
her doctor. The traditional image of the
doctor as both friend and medical adviser of
a family, a person whose professional and
personal knowledge of a patient extends over
many years and whose relationship with a
patient grows stronger and deeper in the
process, is contradicted by the facts of
modern life. A typical GP may now have as
many as 3,500 patients, and many of these
patients may be living within the GP's area
for only short periods of time. The waiting
room for the surgery is constantly crowded,
yet the GP must also find time to keep
abreast with the ever-increasing
developments in medical treatment. In these
circumstances it is understandable that
sometimes a patient may be recognizable to
the GP only as a name on a list: a person
who arrives in the surgery demanding
immediate treatment, only to disappear again
until some other problem arises.

The resulting problems for both patient
and GP are immense, but emphasis is placed
here on the need for the patient to make the
best use possible of the resources available,
and the ways in which he or she can do this.
The patient should perform an active role in
all consultations with the GP: he or she
should be prepared to tell the GP all relevant
information concerning an injury or disorder,
and, if the GP gives a diagnosis or prescribes
treatment that the patient cannot readily
understand, should ask for it to be explained.

Everyone, whether ill or not, should make an effort to learn about his or her body and how it works. This not only makes a doctor's diagnosis easier to understand, but also enables a person to protect his or her body from the many disorders and illnesses that can result from carelessness, neglect, or ignorance. Knowledge of the normal functioning of one's own body is the most important factor in preventative medicine.

The next pages in this section are concerned with the medical care that is given in hospitals. In **Hospitals**, background information is given about the administration, organization, and staff of hospitals. The different procedures by which a patient may be admitted to hospital are explained, and details are given about the tests and physical examinations that a patient in hospital may undergo. **Undergoing surgery** outlines the sequence of events that are experienced by a patient who is admitted to hospital for an operation, and gives information about the consent form that must be signed by every patient undergoing surgery. **Hospital routine for a patient** describes a typical day's timetable of events in a hospital ward, from the waking of the patients by the night staff in the early morning to the lights being put out in the evening. It includes information about doctors' rounds, special diets, visiting hours, and the procedure for discharging the patient from hospital. The patient's rights to discharge himself or herself from hospital against medical advice are explained. Finally, information is given about the special facilities that are available for **A child in hospital**. Hospital nursing staff make special efforts to relieve a child's natural anxiety, and a parent may be allowed to stay overnight with a child in hospital if the facilities are available.

All the information concerning hospitals is designed to be read by patients before, rather than after, they enter hospital. Knowledge about what happens in hospital, and an understanding of why the various procedures are necessary, can greatly reduce the anxiety and fear that most people feel when they are admitted to hospital.

Social security benefits describes the various financial benefits that are available from the Department of Health and Social Security in cases of illness, disablement, pregnancy, and death. The whole subject of social security benefits is notoriously complicated and difficult to understand, and this book can offer only a brief and selective guide. Anyone who wants further information, or who wants to claim any of the benefits or find out if he or she is eligible for them, should visit or telephone a local social security office and obtain the relevant leaflet. A citizen who is denied a benefit to which he or she feels entitled may obtain advice and, in certain circumstances, legal aid, from a local Citizens Advice Bureau office.

Specialized hospitals, clinics, and specialists describes some of the hospitals and clinics that provide specialist medical care and also describes the treatment that may be available from qualified specialists such as chiropodists, opticians, and psychiatrists and psychologists. The normal procedure for obtaining a consultation with many types of specialist is for the patient to be referred by the family doctor. Unless a patient has strong reasons for preferring a particular specialist, it is usually wise to accept the specialist chosen by the GP. Fees for private treatment by specialists may be high.

Other sources of medical care lists the names and addresses of a few of the many independent organizations and societies that provide help for patients with particular disorders and conditions. As well as providing medical advice and social contact with other patients with similar problems, some of these organizations also provide financial assistance and practical help with transport, holidays, education, and accommodation. The type of help provided depends on the particular problems that confront patients with different disorders.

This entire section has been designed to enable the patient to make the fullest possible use of the professional medical care available in Britain. Many people are confused by the vast scale and complexity of the NHS, and are deeply worried by the scientific and technological developments in medicine that seem to make modern medical knowledge increasingly inaccessible to the layman. Given these circumstances, it is more important than ever for the patient to be informed about the medical resources available, and to have the necessary confidence to express his or her personal needs.

How the NHS works

The National Health Service was founded in 1948, and underwent a radical reorganization in 1974 in an attempt to improve its administration. Its original goal of supplying free medical care to all those in need has never been fully achieved, and inequalities in the pattern of provision of health care inherited in 1948 have never been completely eradicated. The pressures exerted on the system by rising professional and public expectations and by the development of medical knowledge are constantly increasing. However, despite the current restrictions on NHS resources, it is planned that growth should be fostered in those areas whose health resources have been, until recently, less adequate than those of other areas.

The services of the NHS are provided almost completely by the government and by local authorities. The ultimate responsibility for provision of these services lies with the Secretary of State for Health and Social Services, and carried out through the Department of Health and Social Security (DHSS). The responsibility for the actual running of the NHS is organized through three levels of management committees. In England, the first level consists of fourteen Regional Health Authorities (RHAs); Scotland, Wales, and Northern Ireland each

have a separate Department of Health. The RHAs are responsible for the general strategic planning and allocation of resources within their regions, and their members are appointed by the Secretary of State. The next level consists of 90 Area Health Authorities (AHAs); these are responsible for the planning, development, and management of services within their areas, and their members are appointed by the RHA or by local authorities. The third layer consists of the District Management Teams, of which there are between one and six responsible to each AHA. These teams are responsible for the day-to-day running of the hospital and community health services within their areas, which normally cover between 100,000 and 500,000 people. The District Management Team includes a Community Physician (in place of the old Medical Officer of Health), who is responsible for maintaining community health through efficient immunization, health services in schools, and other resources. He also co-ordinates the care of the patients leaving hospital and returning home, where they will require continued treatment by their general practitioners and ancillary workers such as district nurses and health visitors.

Family Practitioner Committees, responsible to the Area Health Authorities,

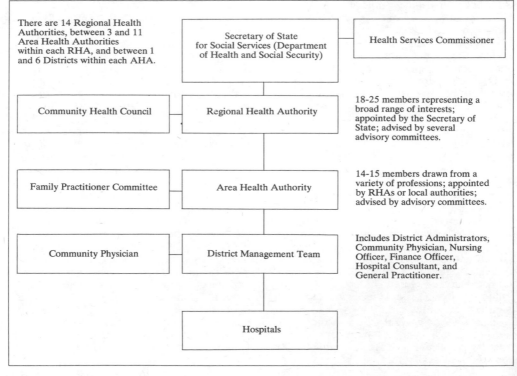

There are 14 Regional Health Authorities, between 3 and 11 Area Health Authorities within each RHA, and between 1 and 6 Districts within each AHA.

Secretary of State for Social Services (Department of Health and Social Security)

Health Services Commissioner

Community Health Council — Regional Health Authority

18-25 members representing a broad range of interests; appointed by the Secretary of State; advised by several advisory committees.

Family Practitioner Committee — Area Health Authority

14-15 members drawn from a variety of professions; appointed by RHAs or local authorities; advised by advisory committees.

Community Physician — District Management Team

Includes District Administrators, Community Physician, Nursing Officer, Finance Officer, Hospital Consultant, and General Practitioner.

Hospitals

arrange the general practitioner, pharmaceutical, dental, and ophthalmic services for each Area.

Community Health Councils, of which there is one for most districts, represent the patients' interests. A Health Service Commissioner, who performs the function of ombudsman, has recently been appointed to investigate complaints about the National Health Service. Although he can easily make enquiries about hospitals, it is more difficult for him to do so about the part of the NHS organized by the Family Practitioner Committees, as there is a more formal complaint procedure that is dealt with by them. It is only after they have reached their own conclusion that the ombudsman can become involved.

The National Health Service is financed almost completely by taxation. Patients are normally required to pay certain charges for drugs on prescription, dental treatment, and glasses, but these charges represent only about two per cent of the total cost of the services provided by the NHS. Certain groups, such as children, the elderly, and those with low incomes, are exempt from these charges. All people resident in Britain can normally receive NHS treatment without need to prove their entitlement; administration is thus kept to a minimum, and represents less than 5 per cent of total expenditure. In contrast, wages and salaries represent about 75 per cent of the total costs of the NHS.

The services provided by the NHS can be roughly divided into hospital services, community health, and general practitioner services. Hospital and community health services provide acute, long-term, psychiatric, geriatric, and maternity care. In England (population about 46.5 million), there are approximately 6 million in-patient attendances in hospitals each year. Two-thirds of these patients receive acute medical or surgical treatment; two-thirds of all hospital beds in use at any given time, however, are occupied by the chronically ill, the elderly, or the mentally ill or handicapped. Hospitals are staffed by approximately 800,000 employees of the NHS; these include technical, administrative, and clerical workers as well as medical and nursing staff.

Family practitioner services include the services of doctors, dentists, opticians, and pharmacists. They all have independent contracts with the NHS, and are not direct employees. In England, there are approximately 21,500 general practitioners; on average, they are consulted by each of

their patients about three times a year.

These main services of the NHS are complemented by other services provided by the Department of Health and Social Security and by local authorities. These include social security cash benefits, and the provision of residential homes or day-care facilities for the elderly and the mentally and physically handicapped. Health visitors and other social workers can relieve general practitioners of many routine tasks, allowing them thus to concentrate on medical work only. Local authorities are also responsible for the maintenance and testing of the public water supply; for the provision of ambulance services (except in London, where ambulances are run by the Greater London Council); for mobile X-ray units; and for the enforcement of many regulations concerning refuse disposal, sanitary facilities in factories and public places, and other matters relevant to public health.

The total cost of the NHS currently represents around six per cent of the gross domestic product, and the figure is steadily rising. It was originally thought that once a higher general standard of health for the nation had been achieved the demand for health services would stabilize at a manageable level. Unfortunately, this has not proved to be the case.

Private practice

The main reasons for the increasing amount of private medical practice in Britain are increasing prosperity, the wish to choose a particular doctor or surgeon, and the need to choose a convenient time for consultation or hospital admission, which the National Health Service can rarely achieve.

Both general practitioners and specialists can work privately, but because many choose to work full-time for the NHS not all doctors can be consulted privately. Fees for private treatment are the responsibility of the patient, but they will normally not include the full cost of all medicines and appliances supplied or used. Private patients may be treated in private rooms of some National Health hospitals if their doctors so arrange, and they will be charged for accommodation.

To help cover the considerable expense of private treatment, many people take out insurance with one of the private medical insurance schemes such as Private Patients' Plan (PPP) or British United Provident Association (BUPA). A person with private medical insurance does not lose any rights to treatment under the National Health Service, but he or she gains no tax concession and must continue to pay the NHS contributions.

The patient and the GP

Many people recognize that the maintenance of good health is an important feature in their lives, but are unwilling to spend time and money in an effort to stay healthy. Yet most people also feel that the relationship between a patient and his or her GP should be something more than a business relationship, such as that which exists between a customer and a shopkeeper. In a patient-doctor relationship, trust, confidence, and communication of knowledge and feelings are also involved.

A patient's first requirement of any doctor is one of competence and ability to treat the patient's illnesses skilfully and effectively. For patients who go to their GP with minor ailments or disorders, this may be all that is necessary. However, there are times when a patient's illness may be associated with emotional stress or anxiety; there are also times when sexual problems, or problems at work or at home, may cause depression and a general feeling of being unwell, even though the patient may be unaware of any obvious physical symptoms. In situations like these, it is natural to look for a responsible, detached, and trustworthy person in whom to confide, and many people look to their GP to fulfil this role. Whether or not this role should be a recognized part of a doctor's job is incidental: the fact remains that patients often make emotional as well as professional demands, and the doctor has to deal with them both.

In some rural areas, where a GP may be looking after relatively few patients, and in certain situations in which the GP has known the patient's family for a long time, there is likely to be a greater understanding of the emotional strains for a patient, an understanding that may make it easier for the doctor to help. These situations, however, are exceptions to the general rule. Many GPs have as many as 3,500 patients in their care, and simply have not got the time to give each patient the amount of attention that the patient or the doctor may feel is necessary.

The patient, therefore, has to make the best use of the GP's time that is possible in the circumstances. All doctors, through their training and professional experience, have considerable knowledge and skills; the patient, however, should not be overawed by this, but should attempt to gain maximum help from the resources that are available through the doctor. All consultations between doctor and patient should involve an exchange of information: the patient's role should be active rather than passive, for the more accurate the information is that the patient gives about his or her symptoms,

feelings, and personal history, the more help the doctor is likely to be able to give. Before a patient visits the GP's surgery, he or she should decide what to say and what to ask. If the patient does not understand what the doctor says, there is every reason to ask for clarification. Understanding the diagnosis and the treatment prescribed may help the patient to benefit from the treatment; it can also increase the patient's trust and confidence in the doctor, and so improve the professional relationship between them.

Most of the information on these pages is given in the form of answers to questions that are often asked by people when they are moving to a new area, choosing a GP, or feeling unsatisfied with their relationship with their GP.

How do I find a general practitioner?

Lists of local GPs are available at the Post Office, local Library and Town Hall. But this is an impersonal way of finding a new doctor, and it is sensible also to ask your neighbours, local chemist and even other shopkeepers for the names of doctors in the neighbourhood. In this way you can get personal advice on the doctor's personality and his particular interest in certain aspects of medicine. Some doctors are particularly good with children for example, while others may be better with the elderly. Find out whether the local doctors work alone or in partnership. Neighbours may give an idea of the way that the practice is organized but it is generally worth an exploratory visit to the doctor's surgery too to see what the practice premises are like.

What should I do if I cannot find a doctor?

If you are unable to find a local general practitioner you should write to the Family Practitioner Committee, giving your NHS number, asking them to put you on the list of a local general practitioner. The Family Practitioner Committee have the power to allocate a doctor to you for a limited period of time: it is the Family Practitioner Committee's legal obligation to supply a medical service. The doctor may, however, if he so wishes, remove you from his or her list at the end of this time; you may then have to go through the whole process of finding another doctor. Fortunately, this rarely happens.

How do I register with a GP?

When you have decided on the doctor you would like to be your GP, visit or telephone the surgery asking if the doctor will accept you as a new patient. General practitioners have the right to refuse to accept a new patient. They may do this if the prospective patient does not live within the area in which they practise; if their list of patients is already full (a doctor is only allowed to have a certain number of NHS patients); or if the doctor simply does not wish to accept the patient. When you have found a doctor who will accept you as a patient, you should fill in Part A, on page 3 of the medical card, applying to be placed on the list of the new doctor, with your signature and your address. The doctor will sign in the space below this and send your card to the Family Practitioner Committee to register your name formally on his or her list. The doctor then receives a fee for undertaking your care. The Family Practitioner Committee will write to your previous doctor asking for your medical records which can then be forwarded to your new doctor. Your name will be removed from your previous doctor's list (so that he or she no longer receives a fee for looking after you), and you will eventually receive a new medical card with your name and address on it, and with the name and address of your new doctor.

Do I have to fill in any forms when I visit the doctor?

On the whole, most consultations with a doctor do not entail any form-filling but, from time to time, your doctor may ask you to sign a form, such as that for a night visit, so that he or she can claim an extra payment for some service that has been done for you. These forms are simple to complete and need not cause you any anxiety.

What should I do if I have lost my card?

This is a common occurrence. Doctors keep a special form, like a small medical card, that can be filled in by the patient and countersigned by the doctor, in the same way as the normal medical card, before it is forwarded to the Family Practitioner Committee.

Special coloured cards – pink in England, Scotland and Wales, and orange in Northern Ireland – are given to the mothers of newborn infants so that the children can be registered with a general practitioner. People leaving the armed forces are also given a special form which should be completed and given to the doctor when registering.

How do I see my GP?

On registering with a doctor, find out the surgery times and whether it is necessary to make an appointment to see him or her. The times of the surgery hours are usually also posted up outside the surgery. Some practices have special clinics for particular conditions or forms of medical attention, such as immunizations, antenatal examinations, or diabetes or high blood pressure clinics.

What is a practice or surgery like?

Practices vary greatly in size. Some comprise only one doctor working with a part-time secretary; others a partnership of several doctors with ancillary help. The number of doctor's assistants in a practice depends in part on the size of the practice. The doctor may have several partners (for legal reasons, a common arrangement is for several doctors to make a business contract between each other) and one or two medical assistants who work part-time (they may be general practitioners in training).

In addition to such medical help, a practitioner may employ a nurse to help with wound dressing, weighing of patients, helping them to undress, assisting with immunization injections, taking blood pressures and examining urine in diabetic clinics. In practices that still do home deliveries of babies, doctors frequently have a midwife to help with antenatal clinics. In areas where there is a large elderly population, a health visitor may be associated with the practice, in conjunction with a community health physician, to visit them. In large practices, a district nurse may have a similar association and will help visit the chronically sick at home who require dressing, injections and home bathing, etc. All these people have some form of professional or nursing qualification.

In addition to qualified help the practice may employ a receptionist, secretary, and filing clerk to help with the day-to-day surgery organization. In practices such as those with six or more doctors, a practice manager may be employed to ensure the smooth organization of the practice, allowing the doctors time for more medical rather than administrative work.

Answering the telephone is one of the more important details in a practice. In off-duty hours the telephone may be transferred to the partner on call, or answered by a machine giving a number to call or asking you to leave a message.

Many practices in large towns and cities also employ an organization to send a deputy doctor to visit their patients during off-duty hours. This means that an unfamiliar (but properly qualified and properly equipped) doctor may visit you when your own doctor is not on duty. In suburban and country areas more practices organize their off-duty hours so that one of the partners, or assistants, is on duty to deal with emergency calls.

Do I have to pay a general practitioner?

No. The only time that a patient may be charged is (1) when the doctor does not want to treat the patient under the NHS and both the patient and doctor are prepared to accept the consultation as a private one; or (2) if a patient claims to be on another doctor's NHS list but is unable to produce a medical card. In this second situation the doctor usually explains to the patient that a charge will be made and a receipt issued. The patient should then send the receipt to the local Family Practitioner Committee who will refund the money to the patient, and deduct it from the doctor's income.

Will my GP visit me at home?

If you are seriously ill with a high temperature or physically unable to visit the surgery, your GP may see you at home. Ring the surgery before 10 a.m., giving brief details of your illness and your full name and address. You may then be visited sometime during the day by your GP or one of his partners or assistants. Unless you are very seriously and suddenly ill, you should not call your doctor between 8 p.m. and 9 a.m. and if the doctor visits you between 11 p.m. and 7 a.m. you, or one of your relatives, will be asked to sign a form which states that you requested the night visit.

What should I do if I move addresses within the same area?

It is essential to inform your doctor for two reasons. The first is to ensure that he or she is still willing to look after you at your new address, and the second is so that the address can be changed on your records in case there is a need to visit you at your new home. The doctor then sends a notice to the Family Practitioner Committee agreeing to keep you on his or her list. You should send your medical card to the Family Practitioner Committee so that a new and accurate one can be returned to you.

What if I am ill when away from home?

If you are away from home for less than three months you should ask the local doctor to accept you as a temporary resident but not actually register you. The doctor will give you a form to complete and sign, and you will be expected to give him your NHS number (on the front of your medical card).

If the doctor treats you on only one or two occasions, or if the doctor does not wish to take you on either as a temporary resident or on his permanent list, a different form will have to be completed acknowledging that you have received treatment from the doctor.

Can I ask my NHS general practitioner to send me to a private specialist?

Yes, the GP first writes a letter to the specialist and either you or your doctor then makes an appointment at the specialist's private consulting rooms. Remember that you will have to pay a fee and it sometimes takes longer to get an appointment with an internationally known specialist in his private rooms than it does with the same specialist at a hospital.

As an NHS patient, can I choose my own specialist?

Yes, but the choice should be made in consultation with your doctor. Unfortunately, the length of the waiting list at the local hospital may be so long that it is often advisable to take the first available appointment with any consultant in the specialty that you require. (If an appointment is really urgent your doctor may be able to get one within a few days provided he is able to give good medical reasons.)

How can I get another medical opinion?

If your doctor suggests, while you are ill, that a further opinion is necessary, he or she usually makes arrangements for you to be seen (as an NHS patient) at the local hospital. However, there may be occasions when, for many understandable reasons, you yourself may want another opinion and may be hesitant about asking for it in the fear that it may upset your doctor.

In fact, though, most doctors do not mind being asked about a second opinion. But the manner in which the approach is made is important: you do not want to give your doctor the feeling that you have lost confidence in his professional ability. A second opinion, if it confirms your doctor's original diagnosis, can be reassuring to both patient and doctor. Even if it differs from your doctor's, treatment can then be modified to prevent any more serious condition occurring.

Can I complain if I think I have been badly treated?

Yes, but a discussion about the problem, with

the doctor, is usually the best way of resolving the problem. Understandably, however, most patients resolve the situation by simply changing to another doctor without explaining their reasons. Complaints about doctors are rare.

If the complaint is serious, the patient may write to the local Family Practitioner Committee, within six weeks, explaining the problem. Complaints can very often be dealt with informally by the chairman of the Family Practitioner Committee who can act as an intermediary, having heard both sides of any set of circumstances. More serious complaints are dealt with by the Committee as a whole, with the patient and doctor present explaining their positions. Although the Community Health Council may help a patient in writing the letter of complaint and in general advice, it can do nothing to influence the complaints procedure before the Family Practitioner Committee.

The Family Practitioner Committee gives a verdict and, if the doctor is found to be at fault, a fine will be imposed on the doctor.

Complaints about hospital treatment and service are dealt with by the hospital administrator.

If a patient still feels that the answer given to the complaint is unsatisfactory, then a further appeal to the Health Service Commissioner, the ombudsman, may be made.

Complaints about a doctor's professional ability and skill involve a much more complex procedure; they cannot be considered by the Family Practitioner Committee. Further medical opinion may have to be sought before legal action for damages, if damage can be proved, may be started.

Rarely, a complaint may be made to the General Medical Council (not the British Medical Association) about a doctor's ethical behaviour. The complaint has to be fully substantiated by the patient before any action is taken.

Understandably, complaints against a doctor almost inevitably lead to the doctor's removing the patient from his or her list, and the complaining patient's having to find another doctor in the area.

Can I change doctors within the same district?
Yes, but you must first ensure that the new doctor will accept you, and you should ask your original doctor to sign Part B on the back of your medical card, stating that he or she agrees to the transfer. When your original doctor has signed the card, you can complete Part A of the medical card in the same way as you would do when transferring to a doctor after moving to a new address.

Prescriptions
A prescription represents an instruction from a doctor to a pharmacist, detailing the type of preparation or drug, the frequency with which it is to be used or given, and any other points that may be necessary for the pharmacist to know.

Some drugs, such as aspirin, do not require a doctor's prescription. Other drugs, such as antibiotics and most commonly prescribed drugs, are legally controlled and require a doctor's prescription with both the patient's and the doctor's name and address. There are a few drugs, such as morphia, amphetamines and a few sleeping pills, that are very strictly controlled by the Misuse of Drugs Act to prevent addiction: these can be dispensed only if the doctor completes a prescription in a particular manner.

Drugs for treatment under the National Health Service are prescribed on a particular form, supplied to the doctor by the Family Practitioner Committee, so that the pharmacist knows that the NHS regulations (for payment of fees, etc.) will apply.

Prescription charges are payable for each item on the prescription. The amount paid varies from time to time.

On the back of the prescription form there is a list of people who are exempt from payment of prescription charges. Children under the age of 16, adults over the age of 60 (women) or 65 (men), and any people who are receiving social security benefits do not have to pay. There are some patients, such as diabetics, who require frequent prescriptions and can obtain a certificate exempting them from further prescription charges on payment of a lump sum for the year.

If you are not sure whether you are exempt from charges, obtain a receipt from your chemist so that if you find you should not have been charged, you can make a claim for a refund using a form obtainable at a post office.

Emergency
In the event of an accident it is usually advisable to dial 999 and call an ambulance. In the event of someone being taken seriously and suddenly ill you should ring your general practitioner and explain what has happened. The doctor may visit you at once or tell you to call an ambulance to take the patient to hospital. In this event the doctor may ring the hospital to forewarn them that a seriously ill patient is arriving.

Hospitals 1

Administration

The practical day-to-day administration of an individual hospital is the responsibility of the Administrative Officer, sometimes known as the Hospital Secretary (and formerly known as the House Governor), who works in co-operation with the Chief Nursing Officer (Matron) and the Medical Staff Committee. Although a large district hospital obviously requires a larger staff than a small children's hospital, the basic administrative structure remains the same for all hospitals.

The Clerk of Works is responsible for the electricians, plumbers, and painters who maintain and repair the hospital buildings, as well as for the specialist technicians who maintain the many different types of specialist medical equipment that are used in a hospital. The Domestic Superintendent is responsible for employing domestic staff, and for maintaining basic standards of cleanliness throughout the hospital. The Catering Manager works with the kitchen staff and dieticians to prepare and cook the food. The Head Porter is responsible for the transporting of both equipment and patients. A special transport office is responsible for the transporting of equipment and patients between hospitals, and also for the ambulance service that brings patients to hospital on admission and takes them home on discharge. Although most hospitals keep a store of essential equipment, each District Management Team or Area Health Authority maintains a supply of special equipment that can be transported to individual hospitals when required.

A Senior Office Administrator supervises the typists and clerks who work with the administrators and medical staff in the hospital, as well as the ward clerks who help with the day-to-day administration of the wards. A special administrative office is responsible for the organization of the admission of patients to the hospital and of the waiting list of patients due to be admitted. The waiting list is commonly divided into two groups: those requiring urgent admission, such as patients with cancer, and those requiring routine admission, such as patients with hernias, or patients requiring tonsillectomy or special investigations.

The efficient running of a hospital depends on good co-ordination between the different departments and much routine hard work that is carried out day and night. However, if the hospital administration is efficient, most patients, as well as most doctors and nurses, remain unaware of the many different background activities involved.

Departments and special units

The most familiar hospital departments are the out-patients department and the accident or emergency department. Efficient appointment systems can greatly reduce unnecessary delays and waiting time in out-patients departments. Emergency departments are for patients requiring immediate treatment, often for injuries sustained in road or other accidents, and are not for patients with minor illnesses or complaints. Most emergency departments have a small X-ray unit attached to them.

Although some medical tests and investigations can be carried out in the patient's ward (*see* **Wards,** p.718), most investigations have to be done in special departments. These departments are under the control of senior doctors, but most of the tests and investigations are carried out by skilled technicians. These technicians are usually prepared to discuss with the patient what they are doing, but only the consultant, or other senior medical staff, has the responsibility to inform the patient of the results of the investigations.

There are special departments for X-rays, electrocardiograms, electroencephalograms, and specialized hearing and eye tests. In larger hospitals, there is often a department of nuclear medicine that uses radioactive isotopes in the investigation and, sometimes, treatment of diseases. Special departments concerned with treatment in a hospital include physiotherapy and occupational therapy departments, speech therapy, and, in psychiatric hospitals, group therapy departments. In hospitals concerned with the treatment of cancer, the radiotherapy and the allied department in nuclear medicine help in treatment of malignant diseases.

Patients who are seriously ill, or badly hurt in an accident, and who require all the facilities of a hospital in addition to highly skilled nursing in one place, are admitted to the intensive therapy unit (ITU), also called the intensive care unit. In larger hospitals a similar unit, the coronary care unit, specializes in the treatment of patients with myocardial infarctions, or heart attacks.

Patients needing an operation are taken to the operating suite, where an anaesthetic will be administered in the anaesthetic room before they are taken to the operating theatre. After more serious operations, patients often spend a short time in the intensive therapy unit before returning to the ward. This ensures specialized treatment during the most hazardous time following an operation.

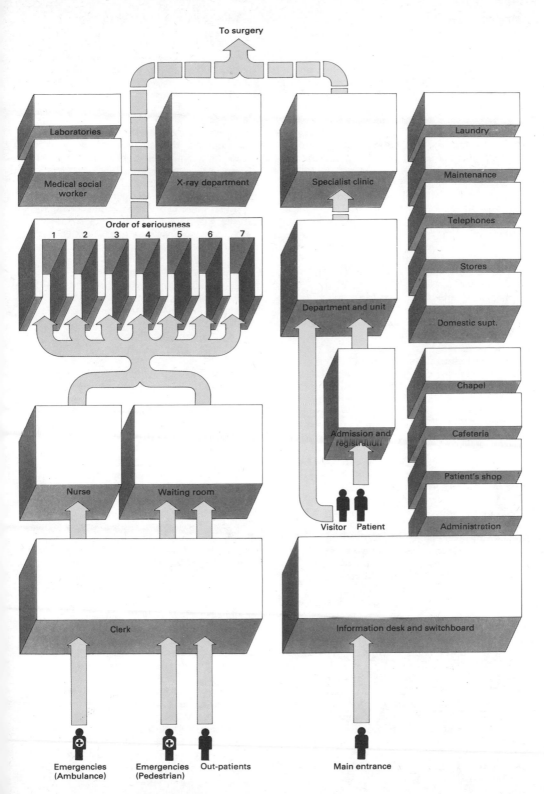

To surgery

Laboratories

Medical social worker

X-ray department

Specialist clinic

Laundry

Maintenance

Telephones

Stores

Domestic supt.

Order of seriousness

1 2 3 4 5 6 7

Department and unit

Chapel

Cafeteria

Patient's shop

Administration

Nurse

Waiting room

Admission and registration

Visitor   Patient

Clerk

Information desk and switchboard

Emergencies (Ambulance)

Emergencies (Pedestrian)

Out-patients

Main entrance

Hospitals 2

Medical staff

The senior medical specialists on the staff of a hospital are the consultants, who are usually appointed at about the age of 35 and remain on the hospital staff until retirement at the age of 65. These senior doctors may be responsible for a large number of patients in two or three hospitals in the same area, and usually visit each hospital about two or three times a week.

More junior doctors, known as Registrars, are responsible for the day-to-day care of patients in a hospital. Registrars are doctors who are in training for the medical specialty (such as heart or intestinal disorders) that is the particular interest of the consultant with whom they work. Senior Registrars, who are completing their training, are appointed to a hospital for four years; Junior Registrars are appointed for two years.

The doctors whom a patient will see most frequently are called House Officers (or Housemen), and are resident in a hospital. In the United Kingdom, a doctor may not legally start in practice until he or she has worked as a House Officer for two periods of six months each in hospitals approved by the General Medical Council as suitable for completing a doctor's training. When these posts have been completed, the provisionally qualified doctor can obtain full registration. Many House Officers, therefore, are junior doctors who have recently qualified, although there are others who are fully registered doctors.

Every patient in a hospital is cared for by a team of doctors consisting of a consultant and one or more Registrars and House Officers. This team is commonly known as a "firm". In teaching hospitals the "firms" are usually larger than in non-teaching hospitals, as they include the professor, research assistants, lecturers, and associated medical students.

In hospital departments with which patients may have little immediate contact, such as the X-ray and pathological departments, the staffing structure is similar.

Nursing Staff

The Principal Nursing Officer (PNO) is a senior nurse who is responsible for several hospitals within a district. Within each hospital there is a Chief Nursing Officer (CNO), ordinarily known as the Matron, and each ward or department is under the supervision of a Nursing Officer, generally called the Sister, or a Nursing Officer of a lower grade, called a Staff or, if male, a Charge Nurse. Every Nursing Officer has qualified as a State Registered Nurse (SRN).

Most ward sisters work with a team consisting of at least one other SRN and other nurses who are in training. There are two forms of training that a nurse may follow: one is a three-year course leading to qualification as an SRN, and the other is a two-year course leading to qualification as a State Enrolled Nurse (SEN). All nurses may be distinguished by the differences in their uniforms.

The sister is responsible for the organization of the nurses within each ward, and for arranging their duty hours, their days off, and, where necessary, their times for studying. The sister tries to ensure that only a limited number of nurses care for each individual patient, so that there is as much continuity of personal care as posible.

Psychiatric nurses may follow similar three- and two-year training courses to qualify as Registered Mental Nurses or State Enrolled Nurses (M). Further specialized training is necessary for the care of the mentally handicapped and the mentally subnormal. Midwives need the basic SRN qualification before they continue their training to qualify as a State Certified Midwife (SCM).

Paramedical staff

In addition to doctors, surgeons, and nurses, there are many other workers with specialist training who are part of the staff of any hospital. These may include physiotherapists, radiographers, laboratory and ECG technicians, occupational and speech therapists, and, in mental hospitals, psychiatric social workers and academically qualified psychologists. Radiographers, who take X-rays, can usually be identified by small rectangular badges worn on the lapel that record the amount of radiation to which the individual has been subjected.

Attached to most "firms" there is a Medical Social Worker (formerly known as an Almoner), who is responsible for the social care of the patient. The MSW helps with any financial or domestic problems that a patient may have, and acts as a link between the hospital and the Community Health Officer. In this way arrangements can be made for home helps, visits by district nurses, and structural alterations to a handicapped patient's home.

Other visitors to patients in hospital wards may include priests of various denominations, members of the Red Cross and St John Ambulance Brigade, and members of the League of Friends of the hospital. Voluntary organizations also help with the hospital's library service and with trolleys containing toiletries and sweets.

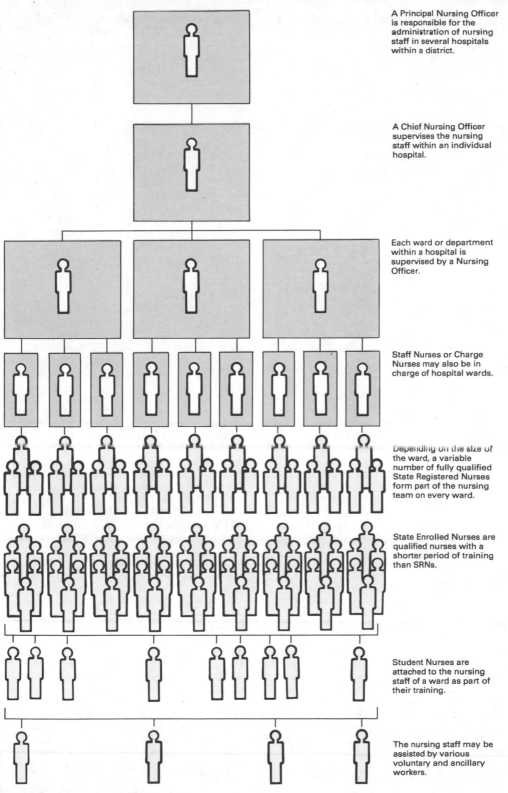

A Principal Nursing Officer is responsible for the administration of nursing staff in several hospitals within a district.

A Chief Nursing Officer supervises the nursing staff within an individual hospital.

Each ward or department within a hospital is supervised by a Nursing Officer.

Staff Nurses or Charge Nurses may also be in charge of hospital wards.

Depending on the size of the ward, a variable number of fully qualified State Registered Nurses form part of the nursing team on every ward.

State Enrolled Nurses are qualified nurses with a shorter period of training than SRNs.

Student Nurses are attached to the nursing staff of a ward as part of their training.

The nursing staff may be assisted by various voluntary and ancillary workers.

Wards

The typical main hospital ward has about twenty beds, or may be subdivided into small wards containing two or four beds each. In most wards there are one or two single rooms for the more seriously ill patients.

In addition to the main part of the ward, there is an office for the sister and the other nursing staff, a room for the use of the doctors, a treatment room, a kitchen, and a sluice where bedpans can be washed out. In modern hospitals there is often a separate day room for the use of patients who are able to walk around. This room contains comfortable chairs and usually a television set.

Some hospitals have mixed-sex wards, but place patients in separate wards if they prefer this.

Children's wards often have special facilities and are brightly decorated to relieve a child's anxiety. Visiting hours for parents in children's wards are very flexible, and it is usually possible for one parent to stay overnight with the child.

After admission to the ward, the patient is cared for by the nursing staff responsible for that ward and a consultant, who is assisted by a team of more junior doctors.

The bed

The modern hospital bed is specially designed so that the doctor or the nurse can adjust the height of the bed, and the angle of either the foot or the head of the bed.

The bed should be low enough to enable the patient to sit on the edge and touch the floor with the flat of the feet. It is then safe for the patient to assume a standing position, especially if he or she is weak or elderly. On the other hand, the nurse may prefer to raise the height of the bed for bathing the patient, changing dressings, or making the bed when the patient is sitting in his or her chair.

Hospital mattresses are, for several reasons, firmer than mattresses sold commercially. A soft mattress allows the hip and abdomen to sink downward, causing an appreciable curvature of the spine. A firm mattress not only alleviates backache, but makes routine examination easier for the doctor.

Bedsores are difficult to avoid when nursing a patient who cannot move because of paralysis, coma, or pain. A soft mattress encourages bedsores because the part of the body that sinks downward sweats more and receives less air. The skin can quickly become damp and soft, making it more susceptible to ulceration.

On the console near the bed is a push-button bell which is used to summon assistance. There is often a bell to call the day staff, and one to call the night nurse. The console may also be equipped with headphones and a radio and television tuner that enables the patient to listen to the radio and watch television. There are some other devices and aids on the console, some for the benefit of the nursing staff, and some for the patient.

Next to the bed is a bedside table with drawers and compartments for personal possessions. The table is usually on rollers to make bedmaking easier for the nursing staff, so the patient should not use the table as a support when getting out of bed.

Above the bed is a variable-angle wall lamp for reading, but after 9 o'clock in the evening, the wall lights are dimmed to a night light. The night lights allow the nursing staff to give necessary medications during the night.

Toilet facilities

Some hospitals provide a small washbasin with taps next to the bed to allow the patient to sit on the edge of the bed to wash, brush his or her teeth, or shave. The hospital may provide facilities to enable the patient to buy small toilet articles such as toothpaste and soap.

The bathroom is usually near to the beds, and is provided with a toilet, shower, and washbasin with bars on the walls placed in strategic positions to help the patient use the facilities. There are no locks on the doors of the bathrooms, and patients must use the "occupied" notice for privacy. The reason for this is if a patient faints, or falls in the bathroom, the nursing staff needs free access to the room. Sometimes the bathroom partitions do not reach to the full height of the ceiling. Again, this is to enable a member of the staff to get over the partition if a patient falls across the door on the inside. If a patient is not well enough to use the bathroom, the nursing staff may bathe the patient in bed. Similarly, the patient can use a bedpan and urine bottle if he or she cannot get to the bathroom.

Restraints

The use of restraints in the hospital often shocks and angers relatives and friends of the patient, but there is sometimes reason for the use of restraints. If a patient is confused for any reason, particularly during the night, he or she may be restrained in bed with a device other than the bedrail. This is because the risk of the patient injuring himself or herself is high if he or she is able to wander around the ward.

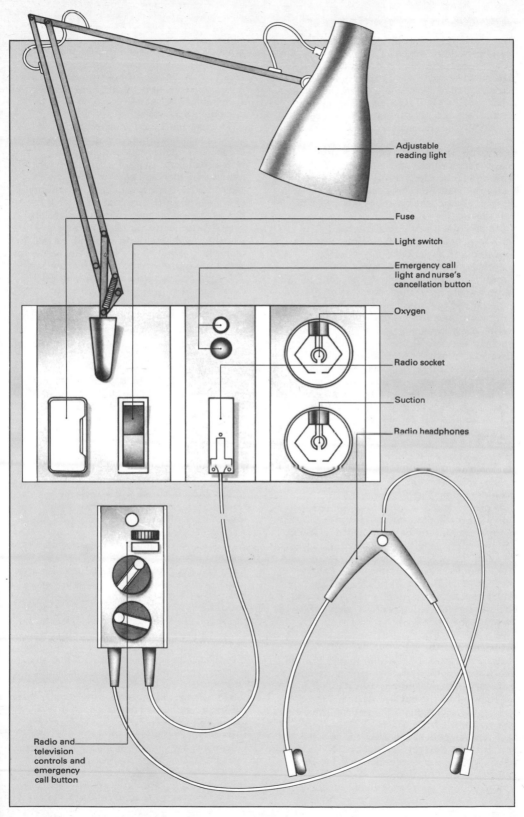

Adjustable reading light

Fuse

Light switch

Emergency call light and nurse's cancellation button

Oxygen

Radio socket

Suction

Radio headphones

Radio and television controls and emergency call button

Admission and routine tests

There are three ways in which a patient may be admitted to a hospital.

The usual admission procedure is for the patient to be referred to the hospital outpatients department by a GP for specialist advice, and then, if the hospital specialist decides that an operation or specialized investigations are necessary, the patient's name is placed on the waiting list for hospital admission. If the condition is very serious, the patient's name is placed on the urgent waiting list for admission as soon as a bed becomes available; if the condition is less serious, the patient's name is placed on the routine waiting list.

At any one time there are about half a million people on hospital waiting lists in England and Wales. Waiting times vary greatly between different areas of the country, and according to whether the patient requires surgery or other forms of treatment. When a bed becomes available, the patient will be sent a letter or telegram asking him or her to come to the hospital at a certain time on a certain date. If the hospital does not send a list of what clothes to bring, the patient should take pyjamas or night-dress, slippers, a dressing gown, and toilet articles.

The other two ways in which a patient may enter hospital as an in-patient involve direct admission through the emergency department. Either the patient is taken directly to the emergency department following an accident, or the patient's GP decides that the patient's illness requires urgent treatment and arranges for the patient's immediate admission.

Whichever way a patient is admitted to hospital, certain formalities have to be completed. A form has to be filled in giving the patient's name, sex, age, address, and religion, as well as the name and address of the patient's nearest relative and of the patient's GP. A copy of this form is kept by the admissions office, and a further copy is included in the patient's notes when taken up to the ward.

Routine tests

After a person has been admitted to hospital, there are several routine tests that are done on every patient. These tests are usually carried out by the nursing staff, and the results are recorded on the patient's chart at the end of the bed.

After the patient has reached the ward and has undressed to get into the bed, he or she is asked to produce a specimen of urine. A nurse will test this to detect any abnormalities, such as albumen, sugar, or blood, as well as the degree of acidity and,

sometimes, the concentration (specific gravity). These tests are simple to carry out, and are usually done in the sluice or ward lavatory. The nurse will use specially prepared strips of paper that are covered with patches of chemicals which react to constituents in the urine.

The patient is then weighed and, sometimes, measured. The measurements are recorded in metric units; all hospital instruments and drugs now conform to the metric system. The height and weight measurements show whether the patient is over or under the expected weight for his or her particular height and age, and are also useful for certain tests and treatments. The measurements are particularly important for children and babies, for whom the dosage of drugs is adjusted to the individual's weight.

Height and weight measurements also enable doctors to assess the effects of treatment. For example, treatment of patients with heart failure, who have an excessive amount of fluid in the body, with diuretic drugs (which increase the volume of urine) causes not only a lot of urine to be passed, but also a rapid loss of weight.

As well as weighing and measuring the patient, a nurse will also take the patient's blood pressure. If this is normal, there will be no need to take it again, unless the doctor requests it. If there is any abnormality, the pressure being higher or lower than usual, the blood pressure test has to be repeated regularly, usually every four hours, to see if the abnormality remains constant. At the same time, the nurse will record the temperature, pulse, and breathing rates, and this procedure is repeated every four hours, or twice a day.

The above routine tests are done on all patients admitted to hospital. There are, however, many other tests that may be done as a routine when patients are admitted to hospital with particular illnesses or conditions. These tests are done to provide the specialist with basic information about the patient before any treatment is given.

Some hospitals carry out a large number of blood tests on every patient admitted as a matter of routine, but this is the exception and not the rule in Britain.

Many surgeons automatically require tests for haemoglobin (to detect anaemia), blood group and Rhesus factor, and electrolytes (blood salts) to be carried out on all patients before any big operation. In most patients over the age of forty an electrocardiogram (ECG) and a chest X-ray are taken so that the normal, pre-operative appearance is known in case any complications follow the operation. None of these investigations indicates that the surgeon considers that there is something wrong, and the patient should have no cause to feel frightened. Rather, the patient should feel reassured by these investigations that every possible care is being taken.

Hospital tests inevitably vary from patient to patient: different disorders require different investigations. Although every patient has the right to know why a particular test or investigation is being carried out, most patients accept routine tests without asking for precise details of the reasons. While they are carrying out tests, nurses and technicians often talk to patients and explain what they are doing in simple terms, and many patients find this reassuring.

Technicians are not allowed, however, to tell patients the results of the tests they carry out: this responsibility lies with the consultant or another senior doctor.

Details of some of the more common tests and investigations that may be experienced by patients in hospitals are given below. This section is unable to consider all the possible tests a patient can have done, but by explaining the significance of the most common tests in a diagnosis, it is hoped that a patient will submit to the tests with interest, not impatience. A test is less alarming if the patient knows what to expect beforehand.

Blood samples

You can be certain that during a stay in a hospital you will receive many visits from a laboratory technician who will take a sample of blood. You will notice that the technican who draws your blood will collect it in glass tubes with rubber stoppers of different colours. For a full blood count (FBC) the stopper is usually a red colour because there is a chemical in the tube which stops the blood from clotting. For many other tests the stopper is white and the tube is plain glass. The blood is allowed to clot and the clear yellowish fluid known as serum is used for testing. With modern needles and experienced technicians the discomfort of having your blood taken is minimal.

Full blood count

When a FBC is done the technicians calculate the number of red blood cells per cubic millimetre of blood. They also look at the size and shape of the cells, the proportion of red cells to the total amount of blood (the haematocrit), and the amount of haemoglobin (protein in the red cells that carries oxygen to the tissues) in the sample. A low red blood cell count is called anaemia.

If you are anaemic your body cells may not receive an adequate supply of oxygen. A common cause of anaemia is loss of blood, or lack of iron in the diet, but it may also be caused by a malfunction of the bone marrow that produces the cells, or an increased rate of destruction of the red cells which should survive for about four months before being broken down.

The technicians also look at the white cells. Although there is only one variety of red blood cell, there are several different types of white blood cell. They are one of the main body defences against infection and disease. An increase in the number of normal white cells is often seen if the body is fighting an infection such as appendicitis or pneumonia. Although a normal white blood count (WBC) would not exclude the condition, it would make it less likely. An excessive number of abnormal white cells may indicate leukaemia.

The technicians also investigate the blood's ability to clot. If there is a break in a blood vessel wall, it is plugged by small components in the blood known as platelets, which release a chemical and start the process of clotting. A platelet count is part of the automated FBC now used universally.

Continuous flow analysis

Another test that requires a blood sample is run on a machine called a continuous flow analyser. With barely 20ml. of blood the technicians can run twelve to twenty different tests at appreciably less cost than if the various chemical tests were ordered individually. Several different body functions are screened, and if a result is abnormal it may provide a useful clue to some disorder or condition. Sometimes the routine screening picks up an elevation of blood sugar long before any symptoms of diabetes have developed, and although no treatment is needed, the patient can be advised to alter his or her diet.

Blood clotting tests

In addition to the many blood tests used to help in diagnosis, there are other tests which are used to gauge the severity of a disease, or the effectiveness of treatment. For instance, the victim of a heart attack has daily blood tests taken to measure the level in the blood of chemicals released from damaged or dead heart cells. The more extensive the damage the higher the proportion of chemicals in the bloodstream.

Some conditions, for instance thrombophlebitis of the deep veins, are treated with agents to slow down the rate of clotting. Tests are done daily before drugs

Electrocardiogram (ECG)

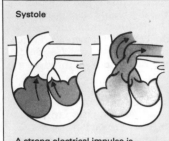

Systole

A strong electrical impulse is produced causing a strong systolic contraction.

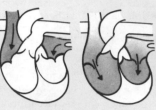

Diastole

A weaker electrical impulse is recorded prior to atrial contraction or diastole.

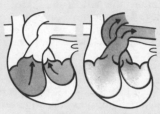

Systole

A small presystolic contraction stimulates the strong systolic contraction.

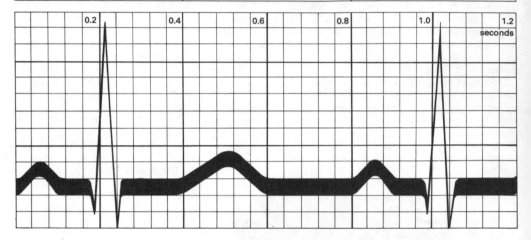

0.2	0.4	0.6	0.8	1.0	1.2

seconds

NORMAL

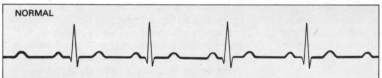

ATRIAL FIBRILLATION

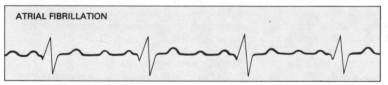

RECENT INFARCTION

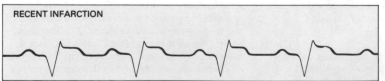

OLD INFARCTION

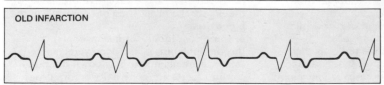

As the breakdown of the ECG chart shows, each impulse of the heart is accurately recorded through the sensitive electrodes placed on the patient's body. The doctor is able to study the strength and the quality of each phase of the heartbeat and identify disorders such as atrial fibrillation. On this recording, the doctor can see that the atrial impulse is weak and irregular, thus preventing adequate systolic impulses. Similarly, the recording of a patient who has had an infarct recently, or a patient who has suffered an infarct some time before, is easily identified by the unusual ECG recording.

are given to ensure that the interference with the clotting is not too great.

Frequent taking of blood can be tedious for the patient. But it makes everything more interesting if you ask the technician what the tests are for. The technician may welcome the chance to explain. Remember, he or she cannot tell you why a test has been ordered, or talk about the result. This is the responsibility of the consultant.

Electrocardiograph

An electrocardiograph (ECG) records the electrical activity of the heartbeat. The test is safe and painless because the electrical impulses flow from the patient to the machine, not the other way around. Electrodes are placed on the patient's wrists, ankles, and chest, and adequate contact is achieved by moistening the skin with jelly before applying the electrodes. The resulting graph is useful even if it is a normal recording, because it is changes in the ECG that are important. When a doctor is faced with an ECG recording with questionable changes, it is a great help if there are previous normal tracings for comparison. It should be emphasized that repeated ECG tests do not imply that there is something seriously wrong with your heart.

Stress test

A common test of cardiac efficiency is the stress test, which is usually done as a "screen" for coronary artery disease before any disease is obvious. Although it is more commonly an out-patient procedure, it is usually done in a hospital cardiac department. Electrodes are attached to the patient, who walks slowly on a revolving rubber treadmill. The speed is gradually increased, and the heart rate is kept under constant observation for any signs of strain.

X-ray photographs

A chest X-ray used to be routine for any patient in the hospital. Today there is evidence that routine chest X-rays performed on people under the age of thirty with no respiratory or cardiac symptoms are no longer justified. The amount of radiation received during a chest X-ray is negligible, but any unnecessary exposure to radiation is now avoided.

X-ray photographs of the stomach, the bowel, the gall bladder, and the kidneys demand special techniques, and the patient has to be prepared beforehand. The stomach and intestine must be completely empty because any food that is retained reduces the quality and clarity of the X-ray. The patient must fast for at least half a day before the X-ray. He or she is also given laxatives followed by an enema to clear the large intestine.

For a stomach and bowel X-ray the patient has to drink a thick chalky liquid known as a barium meal. It is completely flavourless. The patient lies down for the X-ray, and may have to wait long intervals between films to allow the barium to move through the system before another organ is outlined.

For a kidney X-ray, known as an IVP (intravenous pyelogram), the patient is given a small injection. A similar procedure may be used before X-raying the gall bladder.

Nuclear scanning

Nuclear scanning is a simple and safe procedure. A chemical is injected into the bloodstream. It is called a radioactive tracer, and it is taken up by various organs in the body. The concentration of radioactive material in the various organs is measured with a Geiger-Müller counter, giving an impression of their size and ability to function. The test is often used as a safe screening procedure to determine whether there is an abnormality that might require further, more complicated tests.

Ultrasound and echo-studies

These studies are used mainly for examinations of the heart and abdomen. The procedures are painless and completely safe. They work on the same principle as radar in that the sound waves or ultrasound waves reflect off different tissues at different rates, enabling an image to be formed.

Computerized axial tomography

One of the more dramatic advances in recent years is the CAT scan. Information that formerly could only be obtained by exploratory surgery can now often be gathered with accuracy and safety. For instance, the investigation of certain brain diseases sometimes required a procedure called air encephalography that was painful for the patient, required the services of a neurologist, a radiologist, and a technician, and involved some danger. The CAT scan has made this procedure rarely necessary. From the patient's point of view the scan is no more troublesome than having one's photograph taken.

Respiratory laboratory

This is where the efficiency of a patient's lung function is tested. The test normally involves little more than breathing in and out of a series of machines, but may also include some blood sampling.

Physical examinations and consultations 1

One of the duties of the nursing staff who receive a patient on the ward is to notify a member of the resident medical staff that the patient has arrived so that the resident doctor or houseman (a recently qualified doctor who lives in a hospital) can take a history of the patient's present condition and previous illnesses. The doctor also examines the patient and gives instructions to the nursing staff about treatment and general care of the patient, medication, special diets and whether or not the patient is allowed out of bed.

A doctor usually takes the history soon after the patient has settled into the ward. The interview is likely to be quite long, and some of the questions may be reviewed by other members of the staff. The patient must co-operate to the best of his or her ability, and should never insist that because the family doctor has taken all the details already, repetition is unnecessary. Often the patient forgets to tell his or her own doctor about something, and this comes to light only during the interview in hospital. This medical history is the most important single factor in helping the doctor to make a diagnosis – it is often more important than a physical examination, the tests, or the X-rays even with the sophisticated equipment in modern hospitals.

Giving a history

Doctors vary in their interview technique, but commonly the doctor begins by discussing the patient's main symptoms, because obviously this is causing the patient the most concern. When the doctor asks you what is wrong, you should explain the most prominent symptom or symptoms, such as shortness of breath, or abdominal pain. The doctor does not want to hear your own diagnosis.

The questions that follow relate to the presenting symptom. For example, if you are complaining of abdominal pain, the doctor will ask you to describe the pain; whether the pain has changed position; whether the pain is related to particular foods; and whether the pain has become localized or has spread to other areas of the abdomen. The doctor will ask questions relating to the intensity of the pain (a question commonly asked of mothers is whether the pain is as intense as labour pains). The doctor will also want to know if anything makes the pain worse, such as moving a limb, or whether anything eases the pain, such as sitting up or lying down. The doctor will ask if you notice any other symptoms at the same time as the pain, for instance gas or flatulence.

After the questions concerning the main complaint, the doctor will probably ask about your past medical history. The questions will cover such areas as previous major illnesses (do not forget to mention any childhood illnesses you have had); whether you have undergone surgery (you should mention even the most minor operations, such as removal of a mole); and whether you have been treated for a disorder (remember to mention minor disorders such as indigestion). The doctor will ask a female patient about her menstrual and obstetric history, for example the regularity of menstruation; whether menstruation is painful; the number of children she has had; whether all the pregnancies and labours were normal; and whether there were any postnatal complications. A female patient must remember to mention any blood pressure problems during pregnancy, or complications such as forceps delivery or induced labour. If you have ever been in hospital, you will be asked the year and your home address at the time, the name of the previous hospital, and the doctor in charge of your case.

The doctor will ask what job you do and whether it exposes you to any particular hazards, or emotional stress. A patient's social history can give the doctor valuable clues towards reaching a diagnosis.

The doctor will ask if your parents are still alive – if they are not, he or she will want to know what they died of and at what age. If you are an adopted child, you should mention it. The doctor may also ask direct questions about conditions and illnesses in the family, such as whether any member of the family has suffered from tuberculosis, a stroke, or heart disease.

The doctor will want to know about your drinking and smoking habits. This is not so that he or she can criticize or pry into your habits; such information is relevant to your state of health and can help the doctor to reach the correct diagnosis. Therefore, it is important to answer the questions as accurately as possible.

The doctor will then probably move on to questions related to drugs and other medicines. A patient often denies taking drugs regularly only to admit after closer questioning that he or she has been taking antacids to counteract indigestion for several years, or a laxative every morning. It is most important to think carefully before answering – the doctor will not mind your mentioning something that is irrelevant, but an omission could result in an inaccurate diagnosis. It is essential to mention whether or not you take oral contraceptives – many women do not regard this as regular medication, but during major surgery they can encourage the formation of blood clots that could prove fatal. The doctor will also want to know about drug and other allergies.

At the end of the medical history many doctors make a general survey of all the body's systems, asking direct questions about each. This is a sort of screening that gives the patient a last chance to remember anything that may be important. The questions about the chest may include whether and how much you smoke; whether you ever get out of breath when climbing stairs; and whether you ever cough up mucus. Questions about the bowels may include the frequency of bowel movements; whether you have ever noticed blood in the faeces; and whether you have felt bowel discomfort at any time. Questions about the urinogenital system may include the frequency of urination; whether you have ever noticed pain or burning on urination; whether you have ever noticed blood or cloudiness in the urine; whether you have ever suffered from stress incontinence or abnormally frequent urination; and whether you have ever had difficulty in urinating. A female patient may also be asked about her menstrual cycle.

The examination

After the interview, the doctor will probably give you a thorough examination. Again, the order in which the doctor examines you may vary; he or she may begin by examining the physical signs of the actual condition, or may begin by examining the head and neck and work down the body. The illustrations show the main examinations, and explain what the doctor is looking for in each system. If the disorder is associated with a limb, the doctor always begins by examining the healthy limb. This is to discover what the healthy limb is like in order to give a standard against which the unhealthy limb can be compared. A pelvic or rectal examination may also be included.

At the conclusion of the examination the doctor usually makes some comment about the impression he or she has formed. You must remember however, that the first doctor you see is usually less experienced than the consultant, and will not have any results of tests or X-rays, so it is unlikely that he or she will be able to make an accurate diagnosis at this point. If the first doctor was a houseman, you may have to go through the questions and examination again, this time by a more senior doctor. Finally you will see the doctor in charge. If you ask all three for their opinion you may get three slightly different answers, and many people get worried in this situation because they feel that there is some uncertainty about their case. A patient may worry because one doctor orders a stomach X-ray, whereas another suggests a gallbladder X-ray first. Both have a good reason for their opinion, and the final diagnosis will be achieved either way, but techniques do differ. Another cause of worry is confusion about the terms that a doctor uses. A patient may be told by one doctor that he or she has a peptic ulcer, whereas another may say the patient is suffering from a duodenal ulcer. This is because a duodenal ulcer is a type of peptic ulcer, not because the diagnosis is different. The safest policy to adopt is always talk to the doctor in charge of your case. He or she can give an opinion based on the information from the other doctors and explain any confusion or misunderstandings.

If your condition is rare or unusual in any way, you may be asked if you are willing to be examined by medical students. If your condition is exceptional, you may also be asked to be the subject of a special medical consultation at which the doctor in charge of your case presents the details of your condition to a number of consultants and specialists. During the consultation any of the doctors may ask you questions. You may also be asked to perform certain actions to demonstrate a particular point. For example if you have sustained a mouth injury, you may be asked to talk or whistle.

Preparation

You can prepare information in advance for the medical history. It is often difficult to recall at short notice the exact year that you had a certain operation done, for example, an appendicectomy at the age of six, or a tonsillectomy at the age of ten. You can find out the dates before you are admitted to the hospital. In fact, many patients forget about major operations in childhood, and the doctor discovers that such operations have been performed only when he or she sees the surgical scars. If you are uncertain about the cause of death, or the age at death, of a parent or grandparent, try to get the facts from another family member. If you are taking regular medication, look carefully at the bottles, and write down the name of the drug, and the dosage, or take the drug with you.

Although the outcome of your hospital stay depends on the skill and concern of those who look after you, your own participation should not be entirely passive. A patient's history is vitally important, and you should do everything in your power to ensure that the history and facts that you provide are accurate and concise.

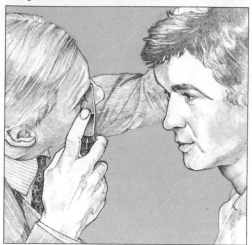

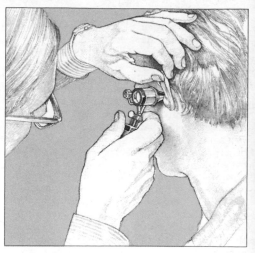

Eye examination

The doctor will ask you to move your eyes in all directions to test the function of the eye muscles. After shining a light into each eye to test the reaction of the iris, the doctor will use an ophthalmoscope to study the retina of the eye. The retina reflects the state of the small blood vessels in the body. Sometimes the doctor may also check the pressure within the eyeball.

Ear examination

The doctor uses an otoscope to examine the outer ear and the eardrum. The otoscope is a cone-shaped instrument with a light that illuminates the canal. The doctor can then see that the canal is healthy, and not inflamed, that the ear is not obstructed by hardened wax that has accumulated at the base of the canal, and that the eardrum is a normal colour and healthy.

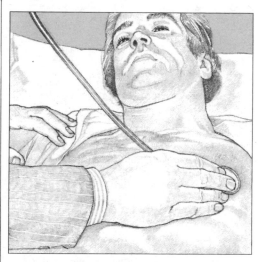

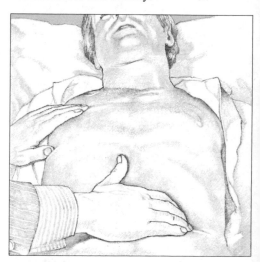

Heart examination

Initially, the doctor assesses the size and position of the heart by percussion, and by placing a hand on the chest wall to feel for the point of the strongest heartbeat. He or she then listens to the heart with a stethoscope to detect any abnormal heart murmurs that may indicate valve disease, abnormal heartbeat, or the presence of fluid in the sac around the heart.

Abdominal examination

The doctor will press each side of the abdomen just below the ribs to detect an enlarged liver or spleen. The mid or lower abdomen is then pressed gently to detect any abnormal masses, such as enlarged kidneys. The doctor may then listen to the abdomen with a stethoscope to detect any abnormal sounds within the abdominal cavity and internal organs.

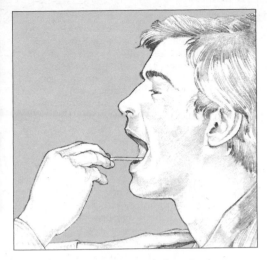

Mouth and throat examination

The doctor will ask you to open your mouth wide so that he or she can see inside the mouth and throat. The doctor will also press your tongue down with a wooden spatula, and ask you to say "Aaah". This moves the tongue out of the way, and moves organs in the back of the throat, such as the tonsils, into view. The doctor can then see that there is no throat inflammation.

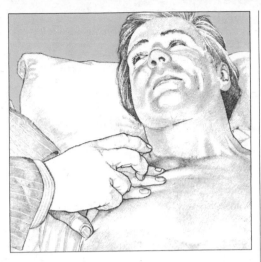

Chest examination

First, the doctor will ask you to take a few deep breaths to see that both sides of the chest move normally. He or she will then tap on the chest with the fingers. A normal chest has a faint, hollow sound when examined in this way (percussed) and the presence of solid tissue changes the sound. The doctor will then listen to the movement of air in and out of the lungs with a stethoscope.

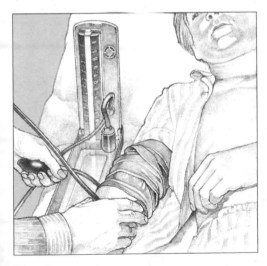

Blood pressure

The doctor measures your blood pressure with a sphygmomanometer. A cuff is wrapped around the upper arm, and inflated to stop the blood flow. The doctor places a stethoscope over the front of the elbow, and listens while the pressure in the cuff is gradually released, and determines the level at which blood flow first restarts (systolic) and is continuous (diastolic).

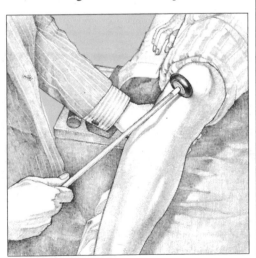

Reflex examination

The doctor will test the reactions of the nervous system by noting the speed with which the body responds when muscle tendons are suddenly stretched. This is done by gently tapping them with a special hammer. The reflexes are tested at the elbow, wrist, knee and ankle. The big toe reflex is tested by stroking the outer side of the foot

Undergoing surgery

Surgery may be necessary for many reasons. It may offer a patient the only chance of survival in an emergency, or slow down the rate of a progressive disease such as cancer. Surgery may be performed to improve the quality of a person's life as in a total hip replacement, or it may be done to improve a person cosmetically. Surgery may also be performed as a diagnostic aid, for instance, the removal of a mole or enlarged gland to test for malignancy, or it may be performed to remove some obstruction or disturbance of normal bodily function.

Your doctor and the consultant surgeon will explain exactly why the operation is being performed, how it will be done, the chances of success, and any possible side effects or complications. You will then be asked to sign a consent form (*see* p.730).

For four hours before the operation you will not be allowed to eat or drink, and if someone mistakenly offers you something, refuse it. The stomach must be empty before the anaesthetic is given, because if there is anything in it the patient may vomit during the operation and inhale the vomit.

The area of the incision is shaved, and shortly before you go to the operating theatre it may be cleaned with an antiseptic soap and covered with a sterile dressing.

About an hour before you are taken to the anaesthetic room, you will be given an injection that makes you drowsy and dry in the mouth. This is called a "premed", an abbreviation of pre-operative medication. It is a combination of drugs that calms you and drys up the secretions of saliva and mucus.

Anaesthesia

Most major surgical operations are performed under a general anaesthetic. Before this is given to you, the anaesthetist injects intravenous anaesthetic into a vein on the back of your hand. While the anaesthetic is slowly injected, the anaesthetist may ask you to count. As the drug begins to take effect, your concentration will fail quickly.

A patient who has an operation may have an intravenous drip put into a vein in the arm. It is inserted while you are under the influence of the anaesthetic, and strapped to your wrist to prevent movement of the needle. The intravenous drip serves several purposes. Fluid can be infused through the vein to prevent dehydration and if a blood transfusion is needed quickly the drip is already set up. Also, the same drip can be used to give muscle-relaxing drugs.

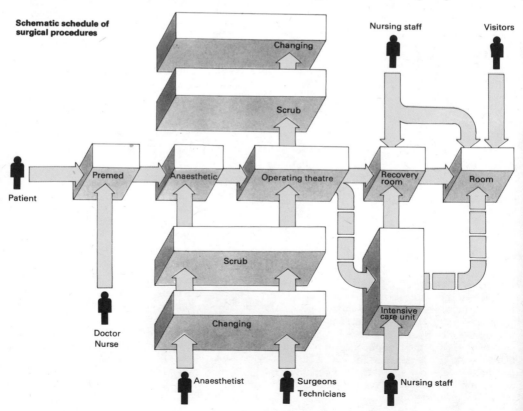

Schematic schedule of surgical procedures

Changing

Scrub

Nursing staff

Visitors

Premed

Anaesthetic

Operating theatre

Recovery room

Room

Patient

Doctor
Nurse

Scrub

Changing

Intensive care unit

Anaesthetist

Surgeons
Technicians

Nursing staff

Operation

During the operation the anaesthetist keeps a constant check on your pulse rate, blood pressure, and breathing. In certain circumstances, it may become necessary during an operation to carry out blood transfusions or intravenous injections.

All the apparatus used during the operation is carefully checked beforehand, and all the gauze sponges are carefully counted before and after the incision is closed.

When the operation is complete the surgeon closes the incision. From the patient's point of view, one of the most important things is a neat scar but the surgeon must always have sufficient room to perform the operation effectively. Because of this the scar may be larger than the patient expected. Initially the surgeon stitches the underlying tissues with sutures that are eventually absorbed by the body tissues, and uses a similar type of material to sew the layer of fat beneath the skin. Finally the surgeon joins the edges of the skin together. This is done either with nylon or silk thread stitches, or metal skin clips.

If the incision is in an area under a great deal of pressure, for instance, a large abdominal incision, the surgeon may insert large-tension stitches to support the skin stitches, particularly if the patient has a chest problem and may strain the incision by coughing. Clips tend to mark the skin less than stitches, but cannot be used if the area of the incision is under great tension.

It is sometimes necessary to leave a drain in the incision to allow blood and other secretions to escape either into the dressing or into a special bottle. The drain is either a tube or a piece of plastic or rubber. This is normal procedure following an operation such as a cholecystectomy.

If an incision has hardly any pressure exerted on it, for example on the face, the surgeon can use butterfly sutures. These are pieces of adhesive tape shaped like a butterfly that are stuck on to the skin to hold it together. The incision is supported by the dissolving stitches in the deep tissue layer, and the butterfly sutures have only to exert a slight pressure to keep the skin edges together until the skin heals. This method leaves no stitch marks at all. Another type of suture that leaves the skin free of stitch marks is the subcuticular suture. A silk thread is run, just below the skin, from one side of the incision to the other. This pulls the edges together until they heal, when the thread is drawn out.

Post-operative care

After the operation, you will be taken to the recovery room where you will be nursed until you wake up from the anaesthetic. A nurse will talk to you to help you regain consciousness. You will be kept under close observation before you wake up, and your pulse, respiration, and blood pressure will be recorded at frequent intervals. The nurse will ask if you have any pain and, if necessary, he or she will give you an injection of a painkilling drug. You will be kept in the recovery room until you are fully awake, and your pulse, temperature, blood pressure, and breathing are all stable. Some people feel nauseated after the anaesthetic, and may even vomit, although this is increasingly uncommon with modern anaesthetics. The nurse will watch for any indications of potentially serious post-operative complications such as shock, bleeding, or discharge from the incision.

You will be taken from the recovery room to the intensive care unit or your ward. Again, a nurse will attend you during the journey. If you are taken to the intensive care unit it does not indicate that something has gone wrong during the operation, or that you are in any danger. After certain operations careful monitoring is essential. This is easier to do in the intensive care unit with special equipment than in a bed on a ward.

Pain relief

A patient is naturally concerned about post-operative pain. It is impossible to predict how much pain a patient will have because awareness of pain and tolerance of pain vary from person to person. Powerful narcotics relieve pain efficiently and are given to most patients for the first four or five days after major surgery. The surgeon, during the preparation for the operation, should have given you some idea of what to expect in terms of soreness. However, in the unlikely event of him or her not doing so, you should ask because if you know what to expect, you will find it easier to cope with your aftercare and will not be unduly anxious about the type of discomfort that is normal for your operation.

In modern post-operative care every effort is made to get the patient out of bed and moving around as soon as possible. This practice has proved to be beneficial to the patient because it has reduced the occurrence of complications such as lung infection, lung collapse, thrombophlebitis (clotting in the veins), and emboli (movement of clots to the heart or lungs).

Consent

Before any surgical operation, the patient must sign an official consent form stating that he or she agrees to the operation being performed. This consent must be based on the patient's reasonable understanding of what is being agreed to, and the doctor or surgeon must explain clearly the nature of the operation and the risks involved before the patient is asked to sign the consent form.

At the time of giving consent, the patient may be asked to consent also to any further operation that the doctor or surgeon may consider necessary if complications arise during the operation.

If a patient is under 16 years old, consent must be given by the patient's parent or guardian. If a patient is unconscious or mentally ill, consent must be obtained from the patient's nearest relative or legal guardian. If a patient is compulsorily detained under the Mental Health Act, medical or surgical treatment may be carried out without the patient's consent.

The rights of consent are the same for both married and unmarried patients.

To the Medical Staff and Board of Governors

CONSENT BY PATIENT

I   JEREMY ROBINSON   of   17, THE CLOSE, REDHILL

hereby consent to undergo the operation of   INJECTION OF VARICOSE VEINS

the nature and effect of which have been explained to me by Dr/Mr   PARKER

I also consent to such further or alternative operative measures as may be found to be necessary during the course of the operation and to the administration of a local or other anaesthetic for any of these purposes.

Date   24th MARCH 1981   Signed   J Robinson

I confirm that I have explained to the patient the nature and effect of this operation.

Date   24th MARCH 1981   Signed   G Parker

Intravenous infusions (drips)

If you have had surgery involving the digestive tract you will not be able to eat for several days. You will have to rely on an intravenous drip for nutrition. It may also be necessary to remove the secretions to your stomach and intestines with a tube which passes down one nostril to the stomach.

After an abdominal operation the intestines tend to lose their normal function temporarily and instead of continually contracting and relaxing to pass on the contents, they become inactive. This is why you may not be allowed foods or fluids by mouth. The surgeon will listen to the abdomen with a stethoscope because it is possible to hear sounds of returning function. It is common for the return of intestinal movement to be accompanied by several hours of uncomfortable swelling which is relieved by passing flatus. This may be followed by several loose bowel movements. The nurse will want to know when you first pass gas after the operation.

Post-operative exercises

After any type of surgery under a general anaesthetic and particularly if the operation involves the chest or abdomen, it is difficult to take deep breaths or to cough. The air is distributed to the lungs by a system of tubes which subdivide into increasingly smaller tubes, ending in grape-shaped alveoli. The tubes produce mucus which forms a thin sticky, coating that traps tiny particles of dust or bacteria. The mucus is constantly moved toward the larger tubes and coughed up. If you cannot take a deep breath, then the mucus accumulates in the base of the lungs blocking the smaller tubes. Once this has happened the area of blocked lung collapses and becomes highly susceptible to infection. For this reason, a physiotherapist will visit you after your operation to help you to breath deeply and cough up any sputum. You will be given adequate pain relief and shown how to make the coughing less painful. It is important to continue with these breathing and coughing exercises.

Muscular exercises

It is essential to keep the circulation in the legs moving to prevent deep vein thrombosis and possible embolism. Before the operation the physiotherapist will teach you exercises such as bending the knees, or forcefully contracting the leg muscles.

Painkilling drugs sometimes suppress a patient's urge to empty the bladder. This is more common in men than women, and may cause problems with passing urine.

Convalescence

After the first day or two, you will begin to feel better and the drains and intravenous drips will usually be removed. You will be encouraged to sit in the chair by the bed as much as possible, and go for short walks around the floor.

Silk stitches and clips are usually removed after eight to ten days. On a large abdominal scar every second stitch is removed on one day, and the rest are removed a day or two later. The stitch is cut below the knot and pulled out with a pair of forceps. It is no more uncomfortable than having a hair plucked out. To remove clips the nurse uses a special pair of forceps which are placed under the clip and squeezed to open it. Again, the discomfort is minimal. Butterfly sutures are removed like a piece of adhesive tape.

The scar is cleaned with an antiseptic solution and re-covered with an ordinary dressing. A deep scar does not fade completely for up to a year, although by the time the stitches come out the wound is stable enough for normal daily activities. At first the scar is a raised, red line but as the line fades to white, the swelling slowly reduces and the scar shrinks. You may experience a slight tingling sensation or numbness in the skin surrounding the scar, but this usually disappears after a few months.

If you have had tension sutures placed by the wound, these are removed usually a few days after the stitches in your skin. The tension stitches are clipped on one side and pulled through on the other side.

Once the sutures are removed you are usually ready to go home. After some operations it is possible to return home before the stitches are removed. Ask the surgeon what activities you are allowed to do at home, and when it is safe to resume normal physical activities. For some operations the patient is given a written list of instructions to follow.

While you are in the hospital there are a number of milestones that help you to gauge your rate of recovery – the first time you walk to the bathroom unaided, the first walk outside your ward, or the first time you can cough without pain. Many patients find that once they arrive home and are in familiar surroundings they realize they need more time to recuperate before they are completely back to normal. A patient may feel weak after walking up a few steps and may suffer from depression during the first days at home. It is important to realize your limitations. If you have any worries about your rate of progress, the best person to talk to is your family doctor.

Hospital routine for a patient

Most hospitals have a strict routine that begins early in the morning, usually before 7 a.m. when the patients are woken by the night staff. Shortly afterwards, the night staff take the patients' temperature, breathing and pulse rates, before going off-duty. These are taken at intervals throughout the day and the results are recorded on the patients' charts, which are at the end of the beds. After this, patients are usually offered tea and are allowed out of bed to wash. Patients who are confined to bed or who are unable to wash themselves are washed by a nurse. The beds are also made before breakfast, which is usually served at about 7.30 a.m.

After breakfast, the nurses in surgical wards change the patients' dressings before the ward is cleaned. This is to prevent the wounds from becoming contaminated by dust that is disturbed by the cleaning. Most of these procedures are finished by 9 a.m. After the wards have been cleaned, patients usually return to bed in preparation for the doctor's rounds, during which most patients are examined and questioned by the doctor.

In the middle of the morning the patients may be offered tea, coffee, or cocoa. Lunch is usually served at about 12.30 p.m. In the afternoon most patients are encouraged to rest before visiting time. At about 4 p.m. tea is served; supper is usually served at about 6 p.m. After supper, many hospitals allow evening visitors, usually from about 7 p.m. to 8 p.m.

After the visitors have left, the beds may be remade, and the patients may wash before settling for the night. The main ward lights are turned out at about 9 p.m., but many hospitals allow patients to listen to the radio with headphones or to read for a short time before going to sleep.

A patient who has difficulty in sleeping may be given a sedative drug that helps to overcome sleeping problems. For certain patients, however, there may be medical reasons that preclude the use of such drugs.

Throughout the day, patients are given drugs, intravenous fluids and any other treatment that is necessary. Various investigations, such as barium meals and electrocardiograms, may also be performed. In surgical wards operations are usually performed only on particular days. Each specialist has certain days for operating. The wards are often very busy on such days as patients are taken to and from operating theatres.

Meals and special diets

Some hospitals offer a selection of food for the main meals. But this is not the case in all hospitals, although great efforts are being made to increase the quality and variety of food in hospitals. All hospitals cater for vegetarian and various religious diets. If a selection is available, the choice a patient is offered may be limited by special dietary restrictions imposed by the doctor. Apart from regular meals, there are usually provisions for small snacks for the patients to make themselves.

Special diets are used in the treatment and management of certain disorders. For example, if a patient is suffering from an acute liver or kidney disorder, a low-protein diet may be prescribed. A low-fibre diet may be prescribed for some intestinal disorders, and a high-fibre diet for diverticular disease. Obese patients may be given a low-calorie diet to encourage loss of weight. Diabetics are maintained on a carbohydrate-controlled diet. The hospital's catering department can provide special diets for patients who need them. Details of other special diets that a doctor may prescribe are described in **Special diets,** pp.684–691.

A patient should consult the doctor in charge of his or her case before accepting food or drink brought in by visitors. If a visitor is uncertain as to what is allowed, he or she should consult the staff nurse of the ward. It may be detrimental to a patient's health to supply him or her with extra food.

Ward routine

Doctors usually make their ward rounds during the morning. During these rounds the patient is examined and questioned by the doctor in charge of his or her case. The doctors are accompanied by the staff nurse, who reports on the progress of each patient. If the consultant wants a second opinion, or if a patient's condition is medically interesting, a consultant who specializes in that condition may also examine the patient. In teaching hospitals some patients may be used in demonstrations to students about their particular disorder. Most hospitals give patients the choice of refusing to be examined by students, but some make it a condition of admittance that any patient can be examined if necessary. It is reasonable for anybody who enters a teaching hospital to expect to be examined by students, and by co-operating in this way, the patient is helping to train future doctors. Patients who do not wish to be seen by students should ask their GP to send them to a different hospital.

It is during the doctor's rounds that patients should ask any questions they may have. The doctor will try to answer in terms that the patient can understand. Doctors are

TEMPERATURE CHART

Patient's Name: ENTHOVEN, ADRIAN

Hospital No. 107216

Floor: 10

Room No. 14

MONTH	DATE											
FEB	17	18	19	20	21	22	23	24	25	26	27	28

Body temperature varies daily. The highest temperatures are usually recorded in the evening, and the lowest in the morning. A patient's temperature is usually measured four times each day.

Pulse (in beats per minute) is also recorded four times each day, at the same times as the patient's temperature.

DISCHARGED

AMOXICILLIN 250mg 6 HOURLY ORAL

A note is kept of any medication that the patient receives during his or her stay in the hospital.

Respiration is measured and recorded.

A record of the patient's bowel movements, and of weight and blood pressure is also made on a daily basis.

In some cases, urine tests are made and details of the analysis are recorded.

	17	18	19	20	21	22	23	24	25	26	27	28
BOWEL ACTION	0 0 1 0	1 0 0 0	0 0 0 1	0 0 1	0 0 0 0	0 0 0 0	0 0 0 0	1 1 0 0	0 1 0 0 0			
WEIGHT	126	124	120	121	120	120	120	119	119			
BLOOD PRESSURE	160/90	168/84	170/80	140/84	136/80	123/74	118/70	110/70	116/72			
URINE SG	1018	1018			1008			1004				
BLOOD	N.I	N.I			N.I			N.I				
BILIRUBIN	N.I	N.I			N.I			N.I				
KETONES	Trace	N.I			N.I			N.I				
GLUCOSE	N.I	N.I			N.I			N.I				
PROTEIN	Trace	Trace			N.I			N.I				
pH	Acid	Acid			Acid			Alk.				

733

not encouraged to discuss the case in front of the patient. For a person without medical knowledge, it may be alarming to hear doctors discussing medical matters that the patient does not fully understand. If a patient is worried by a remark made between doctors, he or she should ask for clarification immediately.

Visiting

Most hospitals have certain visiting times each day. The precise times vary from hospital to hospital, but few permit afternoon visiting before about 2 p.m. and evening visiting usually finishes at about 8 p.m. Some hospitals allow evening visiting only on certain days. Many hospitals extend the visiting times at weekends.

Visiting is restricted to the permitted times to enable the hospital staff to carry out their work with the least disturbance. Visiting may be allowed outside the normal times in certain circumstances, however; for example if a patient is seriously ill, or if a relative has travelled a great distance to see a particular patient.

There may be a limit on the number of visitors allowed to see a patient at any one time. This rule may not be strictly enforced unless, as occasionally happens, the system is abused and patients in nearby beds are disturbed by a crowd of noisy visitors.

Before entering a ward, a visitor should always ask the nurse in charge of the ward whether he or she may visit a particular patient. This is necessary as the patient may not be in the ward, perhaps because he or she is having a special test in another part of the hospital, or, occasionally, because the patient is too ill to receive visitors.

Visitors can be a positive help to the patient in several ways. They can boost the patient's morale, encourage a patient with a poor appetite to eat and drink, and, if the doctor consents, can help to take the patient for a short walk. But visitors should also remember that the patient is a captive audience and may tire easily. A few short visits are less tiring than one long visit.

Patients who find that they are getting unduly tired by visitors, or who do not want to be visited by certain people should inform the nurse in charge of the ward: there are various ways of protecting a patient from unwanted visitors without causing embarrassment.

Children's hospitals and wards often have different visiting times and other routines. Most allow visiting at any time of the day or night, and for extended periods; many allow

Sample diets	Bland diet	Low-fat diet	High-fibre diet
Breakfast	Fruit juice Cereal, milk and sugar Eggs (boiled or poached, not fried) Toast and butter	Fruit juice Cereal, milk and sugar Egg (boiled or poached, not fried) Tea with skimmed milk	Fruit juice Whole-grain cereal or bran, milk and sugar Whole-grain bread Weak tea
Lunch	Cream soup White fish Creamed potatoes Cooked vegetables Stewed fruit and custard Milk or weak tea	Liver or veal or white fish Boiled potatoes Cooked vegetables Fruit Skimmed milk	Lean meat Potatoes Vegetables such as spinach or cabbage Stewed fruit Buttermilk
Supper	Chicken or lean meat Cooked vegetables Sponge cake or jelly Milk or weak tea	Cottage cheese Salad (without oil or dressing) Fruit or cake Skimmed milk	Cheese or lean meat Salad Whole-grain bread Fresh fruit Weak tea

Sample meals

A large number of special diets are prescribed as part of the treatment of certain disorders (see **Special diets,** p.684). The chart above gives sample meals for three diets commonly prescribed in hospitals. The bland diet is often prescribed for patients who have fever or who are convalescent. The low-fat diet is suitable for patients suffering from gall bladder disease. The high-fibre diet is for patients suffering from constipation.

a mother to sleep with a seriously ill child. The different procedures are discussed more fully in **A child in hospital,** p.736.

Hospital facilities
The facilities that are available to patients vary considerably between different hospitals. Most hospitals provide a radio relay: a set of headphones by each bed, so that other patients are not disturbed. The relay usually has only a limited selection of stations. Many hospitals also provide a television set, usually in a separate room to minimize the disturbance to other patients. A mobile telephone is usually available for patients in bed: the telephone is on a trolley and can be connected by the side of the patient's bed. Most hospitals also offer library facilities, usually run by a volunteer who goes round the wards with a library trolley. A mobile shop may also be taken around the wards, selling such items as magazines, toiletries, and stationery. In most hospitals, newspapers must be ordered and collected from the porter's lodge; patients who are fit enough usually collect the papers for all of their own ward. It is a good idea for patients to keep a small amount of money to buy papers and other items, and to ask visitors to bring in books and magazines if the hospital does not have an adequate library service.

Smoking is prohibited in most parts of a hospital but there may be a separate room in which smoking is permitted. Any room that uses oxygen has a sign forbidding smoking.

Talking to a consultant
The time for a patient to talk to the doctor in charge of his or her case or a specialist is during the ward rounds. The doctor will give an explanation of the patient's condition and answer any questions. This gives the patient the opportunity to keep relatives and other visitors fully informed as to his or her progress. However, if the relatives are anxious about the patient's condition, they should talk to the nurse in charge of the ward who is familiar with the patient's case and who can usually explain what is happening. If the relatives are still worried, they can ask the nurse to make an appointment to see the consultant.

If the patient is seriously ill, or develops an unexpected complication, the nurse in charge of the ward usually makes an appointment for the nearest relatives to see the specialist without a specific request from them. The consultant will discuss the patient's condition and, if possible, explain the likely outcome of the illness. Occasionally, however, a patient may ask the doctor not to divulge his or her condition, and, in this situation it is not possible for the doctor to talk to the relatives.

Discharge
The doctor in charge of a patient's case usually decides when the patient is fit enough to leave hospital. The patient is informed a day or two before the scheduled date so that relatives can be told and make arrangements to collect the patient.

Before discharge, the houseman who has been caring for the patient arranges for drugs, dressings, and any other necessary equipment to be taken by the patient on leaving. The patient is also given an appointment to visit the consultant in the out-patients department a week or two later. The junior doctor (houseman) sends a brief note of the patient's condition and any prescribed drugs to the family doctor.

If the patient is unable to arrange for collection on the day of discharge, an ambulance will be arranged to take him or her home. It is usual for relatives to bring a suitcase and help the patient to pack. It is important to ensure that nothing is forgotten because it is difficult for the nurses to identify a patient's personal belongings and arrange for them to be forwarded.

Some patients may be transferred from hospital to a convalescent home for further recuperation before returning home. In such cases, the hospital arranges transport to the convalescent home. As with a normal discharge, the patient is given drugs and other necessary equipment before leaving hospital, and a letter is sent to the doctor at the convalescent home informing him or her of the patient's condition and treatment.

When a patient is discharged, a nurse accompanies him or her to the hospital entrance to say goodbye and to give the porter or admissions office a note that states the bed is empty.

Discharge against medical advice
Any patient is entitled to discharge himself or herself from hospital at any time, unless detained for compulsory treatment under the Mental Health Act. Patients are asked to sign a form stating that they have refused treatment and are discharging themselves. This form is countersigned by a doctor or the nurse in charge of the ward. If a patient refuses to sign the form, the doctor or nurse still sign it and add a note to the effect that the patient has refused both to be treated and to acknowledge that fact. This is a legal requirement to prevent the patient from suing the hospital for inadequate treatment.

A child in hospital

Fortunately for young patients there have been enormous advances in the technical and professional aspects of child care as well as in the understanding of the emotional needs of hospitalized children. Twenty or thirty years ago there was a general feeling that small patients were easier to handle if their parents did not visit them too often. Now it is recognized that although a stay in the hospital is a worrying period for any child, the experience can be less frightening and traumatic if the parents are actively involved in the child's care and recovery.

Before admission

It is probably kinder to delay telling a child under the age of six they are going into the hospital until a few days before the event. This means that the child does not face weeks of worry. However, an older child, particularly one of late school age, may find it easier to know in advance.

Before any child goes into the hospital for surgery, you should make sure that he or she understands which part of the body is going to be operated on, and how the surgeon is going to get there. You must be receptive to any questions the child wants to ask, because often what seems like a thorough explanation to an adult summons up horrific ideas in the mind of a child. For instance, a child may be convinced that the only way a surgeon can reach the adenoids is by taking off the nose. The child will want to know if the operation is going to hurt, and you can explain that an anaesthetic is given before the operation, which makes you go to sleep. Explain that if the child is sore after waking up, the doctor or nurse will give something to ease the soreness.

Older children require detailed answers to questions, and may even want to read about the condition and operation themselves. If your child asks a question which you cannot answer with confidence, discuss it with your family doctor.

Admission

Take the child's immunization record with you, and if your child is adopted or you are a legal guardian, the hospital may require you to show the necessary papers. Some hospitals send pre-admission papers to you ahead of time so that you can prepare.

The pre-admission testing may be done before you and your child are taken to the hospital ward. With a small child the blood sample can be obtained by pricking the heel or finger, which is less painful and frightening than the application of a tourniquet and a needle.

Modern hospitals try to make the surroundings attractive and reassuring, and this is particularly evident in children's units.

The child should not be deprived of any favourite toys or books during his or her stay. The nursing staff is aware of this need.

A child under the age of six is more likely to be frightened by separation from his or her parents than by the actual experience of a stay in the hospital.

Visiting hours

Visiting hours for parents in nearly all hospitals are now unlimited. If you want to stay overnight with your child, the hospital may be able to arrange this. Visits by other people are more subject to general hospital rules, but ask the nurse in charge of the unit if you would like to bring other children in to see the young patient.

When you are at the hospital you may be encouraged to help with the care of the child, by bathing him or her, and helping to give medicines. If you have any questions to ask, talk to the senior nurse on the ward, or the doctor during one of the rounds.

Convalescence

A child is well enough to be out of bed when he or she feels like it. Children's wards are very different from an adult ward – play is actively encouraged, and the children spend most of their time out of bed. They sometimes eat their meals at a communal table, and the children who are too unwell to be up can be wheeled into the main play area so that they can watch the other children. Very sick children do not mind a noisy atmosphere because it relaxes them.

Some hospitals employ a play therapist who works with the nursing team. The therapist encourages and organizes play, and is often able to identify signs of emotional worry through the child's play. The child is also encouraged to learn about his or her experience of being in a hospital.

Discharge from the hospital

Despite the efforts to make a child's experience of hospitalization as free from fear and pain as possible, the child is bound to be affected in some way. Children under the age of four may refuse to let the parent out of sight for a moment when they are home again, and cling as if afraid of losing the parent again. Some children revert to bed-wetting, or may have sleeping and eating problems. All these should be temporary, but need to be handled with sympathy. If the child keeps coming downstairs in the evening, indulge the whim for a few days.

During an out-patient
visit a parent's
participation is important,
particularly with a child
under the age of three who
may be frightened by
having a routine
examination. When the
doctor wants to examine
the child's eyes, nose, or
mouth the parent should
hold the child firmly (but
not roughly). Place one
hand on the child's
forehead, and the other
around the arm. The child's
legs can be firmly held
between the legs. If the
doctor wants to look at the
child's ear, the child can be
held facing to one side,
and the head held firmly
against the parent's chest.
Talk to the child during the
examination, and never
grip him or her tightly if
struggling begins. The
doctor will gain the child's
confidence during the
examination by being
completely honest when
something is going to hurt.
The parent must not try to
distract the child's
attention or tell him or her
to look the other way if
something uncomfortable
is about to take place,
because the child will not
trust the doctor during the
rest of the examination.
The doctor usually decides
whether or not to discuss
the child's case in front of
him or her, but if you feel
strongly against it, talk to
the doctor who can
arrange to discuss the case
with you in private.

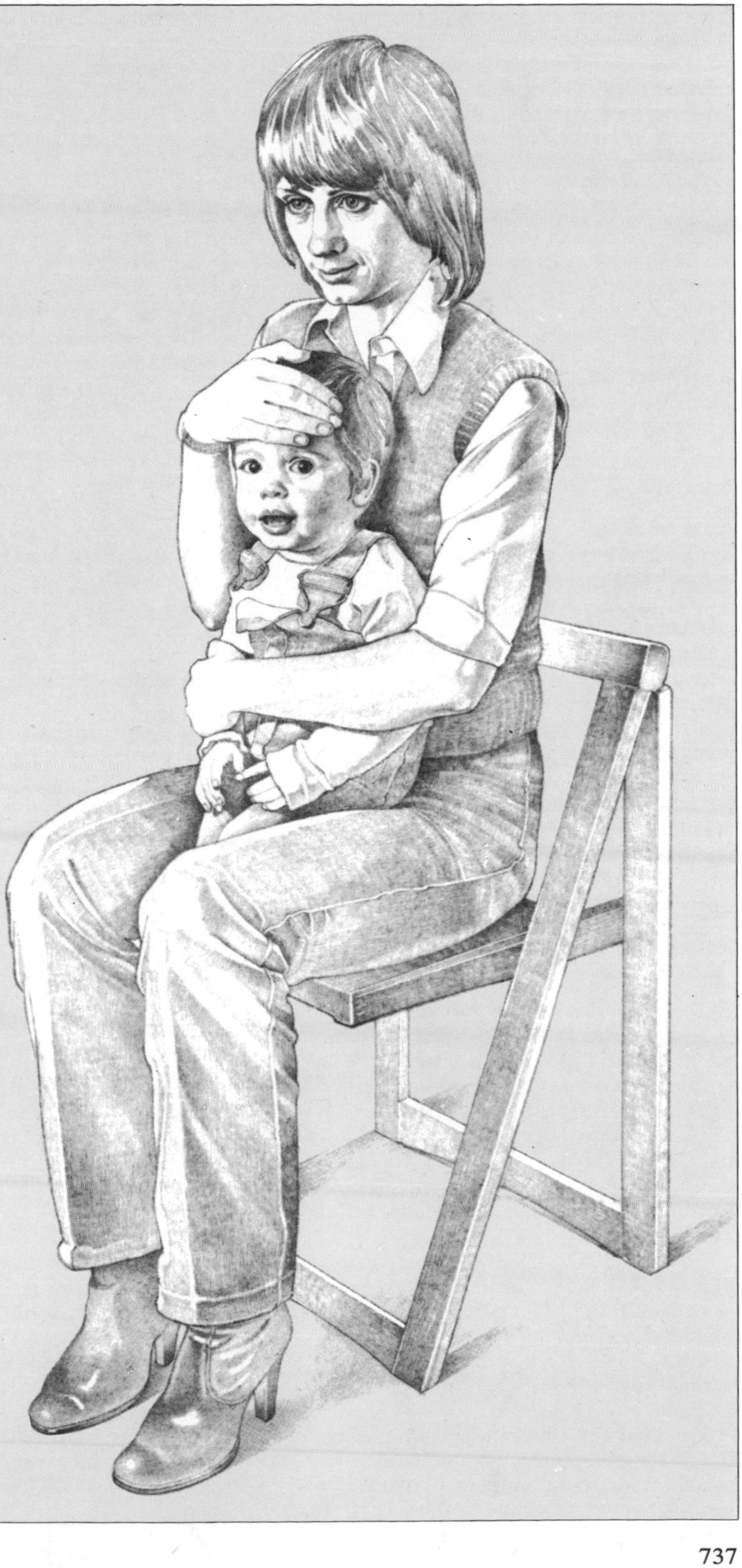

Social security benefits

This section explains some of the social security benefits and welfare services to which a person, or his or her dependants, may be entitled. For some of these benefits and services, a person's entitlement may depend upon the number of national insurance contributions he or she has paid. Generally, it is also necessary to be resident in the United Kingdom. In many cases, the amount of benefit that a person receives is affected by the payment of other benefits, or by a change in his or her circumstances or those of a dependant.

Social security benefits are subject to alterations regarding the amount payable and the criteria for entitlement. Consequently, if a person has any doubt as to whether or not he or she is entitled to a particular benefit or service, or thinks that he or she may qualify for a benefit that is not described in this section, then the person should contact the local social security office.

Cash benefits

The attendance allowance is a weekly payment for people who are so severely handicapped, either physically or mentally, as to require continual supervision or frequent attention throughout the day or night or both, either in connection with bodily functions, or to avoid personal danger or danger to others. The claimant must be examined by a doctor before the Attendance Allowance Board can decide whether or not the claimant satisfies these medical conditions. Children under sixteen must satisfy the additional requirement of needing substantially more supervision than normal for a child of the same sex and age. Children under two are ineligible for this allowance. Before the allowance is payable, the claimant must have satisfied the entitlement conditions for at least six months. A person's entitlement does not depend upon his or her national insurance contributions.

There are two rates of this allowance: a higher rate for those who need supervision during the day and at night; and a lower rate for those needing supervision either during the day or at night.

The attendance allowance is normally paid in full in addition to other national insurance benefits. However, in certain circumstances, such as a constant attendance allowance being paid under the industrial injuries scheme, the attendance allowance may be affected.

The death grant is a lump sum payable on the death of a person who has paid a specified minimum number of national insurance contributions, or the wife, husband, or child of a contributor. In certain circumstances, such as the death of a handicapped person who has never been able to work, the contributions of a near relative may be used to satisfy the contribution requirements, thereby enabling the grant to be paid.

When the deceased has left a will, the grant is usually paid to the executors. In other cases, it is normally paid to the person who pays the funeral expenses, or to the next of kin. The amount of the grant depends upon the age of the deceased.

The industrial death benefit is a pension, allowance, or gratuity for a death that resulted from an industrial accident or disease. If the deceased was entitled to a constant attendance allowance under the industrial injuries scheme, death is presumed to have resulted from the effects of the accident or disease.

Industrial death benefit is normally paid to widows and dependent children but, in certain circumstances, other dependent relatives and women having care of a child of the deceased may be entitled to payment. Entitlement to the basic rate of benefit does not depend upon national insurance contributions.

Industrial widow's pension is paid to the wife of the deceased. There are three rates of this pension. The highest rate is paid for the twenty-six weeks following death; an earnings-related supplement may also be payable during this period. After twenty-six weeks, either of two lower, permanent rates are paid, according to individual circumstances.

For other dependants, industrial death benefit is in the form of a pension, allowance, or gratuity, according to their relationship to the deceased and the extent to which they were being maintained by him or her at the time of death. For dependent children of the deceased, there is an allowance payable in addition to child benefit. There are two rates of this allowance: the higher rate if they are cared for by the widow; the lower rate if cared for by somebody else.

The industrial disablement benefit is a pension or lump sum gratuity for disablement that results from an industrial accident or disease. It is payable from the time injury benefit stops, or after three days if the claimant has not been prevented from working. In the latter case, the claimant is ineligible for injury benefit. Disablement benefit can be paid in addition to certain other national insurance benefits, such as sickness, invalidity, or unemployment benefit.

To qualify for disablement benefit, the claimant must have suffered a loss of physical or mental faculties. This includes disfigurement, even where this causes no bodily handicap. It is not necessary to have paid national insurance contributions to qualify for disablement benefit. It is not payable, however, if the disablement was caused by an accident or disease resulting from employment before 5 July 1948. In such cases, an allowance may be payable under other compensation schemes.

The amount of benefit depends upon the extent of disablement (measured as a percentage) as assessed by a medical board. For disablement of under twenty per cent, the benefit is normally paid as a lump sum; those with a greater degree of disablement usually receive a pension. The pension is usually awarded for a definite period, after which the claimant's medical condition is reassessed. In addition to the basic benefit, the claimant may also qualify for a special hardship allowance, constant attendance allowance, hospital treatment allowance, or unemployability supplement.

The industrial injury benefit is a weekly payment to employees who cannot work because of an accident at work or because of certain industrial diseases resulting from work. Entitlement does not depend upon national insurance contributions.

Injury benefit is paid whether the effect of the injury is immediate or delayed. It is not payable, however, if the injury or disease resulted from employment before 5 July 1948. Generally, an accident at work is considered to have occurred as a result of work, unless there is evidence to the contrary. If the injured person cannot work, he or she should send a medical certificate to the local social security office.

Injury benefit is payable for a maximum of twenty-six weeks from the date of the accident or development of the disease, but not usually for the first three days of incapacity. In some cases, a person receiving injury benefit may also qualify for an earnings-related supplement and an increase for dependants. Injury benefit is discontinued if a person becomes fit for work within twenty-six weeks, or claims disablement benefit, or both. A person who is unable to work after twenty-six weeks may qualify for sickness or invalidity benefit.

Injury benefit is not affected by the payment of salary, wages, or sick pay from an employer. But, while a person is receiving injury benefit, he or she cannot normally also receive certain other benefits, such as widow's benefit or retirement pension.

The invalid care allowance is a taxable weekly payment to men and single women of working age who cannot work because they have to remain at home to care for a severely disabled relative. Entitlement does not depend upon national insurance contributions. However, married women normally cannot qualify for this benefit.

To qualify for invalid care allowance: (1) the claimant must spend at least thirty-five hours per week in caring for the relative; (2) the relative must be so severely disabled as to be entitled to attendance allowance or constant attendance allowance; (3) the claimant must not earn more than a certain amount each week; and (4) the claimant must satisfy certain residence conditions.

If the claimant is already receiving certain other benefits, such as unemployment or injury benefit, he or she is not entitled to invalid care allowance. If the other benefits amount to less than the invalid care allowance, however, the claimant can receive the difference. The basic allowance may be increased if the claimant has dependants. A woman is not entitled to the allowances if she is married and living with her husband; separated but receiving at least the amount of the allowance towards her maintenance; or cohabiting with a man.

The invalidity benefit comprises an invalidity pension and an invalidity allowance. Invalidity pension is paid in place of sickness benefit if a person is still incapable of work after six months. Invalidity allowance is paid in addition to the pension to those who become chronically ill before reaching sixty (men) or fifty-five (women) on the first day of becoming incapable of work. The medical and national insurance contribution conditions that must be satisfied to qualify for invalidity benefit are the same as those for sickness benefit.

A person who qualifies for invalidity benefit may also be entitled to certain other benefits, such as an increase for dependants and free prescriptions.

A person who is not entitled to invalidity benefit may qualify for a non-contributory invalidity pension. This is primarily for people of working age who have been continuously incapable of work for at least six months and who have not paid sufficient national insurance contributions to qualify for invalidity benefit. A married woman can claim non-contributory invalidity benefit only if, in addition to being incapable of paid employment, she is also unable to do normal household work.

Several maternity benefits are available to which a woman who is pregnant or has recently had a baby may be entitled.

The maternity grant is a lump sum payment for the birth of each child. To receive the grant it is necessary for the woman (or her husband if she is married) to have paid a specified minimum number of national insurance contributions. The woman must also claim within the period from fourteen weeks before the expected date of birth to three months after the birth.

Maternity allowance is a weekly payment to pregnant women who have themselves paid full-rate national insurance contributions in the tax year related to the claim. It is payable for a maximum of eighteen weeks, starting eleven weeks before the week of the expected date of birth. This allowance is not paid, however, for any period during which the woman works. The woman may also be entitled to an earnings-related supplement and an increased allowance for dependants. To receive the full allowance the woman must claim between the fourteenth and eleventh week before the expected date of birth.

Paid maternity leave is a weekly payment to a woman who stops work to have a baby. To receive this benefit the woman must have worked for the same employer for at least two years and must continue to work up to the eleventh week before the expected date of birth. Entitlement to this benefit does not depend upon the national insurance contributions of either the woman or her husband. This benefit is paid for the first six weeks that the woman is away from work. A woman who wishes to claim this benefit should tell her employer at least three weeks before stopping work and should produce her certificate of confinement.

Pregnant women and mothers with babies under one year old may also be entitled to free milk and vitamins, free prescriptions, and free NHS dental treatment.

The mobility allowance is a taxable weekly payment for severely disabled people between five years old and retirement age.

To qualify for this allowance: (1) the claimant must be unable, or almost unable, to walk because of physical disablement; (2) the disablement must be likely to persist for at least one year; and (3) the claimant must be able to make use of the allowance. A person who cannot be moved for medical reasons therefore cannot qualify. Entitlement does not depend upon national insurance contributions. A medical examination may be required before a claim can be decided.

The allowance is awarded for a definite period (normally at least one year and often up to retirement age), after which a further

medical examination is required. In most cases, mobility allowance is payable in addition to other social security benefits. A person who receives a private car allowance, an invalid vehicle, or a car supplied by the NHS, cannot receive mobility allowance as well.

Sickness benefit is a weekly payment to people who are usually employed or self-employed but who cannot work because of illness or disablement. It is payable for a maximum of twenty-eight weeks. If after this period a person is still unable to work because of illness or disablement, he or she can normally claim invalidity benefit. Sickness benefit is not payable for the first three days of illness.

To qualify for sickness benefit, the claimant must have paid a specified minimum number of national insurance contributions. The claimant must also send a medical certificate to the local social security office within six days of becoming ill.

A person who qualifies for sickness benefit may also be entitled to an earnings-related supplement, an increase for a wife or one other adult dependant, and an increase for each child. The entitlement of a married woman to these additional payments depends upon her individual circumstances. She cannot get sickness benefit if she has only paid reduced-rate national insurance contributions in the relevant tax year. If the claimant has just started to pay national insurance contributions, is a divorced woman, or is a widow who does not qualify for widow's pension, special arrangements may be made.

Sickness benefit is taxable (from 1982) and is, therefore, affected by the payment of salary, wages, or sick pay from an employer.

Three main widow's benefits are available: widow's allowance, widowed mother's allowance, and widow's pension. All of these benefits are taxable and all depend upon the national insurance contributions of the woman's late husband. The widow may also be entitled to a death grant. If death resulted from an industrial accident or disease, the widow may be entitled to industrial death benefit. If a woman is divorced or the marriage was annulled and her former husband dies, she cannot obtain any of the widow's benefits. But if she has not remarried and has a child towards whose maintenance her former husband was liable to contribute, she may be entitled to a child's special allowance. All widow's benefits, apart from the death grant, stop if the widow remarries or cohabits with a man.

Widow's allowance is a weekly payment to

a widow who was under sixty when her husband died, or whose husband was under retirement age. In addition to the basic allowance, a widow may be entitled to an earnings-related addition and an increase for each dependent child. She may also be entitled to the earnings-related addition if she receives an industrial injuries widow's pension instead of the widow's allowance. Widow's allowance is paid only for the first six months of widowhood, after which the widow may be entitled to widowed mother's allowance or widow's pension.

Widowed mother's allowance is a weekly payment to a widow of any age with at least one dependent child under nineteen. It is also payable to a widow who is pregnant by her late husband, in which case an increase is normally paid on the birth of the child. Widowed mother's allowance is payable from the time widow's allowance stops. If a woman's late husband did not pay sufficient national insurance contributions, she may still qualify for a reduced-rate allowance. A widow with several children may also be entitled to an increase for each qualifying child.

Widow's pension is a weekly payment to a woman who was at least forty when widowed and who does not qualify for widowed mother's allowance. It is payable from the time the widow's allowance stops. A woman may also qualify if she is at least forty when her widowed mother's allowance stops. The amount of widow's pension depends upon the woman's age at the time of her husband's death, or her age when the entitlement to widowed mother's allowance ends. If her late husband did not pay sufficient national insurance contributions, she may still qualify for a reduced-rate pension.

Other social services and benefits

In addition to cash benefits, there are various other services that a person who is ill or disabled may be able to obtain. Some of the services and benefits are also available to other categories of people, such as those with low incomes, whether they are ill or not.

Free NHS dental treatment is an automatic right for those who qualify for supplementary benefit or family income supplement; those entitled to free milk or prescriptions because of low income; pregnant women; women with children under one year old; and everybody under twenty-one years old (but those between sixteen and twenty-one who have left school must pay for dentures). Some people with low incomes who do not have an automatic right may qualify for help with the charges.

Free hospital medicines and appliances are an automatic right for hospital patients who qualify for supplementary benefit or family income supplement; those entitled to free milk or prescriptions because of low income; young people undergoing full-time education; and war pensioners. Some people with low incomes who do not have an automatic right may qualify for help with the charges.

Free NHS spectacles are an automatic right for those who qualify for supplementary benefit or family income supplement; those entitled to free milk or prescriptions because of low income; and young people undergoing full-time education. Some people with low incomes who do not have an automatic right may qualify for help with the charges.

Free prescriptions are an automatic right for those who qualify for supplementary benefit or family income supplement; pregnant women; women with children under one year old; children under sixteen; old-age pensioners; and people with certain medical conditions. Some people with low incomes who do not have an automatic right may also obtain free prescriptions.

Free milk and vitamins are an automatic right for children under school age in families receiving supplementary benefit or family income supplement; pregnant mothers with two children under school age; and the third and subsequent children in families with three or more children under school age. Milk only is free for handicapped children between five and sixteen who are not registered at school. Some people with low incomes who do not have an automatic right may also qualify for free milk and vitamins.

Other services are available for people who are disabled, chronically ill, or mentally retarded. These additional services are intended to help such people live as normally as possible within the community. Some of the services, such as home helps, are also available to people who are only temporarily incapacitated.

The services that may be available include alterations to the home for the disabled; antenatal and postnatal clinics; adult training centres; alarms to alert neighbours; appliances, such as rubber sheets and hearing aids; car parking concessions; cheap travel; help with the cost of heating the home; day centres and day care; home helps; home nurses to provide skilled nursing at home; meals on wheels; help with the cost of telephone installation and rental; visits from social workers; and residential homes for those who cannot be cared for in their own homes.

Specialized hospitals, clinics, and specialists

This section discusses some of the common types of special hospital, and also some of the specialists and specialist services outside hospitals which you may be referred to by a GP or may consult privately.

Specialized hospitals

Artificial limb fitting centres are special hospitals where amputees are fitted with artificial limbs. The centres employ craftsmen to make the artificial limbs (prostheses) to the exact requirements of each patient. There are also physio- and occupational therapists who then teach patients how to use the prostheses and help with general rehabilitation.

Children's hospitals specialize in the treatment of diseases and disorders of children from birth until the early teens.

Going into hospital can be a frightening experience for a young child, so many hospitals allow one parent to board at the hospital during the child's stay, particularly if the patient is very young or seriously ill. Visiting times are usually very flexible, and may even be unrestricted, to allow others as much time as possible with the child. Every effort is made to ensure the child's stay is pleasant; the child may usually bring in favourite toys. Many hospitals have special play and teaching facilities.

Dental hospitals, separate from a general hospital but often the dental department of a teaching hospital, are found in many large cities.

Patients may be referred to a dental hospital by a doctor or dentist for specialized treatment, or they can go directly to the hospital. A few dental hospitals do not charge for treatment: if the hospital is used for teaching, the treatment may be done by a dental student in the final year of training and no charge is made. All such treatment, however, is under the close supervision of a dental surgeon.

Maternity hospitals provide essential and comprehensive facilities to care for childbirth and to deal with any complications that may arise. In addition to the basic ward, delivery, and nursery units, all maternity hospitals have facilities such as antenatal and post-natal clinics, and family planning clinics. The specialist staff includes obstetricians, paediatricians, anaesthetists and midwives.

Modern obstetric care aims to prevent complications from occurring before and during childbirth, as well as to treat and deal immediately with any that do arise. Consequently, obstetricians prefer to look after their patients in a maternity hospital or units where these specialized skills and equipment are available.

Mental hospitals are where about one person in every nine is treated for a mental disorder at some time during his or her life. Some spend a considerable time in a mental hospital, although the modern trend is away from hospital treatment and towards treatment at home or at special day clinics.

Psychiatrists, psychologists, and specially-trained psychiatric nurses work in mental hospitals to provide the specialized treatment and care required by the mentally ill.

If a GP feels that a patient has a serious mental disorder, he or she tries to persuade the patient to be admitted to a hospital for treatment. If, however, the patient refuses to take his advice and the doctor considers the patient is a danger to himself or herself, or to others, the patient can then be compulsorily made to go to hospital for treatment.

Clinics

A Family Planning clinic's main purpose is to provide contraception; they may also offer other services, such as advice about sexual problems and venereal diseases. Some clinics are run by local authorities and others by the Family Planning Association, a voluntary organization.

Contraceptive advice is free, but voluntary organizations often ask for financial help.

Venereal disease clinics are special departments, often in general hospitals, that provide treatment for sexually-transmitted diseases. A patient may be referred to a clinic by a GP, or may go directly for treatment.

The patient registers before being seen by a doctor. Initially, the doctor takes the patient's medical history, then asks about the patient's sexual partner(s) so that, if the patient has a venereal disease, the partner(s) can be contacted. Many clinics, however, rely on the patient to inform his or her partner(s) by giving them a card asking each contact to report to the same clinic as the patient (or one at the nearest hospital), taking the card with him or her.

Finally, the doctor examines the patient. A blood test is taken from all patients. In female patients, samples are taken from the cervix, vagina, and urethra for testing. In men, a sample of the secretions from inside the penis is taken. The samples are examined at once, in an attempt to make an immediate and definite diagnosis. If the diagnosis is confirmed, the patient is also treated immediately. If the preliminary tests are inconclusive, the samples are sent to a laboratory for further testing, which may take several days. If a positive diagnosis is suspected, treatment is usually given during this time. All information that the patient gives to the clinic is in the strictest confidence. The doctors and nurses may not know even the patient's name, for the registration procedure gives the patient merely a card with a number.

Specialists

Chiropodists are non-medical specialists in the treatment of minor disorders of the feet. In addition to treating such disorders as athlete's foot, calluses, and corns, some chiropodists also perform minor surgery, such as the removal of an ingrowing toe-nail.

State-registered chiropodists have undergone a special training course and are professionally qualified. Only state-registered chiropodists are permitted to work for the NHS. But most patients have to pay for a chiropodist's treatment, although some people, such as the elderly, are entitled to free care.

Most **dentists** work for the NHS, and many also treat patients privately. It is not necessary to register with a dentist as it is with a doctor, and you can change dentists at any time. It is advisable, however, to see the same dentist regularly to obtain treatment when needed. Your dentist is then able to keep a dental history and so to be more familiar with your teeth.

A dentist has the right to refuse treatment, without giving an explanation. If a dentist agrees to accept you as a patient, you must sign an application form at the beginning of the course of treatment. This contract finishes when the treatment is complete, after which you must sign the form again. Most adults have to pay for dental treatment; under the NHS, the fee is a proportion of the total cost of the treatment. Certain categories of patients, however, such as children and full-time students, the elderly, pregnant women, and those receiving supplementary benefits, are exempt from dental fees.

District nurses and private nurses are qualified nurses who provide skilled services for the patient at home. If you need regular skilled help that does not require a doctor (for example, in changing dressings), your GP may send a district nurse.

If a patient requires full-time nursing at home, it is possible to employ a private nurse. These can be obtained through a nursing agency and are often very expensive. Full-time nursing at home is not available through the NHS.

Midwives are nurses who have been specially trained to deliver babies and to undertake antenatal and postnatal maternal care, as well as looking after the newborn baby. Most midwives work in hospital, but many are employed by local authorities, working under the supervision of the Community Health Physician, and deliver babies in the home. They usually work in close co-operation with general practitioners, who are responsible for these home deliveries.

Opticians are of two main types. An ophthalmic optician is qualified to test the eyes, and may then prescribe and supply spectacles and contact lenses. A dispensing optician makes lenses to the prescription of an ophthalmic optician.

Anybody can have his or her eyes tested for a fee, and there is a further charge for supplying spectacles. Generally, the patient has to pay a proportion of the cost of the lenses, and of the frames when one of the frames available under the NHS is chosen. Certain categories of patients, such as children and the elderly, are exempt from these charges. But all patients must pay the full cost of frames not supplied by the NHS. The patient has to pay the full cost of contact lenses, except where these are prescribed by a consultant for certain rare medical conditions.

Adults should have an eye test once every two years.

Psychiatrists and psychologists are not the same thing. A psychiatrist is a qualified doctor who has further specialized in mental disorders and illnesses. He or she works in a mental hospital, and may have a separate private practice. A GP may refer a patient to a psychiatrist, who diagnoses the patient's illness, decides the best form of treatment, and judges whether this should be as an out-patient or in hospital.

A psychologist is not necessarily medically qualified, but is trained in measurement and assessment of human behaviour. Within the general field of psychology there are several specialities, such as clinical psychology, which, like psychiatry, is concerned with mental disorders; educational psychology, which is concerned with educational achievement and potential in an individual; and social psychology, which is concerned with the aspects of social behaviour.

A clinical psychologist may work in a mental hospital, in co-operation with psychiatrists in the assessment and treatment of patients. An educational psychologist may be employed by a local educational authority to advise on general educational matters and also on individual children who have specific educational requirements (such as remedial teaching) or problems (such as dyslexia or dysphasia).

743

Other sources of medical care

There are a large number of organizations in Britain that supplement the resources of the NHS by providing practical help and medical advice for patients who suffer from particular disorders or whose condition requires specialist attention. Many of these organizations are registered charities, and are financially supported by voluntary donations from the general public. Most of these organizations provide medical advice and moral support in the form of personal counselling, contact with other patients with similar problems, and information booklets and newsletters. In many cases, these organizations also provide practical help with a wide range of problems that may confront patients suffering from particular disorders. The services they provide vary according to the organization's particular area of concern, but they may include help with education, transport, holidays, sports and other leisure activities, diets, housing and temporary accommodation, and employment and working conditions.

The list of names and addresses given on these pages is only a small selection from the many organizations and societies that exist. Many of the organizations have local branches, and patients are advised to look in their local telephone directory to find out if an organisation has an office in their area. Any patient who wishes to contact a society is advised to consult his or her GP, who will be able to recommend the most suitable society for the patient's needs.

As well as the organizations concerned with particular disorders, there are a number of organizations that provide more general services for patients or other people in need of help. All these organizations have a network of local branches throughout the country. They include the British Red Cross Society (9 Grosvenor Crescent, London SW1), whose services include transport and holidays for disabled or housebound people; St John Ambulance (1 Grosvenor Crescent, London SW1), which provides first aid services at public events and also organizes visits to disabled and housebound people and practical help in hospitals, clinics, and private homes; the National Marriage Guidance Council (Herbert Gray College, Little Church Street, Rugby, Warks.), which provides help with all problems concerning marriage and family relationships; and the National Association of Citizens Advice Bureaux (110 Drury Lane, London WC2), which provides confidential advice and help on all subjects, and has particular experience in dealing with housing and legal problems and welfare benefit entitlements.

Abortion
British Pregnancy Advisory Service,
Austy Manor,
Wootton Wawen,
Solihull, West Midlands.

Pregnancy Advisory Service,
40 Margaret Street,
London W1.

Alcoholism
National Council on Alcoholism,
3 Grosvenor Crescent,
London SW1.

Alcoholics Anonymous,
11 Redcliffe Gardens,
London SW10.

Autism
National Society for Autistic Children,
1a Golders Green Road,
London NW11.

Blindness
Royal National Institute for the Blind,
224 Great Portland Street,
London W1.

Cancer
National Society for Cancer Relief,
30 Dorset Square,
London NW1.

Coeliac disease
Coeliac Society of the United Kingdom,
P.O. Box 181,
London NW2.

Colostomy
Colostomy Welfare Group,
38-39 Eccleston Square,
London SW1.

Deafness
Royal National Institute for the Deaf,
105 Gower Street,
London WC1.

Diabetes
British Diabetic Association,
10 Queen Anne Street,
London W1.

Disablement
Royal Association for Disability
   and Rehabilitation (RADAR),
25 Mortimer Street,
London W1.

Epilepsy
British Epilepsy Association,
Crowthorne House,
New Wokingham Road,
Wolingham, Berks.

Haemophilia
Haemophilia Society,
16 Trinity Street,
London SE1.

Ileostomy
Ileostomy Association of Great Britain
23 Winchester Road,
Basingstoke, Hants.

Infertility
National Association for the Childless,
318 Summer Lane,
Birmingham B19.

Kidney Disorders
British Kidney Patient Association,
Bordon, Hants.

Leukaemia
Leukaemia Society,
186 Torbay Road,
Rayners Lane, Harrow.

Mastectomy
Mastectomy Association,
1 Colworth Road,
Croydon, Surrey.

Mental handicap
National Association for Mentally
   Handicapped Children,
117 Golden Lane,
London EC1.

Mental illness
National Association for Mental
   Health (MIND),
22 Harley Street,
London W1.

Psychiatric Rehabilitation
   Association,
21a Kingsland High Street,
Dalston, London E8.

Migraine
Migraine Trust,
45 Great Ormond Street,
London WC1.

Multiple sclerosis
Multiple Sclerosis Society,
4 Tachbrook Street,
London SW1.

Parkinson's disease
Parkinson's Disease Society of the
   United Kingdom,
81 Queen's Road,
London SW19.

Polio
British Polio Fellowship,
Bell Close, West End Road,
Ruislip, Middlesex.

Pregnancy
Brook Advisory Centre,
233 Tottenham Court Road,
London W1.

Rheumatism
British Rheumatism and Arthritis
   Association,
6 Grosvenor Crescent,
London SW1.

Sexual problems
Albany Trust,
16 Strutton Ground,
London SW1.

Spastics
Spastics Society,
12 Park Crescent,
London W1.

Suicidal depression
Samaritans,
17 Uxbridge Road,
Slough, Berks.

Widows in bereavement
Cruse,
Cruse House,
126 Sheen Road,
Richmond, Surrey.

Hospital in-patient checklist

Things to take when going to stay in hospital

Personal cleanliness and appearance

towels	comb	mirror
face-cloth	hairbrush	razor and blades
soap	cosmetics	shaving cream
toothbrush	nail scissors	aftershave
toothpaste	nail file	
mouthwash		handkerchiefs
deodorant	sanitary towels	box of tissues

Clothing

bedwear

dressing-gown

bed slippers

bed jacket

underwear

Documents

letter of admission

health service details

health insurance details

note of any special diet

Miscellaneous items

reading material	small change (for telephone, newspaper, etc.)
pen and pencil	
writing paper	radio programmes
envelopes, stamps	pack of cards
address book	bottle of cordial
regular medicine	Bible and prayer-book

Emergency information chart – home

Home address: _____
 _____
 Telephone number: _____
	What service is required?
	                 AMBULANCE
	                 POLICE
	                 FIRE

In case of emergency, inform also (relatives):	Medical insurance details:

Service	Name	Address	Telephone
Local casualty hospital	_____	_____	_____
Maternity hospital	_____	_____	_____
Local doctor/health centre (day)	_____	_____	_____
(night)	_____	_____	_____
Alternative doctor	_____	_____	_____
Dentist	_____	_____	_____
Specialists – gynaecologist	_____	_____	_____
– paediatrician	_____	_____	_____
– psychiatrist	_____	_____	_____
– other	_____	_____	_____
Nearest dispensing chemist	_____	_____	_____
Priest/Minister/Rabbi	_____	_____	_____
Samaritans	_____	_____	_____
Other welfare services	_____	_____	_____
	_____	_____	_____
	_____	_____	_____
	_____	_____	_____
Electricity authority	_____	_____	_____
Gas authority	_____	_____	_____
Water authority	_____	_____	_____
Solicitor/Lawyer	_____	_____	_____
Town Hall	_____	_____	_____
Citizen's Advice Bureau	_____	_____	_____
Local information service	_____	_____	_____
Local newspaper office	_____	_____	_____
24-hour taxi service	_____	_____	_____
Employers	_____	_____	_____
	_____	_____	_____
	_____	_____	_____
	_____	_____	_____
Employees	_____	_____	_____

Emergency information chart – work

Work address: _____ _____ Telephone number:_____	What service is required? **AMBULANCE POLICE FIRE**
In case of emergency, inform also (relatives):	Medical insurance details:

Service	Name	Address	Telephone
Local casualty hospital	_____	_____	_____
Maternity hospital	_____	_____	_____
Local doctor/health centre (day)	_____	_____	_____
(night)	_____	_____	_____
Alternative doctor	_____	_____	_____
Dentist	_____	_____	_____
Specialists – gynaecologist	_____	_____	_____
– paediatrician	_____	_____	_____
– psychiatrist	_____	_____	_____
– other	_____	_____	_____
Nearest dispensing chemist	_____	_____	_____
Priest/Minister/Rabbi	_____	_____	_____
Samaritans	_____	_____	_____
Other welfare services	_____	_____	_____
	_____	_____	_____
	_____	_____	_____
	_____	_____	_____
Electricity authority	_____	_____	_____
Gas authority	_____	_____	_____
Water authority	_____	_____	_____
Solicitor/Lawyer	_____	_____	_____
Town Hall	_____	_____	_____
Citizen's Advice Bureau	_____	_____	_____
Local information service	_____	_____	_____
Local newspaper office	_____	_____	_____
24-hour taxi service	_____	_____	_____
Employers	_____	_____	_____
	_____	_____	_____
	_____	_____	_____
Employees	_____	_____	_____

Medical history chart

Name of family member: Date of birth: Blood type:		
Health service number/category/ registration, etc.:		
Medical insurance details:		
Serious illnesses, disorders and injuries, with dates:		
Last hospital treatment – for:* – date:*		
Chronic or permanent illness:		

X-rays: date of last of*
  chest
  head
  teeth
  abdomen
  other		

Immunization: date of last for*
  smallpox
  polio
  typhus
  diphtheria
  tetanus
  whooping cough
  other		

Medicine taken regularly:*
  frequency of dose:
  prescribed by:
  prescription runs till:		

Known allergies – to (condition)
            – to (food/drink)
            – remedy		

Additional gynaecological information:		
Additional dental information: date of last dental check:		
Additional psychiatric information:		
Other information:		
Date this record last checked:*		

*Write in pencil

Medical history chart

Name of family member: Date of birth: Blood type:		
Health service number/category/ registration, etc.:		
Medical insurance details:		
Serious illnesses, disorders and injuries, with dates:		
Last hospital treatment – for:* – date:*		
Chronic or permanent illness:		

X-rays: date of last of*
   chest
   head
   teeth
   abdomen
   other		

Immunization: date of last for*
   smallpox
   polio
   typhus
   diphtheria
   tetanus
   whooping cough
   other		

Medicine taken regularly:*
   frequency of dose:
   prescribed by:
   prescription runs till:		

Known allergies – to (condition)
           – to (food/drink)
           – remedy		

Additional gynaecological information:		
Additional dental information: date of last dental check:		
Additional psychiatric information:		
Other information:		
Date this record last checked:*		

*Write in pencil

Medical history chart

Name of family member: Date of birth: Blood type:		
Health service number/category/ registration, etc.:		
Medical insurance details:		
Serious illnesses, disorders and injuries, with dates:		
Last hospital treatment – for:* – date:*		
Chronic or permanent illness:		

X-rays: date of last of*
    chest
    head
    teeth
    abdomen
    other		

Immunization: date of last for*
    smallpox
    polio
    typhus
    diphtheria
    tetanus
    whooping cough
    other		

Medicine taken regularly:*
    frequency of dose:
    prescribed by:
    prescription runs till:		

Known allergies – to (condition)
                      – to (food/drink)
                      – remedy		

Additional gynaecological information:		
Additional dental information: date of last dental check:		
Additional psychiatric information:		
Other information:		
Date this record last checked:*		

*Write in pencil

Medical history chart

Name of family member: Date of birth: Blood type:		
Health service number/category/ registration, etc.:		
Medical insurance details:		
Serious illnesses, disorders and injuries, with dates:		
Last hospital treatment – for:* – date:*		
Chronic or permanent illness:		

X-rays: date of last of*
  chest
  head
  teeth
  abdomen
  other		

Immunization: date of last for*
  smallpox
  polio
  typhus
  diphtheria
  tetanus
  whooping cough
  other		

Medicine taken regularly:*
  frequency of dose:
  prescribed by:
  prescription runs till:		

Known allergies – to (condition) – to (food/drink) – remedy		
Additional gynaecological information:		
Additional dental information: date of last dental check:		
Additional psychiatric information:		
Other information:		
Date this record last checked:*		

*Write in pencil

Pregnancy progress chart 1

The information in these charts is presented as concisely as possible. More detailed information is given on pp.746-770.

Wait until period is overdue by twelve days before consulting doctor for gynaecological examination and/or pregnancy test.

Pregnancy test POSITIVE

Pregnancy test NEGATIVE

ANTENATAL CARE
Precautions:
— stop smoking
— avoid all drugs and . medications unless prescribed by a doctor

Repeat test again after one week. If again negative, pregnancy is unlikely but not impossible. Ultrasound test after two months if necessary.

Common symptoms
  of early pregnancy:
Frequent urination
Fatigue
Breast tenderness
Nausea (morning sickness)

Common problems
  of early pregnancy:
Vaginal bleeding
Abdominal pain
Fever
Painful urination
Any of these problems must be reported to a doctor immediately.

Pregnancy Progress chart 2

MONTH	3	4	5
SYMPTOMS		"Quickening" (16-18 weeks)	Constipation————
MAJOR PROBLEMS		Bleeding———————— (due to placenta praevia)	
MEDICAL CARE	Monthly antenatal visit—————————————— (unless reason for more frequent visits)		
TESTS	Amniocentesis (for possible congenital abnormality) Ultrasound test (for correct dating and multiple pregnancy) Blood test (for alpha feto-protein)		
TREAT- MENTS	Vitamin and iron pills————————————————		
PRE- CAUTIONS	Stop smoking; avoid all medications——————— unless prescribed by doctor		

6	7	8	9

Ankle swelling ————————————

Backache ————————————

Insomnia ————————

Heartburn ————————

Haemorrhoids ————

Leg cramps ————

"Lightening" (36 weeks)

Intra-uterine death ————————————

Premature rupture of membranes ————————————

Diabetes mellitus ————————

Toxaemia of pregnancy ————————

Premature labour ————————

Abnormal foetal position ————

Onset of labour: regular, strong contractions lasting at least 40 sec. and occurring every 15-20 min.; "show" of blood and mucus; "breaking of waters" (rupture of amniotic sac). The woman should be taken to hospital, or a doctor should be contacted, when any of the above symptoms occurs.

2 weekly ————— Weekly ————
antenatal visits   antenatal visits

Foetus changes position
from breech to vertex

Haemoglobin

Rhesus antibodies

Antenatal exercises ————————————

Mothercare classes ————————————

Adequate rest ————————————

Avoid excessive exercise; avoid intercourse

Pregnancy and childbirth

Section contents

Introduction

Having a baby can be one of the most rewarding experiences in a woman's life. Many women, particularly those who are pregnant for the first time, know very little of what happens to their bodies: the causes and effects of the changes during pregnancy; normal and abnormal symptoms; and the problems that may develop. Ignorance of the changes involved may lead to anxiety, which not only makes pregnancy mentally stressful, but also increases the physical discomfort. The aim of this section is, therefore, to explain the processes and events that occur during pregnancy and childbirth. The section is arranged chronologically, to give an overall view of the developments during pregnancy, and so that the changes, problems and precautions for each stage of pregnancy are described at the most appropriate times.

An outline of the development of the baby from conception to birth is given in **The course of pregnancy**. The remainder of this section of the book describes pregnancy and childbirth from the mother's point of view.

The different stages of pregnancy are accompanied by varying physical and emotional changes in the mother. Sometimes, unfortunately, problems and complications may develop; the ways in which these potential problems are prevented or treated are discussed. In most women, however, pregnancy develops without major problems and leads to the birth of a normal, healthy baby.

Each pregnancy is different and the changes that take place vary in minor ways in each woman. Similarly, doctors and midwives may use different methods in the care of a woman's pregnancy. If your doctor's advice differs from that given in this section, there is no need to have any less confidence either in the doctor or in the book.

The section also gives advice about a sensible regimen of diet, exercise, and rest during pregnancy, and explains the importance of regular antenatal visits to ensure that both the mother and her unborn baby remain healthy. The section goes on to cover several special aspects of pregnancy and childbirth that may cause particular concern, for example abortion, congenital abnormalities of the baby, sexual intercourse during pregnancy, the process of birth itself, artificial induction of labour, and care for the mother after the birth.

The course of pregnancy

Conception occurs when a single sperm penetrates the cell wall of an egg (ovum) and the nuclei of both cells join together. This usually takes place in one of the fallopian tubes. After conception this single cell divides repeatedly to form a ball of cells called a blastocyst, and moves down the fallopian tube to the womb. This takes four to five days.

When the blastocyst reaches the womb, it becomes embedded in the cells of the uterine wall (endometrium) – a process called implantation. The outer layers of the blastocyst produce a hormone (human chorionic gonadotrophin) that stimulates the continued production of the hormones oestrogen and progesterone, which have been under the stimulus of the two pituitary hormones, follicular stimulating hormone (FSH) and luteinizing hormone (LH). Oestrogen and progesterone keep the body in a "state of pregnancy" – they prevent ovulation and menstruation, and maintain the thickness of the endometrium.

After implantation, the blastocyst receives food and oxygen through the endometrium, and develops very rapidly. Two weeks after conception the blastocyst has developed into two layers of cells, the ectoderm (outer layer) and the endoderm (inner layer), and the fluid-filled amniotic sac has appeared.

The embryo

From the moment of conception until the end of the third month the developing individual is called an embryo. It continues to grow so that a third (central) layer of cells appears, the mesoderm. At this stage the cell layers are relatively undifferentiated, but later the ectodermal layer develops into nervous tissue and skin; the mesodermal layer develops into bones, muscles, blood vessels and connective tissue; and the endodermal layer develops into the lining of the digestive system and the various organs attached to it.

The amniotic sac grows until it completely surrounds the embryo, which floats in the amniotic fluid. The placenta and umbilical cord also develop. These contain blood vessels that are a continuation of the embryo's circulatory system. The placenta is attached to the uterine wall and is a disc-shaped structure through which food and oxygen pass into the embryo's bloodstream and waste substances pass out. There is no direct connection between the blood circulations of the mother and embryo; the placenta thus acts as a filter. The placenta produces increasing amounts of oestrogen and progesterone so that, by the end of the fourth month of pregnancy, the ovary no

longer produces these hormones.

By the end of the third month, the embryo has grown to a length of about 8cm (3in) and has just become recognizable as a human being.

The foetus

From the end of the third month of pregnancy until birth, the baby is called a foetus. During this period, the foetus grows and matures rapidly. About the 18th week of pregnancy, when it is large enough, the mother notices foetal movements. After about the 28th week, the foetus has usually matured sufficiently to have a chance of survival if it is born prematurely.

Although most of the internal organs and body systems of the foetus develop fully before birth, many of them are not needed until after birth. The blood circulation in the embryo and foetus is designed to largely bypass the lungs through a hole in the heart and a special blood vessel called the ductus arteriosus, which joins the artery supplying the lungs and the aorta. This enables the blood to flow through the placenta in close contact with the mother's blood vessels and permits the exchange of oxygen, nutrients, and waste products. This foetal circulation changes to the normal adult circulation shortly after birth – the baby's lungs expand and breathing starts; the hole in the heart and the ductus arteriosus close, diverting blood to the lungs; and blood stops flowing through the placenta.

By the end of pregnancy, the foetus has grown to about 50cm (20in) long and weighs about 3kg (7.5lb). It has also changed to a position in which the head presses downwards against the cervix.

The onset of labour

Towards the end of pregnancy various changes take place in the mother's body, such as a gradual deterioration in the function of the placenta, and an increased production of pituitary hormones that help to stimulate the onset of labour and the secretion of milk. Milk production seldom takes place until after delivery because it is suppressed by the placental hormones.

It is not known exactly what initiates labour but it appears to be a combination of several factors that allow the rhythmic contractions that occur throughout pregnancy to increase and eventually become strong enough to burst the membranes and expel the mature foetus from the womb. This is followed by expulsion of the placenta, and of the surrounding membranes.

Becoming pregnant

The menstrual cycle

Each ovary in a woman contains up to 250,000 immature eggs (ova); these are formed before birth but only develop when the ovaries are stimulated at puberty by the pituitary gland, when follicular stimulating hormone (FSH) and luteinizing hormone (LH) are produced in increasing amounts. These hormones stimulate the ovaries, causing the first menstruation (menarche), and continue in a monthly cycle until the menopause, when the ovaries no longer respond to the pituitary hormones and menstruation ceases. Under the influence of FSH and LH, an ovum matures in one of the ovaries and is usually released every month. The release of the ovum (ovulation) occurs about two weeks before the start of menstruation.

The hormones FSH and LH also indirectly affect the womb by controlling the production of oestrogen and progesterone by the ovaries. Oestrogen is produced mainly during the first half of the menstrual cycle, and progesterone in the second half. The effect of these hormones on the womb is to prepare the endometrium for a fertilized ovum. If the released ovum is not fertilized, there is a decrease in oestrogen and progesterone, and menstruation occurs, with the loss of the ovum and endometrium. If the ovum is fertilized, the amount of oestrogen and progesterone remains high, menstruation does not take place, and further ovulation is prevented.

Conception

During sexual intercourse, a man ejaculates between 200 and 400 million sperm. These are chemically attracted into the cervix and they swim into the womb. Relatively few sperm manage to reach the womb, and fewer still are able to progress from the womb along the fallopian tubes to reach the ovum. Conception usually occurs in one of the fallopian tubes when a single sperm penetrates the cell wall of the ovum and the two nuclei unite. The nucleus of each sex cell (sperm and ovum) contains 23 chromosomes, which is only half the number in a normal body cell. When the nuclei join, a cell is produced that contains 46 chromosomes.

There is only a limited period during the menstrual cycle in which a woman can become pregnant. This fertile period lasts about three days around the time of ovulation. This is because sperm can only survive for about two or three days in the womb and fallopian tubes, but the ovum must be fertilized within a few hours of ovulation.

The time of ovulation can be calculated by the change in a woman's body temperature. If a woman takes her temperature every morning before getting out of bed, there will be a rise of about 0.5°C(1°F) above her usual morning temperature on the morning after ovulation. Other changes that may indicate ovulation include a slight increase in the normal vaginal secretions; mild abdominal pain, which usually lasts only an hour or two; or, rarely, slight bleeding from the womb.

Length of pregnancy

The average length of pregnancy is about 265 days from the date of conception. However for practical purposes, the length of pregnancy is considered to be about 280 days from the first day of a woman's last normal period. This is because ovulation, and therefore conception, occurs about two weeks before the start of menstruation.

The expected date of delivery (EDD) is nine calendar months and one week from the last period; for example, the EDD of a woman whose last period started on 25th May is 4th March in the following year. This calculation has to be modified for women whose periods are irregular. Slight bleeding may sometimes occur in the first two months of pregnancy and this also causes difficulties in calculating the EDD. Such minor bleeding may be due to a form of menstruation, as the interior of the womb is not completely filled by the foetus. In some cases however, it may be caused by a threatened miscarriage.

Although the average length of pregnancy is about nine months, it is usual for labour to begin a few days late or early. A pregnancy that ends more than about three weeks early usually produces a small or immature baby that is less able to survive independently and so needs specialized nursing. Any baby that weighs less than 2.5kg (5.5lb) at birth is defined as premature, even if the baby is born near the expected date. A baby may be underweight for any of several reasons, such as pre-eclampsia, which is a condition peculiar to pregnancy, causing high blood pressure and fluid retention in the mother; twins; bleeding due to premature separation of the placenta (antepartum haemorrhage); or congenital malformation. In many cases however, the cause of prematurity is not found.

Likelihood of becoming pregnant

Many couples believe that pregnancy will occur within a few weeks of stopping contraception. However, this is not necessarily true. The probability of becoming pregnant depends upon several factors, such as the frequency of sexual intercourse; the ages of the couple, particularly of the woman; and whether or not the woman has been pregnant before. Generally, the chance of becoming pregnant on any one occasion is about 1 in 100.

For a fit couple under 30 years old having intercourse two or three times a week, there is a 50 per cent chance of conceiving within six months, and an 80 per cent chance within a year. The probability of becoming pregnant is lower in women over the age of about 30, when fertility begins to diminish.

It is advisable for a young couple to wait about a year before consulting a doctor about failure to conceive. Older couples should consult a doctor after about six months if the woman does not become pregnant.

Many couples who are planning a pregnancy can increase their chances of success by first consulting their doctor, who can give advice about removing or treating possible causes of infertility, such as obesity, diabetes, or disorders of the reproductive system. The doctor may also advise the couple to improve their general health by stopping smoking and reducing alcohol consumption. Apart from detecting diseases of the woman's reproductive system, a gynaecological examination can also reassure her that she is fit to proceed with pregnancy.

If the woman has been using the contraceptive pill or an intra-uterine contraceptive device (coil), the doctor may advise the couple to use another form of contraception, such as sperm-killing creams or a sheath, until the woman has had a period.

If the treatment of these minor disorders is not successful, the doctor may recommend further investigations to discover the cause of infertility.

Care before pregnancy

Any woman who has not had German measles (rubella) or not known to have had the immunizing injection should have a blood test to discover if she is immune. If she is not immune, she should have an injection of rubella vaccine, and contraception must be continued for at least three months. This will prevent conception while the rubella virus is still alive in the woman's body and capable of causing congenital malformations in the embryo.

During the interval between ovulation and the expected date of the onset of menstruation a woman does not know whether or not she has conceived. It is, therefore, particularly important that she takes care not to damage an embryo that may be developing during this time.

Since the thalidomide tragedy, women are advised not to take drugs without medical approval. Although this is probably being over-cautious, it is nevertheless a safe precaution because other drugs may cause congenital abnormalities. However, many drugs are known to be safe, for example, the drugs that are used to treat nausea and vomiting during pregnancy. A woman should tell her doctor that she wishes to become pregnant so that her regular prescriptions can be changed if these drugs might damage a developing embryo.

Among women who smoke there is an increased incidence of underweight babies, miscarriages and stillbirths. There is also an increased likelihood that the child will be less well developed, both physically and mentally, than children born to mothers who do not smoke.

A developing embryo may be damaged by X-rays, and it is for this reason that women are asked the date of their last period before an X-ray examination. The X-rays can then be taken during the first half of the menstrual cycle when it is certain that the woman is not pregnant. Women who use a reliable form of contraception, such as the contraceptive pill, can safely be X-rayed at any time. Although the risk to a developing embryo is minimal, many dentists prefer to X-ray a woman's teeth during the first half of the menstrual cycle, or after the first three months of pregnancy when the foetus is less vulnerable.

Congenital abnormalities

Most couples are understandably concerned about the possibility of their child being born with a congenital deformity. Fortunately, congenital abnormalities are comparatively rare, and most of them are minor deformities, such as webbed fingers, a hare lip, or a squint, which can easily be treated by surgery.

Couples who have previously had a child with a congenital abnormality or in whose families a congenital abnormality has occurred should consult a geneticist (a specialist in the field of inherited characteristics, including congenital abnormalities) recommended by their doctor.

The Department of Health and Social Security produces a booklet entitled *Human Genetics* which may help a couple to decide whether or not they need expert advice.

The incidence of congenital abnormalities is higher among babies born to women over 30 years old. The reason for this is not known.

The first three months

Confirmation of pregnancy

It is difficult for a doctor to diagnose pregnancy during the first two weeks after a period is missed. This is because the womb is not noticeably larger until the woman's period is three or four weeks overdue.

Pregnancy tests depend on the presence of human chorionic gonadotrophin (the hormone produced by the placenta) in the urine. The hormone concentration is not high enough to be easily detectable until the woman's period is about 12 days overdue, so these tests do not give reliable results if performed before this time. If an early test is negative, another test should be done a week later. Pregnancy tests that use hormone pills must be avoided because there is evidence that the hormones can cause congenital abnormalities.

A free NHS pregnancy test can be arranged by the woman's doctor. Alternatively, many chemists can arrange for a test to be performed for a small fee, or you can buy a do-it-yourself testing kit that is easy to use and has a high degree of accuracy.

Although the different types of pregnancy test are highly accurate, none of them gives completely reliable results. A woman near the menopause or taking certain drugs, particularly antidepressants, may produce a false positive result. If a woman has any doubt as to whether or not she is pregnant, she should consult her doctor.

Symptoms of early pregnancy

The most obvious symptom of pregnancy is the absence of a period. Other symptoms may occur around the time that a period is due. They include swelling and tenderness of the breasts, and a feeling of lethargy. These symptoms gradually become worse and, after a week or two, are often accompanied by nausea and vomiting in the mornings (morning sickness). There may also be frequent, painless urination, caused by pressure on the bladder by the enlarging uterus. The severity of symptoms varies from woman to woman and, apart from the absence of periods, may not occur.

If it is a woman's first pregnancy, the pink disc of tissue around the nipple gradually darkens and becomes covered with small protuberances, which are similar to those that often appear before a period.

Morning sickness can often be helped by eating a few plain biscuits with a glass of milk before getting out of bed. If the symptoms persist, a doctor may prescribe antinauseant drugs. Rarely, vomiting is extremely severe, causing dehydration and weight loss. This condition is called hyperemesis gravidarum and is a serious complication of early pregnancy. It requires hospital treatment.

Breast tenderness may be helped by wearing a firm, supportive brassiere during the day and, if necessary, at night. The increased frequency of urination cannot be reduced, but it usually improves during the fourth month of pregnancy when the womb rises out of the pelvis, reducing the pressure on the bladder.

Emotional changes

Most women are happy when they find that they are pregnant. At the same time it is common for a woman to be apprehensive about the physical effects of pregnancy and the prospect of looking after a totally dependent baby. The woman's husband can be of immense help by soothing such natural anxieties and maintaining her morale. The doctor can also help by explaining the changes that occur during pregnancy.

Some women are distressed to discover that they are pregnant. In such cases, the woman's husband has a crucial role to play in reassuring and supporting her. Occasionally, a woman is so severely depressed that her doctor may advise her to have an abortion.

Sexual intercourse

Intercourse can usually be continued until the end of pregnancy, unless the woman has miscarried during a previous pregnancy. If this has happened, her doctor may advise against intercourse around the time of an expected period in the first three months of pregnancy. In many women, fatigue and nausea reduce sexual interest during early pregnancy. It usually returns and may even be increased during the middle of pregnancy. In the last month, intercourse is usually less frequent because of the physical difficulties involved. There is some evidence that intercourse during the last month may be associated with an increased risk of uterine infection after childbirth.

General care

Throughout pregnancy a woman should take a reasonable amount of daily exercise, but she should avoid excessive strain and should ensure that she has enough sleep. Her diet must include plenty of protein foods, fruit, and vegetables. It is also advisable to drink additional milk to maintain an adequate intake of calcium, the bone-building mineral. If large meals cause nausea, small amounts eaten at frequent intervals reduces the chance of vomiting and maintains adequate nutrition.

Pregnant women should avoid contact with people who are suffering from infectious diseases. Some viral illnesses, particularly German measles, are known to cause congenital deformities.

All drugs should be avoided, unless prescribed by a doctor, because of the danger that some may cause congenital abnormalities. A small amount of alcohol is unlikely to be harmful. Regular dental examinations are important because foetal demands on the woman's body may lead to dental problems.

Specialist antenatal care

It is important to be under skilled, specialist care early in pregnancy to enable potential complications or foetal abnormalities to be detected. A woman is usually given a letter of referral by her doctor to a specialist at a hospital before the 12th week of pregnancy.

On the first visit to the hospital antenatal clinic, the woman is asked to give her personal details, such as her full name, age, address and religion. She is also asked about her medical history, particularly about high blood pressure and kidney disease; details of previous pregnancies, including the number of living children, miscarriages and other complications; and any conditions that may occur in the family, such as diabetes or multiple pregnancies.

The woman is then given a general physical examination, including urine and blood pressure tests, and measurement of her height and weight. This examination helps the obstetrician to anticipate any potential problems. Special antenatal care may be needed by women who are overweight; are under 1.8m (5ft 2in) tall; have high blood pressure; or who have kidney disease or diabetes. The obstetrician also examines the woman's breasts to ensure that she will not have problems with breast-feeding. Unless there is a history of miscarriage, the specialist usually performs an internal gynaecological examination to assess the size of the womb, and to ensure that the opening of the pelvis is large enough for the baby to pass through during labour. A cervical smear is usually taken to test for cancer of the cervix.

Finally, various blood tests are done. These include tests for anaemia and, in coloured women, for sickle cell anaemia; the woman's blood group and rhesus factor; and immunity to infections, such as German measles. Chest X-rays are usually only necessary for women with a history of chest or heart disorders.

When the examinations have been completed, the specialist discusses the findings with the woman. Later,

arrangements are made to show her around the wards and delivery rooms, and for her to join antenatal and mothercare classes. Unless there are any problems, she is usually given an appointment to visit the clinic a month later.

Common problems

At least one in ten pregnancies end in a miscarriage, and it is relatively common for a woman to have had two or three miscarriages without there being a serious underlying cause. However, women who have miscarried more than twice are usually given special antenatal care. These women may be given hormone injections or, if the cervix has been damaged by a previous labour, a special surgical stitch may be used to keep the cervix closed until immediately before labour, when the stitch is cut.

An ectopic pregnancy is a rare but serious complication in which the fertilized ovum implants in one of the fallopian tubes or on an ovary. In early pregnancy this condition causes sudden vaginal bleeding and abdominal pain. An ectopic pregnancy is very difficult to diagnose and, in most cases, remains undetected until the growing embryo bursts the fallopian tube, causing severe internal bleeding, severe shock and pain that needs an emergency operation.

Multiple pregnancies are associated with an increased risk of premature labour and other complications, such as pre-eclampsia.

Termination of pregnancy

An abortion can be performed legally only if two doctors agree that the continuation of pregnancy will endanger the woman's physical or mental health; or that the baby is likely to be deformed; or that the birth of another child will seriously affect other members of the family. The earlier an abortion is performed, the safer it is for the woman. If possible, it should be carried out before the end of the third month, although it can be done later in pregnancy. However, it should be remembered that, although her doctor may recommend an abortion, the final decision rests with the woman herself.

There are several methods of terminating a pregnancy. In a dilatation and curettage (D and C) the cervix is enlarged and the embryo is scraped from the uterine wall. In a vacuum aspiration, the embryo is removed by suction through the cervix. These methods are only suitable for use before the 14th week of pregnancy. After this time, a hysterotomy (an operation to open the womb through the abdomen) or special methods involving the use of drugs may be used.

Antenatal exercises 1

It is important for women to learn about pregnancy and prepare themselves mentally and physically for childbirth, because knowing what is involved reduces fear and tension. This section describes some of the antenatal and breathing exercises to practise at home. The woman's concentration on breathing is a positive help in reducing the awareness of pain during labour.

Correct posture during pregnancy can relieve strain on the body and help to prevent the ligaments from overstretching. This, in turn, reduces backache and fatigue and later makes normal posture easier to regain.

Relaxation techniques help to overcome tiredness during pregnancy, and should include an hour's rest every day. Relaxation during labour prevents excessive tension and enables the woman to regain strength between contractions. To begin relaxation, the woman should lie in a comfortable position with eyes closed. She should imagine each limb slowly spreading sideways, then concentrate on relaxing each part of the body in turn. When the body is relaxed, the woman should breathe deeply and rhythmically, with the outward breaths accentuated.

Exercise maintains physical well-being and may alleviate some of the minor problems of pregnancy. One valuable exercise is contraction of the pelvic floor muscles. For this exercise the woman should imagine that an internal tampon is coming out and that the bowels need to move. She should try to prevent these from happening by pulling up the appropriate muscles and keeping them tight for a few moments. This exercise should be done while standing and should be repeated several times daily.

The breathing exercises concentrate on accentuating the outward breath. The first level of breathing is done with the lips separated and a gentle, passive intake of breath. The second level still emphasizes the outward breath but breathing becomes shallower and quicker. The third level combines panting and blowing: two shallow, panting breaths (OUT-in OUT-in) followed by two outward blowing breaths (BLOW-in BLOW-in). Practise daily for brief periods but do not force breathing too far from a normal rhythm.

As a contraction starts the woman should focus her attention on a distant object and breathe above the wave of each contraction. Breathing begins with the first level for milder contractions, gradually becoming shallower until finally the third level is needed for the stronger contractions towards the end of the first stage of labour.

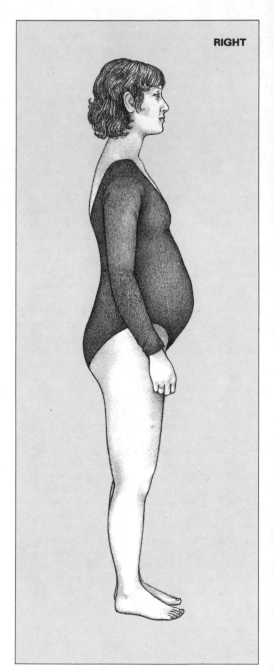

RIGHT

Standing: correct posture

Correct posture helps to prevent fatigue and strain, especially on the lower back.

The knees should be relaxed and the shoulders lowered. The head should be held erect, and the neck and spine should form a straight line so that the weight of the body is on the front of the feet.

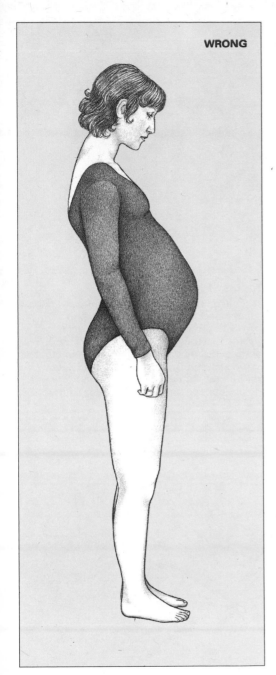

WRONG

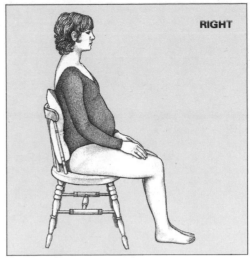

RIGHT

Sitting: correct posture

The correct way of sitting is in an upright position, well back in the chair. The head should be erect, the shoulders lowered, and the hands held loosely in the lap. A cushion in the small of the back helps to maintain correct posture and prevents strain. Women with varicose veins should not sit in a cross-legged position.

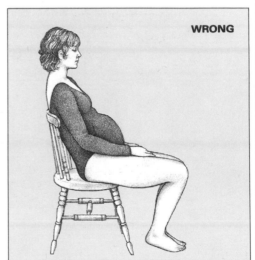

WRONG

Standing: incorrect posture

Many pregnant women stand incorrectly in an attempt to counterbalance the weight of the baby. The usual incorrect posture is with the weight of the body thrown backwards on to the heels, the knees rigid, and the abdomen and chin pushed forwards. This causes overstretching of the abdominal muscles, fatigue and backache.

Sitting: incorrect posture

Sitting in an incorrect position by leaning too far back in the chair with no support for the small of the back causes the spine to curve, which leads to backache from excessive strain on the ligaments of the spine. In this position, the abdomen is pushed forwards, and it is more difficult to hold the head erect.

753

Antenatal exercises 2

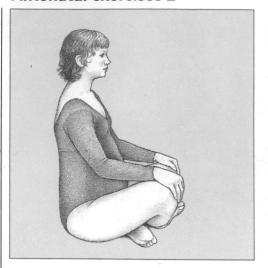

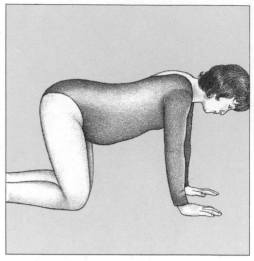

Sitting on the floor

Some women find it restful to sit on the floor in a cross-legged position. The spine should be straight, the head erect, and the hands placed on the knees. The legs should be loosely crossed, but not overstretched. In this position, the abdomen tends to tilt forwards, thereby relieving excessive strain on the spine.

Relief of backache

Kneeling on the hands and knees may help to relieve backache, which is a common complaint during pregnancy. The arms should be straight, but not rigidly tensed. The abdomen should be allowed to sag so that the spine and muscles are relaxed. The neck should also be relaxed. This position should be maintained for a few minutes at a time.

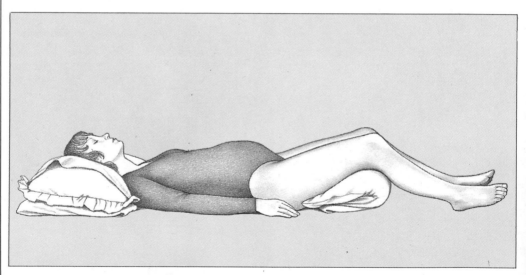

Relaxation: lying on the back

Many women find that lying on the back, either on the floor or on a firm bed, is a comfortable position in which to relax. The head and neck should be firmly supported with two or three pillows. Another two pillows should be placed under the thighs and an extra small pillow placed under the small of the back. The arms and hands should lie loosely at the sides, and the legs should be allowed to become limp and to fall apart.

All of the muscles should be relaxed, including those of the head and face, and the eyes should be closed. Some women, however, tend to become faint when lying on the back and should in this case lie on the side.

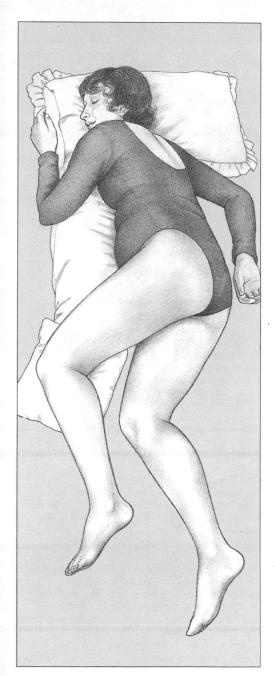

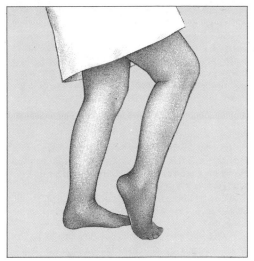

Foot exercise

This exercise helps the leg circulation. Keeping the left foot flat on the floor, rise on to the ball of the right foot. Shift the weight on to the right foot by slowly lowering the right foot and simultaneously rising on to the ball of the left foot. This should be done as a continuous movement. Repeat about twenty times.

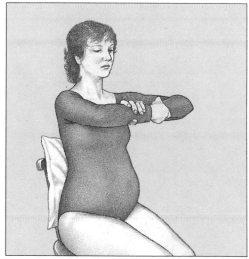

Relaxation: lying on the front

The body should be positioned as shown above, with the knees bent, the lower arm lying limply behind the back, the muscles relaxed, and the eyes closed. The head and neck should be firmly supported with two or three pillows. A small pillow should also be placed under the abdomen to give support, and another pillow placed under the knee.

Exercise for the pectoral muscles

This exercise helps to prevent the breasts from sagging. Sit upright in a chair, with the knees together. Grasp the forearms and raise them to shoulder level. With a rapid, jerking movement, firmly push the skin of the forearms towards the elbows. Repeat the exercise ten times, about three or four times every day.

The fourth to ninth month 1

After the first three months of pregnancy the foetus grows rapidly and the woman becomes aware of the increasing activity of the unborn baby. In most women, this stage of pregnancy is uneventful, with only minor problems that may cause her some anxiety but that are not usually serious. Complications can occur, however, so it is important to visit the antenatal clinic regularly.

Antenatal visits

Antenatal visits usually take place every month until the 32nd week of pregnancy, then every two weeks until the 36th week, and once a week from then on.

At each visit the woman's weight and blood pressure are measured and her urine is tested. A midwife or obstetrician examines her abdomen to assess the enlargement of the womb, and usually also asks if there are any problems with the pregnancy. If necessary an amniocentesis may be performed at about the 14th week of pregnancy. This is a method of testing for foetal abnormalities by analysing the amniotic fluid that surrounds the foetus. It is carried out on women who have had a baby with a congenital abnormality, or who are over 40 years old. A blood test for alpha feto-protein may also be done to detect severe forms of spina bifida. In many hospitals, an ultrasound examination is done during the fourth month to assess the development of the foetus and to detect the position of the placenta. This technique involves passing inaudible, very high-frequency sound through the abdomen; it is painless and does not harm the foetus.

Towards the end of pregnancy, further blood tests are taken to ensure that anaemia is not developing and to test for Rhesus factor antibodies. It is also advisable to have a further dental examination during the last two months of pregnancy.

Physical changes

Apart from the increasing size of the abdomen, there are many other physical changes that occur in the woman's body because of hormonal effects on the various tissues. In many women, the complexion improves during pregnancy. In a few women, the facial skin thickens and acne may develop; these conditions usually disappear after childbirth. Hair growth is normal during pregnancy, but the normal slight hair loss is reduced, causing the hair to thicken. This is followed by an increased hair loss after pregnancy, which causes a temporary thinning of the hair.

Some women develop stretch marks, thin pink lines that appear across the abdomen, buttocks, and breasts. Stretch marks are caused by a change in the elasticity of the skin and cannot be prevented or removed by the use of lotions or creams.

As pregnancy progresses, the increasing size of the breasts may cause slight discomfort. A firm, supportive brassiere gives relief and, if worn at night, may also help to prevent sagging of the breasts after the birth. A slight oozing of clear milk (colostrum) is normal. It may occur at any stage of pregnancy and usually increases just before the baby is born.

An increase in the vaginal secretions is normal during pregnancy but may cause slight discomfort in the vulval area. It is sometimes necessary to wear a small pad of cotton wool during the later stages of pregnancy to prevent soreness from undue rubbing.

Foetal movements

During the early months of pregnancy the small foetus is surrounded by a relatively large amount of amniotic fluid and the woman cannot feel its movements. The first awareness of foetal movement usually occurs about the 18th week of pregnancy, when an occasional slight fluttering is felt in the lower part of the abdomen. This is called the "quickening". The specialist usually asks when it was first noticed because it gives an indication of the maturity of the foetus. Women who have had a previous pregnancy usually notice the quickening a week or two earlier than a woman who is pregnant for the first time.

As the foetus develops, its movements become stronger and can usually be seen and felt through the abdominal wall during the last few weeks of pregnancy. There will be times when the foetus is active, and times when it is still. The resting periods may last for several hours, or even a few days. Long periods of inactivity are normal, but sometimes the woman is naturally anxious and wonders if the foetus is still alive; she should consult her doctor, who will listen for the foetal heartbeat.

Between the 32nd and 36th week the foetus usually moves from a crouched, sitting position (breech position) to a head-down position (vertex position). When the head finally settles into the pelvis, commonly occurring around the 36th week, the abdominal swelling seems to become smaller. This is called the "lightening". In women who have had a previous pregnancy, the lightening may not occur until just before labour. Occasionally, constant kicking by the foetus when it is in the vertex position causes soreness under the diaphragm.

General care
A well-balanced diet should be eaten throughout pregnancy, with plenty of protein, fresh fruit and vegetables, and milk. Many women find milk distasteful during pregnancy; they should discuss this with their doctor, who will suggest other sources of calcium, such as cheese. After the first three months, additional vitamins, iron, and sometimes folic acid must be taken daily. If the woman gains too much weight, she should reduce the amount of carbohydrates and sugar in her diet. It is safe to drink alcohol in moderation, but many women find that their desire for alcohol is reduced towards the end of pregnancy. In the last few weeks, large meals may cause nausea, so frequent, small meals should be eaten.

Regular daily exercise is advisable. Activities such as swimming, riding, and tennis can safely be undertaken during the middle of pregnancy. Towards the end of pregnancy, a woman's increasing size usually makes it difficult to continue these sports. It is also advisable to rest for at least an hour every day, both to relieve fatigue and to allow the softened ligaments to return to their normal shape.

Suitable, loose clothing should be worn during pregnancy. A special nursing brassiere will give good support. Care should be taken in selecting tights because they may rub the vulva, causing soreness and the likelihood of infection.

Antenatal and mothercare classes
The purpose of these classes is to prepare the woman for childbirth and motherhood. During the classes, the course of pregnancy, labour and delivery is explained, the woman is taught ways in which she can help during labour, and advice is given on care of the baby after birth. Women are also shown around the maternity unit and labour wards. Antenatal exercises are an important part of antenatal care because they help the woman to relax and conserve her energy during labour as well as helping the safe delivery of her baby.

Attitudes towards birth and baby care
It is important that a woman is happy and confident about pregnancy. By attending antenatal classes, reading books, and talking to friends who have recently given birth she will realize that complications during pregnancy are rare. She will also learn ways to cope with the problems of looking after a newborn baby. The woman's husband can help by learning to assist her during labour, and by going with her to at least one of the mothercare classes in which methods of baby care and help during labour are taught.

Minor problems
Insomnia is a common problem during the last few weeks of pregnancy. It may be caused by foetal movements, backache, or the increasing size of the abdomen. If necessary, the specialist may prescribe a mild sedative. Palpitations and sweating may also occur, but are rarely severe and do not usually require treatment.

Leg cramps may occur at night. It is advisable to do leg exercises before going to bed and to use a support to hold up the bedclothes, so reducing their weight on the feet.

Backache is a very common symptom that is mainly caused by the normal softening of joint ligaments that occurs during pregnancy; incorrect posture will make the condition worse. Backache can often be prevented by good posture and by wearing low-heeled shoes. If the bed is too soft, a board placed under the mattress will help. Occasionally, a lumbar support corset is necessary.

Headaches are often associated with fatigue and anxiety. They are seldom severe and can usually be relieved with aspirin.

Frequent urination, after temporarily disappearing during the middle of pregnancy, often recurs in the last weeks due to the pressure of the enlarging womb on the bladder. Unless urination is painful, in which case it may be caused by cystitis, treatment is not necessary.

Constipation is caused by the hormonal changes that occur during pregnancy. An increase in dietary fibre often produces an improvement but it is sometimes necessary to take a mild laxative towards the end of pregnancy.

Heartburn may be alleviated by eating small meals at frequent intervals and by avoiding large meals late at night. Additional pillows to raise the head and shoulders in bed may also help. Sometimes, the specialist will prescribe antacids.

Varicose veins are caused by pressure from the enlarged womb preventing the normal drainage of blood from the legs. These produce aching legs and ankle swelling. Elastic stockings may be uncomfortable, but they are the only treatment that relieves the symptoms and may prevent the development of more varicose veins. During the last few weeks of pregnancy, varicose veins may also appear on the vulva. It may help to rest with the legs raised above the level of the hips and to sleep with the foot of the bed elevated so that the blood returns to the circulation more easily. Varicose veins improve after childbirth.

Haemorrhoids may occur for the same reason as varicose veins and are usually made worse by constipation. The specialist may prescribe various ointments.

Ankle swelling commonly appears during the last few weeks of pregnancy and is made worse by hot weather, varicose veins, and the increasing size of the womb. Although ankle swelling is not usually serious, it may be a symptom of toxaemia of pregnancy, which is why the specialist examines the ankles on every visit to the antenatal clinic.

Some women develop a craving for unusual foods, or even for things that are not normally eaten, such as coal. This condition is called pica. It is not usually serious but, occasionally, it may be a sign of anaemia.

Danger signs

Vaginal bleeding, whether it is painful or not, must be reported at once to the doctor. If bleeding occurs after sexual intercourse, it may be the result of the rupture of a small blood vessel in the neck of the womb. Rarely, vaginal bleeding may result from placenta praevia, a potentially serious complication in which the placenta lies in front of the foetus.

Abdominal pain can be caused by any of several underlying disorders. A doctor must be consulted to diagnose the cause, particularly if the pain is intermittent, severe, or accompanied by vaginal bleeding.

A sudden increase in weight, often first noticed by tightness of rings or shoes, may indicate the onset of toxaemia of pregnancy, particularly if this occurs towards the end of pregnancy. A woman must consult her doctor if her weight suddenly increases.

Other illnesses may occur at any time in pregnancy and should be reported to your doctor particularly a fever that persists for more than two days.

Complications

Most pregnancies progress without any serious problems and lead to the successful delivery of a healthy baby. However, complications are more likely to develop in the last two months of pregnancy; they are also likely to be more serious.

The woman's health may affect the progress of pregnancy. If she has high blood pressure, kidney or heart disease, anaemia or diabetes she is more likely to have a small baby.

A woman who is under 1.8m (5ft 2in) tall will have a narrow pelvis. This may lead to difficulties in delivering a normal sized baby and, sometimes, she may need a Caesarean section.

Congenital abnormalities, such as Down's syndrome (monogolism), hydrocephalus, and spina bifida can often be detected early in pregnancy, and an abortion performed if the woman requests it.

Placenta praevia is a condition in which the placenta lies in the lower part of the womb in front of the foetus. It can usually be discovered using ultrasound and frequently needs delivery by Caesarean section to prevent bleeding.

Toxaemia of pregnancy (pre-eclampsia) is a condition peculiar to pregnancy in which there is an increase in blood pressure, the appearance of protein in the urine, and weight gain due to fluid retention. This condition causes placental damage and often leads to the birth of an underweight baby with an increased chance of dying. However, regular antenatal examinations usually detect toxaemia of pregnancy early enough to enable correct treatment to be given and reduce the likelihood of complications.

Premature rupture of the membranes that surround the foetus is potentially serious because the amniotic fluid is lost, thereby reducing the freedom of movement of the foetus and increasing the chance of uterine infection. This condition usually results in spontaneous labour.

Intra-uterine death is relatively common in the early weeks of pregnancy, leading to a miscarriage, but is rare during the later stages. Initially, the woman usually notices that the foetus has not moved for several days and reports this to her doctor, who tests for signs of life. If the foetus is found to be dead, it is usually advisable to wait two or three weeks for spontaneous labour to occur. If labour does not start naturally, it is induced artificially to prevent the development of a serious but rare bleeding disorder.

Foetal positions

The "lie" of the foetus is the way in which it is positioned in the womb. The "presentation" refers to the part of the foetus that is lowest in the womb, just above the cervix.

During the early months of pregnancy the foetus floats freely in the amniotic fluid and may lie in any position. Later, the foetus moves to an upright position with the buttocks in the mother's pelvis (breech presentation). Between about the 32nd and 36th week, the foetus moves to the cephalic

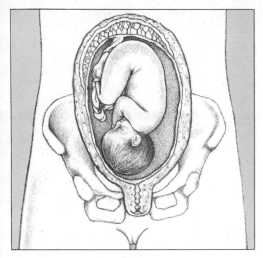

Normal presentation

In most pregnancies the baby moves into the normal head-down (cephalic) presentation between the 32nd and 36th week of pregnancy. In this position, the back of the head (vertex) lies immediately above the cervix and is turned towards the front of the uterus. Occasionally, the face may lie above the cervix (face presentation), which may cause difficulties during labour.

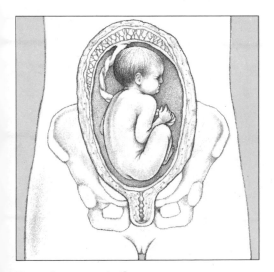

Breech presentation

Until the last two months of pregnancy, most babies lie in the breech position with the buttocks above the cervix. Some babies fail to turn to the cephalic presentation. If this occurs, the specialist will try to manipulate the baby into the cephalic presentation. If this fails, it must be decided whether to allow a breech delivery or do a Caesarean section.

(head) presentation, with its back turned towards the front of the womb and its head above the cervix. This is the best lie and presentation for labour because the back of the head (vertex) is the smallest area that can present, and so is the part of the foetus that can pass most easily through the birth canal during labour.

The specialist checks the lie and presentation at each antenatal visit. If the foetus is still in the breech position after the 32nd week, the specialist usually attempts to turn it to the cephalic presentation by manipulating the outside of the woman's abdomen; this is not painful. If this fails, the specialist will decide whether to allow a breech delivery, or do a Caesarean section near the expected time of labour.

Occasionally, the birth canal may be blocked by a placenta praevia, or the foetus may be disproportionately large. The specialist must decide if a normal delivery is possible, or perform a Caesarean section.

Arrangements for labour

About 95 per cent of women in the United Kingdom give birth in hospital. This ensures that the women receives skilled care and that, if any complications arise, immediate treatment can be given.

It is advisable on medical grounds for some women to have their babies in hospital. For example, if they have had complications with previous pregnancies; are expecting twins; or if they have certain medical conditions, such as high blood pressure, or toxaemia of pregnancy.

Some women may wish to give birth at home. If the general practitioner is trained in home delivery and the midwife is satisfied that the facilities in the home are adequate, they will usually undertake this responsibility. However, if complications arise during pregnancy or labour, they will recommend delivery in hospital.

Most specialists understand a woman's desire for natural childbirth and will try to make this possible. However, most women realize that the use of painkilling injections and epidural anaesthesia (a local anaesthetic given by an injection around the lower part of the spinal cord) can make labour more comfortable without detracting from the experience of childbirth. Few hospitals or antenatal clinics are accustomed to the Leboyer method of natural childbirth. If a woman is interested in this particular method, she should discuss it with the specialist who normally looks after her.

Birth 1

The onset of labour

Throughout pregnancy, the womb gently contracts and relaxes about two or three times every hour. These contractions, called Braxton-Hicks contractions, last between ten and twenty seconds and are not painful. The woman may have noticed them when her hand rests on her abdomen. In the final week or two of pregnancy, the contractions become more obvious and may occasionally become uncomfortable, but are not usually painful.

In normal pregnancies, labour may start at any time between the 38th and 42nd week. What starts labour is not known, but it is probably a combination of hormonal changes in the woman and the maturity of the foetus. It is not true that most babies are born at night; most labours last for about 12 hours and it is therefore probable that some part of labour will occur at night.

When the first stage of labour commences, the Braxton-Hicks contractions become regular, stronger, and more forceful. These contractions are uncomfortable but not always painful. The woman should be taken to hospital, or her doctor contacted if she plans to give birth at home, when the contractions occur regularly every 15 to 20 minutes, or when the membranes break, whichever is first.

Hospital admission

Towards the end of pregnancy, the woman should keep a case packed containing her clothing, toilet articles, and clothing and nappies for the baby, ready for admission to hospital. After admission, a midwife checks the lie and presentation of the foetus, listens for the foetal heartbeat, measures the woman's blood pressure, and examines a specimen of her urine. A vaginal examination is also performed to discover how far the cervix has opened; this indicates the stage to which labour has progressed. The woman may be given an enema to empty the rectum and her pubic hair may be shaved.

If the woman is far advanced in labour, she is usually taken at once to the delivery room. Normally, however, the woman and her husband are put into a side ward until nearer the time of birth.

Some women find that the contractions cease or become less frequent after admission to hospital. If this occurs, the woman is encouraged to walk around and may even be given a strong laxative, a hot bath, and an enema in an attempt to stimulate labour. In some women however, labour has stopped and they are sent home. Although this is disappointing, it is better to be admitted to hospital than to wait too long at home.

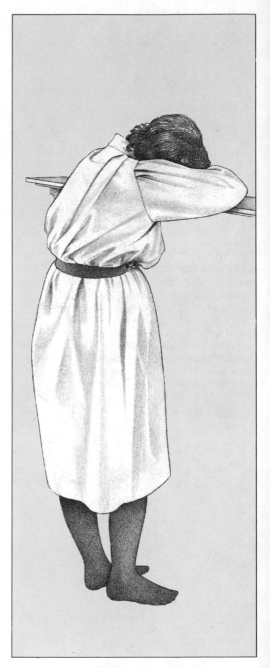

Relaxation during a contraction

When a contraction begins, fold the arms and rest them on a mantelpiece or back of chair: let the head rest on the arms. Bend the knees slightly and relax the chin, face and body muscles. During the early stages of labour this position for relaxation allows full concentration on the breathing exercise.

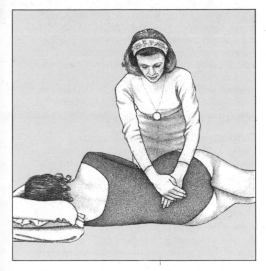

Pain relief during a contraction

The woman should lie on her side with her head supported by pillows. Another person should press firmly over the base of her spine with crossed hands. Continue to press until the contraction has finished. This technique is helpful towards the end of the first stage of labour, when contractions become stronger.

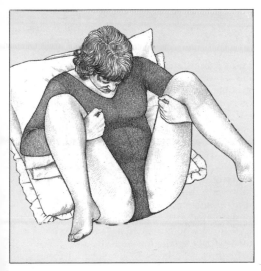

Position for the second stage of labour

When a contraction begins lie in the position shown, back firmly supported, pull the knees up and put the hands around the thighs. When told to push, take a deep breath, hold it as long as possible, round the shoulders, chin on the chest, and give a long, slow push. After the contraction, breathe and relax.

The stages of labour

Labour is divided into three stages. During the first stage, the contractions become stronger, regular and more frequent and the cervix starts to open. This stage lasts until the cervix is fully dilated. The second stage begins when the cervix is fully dilated and ends with the birth of the baby. The third stage ends with the expulsion of the placenta.

The baby cannot be born until the cervix is fully dilated. The contractions may help the cervix to begin dilating a few days before the onset of labour. Normally, the cervix remains closed until labour starts. It is often difficult to know when the first stage of labour begins. The main sign is the regularity and frequency of contractions. If labour has started, they occur at least three or four times an hour; each contraction lasts about 40 seconds. There may also be a deep, dull backache.

At some time during the first stage there is usually a "show": a small amount of blood and mucus from the vagina. This is caused by the discharge of the plug of mucus in the cervix and is a sign that the cervix is opening. Another sign that labour has begun is the "breaking of waters", in which the amniotic sac ruptures and watery amniotic fluid discharges from the vagina. This may vary from a slight trickle to about 250ml (half a pint). Some women also feel nauseous and may vomit.

The first stage of labour lasts between three and fifteen hours, but is usually shorter in women who have had a baby before. The contractions become stronger, more frequent and cause abdominal pain. It is at this stage that the antenatal breathing and relaxation exercises help.

At the end of the first stage of labour the contractions occur about once every two or three minutes and there is a change in the sensation that they produce. The woman has an involuntary desire to push. The midwife or doctor will usually do a vaginal examination to ensure that the cervix is fully dilated and that the second stage of labour has begun. When this has been confirmed, the woman can start to push. Antenatal classes teach her to lie in the correct position and to use the abdominal muscles to help the uterine muscle force the baby down the vagina.

The second stage of labour seldom lasts for more than about an hour, during which time the contractions occur every two or three minutes. Towards the end of the second stage, the midwife or doctor carefully observes the baby's head emerging through the vagina. If there is any danger that the skin around the vagina will tear, an episiotomy is usually performed. This is a cut

761

Birth 2

in the back of the vaginal opening. It is seldom painful, even if performed without a local anaesthetic. In many cases, both tearing and an episiotomy can be avoided by following the midwife's or doctor's instructions so that the baby's head is delivered slowly.

In most births, the membranes that surround the baby in the womb rupture during the first stage of labour. If the membranes are still intact by the second stage, they are broken using forceps.

After the baby's head is delivered, the body, arms and legs follow with the next contraction. It is at this stage that the mother is given an injection of the hormones ergometrine and oxytocin to make the womb contract and prevent excessive bleeding. This marks the end of the second stage of labour. The umbilical cord is then tied and cut.

The third stage of labour is the expulsion of the placenta; this takes about ten to twenty minutes. The uterine contractions, aided by the hormone injection, push the placenta to the upper part of the vagina. The doctor may then help by very gently pulling on the umbilical cord and lightly pressing on the womb through the abdominal wall. When the placenta reaches the vagina, the woman gives a final push and the placenta, with its membranes, is delivered. It is during the third stage that any tear or episiotomy incision is repaired. This operation is usually painless.

Help during labour

Throughout labour both the mother and her unborn baby are kept under close observation. The foetal heart rate is listened to through the mother's abdominal wall. A sudden change in the heart rate may be a sign of foetal distress, which requires a rapid delivery with forceps or by Caesarean section.

The breathing and relaxation exercises taught in the antenatal classes help to relieve the discomfort of the contractions during the first stage of labour. The woman may also find it more comfortable to walk around. Many hospitals allow the woman's husband to be present during labour. He can help by pressing on the lower part of her back during a contraction, and by encouraging her with the breathing exercises during the second stage.

Labour pains can be reduced with an injection of a mild sedative. This produces a twilight state of consciousness, in which the woman is sufficiently alert to help during the contractions but becomes drowsy and relaxed in between. Painkilling injections or anaesthetic gas are often used as well as the sedative. In many hospitals, an epidural anaesthetic may be used during labour. This is an anaesthetic that is given by injection around the spinal cord. It causes loss of sensation below the waist without impairing the woman's consciousness. Usually the woman will have decided before labour starts whether to have an epidural anaesthetic or not.

Complications during labour

Complications occur during labour for three main reasons: the uterine contractions may be too weak; problems may arise with the foetus; or the woman's pelvis may be too narrow.

A prolonged labour with weak or infrequent contractions is very exhausting for the woman and may eventually endanger the foetus. In many cases, there is no apparent cause for labour to be prolonged. Occasionally, a labour that has started normally may slow down. If this occurs during the first stage of labour, drugs may be given to stimulate the contractions. However, if the mother or the foetus become distressed, a Caesarean section is necessary. In labours that slow down during the second stage, it is often possible to do a forceps delivery or a vacuum extraction, in which a suction cap is attached to the baby's skull.

Sometimes the foetus is too large for a normal delivery or is in an abnormal position. If this is the case, the foetus can often be turned to the normal vertex (back of the head) presentation by internal manipulation, and a normal or a forceps-assisted delivery is possible. Occasionally, the specialist may know that problems are likely to develop, but will allow labour to proceed if there is a chance of a normal delivery. When this happens the specialist is prepared to perform a Caesarean section if necessary.

Delivery of twins is usually easy because the babies tend to be small. Sometimes the babies are intertwined or the second baby is in an abnormal position and has to be manipulated into the correct position.

Women who are small also tend to have a narrow pelvis, which is likely to cause difficulties with labour. The specialist may allow labour to proceed naturally, but will be prepared to do a Caesarean section if labour is prolonged.

Occasionally, labour may be accompanied by continuous, excessive bleeding. Rarely, the bleeding may be so severe that an immediate Caesarean section is necessary. Such bleeding is often due to a placenta praevia, in which the placenta lies in front of the baby.

Artificial induction of labour

It is sometimes necessary to induce labour artificially, usually because of problems with the woman's health, such as toxaemia of pregnancy or diabetes, or because of conditions affecting the foetus, such as haemolytic disease or postmaturity. A postmature pregnancy is one that continues for at least a week beyond the expected date of delivery. Postmaturity may endanger the foetus because the placenta begins to deteriorate towards the end of pregnancy, depriving the foetus of food and oxygen.

Labour can be artificially induced either medically or surgically. In a medical induction, the woman is given hormones, either by intravenous injection or in tablet form. In a surgical induction, the woman is given a mild sedative, then a special instrument is passed through her cervix to rupture the membranes that surround the foetus. This releases the amniotic fluid, causing the head of the foetus to press on the cervix and the uterus to contract. If both medical and surgical induction fail, it is usually necessary to do a Caesarean.

Care of the baby after delivery

Immediately the baby is born, the mouth and nostrils are sucked out to remove any mucus or fluid. This clears the airway for the first breath. The eyes are also cleaned.

The appearance of a baby immediately after birth can be worrying. The skin has a wrinkled appearance and is covered with a thick, slightly greasy material known as vernix which, when mixed with the blood that is produced during labour, may give the appearance that the baby is bleeding. The skin is usually bluish, due to the lack of oxygen in the blood, but becomes pink as soon as normal breathing starts. A slightly misshapen head is common. This is known as moulding. A baby's skull bones are not joined together and overlap slightly during childbirth. The moulding gradually disappears in a few days and the baby's head becomes rounded. A baby delivered by Caesarean section does not have a moulded skull. When the baby has been bathed, a fine downy hair (lanugo) may be noticed. This is common in newborn babies and soon disappears.

A baby that has been delivered with forceps or a suction apparatus may have bruising over the area where the instrument has been applied. This soon disappears.

A baby may cry as soon as the head has been delivered and before the rest of the body appears, but does not usually do so until shortly after birth. The initial breaths are often shallower and irregular before a deeper breath is taken and the first cry occurs. Crying and deep breathing are essential to open the lungs and clear them of fluid and mucus. This allows air to enter, and the baby becomes a healthy pink colour. After a few cries, breathing often remains irregular; this is normal.

All these events happen rapidly. Meanwhile, the cord is tied then cut so that the baby can be separated from the placenta. Usually a specimen of cord blood is taken. Occasionally the cord is left uncut, as part of the Leboyer method of delivery, and the baby is given to the mother until the cord stops pulsating.

An immediate assessment of the baby's state of health is made. This is known as the Apgar score. Most babies score nine or ten out of a possible maximum of ten. If there are any problems, a lower score is achieved and particular care of the baby is taken. If the baby is healthy, a label, with name and date of birth, is clipped around one wrist and the baby is weighed and bathed.

The commonest problem in a newborn baby is difficulty with breathing. This may need urgent attention, with breathing tubes to ensure a clear airway, and an incubator to keep the baby warm and in a humid atmosphere. Breathing problems are most likely to occur if the baby is premature, delivered by Caesarean section or forceps, or if the mother has had toxaemia of pregnancy or diabetes mellitus.

Fortunately most babies are healthy, and, after the cord has been tied and cut, the baby is swaddled and given to the mother.

Problems after delivery

There are two main problems that may affect the mother shortly after delivery: bleeding from the womb, and retention of the placenta.

Bleeding after delivery (postpartum haemorrhage) may be sudden and severe or a continual slight loss. Continued bleeding will endanger the mother's life. Postpartum haemorrhage usually results either from relaxation of the womb, which may occur even after the injection of hormones, or from retention of a piece of the placenta in the womb. Immediate treatment is necessary to stop the bleeding, with another hormone injection and, if necessary, a blood transfusion.

Retention of the placenta is a condition in which the placenta has not been delivered after 30 minutes. In such cases, the woman is given a general anaesthetic and the placenta is removed by the obstetrician inserting a hand into the womb.

Postnatal care

The puerperium

The puerperium is the period of recovery from childbirth, which usually lasts about six weeks. Like pregnancy, the puerperium is a healthy state, but care must be taken because complications may occur.

Normal symptoms of the puerperium

Immediately after the safe delivery of her baby, the mother usually spends a day or two in a mood of excitement and pleasure. This is commonly followed by a time of fluctuating moods in which happiness alternates with depression ("post-baby blues"). These mood changes are probably due to a combination of the natural happiness, tiredness and the rapid hormonal changes after childbirth. It may take time for the new baby to become loved as some mothers feel detached, or even dislike the baby for a few days.

The vaginal discharge that continues for three to four weeks after childbirth is known as the lochia. In the first few days it is a bright red colour, which gradually becomes browner, then yellow-brown and finally turns white towards the end of the three weeks. The amount of lochia varies greatly from one woman to another, and often from day to day, but gradually decreases until it turns into the normal vaginal moistness.

If the mother is breast-feeding, the hormonal stimulus that produces slight concentration of the breast tissue also affects the womb, causing it to contract and increase the flow of lochia. This sometimes produces a vague lower abdominal discomfort similar to a mild labour pain, known as an after-pain. After-pains commonly occur for two or three days after childbirth. They are seldom severe enough to require more than a mild painkiller.

The first time that the bowels and bladder work may be painful due to the bruising that has occurred during childbirth, particularly if aggravated by piles that may have developed during pregnancy. If there has been extensive tearing or a large episiotomy, the stitching may cause considerable pain. A mild laxative, or even an enema, will be given to ensure that the faeces are soft and easy to pass for the first bowel movement. Continued discomfort on passing urine is not normal and is usually due to a urinary infection so a doctor must be consulted.

During pregnancy the normal slight hair loss that occurs in all people does not take place. Therefore, by the end of pregnancy, the hair is frequently thick. Hair loss in the puerperium is sometimes heavy until the hair returns to normal.

Mothers hope to return to their normal weight within a few weeks of childbirth. The more weight that a woman has gained in pregnancy the less likely she is to return to her normal weight during the puerperium.

Unless the mother has decided that she does not want to breast-feed, in which case she will be given an injection of the hormone oestrogen to stop milk production, it is common for the breasts to become swollen and tender two or three days after the baby is born. This is known as breast engorgement and occurs when there is a sudden production of milk. Although this is uncomfortable, the combination of breast-feeding and wearing a firm brassiere will control the symptoms until normal feeding starts.

Permanent effects on the mother

There are few permanent effects of pregnancy on the mother. The darkening of the skin around the nipple, which occurs during the early part of the first pregnancy, remains. Unfortunately, stretch marks that may have appeared on the breasts, abdomen and thighs do not disappear. They become pale during the puerperium. Varicose veins appearing during pregnancy usually do not disappear completely. Most specialists advise the woman not to have varicose veins treated by injections or surgery until she has had all the babies that she wants. However, an unusually distended vein may be injected after the puerperium.

Although the breasts enlarge during pregnancy, they return to their normal shape during the puerperium, unless breast-feeding is taking place. Undue sagging can usually be prevented by wearing a firm, supportive brassiere.

Internally, the woman returns to normal size. Although the vagina has been stretched, the only permanent damage that may remain is a scar from an episiotomy or tear. The womb returns to its normal size and position but the shape of cervix remains slightly altered.

Normal care during the puerperium

It is important for the woman to be treated as a normal, healthy individual after the first 24 hours of rest following childbirth. She should be encouraged to get up, move around and look after the baby, even if she has had a Caesarean operation or forceps delivery. She should also have two hours rest each afternoon to compensate for any loss of sleep and to allow the softened ligaments to return to their normal position without strain. It is now that the postnatal exercises, often taught at the antenatal classes, can be started. They help to strengthen the muscles of the pelvis, abdomen and back. While the mother is in hospital, the exercises are supervised by a physiotherapist but they must be continued when she returns home. It takes time and regular exercise for the abdominal muscles, which have been stretched by the large womb during pregnancy, to return to their normal length and tone; until they do so, the abdomen will bulge. Excessive exercising can make the mother tired and, sometimes, strain the muscles.

The vulva will be sore and bruised after childbirth. This discomfort will be increased if the tissues were stitched after a tear or episiotomy. During the first day or two, regular bathing with a warm solution of salt and water helps healing. After this, the mother can bath, with salt added to the water. Vulval cleanliness is essential and frequent changes of external sanitary towels are needed. Internal tampons must not be worn as they are too small and may introduce infection into the womb.

During the first ten days after childbirth the mother is visited at least once a day by a midwife, whether she is in hospital or at home. The midwife examines the vulva and the stitches, and feels the abdomen to ensure that the womb is becoming smaller at a normal rate. Immediately after childbirth the womb can be felt at the level of the navel. It rapidly shrinks until it can no longer be felt by the tenth day. This shrinking is accompanied by the changes in colour of the lochia, so the midwife also examines the sanitary towels. It is important that a regular record of the temperature and pulse rate is kept to detect any fever. During the first few days the blood pressure is taken regularly, as a sudden rise may be due to pre-eclampsia (toxaemia of pregnancy).

Although most mothers wish to lose weight rapidly, excessive dieting should be avoided. Weight loss normally takes place gradually and strict dieting causes fatigue and depression. It is important to drink plenty of fluids, particularly when breast-feeding. A normal diet with fresh fruit and extra protein reduces the need for carbohydrate foods, which tend to increase weight.

The length of time spent in hospital depends mainly on the health of the mother and baby, and also on whether she has had a baby before. If it is the mother's first baby, it is usual to keep her in hospital for about a week to ensure that she knows how to feed and care for it. If she has previously had a baby, she can usually go home in two or three days. The midwife will visit her at home to continue the normal nursing care for ten days, before handing over to the Health Visitor.

A blood test to detect anaemia is usually done before the mother leaves hospital. Most specialists recommend that iron and vitamin pills are continued until the end of the puerperium.

Feeding the baby

Breast milk is the best food for the baby: it supplies all the essential nutrients at the correct temperature, and it contains antibodies that help the baby resist infections.

Some mothers do not wish to breast-feed. Sometimes there are medical reasons why breast-feeding should not take place; the specialist will give advice about this. A mother who does not breast-feed should not feel that she is depriving the baby of some factor that will prevent normal growth and development. However, bottle-feeding has several disadvantages: a lowered resistance to infection in the baby; the possibility of producing dehydration or an imbalance of body salts as a result of incorrect mixing of the milk; and the need to sterilize the bottles, teats and feeding equipment.

The technique of breast-feeding is discussed elsewhere in the book but it is essential that the mother knows how to care for her breasts – keeping the nipples clean and preventing them from becoming cracked – in order to reduce the chance of breast infection. A special pad should be worn over the nipples between feeds; a nursing brassiere that gives sufficient support to hold the enlarge breasts should also be worn.

Complications in the puerperium

In most women, the puerperium progresses without any serious complications. Minor disorders, such as breast engorgement, painful haemorrhoids and "post-baby blues" seldom become a problem. The discomfort of a torn and bruised vulva usually settles within two or three days and is greatly helped by sitting on a rubber ring or soft material.

Unfortunately, more serious complications may sometimes occur. Puerperal fever is due to infection of the womb. This used to be a potentially fatal complication of pregnancy, but it is now rare and can be cured with antibiotics, so that fever is more usually due to a urinary or breast infection. However, the cause of any fever must be discovered by a doctor. Often fever is accompanied by other symptoms. Breast infection usually produces local tenderness and swelling in one breast. Urinary infections commonly produce pain and frequent urination, particularly when due to cystitis. Both breast and urinary infections may produce sudden shivering and a high temperature without local symptoms.

Infection of the womb, particularly if it is mild, commonly produces lower abdominal pain and a change in the colour and smell of the lochia. The womb also takes longer to return to its normal size. This is known as subinvolution and is often detected by the midwife who finds that the womb is slightly tender and is still enlarged by the tenth day. More serious infections are accompanied by a high temperature, severe pain and, sometimes, a haemorrhage.

The stitching of a tear or episiotomy may become infected, producing an abscess between the back of the vagina and the anus. If this occurs, the stitches are cut and the pus allowed to escape.

Women who have diabetes mellitus, anaemia or other medical disorders are more likely to get infections during the puerperium.

A haemorrhage may occur immediately after childbirth, particularly if labour has been prolonged and difficult, and is usually due to either a retained piece of the placenta or membranes, or to a failure of the womb to contract firmly. Immediate injections of the hormones that make the womb contract, blood transfusions and, if necessary, removal of the retained piece of placenta, will stop the haemorrhage. A haemorrhage occurring later in the puerperium is usually due to uterine infection or a retained piece of placenta. If the mother has already returned home, she must be readmitted to hospital so that the appropriate treatment, with antibiotics, blood transfusion or removal of the retained piece of placenta, can be given.

Venous thrombosis (clotting of the blood in the veins) used to be a common complication of childbirth. This is less likely to happen now because mothers are encouraged to get up after the baby is born. However, women with varicose veins may develop thrombosis. This is seldom serious, although the surface vein may be tender. Wearing an elastic stocking is often the only treatment that is required. Thrombosis in a deep vein in the muscles of the leg or pelvis is a serious complication, causing swelling of the ankles and tenderness of the muscle. The danger of a deep vein thrombosis is that a small piece of the blood clot may break off and pass through the circulation to the lung (a pulmonary embolus). A pulmonary embolus may cause few symptoms but, rarely, can be a life-threatening complication, with severe chest pain, breathlessness and haemoptysis (coughing up blood). This requires emergency treatment in hospital with anticoagulant drugs. A deep vein thrombosis may cause a permanent blockage so that the leg will always remain slightly swollen; this is known as "white leg".

Occasionally, pre-eclampsia occurs for the first time after childbirth or, more usually, becomes worse. If it is not diagnosed and treated, eclampsia (a condition in which fits and coma occur) may result.

The two most common complications of the puerperium are anaemia and depression. Anaemia may be the result of excessive bleeding or of failure to take iron throughout pregnancy. It is for this reason that obstetricians usually do blood tests for anaemia before the mother leaves hospital and again at the postnatal examination.

Although most mothers experience a day or two of depression in the few days following childbirth, this is usually transient. However, about one in twenty women develop depression that is severe enough to need medical treatment. This depression is usually a continuation of the "post-baby blues", combined with the normal anxiety and fatigue of looking after the baby and the rapid hormonal and chemical changes that occur after pregnancy. The woman feels increasingly inadequate, with a fear of looking after her baby combined with anxiety and apprehension when separated from him or her. Sleep, already disturbed by feeding, is often worse than normal. Fortunately, treatment with antidepressant drugs for some weeks usually cures postnatal depression.

Baby care

Apart from the initial examination after birth, the paediatrician (child specialist) examines the baby carefully within the first day or two to discover any abnormalities or problems which may not have been noticed on the first occasion. This second examination gives the paediatrician a chance to discuss the baby's health with the mother and for her to ask about anything that she has noticed, and that she thinks may be abnormal.

During the first few days of life the baby usually loses 50-150 grams (a few ounces) in weight but commonly recovers the birthweight between the seventh and tenth day, about the time of discharge from hospital. It is during this time that slight jaundice (yellowing of the whites of the eyes) may be noticed. This is normal. All babies are born with extra haemoglobin in the blood to help during the final days of pregnancy and throughout labour when the extra oxygen-carrying capacity is needed. Breakdown of the haemoglobin causes jaundice because the liver cannot cope with the extra waste products. Jaundice is only serious when there is a Rhesus incompatibility.

The baby's faeces are sticky and dark in colour on the first two or three occasions. This is known as meconium and is due to the substances swallowed by the foetus while in the womb. Meconium is replaced by the normal yellow, porridge-like faeces of the milk-fed baby. The kidneys are unable to concentrate urine, so frequent urination occurs for the first few weeks of life.

The umbilical cord remains as a shrivelled worm-like structure lying on the abdomen. It must be kept dry with spirit and powder until it spontaneously falls off after five to ten days. This may be accompanied by slight bleeding. A scab forms on the umbilical stump, which must also be kept dry and clean to prevent infection. The scab usually falls off within a week.

The PKU (Guthrie test) is done about ten days after birth to detect phenylalanine, a substance that accumulates in the blood in babies suffering from a rare congenital disorder that can cause mental retardation. Blood for the test is obtained from a pinprick on the heel. This disorder can be prevented by a phenylalanine-free diet for the first few years of life.

Most mothers are anxious that a newborn baby is not getting sufficient food and fluid but, because a baby is born with an excess of body fluid, the first 48 hours can safely be a time of relative starvation. Although the baby usually sucks enthusiastically, this seldom gives an adequate feed for the first two or three days. It is during this time that the midwife shows the mother how to handle and feed the baby.

Some hospitals encourage the mother to have the baby beside her all the time, day and night. Other hospitals keep the baby in the nursery during the afternoon rest period and at night. Nursery care is particularly necessary in hospitals where mothers are in a ward, as one baby crying can disturb the entire ward.

Many parents ask about circumcision. There are seldom medical reasons for circumcision but in most hospitals there is a doctor who will do the operation, if asked, before the baby leaves hospital.

After the mother and baby have left hospital, the Health Visitor will see them at home and recommend visits to the local baby clinic.

Postnatal examination

When the mother leaves hospital, she is given an appointment for a postnatal examination about six weeks after the birth of the baby. This enables the specialist to ensure that she is in good health and to deal with any problems. The specialist checks her blood pressure, urine and breasts; examines the scar formed after an episiotomy or tear; and does a vaginal examination to make sure that the womb has returned to its normal shape and size. A cervical smear is also done to check for cancer. The postnatal examination gives the woman an opportunity to ask about any problems that may have occurred and to discuss what type of contraception to use.

Most women ask when menstruation will return. In women who are not breast-feeding, a period may have already occurred before the postnatal examination, or may not occur for a further few weeks without any abnormality being present. Even if the period is delayed, a pregnancy can occur if contraception is not used. Breast-feeding frequently delays the first period until feeding stops but does not prevent conception.

Sexual intercourse

Most specialists advise women not to have intercourse during the puerperium until the postnatal examination has been done. Intercourse in the first few weeks may introduce infection into the womb and may also be painful if an episiotomy was performed or if the skin at the entrance to the vagina was torn. Sexual activity can be resumed during this time, but it is advisable to avoid the penetration of full sexual intercourse. This is safe for the first month of the puerperium but after this time some form of contraceptive cream or pessary should be used.

Registering the birth

This must be done within six weeks (three weeks in Scotland). In many hospitals, the Registrar visits at least once a week so that registration can be done without the need to visit the local office. As the hospital will inform the Registrar of the birth, a letter will be sent to all parents who have not registered within the legal time. You will need to know the date and place of birth, as well as the names and sex of the baby. The father's names, place of birth and occupation are recorded, provided the parents are married or the father accepts paternity; and the mother's names and her maiden name have to be given. The Registrar then provides a card so that the parents can register the baby on the NHS list of their local doctor.

Postnatal exercises 1

The importance of antenatal exercises, with particular reference to breathing and posture, has already been described earlier in this section. Exercises after birth are also important, although the emphasis is slightly different, with the accent on recovery and regaining normal muscle tone and fitness.

Recovery is encouraged by starting the exercises soon after the birth. The antenatal exercises described in this section (*see* **Antenatal exercises**, p.752) should be continued and the postnatal exercises described here are additional. All of these exercises are particularly helpful for the muscles of the abdomen and back, as well as those of the pelvic floor, which have been stretched during pregnancy and childbirth.

The mother should exercise every day, taking care not to strain herself. If she feels overtired after exercising, she should start with a few repetitions of each exercise and gradually build up to the recommended level. In addition, women who suffer from disorders that may be adversely affected by excessive exercise should consult a doctor before starting postnatal exercises. It may take time for the benefit of the exercises to become noticeable, so the mother should not feel discouraged if she seems to be making slow progress in the beginning.

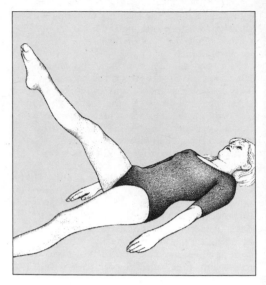

Leg raising
This exercise is for the leg and stomach muscles. Lie on the back with the arms loosely by the sides and the legs together. Keeping the knee straight, slowly lift one leg as high as possible. Gradually lower the leg, then slowly lift the other leg.

Repeat 10 times with each leg.

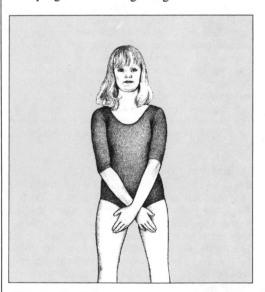

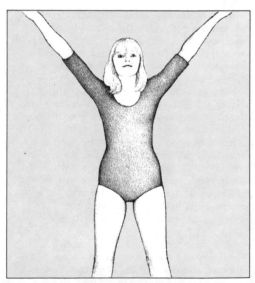

Arm swinging
This exercise benefits the waist, the stomach muscles, and general posture. Stand upright, with the spine straight and the head erect and facing forwards. The legs should be slightly apart, and the knees should be straight. Loosely cross the wrists in front of the body and, keeping the elbows straight, swing the

arms outwards and upwards as far as possible. When the arms are fully extended, the muscles of the abdomen and chest should feel slightly tight. Return the arms to the starting position, also with a vigorous swinging movement.

Repeat 15 to 20 times.

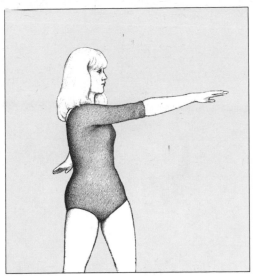

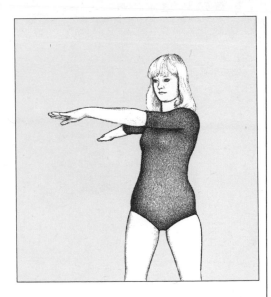

Trunk twisting

This exercise benefits the waist. Stand upright, with the spine straight and the head erect and facing forwards. The legs should be slightly apart with the knees straight. Raise the arms to shoulder height. Swing the head, arms and shoulders to one side so that a slight pull is felt on muscles around the waist.

Ensure that the hips and legs do not move and that the spine remains straight. Then swing to the opposite side; the further you can twist, the greater the benefit. This exercise should be done as a continuous movement.

Repeat 10 times on each side.

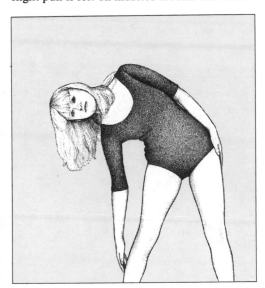

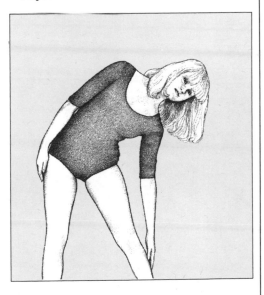

Side bending

This exercise benefits the waist and hips. Stand upright, with the spine straight, and the head erect and facing forwards. The arms should hang loosely at the sides, the legs should be slightly apart, and the knees should be straight. Keeping the legs straight, slowly bend from the waist down one side of the

body. You should keep facing forwards and should reach down as far as possible so that the waist muscles feel stretched. Slowly return to the upright position, then bend to the opposite side. This exercise should be done slowly and smoothly.

Repeat 10 times on each side.

Postnatal exercises 2

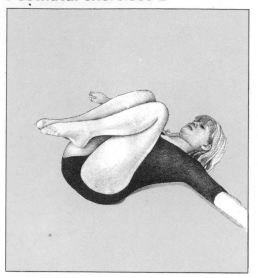

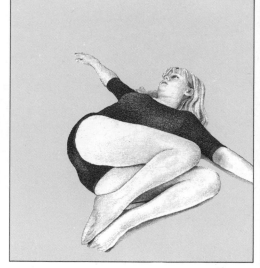

Hip rolling

This exercise benefits the waist and hips. Lie on the back, with the arms stretched out at right angles to the body and the palms of the hands downwards. This position helps to keep the body balanced while the exercise is done. Bend the knees and bring them up towards the chest. Keeping the knees bent and the shoulders firmly on the floor, slowly twist the body to one side until the knees touch the floor and the waist muscles feel stretched. Slowly return the knees to the vertical position, then down to the floor on the opposite side.

Repeat 10 times on each side.

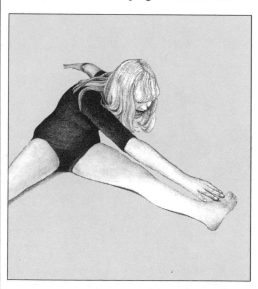

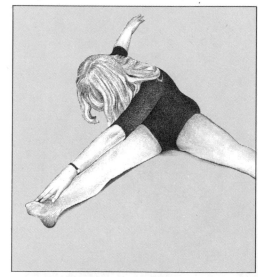

Toe touching

This exercise benefits the waist, legs and stomach muscles. Sit upright on the floor, with the legs straight and stretched wide apart. Swing the body to the left and lean forwards to touch the left toes with the right hand; the left arm should swing outwards behind the body. This should make the muscles of the waist and insides of the thighs feel stretched. Return to the upright position; repeat the procedure on the other side so that the left hand touches the right toes. This exercise should be a continuous movement, swinging from side to side.

Repeat 10 times on each side.

The healthy child

Section contents

Introduction

Good parental care during childhood can prevent many potential problems from occurring, and can help a child grow into a healthy adolescent and adult.

A young child has physical needs, such as food, clothing, and protection from illness; emotional needs; and intellectual needs. It is of the utmost importance that parents understand and try to fulfil these needs.

The most pressing needs of a newborn baby are mainly physical. In the first part of the section, there are clear explanations of how to take care of the routine physical requirements of a baby.

Despite all parental precautions, a young child is likely to become ill. In fact, it is preferable for some diseases, such as chicken-pox, to be caught during childhood rather than during adult life, because certain infections can be much more serious in adults. The second part of the section, entitled The growing child, provides guidance on immunization against serious diseases, and on the action the parents should take when a child becomes ill.

As the child grows older, the parents can help him or her to develop psychologically so that, in this respect, the child becomes increasingly independent. However, a young child still depends on the parents to fulfil emotional needs and to provide guidance in social and intellectual development.

Strong emotional bonds are formed between the parents, particularly the mother, and the baby during the first few days following birth. As the child develops, his or her emotional needs change. Parents should try to recognize these changes and adjust their own behaviour accordingly. They should try to provide an emotionally-secure environment for the child.

As children mature they become aware of themselves as individuals, and may begin to challenge the standards of their parents. This may cause difficulties in the parent-child relationship, particularly over matters of discipline. Children also become aware of their sexuality. The section discusses the common problems that may confront parents during their child's sexual development. It provides guidance on sexuality; on how parents can explain sex to their children; and on the difficulties that may result from the child's increasing independence.

The baby's room

Many newborn infants share their parents' bedroom for the first few months, but whenever possible a separate room should be planned and equipped so that everything is conveniently at hand for the main activities in the baby's life: feeding and playing, washing and nappy changing.

The room itself should be warm and well ventilated. A constant temperature of 20° to 22°C (68° to 72°F) is advisable for any baby who weighs less than eight pounds (3.6kg), but as the baby grows and puts on weight, the night-time temperature may be allowed to fall as low as 15°C (60°F). It is important that the air in the room is not too dry. Place a bowl of water in the room to keep the air moist.

Every baby needs fresh air, but should be protected from draughts, so make sure that the cot is not next to an open window when the baby is asleep. Alternatively a screen can be used if a small window is open. In cold weather, the room should be aired when the baby is not occupying it.

Lighting

For the convenience of the parents the room should be well lit, but newborn infants are unable to adjust their eyes to a bright light. A ceiling light should therefore have a low-power bulb, or a dimmer attachment on the light switch. A small table-lamp is useful, particularly at night when changing the baby.

Even small babies become quickly bored by having nothing to look at. A mobile above the cot or cradle may hold the infant's attention, as may brightly coloured pictures fixed within the baby's field of vision.

Furniture and equipment

The most important piece of furniture in the baby's room is the bed. The most suitable first bed for a newborn infant is a cot, cradle, moses basket, or carrycot because a tiny baby feels more secure in a fairly small space. If the baby is going to start in a big cot, tie bumper pads around the edge, and wrap the baby firmly so that he or she feels secure.

The mattress must be firm and smooth, and should fit the bed snugly. Never use a pillow instead of a mattress. A firm rubberized hair mattress is recommended at least 25mm (one inch) thick, with a well-fitting waterproof cover. If you are using a straw or cane cradle, line the inside with material to prevent the baby catching or scratching the fingers or face on a rough edge. This also helps to prevent draughts. A baby under the age of two should never be given a pillow for sleeping.

A low, comfortable chair without arm-rests and a straight back is an important item in the baby's room. The chair can be used for feeding with the bottle or at the breast, or the parent can sit on the chair and change the baby's nappy on the lap instead of on a changing mat.

All the equipment needed during a nappy change should be within reach so that the parent does not have to leave an infant unattended on the changing surface. A set of shelves above the changing mat is useful for storing equipment needed for changing, but if this is not possible, make sure that there is a working surface at the correct height next to the changing area.

By the side of the changing mat put two buckets with lids, one for dirty nappies and the other for dirty clothing. A waste basket is needed for tissues and cotton wool.

There should be a baby bath on a sturdy stand in the room, and a rack to hang towels and clothing on. It is more suitable to bath a small baby in his or her room because the temperature is more easily maintained than in a bathroom. Even if the room is centrally heated, it may be necessary to boost the room temperature with a heater before bath-time. The heater can be either of the radiator type, or an electric heater placed high on the wall.

An easily cleaned table can be used for feeding and equipment, but a trolley is useful if feeding is sometimes to be done in another room.

A cupboard or chest of drawers is needed so that clean clothing and blankets, towels and nappies are readily available. All articles must be well aired before they are put away.

Safety

When planning and equipping a baby's room, safety factors should always be borne in mind. Babies quickly become mobile, and it is often not until a near-accident occurs that the parents realize with some concern how active the baby is.

All the furniture in the room should be strong and stable so that a crawling infant is not able to overturn it. The windows should have safety catches on them to prevent them opening wide enough for the child to crawl out of. Alternatively, fix bars (vertical ones) over the window. If there are electric sockets at ground level, place a piece of heavy furniture in front of them because a crawling child will soon try poking something into the holes.

Never use an unguarded fire in a baby's room – oil heaters are also dangerous because they may be overturned, and should not be used.

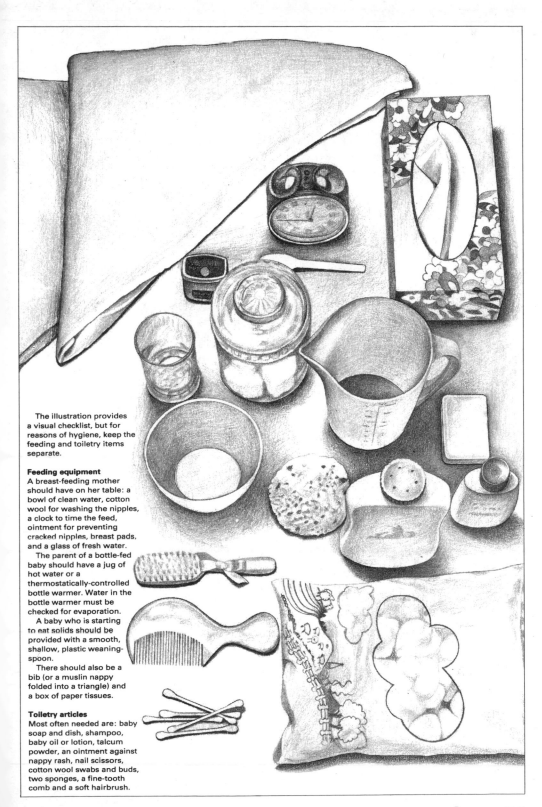

The illustration provides a visual checklist, but for reasons of hygiene, keep the feeding and toiletry items separate.

Feeding equipment
A breast-feeding mother should have on her table: a bowl of clean water, cotton wool for washing the nipples, a clock to time the feed, ointment for preventing cracked nipples, breast pads, and a glass of fresh water.

The parent of a bottle-fed baby should have a jug of hot water or a thermostatically-controlled bottle warmer. Water in the bottle warmer must be checked for evaporation.

A baby who is starting to eat solids should be provided with a smooth, shallow, plastic weaning-spoon.

There should also be a bib (or a muslin nappy folded into a triangle) and a box of paper tissues.

Toiletry articles
Most often needed are: baby soap and dish, shampoo, baby oil or lotion, talcum powder, an ointment against nappy rash, nail scissors, cotton wool swabs and buds, two sponges, a fine-tooth comb and a soft hairbrush.

Clothing and equipment

Clothing

The pregnant mother gets great enjoyment from buying or making the baby's clothes, but the price, laundering time and effort of dressing the baby must also be kept in mind. A baby grows rapidly and there is no need to buy large quantities of clothing since both the size and need are constantly changing. It should be remembered that:

1) clothing should allow growing space;
2) garments should be easy to launder;
3) all items should be comfortable and safe for the baby to wear; and
4) garments should be simple and easy to put on and take off the baby.

Pretty clothes often look smart but are frequently impractical, for most babies hate being dressed and undressed, and cry and struggle. A crying baby is rigid and uncooperative, so ensure that clothing is loose-fitting, easily fastened and does not have to be tugged over the baby's head. All new clothing and nappies, wrapping blankets or similar articles that are to touch the baby's skin should be washed before they are first used. A newborn baby's skin is easily irritated by the sizing, or starchy substance, used in all new materials. Use a mild soap powder and warm water and make sure that all the soap is thoroughly rinsed away. Labels can cause pressure marks on sensitive skin, so all labels (except those giving washing instructions) should be removed.

Nappies

Although only a limited amount of clothing is recommended there should be a plentiful supply of nappies – unless you live in a large city where a commercial nappy service may be available.

Disposable nappies are available in many different types; some are pads which are put inside plastic pants, while others are sold with plastic adherent and do not require pants. They are useful when there is limited washing and drying room or when travelling. But they are expensive and occupy a lot of room.

Muslin nappies are soft, absorb well, and are less bulky than towelling nappies. The large size, 75cm × 75cm (30in × 30in), is more useful than the smaller one. It can be used alone for babies under 8lbs (3.6kg); used inside a towelling nappy; used as a bib or towel; or used over the sheet in the cot.

Turkish towelling nappies are the most frequently used and most absorbent of all.

One-way nappies are non-absorbent nappies that can be put inside towelling nappies when the baby starts to sleep overnight. They protect the skin by preventing it from becoming wet.

Babycare checklist

Essential items
Cot or moses basket
Firm mattress
Cotton sheets
Lightweight blankets

Nappies and pants
36 Turkish towelling nappies (12 if disposable nappies used)
12 muslin nappies
One-way nappies
6 nappy pins
Disposable nappy liners
3 pairs small soft plastic pants
3 pairs medium soft plastic pants

Other clothing
3 lightweight cardigans or matinee jackets
2 heavier ones for outdoors
4 pairs booties
Bonnet and mittens for outdoors
4 nightdresses
4 cotton vests
3 bibs
4 to 6 receiving blankets

Feeding articles
6 8oz (220ml) bottles with teats, discs, screw caps and covers
2 4oz (110ml) bottles for water or fruit juice
Measuring jug with lid
Large plastic spoon
Plastic knife
Bottle brush
Extra teats in 3 sizes
Large plastic container to hold all equipment for sterilizing
Sterilizing fluid

Toiletry articles
Baby soap and dish
Shampoo
Baby oil or lotion
Talcum powder
Ointment for nappy rash
Cotton wool balls
Cotton buds
2 sponges (one for body, one face)
Fine-tooth comb
Soft hairbrush
Nail scissors
Box of paper tissues
Nappy bucket with lid
Antiseptic fluid

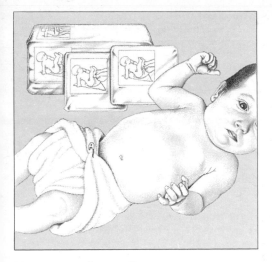

Nappy requirements

12 muslin (gauze) nappies
36 Turkish towelling nappies (or 12 if
  disposable nappies are used)
One-way nappies
6 rounded nappy pins with locking heads
Disposable nappy liners
3 small and 3 medium-sized plastic pants
  of soft material

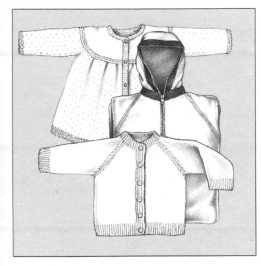

Cardigans and matinee jackets

Three lightweight cardigans for indoor wear
and two heavier ones for use outside (one
with a hood) are needed. Pure wool, cotton
yarn, or synthetic fibres other than nylon are
recommended: these allow the skin to
"breathe".

Buttons, velcro fasteners and press studs
are safer and easier to use than ribbons,
which can be pulled too tightly.

Receiving and wrapping blankets

Blankets in which a baby can be wrapped are
essential to the layette; four, five, or even six
may be required. They should be made of a
soft material, such as cotton knit or
flannelette.

Being wrapped in a receiving blanket has a
calming effect on a newborn baby whose
tendency is to kick and wave. Such a
tendency is generally caused by the baby's
feelings of insecurity: a well wrapped baby
feels more secure.

Babies' nightdresses

Nighties made of cotton or flannelette keep a
baby warm and comfortable. The minimum
number likely to be required is four. For
many parents, nightgowns are the most
popular form of clothing for the baby in the
early weeks because they are not difficult to
put on – certainly easier at that stage than a
stretch suit.

Later, however, the parents may decide to
switch to a stretch suit, either a one-piece or
a two-piece. When buying a stretch suit,
make sure that the baby will have enough
room for the feet as he or she grows.

Vests

At least four cotton vests are essential.
Whether the vests have long or short sleeves
is not as important as their having an opening
down the front, for it is much easier for the
parent (and less troublesome to the baby) to
put this kind on than the kind that goes on
over the head.

If the vests have ribbon ties at the front,
make sure that the ribbons are securely sewn
on. Some babies enjoy sucking them and may
swallow them if they come off.

When buying vests, err on the large side
rather than the small. Cotton vests next to
the skin do not generally cause allergic rashes,
as those made with artificial fibre have been
known to do.

Booties, mittens and bonnet

A baby born during the winter months needs
at least four pairs of booties, of a plain and
simple kind.

The circulation of the blood in an infant
takes time to adjust and adapt to changes in
temperature. A parent should be able to tell
by touch whether the baby's feet need
protection. Do not let the baby's feet become
either too cold or too hot.

The judgement of a parent is similarly
required on the use of mittens and a bonnet.
In general, these articles should really be
used only out of doors, and then only in cold
weather.

Bottle-feeding

There are many different reasons for a mother to choose not to breast-feed her baby. Having decided to bottle-feed, a mother should not then feel guilty about her decision. Millions of infants fed on milk from a bottle have grown up healthy.

Combination feeding

It is important that from birth breast-fed babies learn to drink from a bottle. The baby can be offered plain, boiled water from a small bottle to pacify him or her between feeding times. A baby of three or four months who has never had a bottle may obstinately refuse one when the mother decides to wean. Such a baby's stubborn resistance, against the mother's insistence, can make for a difficult time.

A woman who wishes to breast-feed and to return to work outside the home generally finds this no problem if the baby has had the experience of a bottle. She can then leave a prepared bottle with the baby sitter to give to the baby as a lunchtime substitute for the breast.

A mother's breasts soon adjust to a new schedule; so does the baby. It is important that the bottle is offered at the same time each day. The working mother should eat a nutritious lunch and drink plenty of liquids.

Choice of milk

There are many types of milk powder and evaporated (tinned) milk on the market suitable for a baby's bottle. A mother should continue using the same type that the baby was first given in the hospital, or a doctor may suggest an alternative.

As an aid to the baby's digestion, it is sometimes better to add slightly more water to the milk than the instructions suggest.

Condensed milk is not suitable for babies. Pasteurized cow's milk should be introduced only after the baby is six months old. The milk should then be diluted according to the clinic's instructions.

How much fluid does a baby need?

A baby whose birth weight was from 6 to 9 pounds (2.7kg–4.1kg) must be fed every three or four hours round the clock in the first few weeks. Usually, after three weeks, a four-hourly schedule of five feeds and an eight-hour sleeping gap can be established.

The total amount of bottled milk that a baby should be given each day is based on his or her body weight. In general, for every pound (0.45kg) weight, the baby should be given $2\frac{1}{2}$ fluid ounces (75ml). The total should then be divided by the number of feeds.

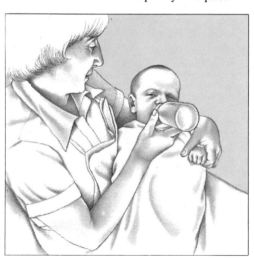

Position of baby

The parent or baby sitter should sit well back in the chair, in a relaxed position, holding the baby close to the body at an angle of about 45°. The bottle should be held from underneath and tilted so that the teat is always filled with milk.

It is important to concentrate on the feeding. If the feeder's attention wanders, the bottle may slip and the teat fill with air.

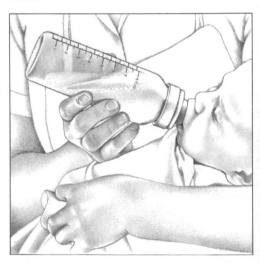

Giving the bottle

Make sure that all the items needed for the feed are nearby, so that the baby's feeding time is not interrupted. Have ready the bottle; a bottle warmer or jug; a box of tissues; and a soft nappy or bib, to cover the baby's arms and front, which stops the baby from fidgeting.

The milk should be given to the baby at body temperature.

Preparing the bottles

When preparing the feeds for your baby it is essential that every piece of equipment is scrupulously clean. Infectious bacteria may grow on stale milk.

There are three methods for sterilizing the feeding equipment and keeping the milk free from infection; the boiling method, the aseptic method, and the terminal method.

In the boiling method, the feeding equipment is completely covered and boiled in water for ten minutes.

In the aseptic method, the equipment is soaked in a chemical solution which must be prepared and used in the way that the manufacturer recommends.

The terminal method, which is rarely used in this country, is a method in which both the milk and bottles are sterilized together.

Feeding equipment

It is easier to make up bottles of milk sufficient to last for 24 hours, and to do this once a day. The following equipment is needed:

6 8oz (220ml) bottles of either transparent plastic or glass, with teats, discs, screw cap and covers.
A measuring jug, with lid, for mixing the feeds.
A large plastic spoon, for mixing the milk powder.
A plastic knife, kept in the tin of milk, for levelling off the powder on the spoon.
A large plastic container which can hold all the equipment totally submerged in a sterilizing solution. A bottle brush, kept in a separate jar. 2 4oz (140ml) bottles, used for giving water or juice between feeds.
A variety of extra teats, small, medium and large.
Household salt for rubbing the teats.

Most teats are not marked for size; it may therefore be impossible to distinguish one from the other once they are in the sterilizing unit. To identify them, mark them with different coloured threads (perhaps white for small, red for medium and blue for large) by sewing the thread into the rim.

Preparing milk for 24 hours

Prepare a clean surface in the kitchen while boiling a kettle of water and then letting it cool for a few minutes while you thoroughly wash your hands. Take the bottles, teats, and discs from the sterilizer and drain them. Put the jug, mixing spoon and plastic knife on a dry surface. Rinse all the equipment with some of the boiled water from the kettle as some babies do not like the smell or taste of the sterilizing solution. Carefully follow the instructions as to the correct quantities that will be required for the amount of milk for the next 24 hours. Pour the boiled water into the jug, checking the exact quantity by holding it at eye level. Next add the required number of scoops of milk powder to the water, levelling each scoop with the knife. Stir the mixture thoroughly with the spoon and then fill each bottle with the required amount. There is usually a little extra milk left in the jug, for the powder added to the water increases the volume. The extra can be added to the bottles or thrown away. Insert the teats upside down in each bottle and cover with a sterile cap and ring. Put the bottles in the refrigerator.

Making individual bottles

If a refrigerator is not available, each bottle must be made up before each feed; it is not safe to leave milk at room temperature. One feed can be made up in the bottle by filling the bottle with the required amount of warm, boiled water, checking the volume at eye level, and then adding the correct number of scoops of milk, levelled off with the knife, before screwing on the teat and cover. It is essential to shake well to ensure the milk is properly mixed.

Washing the feeding equipment

Using the bottle brush, wash all the bottles, caps and jugs etc. in hot water with a detergent, taking particular care to clean the rim of the bottle in order to remove milk particles. Then rinse in cold water. Rub the teats with salt, inside and out, to remove milk particles and then rinse thoroughly before putting all the equipment in the sterilizing container. Sterilizing fluid must be replaced every 24 hours.

Other bottles

Hospitals use ready made-up feeds which come in all-glass bottles accompanied by a sterile teat. The cap is removed and the teat applied when a feed is needed. These bottles are thrown away after use.

Playtex bottles

Playtex bottles, often called disposable bottles, are available but seldom used in this country. The teat is shaped much more like the mother's nipple and breast-fed babies often prefer these bottles for water, juice, and later when changing from the breast to bottle feeds. They are made of a plastic rounded container into which a sterile plastic bag is fitted. The bag can be filled with milk and is thrown away after each feed. The rest of the equipment has to be boiled.

Breast-feeding 1

In the first two to three days after birth, the mother's breasts produce a fluid called colostrum. Colostrum resembles melted butter, is high in protein, and contains antibodies that protect the baby. It helps to empty the bowels of meconium, the faeces in the bowels of all newborn babies. There is no artificial substitute for colostrum.

Breast milk

Breast milk is easily digested by the infant's intestines and helps to prevent allergies. Unlike cow's milk, breast milk leaves an acid residue in the bowel, and prevents the growth of harmful bacteria. Breast-fed babies do not usually suffer from constipation if there is an adequate supply of milk. For the first few weeks bowel movements may be frequent, but these may decrease to once or twice a day.

Most women find breast-feeding a pleasure, once it is established, although initially it may be difficult. Emotionally, it ensures closeness with the baby; physically, it helps the womb to return more quickly to its normal size. Successful breast-feeding depends on the mother's attitude; antenatal preparation of the breasts and nipples, and their postnatal care; a good, balanced diet, with plenty of fluids; rest; and patience.

Antenatal breast care

A well-fitting bra should be worn, both day and night, from the seventh month of pregnancy. From this time, the nipples should be washed well each day and gently rubbed with a towel. Some doctors advise applying a bland ointment.

Flat nipples should be drawn out and rolled between thumb and forefinger. At about the eighth month, the breasts should be gently massaged, so that a little colostrum appears from each nipple. This helps to open the milk ducts.

Women with inverted nipples should wear devices popularly known as "shells" inside the bra for a few hours daily during the last three months. If no improvement occurs, a Natural Nursing Nipple Shield is helpful when breast-feeding.

Breast-feeding

Before putting the baby to the breast, clean the nipple with a cotton wool swab dipped in warm water, to remove any ointment. Start each feed on the opposite side from the last.

After the feed, wipe the nipples with cotton wool dipped in warm water and apply an ointment or spray. Try to avoid the use of plastic-backed milk-retaining pads inside the bra because they can make the nipples sore.

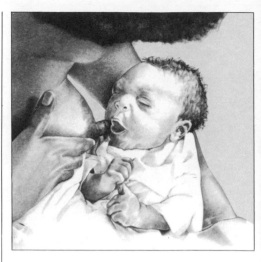

The first time

A newborn infant does not immediately know how to find the mother's nipple. The mother should support her breast from underneath and gently guide the nipple towards the baby's mouth.

Restless babies feed better if firmly wrapped in a receiving blanket with the arms and hands tucked inside.

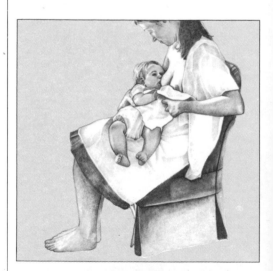

Breast-feeding at home

Once home from the hospital, the mother's early discomfort after the birth will quickly go. She can now sit well back in a low chair, feet flat on the floor, to nurse the baby. While feeding, a towel on the lap is comfortable for the baby. When the baby starts to suck, the other breast may leak. Control this by firmly pressing a paper tissue against the nipple.

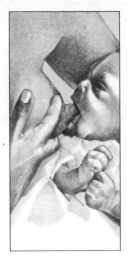
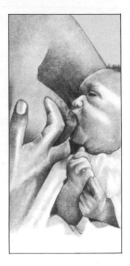
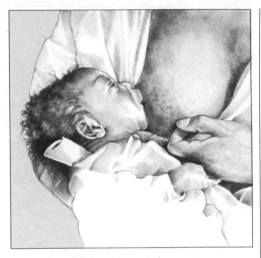

On the breast

The nipple and areola are now in the baby's mouth and the baby's head is resting in the crook of the mother's elbow. The mother can depress the breast above the nipple with her finger so as not to smother the baby.

The baby's hands are clenched at the start of feeding. Satisfied by the milk, the baby relaxes and may touch and pat the breast.

Asleep on the breast

Often a baby falls asleep on the breast in contentment from the warmth and the closeness to the mother. Delightful as this may be, it is better to encourage the baby to continue feeding.

In order to do this slip your middle finger under the baby's chin, and close the mouth. This should restart the sucking reflex.

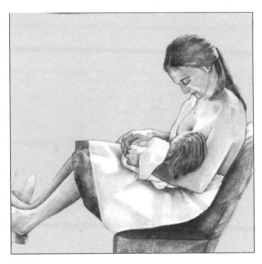
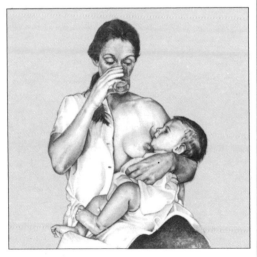

Feeding position

It is important for the breast-feeding mother to be relaxed and comfortable.

Another excellent position for feeding is sitting in a low chair, facing the side of a bed, and resting the feet between the mattress and the base of the bed. The thighs should be raised slightly to prevent the baby from slipping off the lap. Do not hunch the shoulders.

The importance of fluids

Half an hour before feeding the baby, drink a glass of liquid such as milk, water, tea, or weak coffee.

Make it a practice to have a glass of water on the feeding tray. It is usual to feel thirsty while feeding. Do not drink anything hot: it could spill on the baby. A breast-feeding mother should increase her fluid intake by at least 1 litre (2 pints) a day.

Breast-feeding 2

Patience and perseverance are needed during the first week of breast-feeding when difficulties may arise. Breast-feeding mothers should be aware that it can take six weeks before a steady milk supply is established.

In the first two to three days, the baby sucks colostrum. At this stage the mother does not experience much change in her breasts. Usually between the third and fifth day milk "comes in" and, as the breasts enlarge, there may be some discomfort or even pain. Should the milk come in with a rush, the baby should be allowed to feed frequently and this will prevent engorged breasts. Different babies have different needs, and you will have to work out the best schedule for your baby by trial and error.

Breast-feeding problems

Some women do not produce much milk while in the hospital, but produce more when they return home. Until there is enough milk for the baby's needs, a supplementary bottle may be given, but only after (never instead of) breast-feeding. The baby's sucking stimulates the breasts to produce more milk, and frequent feeding helps to increase the supply.

It is useful to know before the baby's birth how to press out ("express") milk from the breasts. Have a sterilized cup ready. Wash your hands and make sure that they are warm. Sit comfortably at a low table with the cup on the table just under your breast. Massage the whole breast with both hands. Then, with thumb and forefinger of one hand, squeeze the milk reservoir deep behind the areola. Slide thumb and forefinger through ninety degrees round the areola, and squeeze again, making sure that all the milk sacs are emptied. Meanwhile, with the other hand, massage the breast gently from top, side, and bottom toward the areola.

Engorgement may occur at the beginning of the milk-producing cycle. The milk-making cells enlarge following hormonal stimulus and an increase in the blood supply. The process lasts for two to three days, and in many women causes the breasts to swell painfully. Cold compresses and a mild painkiller should relieve the condition. Feed the baby frequently, applying warm compresses before feeding. Put a little oil on the breast and express gently.

In the hospital, a hand pump may be supplied and instructions on how to use it. Some hospitals use electric pumps. A close-fitting funnel is placed over the nipple, areola, and breast tissue, and milk is withdrawn by suction produced by the pump.

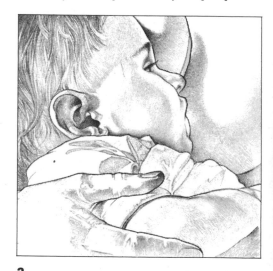

1
Prepare a feeding tray before settling down to feed the baby. Have warm water and cotton wool swabs for cleaning the breast before and after; a clock; ointment or spray; clean breast pads; and a glass of water. Feeding time should be two to three minutes on each breast the first day, gradually increasing to ten minutes.

2
The position illustrated is comfortable for both the baby and the mother throughout the feeding session. Held like this, the baby is able to empty the milk sacs that lie at the top of the breast. Note how much of the nipple and areola is taken into the baby's mouth.

A relaxed mental attitude is important to correct any lack in the supply of milk. Follow a sensible diet and eat a little more than was necessary during pregnancy. Let the baby feed frequently, emptying the breasts at every feed. Drink plenty of liquids, at least five pints a day, especially before and during feeding. Get enough sleep and rest whenever possible, so as not to become tense or anxious.

To prevent excess milk from flowing out, splash the breasts with cold water before feeding, then express a little milk before putting the baby to the breast. Slow the flow of milk to the baby by pressing against the areola with your forefinger and middle fingers. Removing the baby at frequent intervals increases the duration of the feed without giving further stimulus to milk production by rapidly emptying the breast.

The milk may begin to "let down" when you hear your baby crying, or when you are out and think about the baby. Fold your arms and press your fists firmly against the nipple and areola area until the tingling sensation stops. Lack of muscle firmness can also cause leaking. Splashing the breasts with hot and cold water before each feeding period can improve muscle tone. Make sure your bra fits firmly and always wear it.

Soreness, or even cracks that bleed, may develop if a baby sucks hard or chews the nipple. If this happens, feeding must stop temporarily, and milk from the breasts must be expressed (pressed out) into a sterile container at regular intervals. The milk expressed from the breast is preferably given in a spoon to prevent the baby becoming used to a bottle. A mother's sore nipples heal quickly if the baby does not feed for about forty-eight hours. Expose the nipples to the air and to the warmth of the sun or of an electric light whenever possible. Take a mild painkiller, and use an ointment or spray as recommended by the doctor. When the cracks have healed, usually within forty-eight hours, the baby may be breast-fed again, but only for short periods initially. Express a little milk first so that the baby starts sucking at once.

Consult the doctor if a hard area persists in the breast after feeding and massaging; if a red, painful area, like a boil in the early stages, appears; or if your temperature rises suddenly and you start shivering. Doctors do not agree on whether a mother taking antibiotics should continue to breast-feed. Each situation is different so it would be wisest to follow your own doctor's instructions.

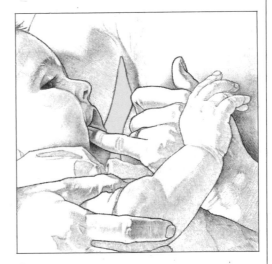

3
When the baby has emptied the front, or top, of the breast, it is important to massage gently the underarm area of the breast and also under the breast itself, directing the milk toward the nipple. If any lump is felt, use a circular massage movement; this helps to disperse congested milk and prevent infection occurring.

4
To remove the baby from the breast without hurting the nipple, slip the little finger of your free hand into the corner of the baby's mouth. Newborn babies become sleepy on the breast. It is therefore advisable to leave the baby a shorter time on the first breast, so that he or she is still interested in feeding when put on the second one.

Winding a baby

All babies swallow air when they suck, whether fed at the breast or on the bottle. The air collects as a bubble in the baby's stomach, and causes discomfort and sometimes pain. The baby stops feeding and begins to cry. To avoid this happening, pause about half-way through the feeding in order to wind the baby.

The amount of air a baby swallows depends on both the flow of milk from breast or bottle, and on the baby's sucking ability.

It is important that all air bubbles are expelled at the end of the feed as well, or the baby will cry soon after being put in the cot.

There are many different kinds of teat available for baby bottles. Some are long, some short; some are made of hard rubber, some of soft. The teats can have a small, medium, or large hole. By buying a selection, the one that is most comfortable and most effective in your baby's mouth can be found. The ability to suck also varies according to the baby's age and whether the baby is hungry. A one-week-old baby who is slightly jaundiced and sleepy, for example, needs a medium-hole or large-hole teat. A jaundiced baby, sucking through a small hole, swallows a lot of air in an effort to get the milk, and falls asleep exhausted and uncomfortable. But if the hole is too large, the milk gushes through so fast that the baby may choke or vomit afterwards.

Controlling the milk flow is more of a problem when the baby is breast-fed. If the flow of milk is too fast, first follow the suggestions given in **Breast-feeding 2,** pp. 780–781. If this does not help, and the milk is still coming so fast that the baby is gulping, take him or her off the breast after two or three sucks. Allow the baby then to take one breath without disturbing the position. Do not sit the baby up for winding too often: it only makes the infant cry, and disrupts the feeding.

Posseting

A baby who feeds too quickly may vomit a little after the feed. Bringing up a small amount of milk is often called posseting and is nothing to worry about. Even if the baby occasionally brings up the entire feed, there is no need for alarm. If the vomiting occurs repeatedly, however, consult a doctor.

When winding a baby in the upright position, the baby's chin resting on your shoulder, be sure to protect your clothing in case the baby should posset.

Wind pains

A baby who has swallowed a lot of air may be unable to expel the wind by belching immediately after being fed. The resulting discomfort can last for a few hours, and demands a great deal of patience. A reliable sign of wind is that the baby may take two or three gulps of milk, draw away from the breast or bottle, and arch the back.

Feed the baby slowly and try to be relaxed. Walking slowly round the room with the baby in your arms sometimes helps to start him or her feeding again. Another method is to change the baby to a different feeding position: so that he or she is in a more upright or flat position. When the condition improves, make sure that the baby returns to the usual feeding position.

Inexperienced parents or baby sitters commonly try to bring up a baby's wind by thumping the baby sharply on the back. But this only makes the baby tense and even less able to release the air. Sometimes such patting on the back may actually cause the baby to bring up some milk.

The illustrations on these pages show some of the best ways to wind the baby during the process of feeding, but if no wind comes up within a few minutes, continue with the feed, unless the baby refuses.

Reluctant feeding

Because the liver does not work normally until some time after birth, some babies may become slightly jaundiced. This condition makes a baby sleepy and disinclined to suck during the first week, when it is important that a baby should drink enough. To encourage a baby to feed, apply gentle pressure under the baby's chin with the little finger. Continue even if the baby is sleepy; it is essential to give enough fluid.

Restless feeding

Some babies for one reason or another fidget and are restless at feeding time. If they can, they wave their arms about, scratching at the bottle, or hitting the breast. Such a baby should be held close to the body and wrapped in a blanket from the waist down. The baby's arms may be left free if they are kept out of the way. One arm can be tucked behind the feeder's back, while the other hand can be held. Hold the baby firmly, but not roughly, because this may make the baby struggle even more.

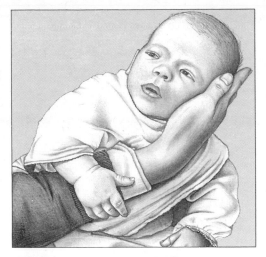

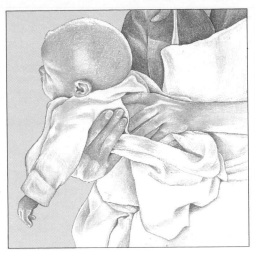

Winding the newborn baby

Sit the baby up in your lap, facing to one side, with your forearm across his or her chest and stomach. Tilt the baby slightly forwards, and diagonally away from you. Slide your forearm up the baby's chest until the baby's head rests in the palm of your hand. Then place your other hand in the middle of the baby's back, stroking gently upwards.

Winding an "older" baby

An older baby needs to be supported only by one hand under the armpit. Again the baby's head should be tilted slightly to the side and the body bent forwards. It is useless to continue to wind the baby, however, if air has not come up after a few minutes. Some babies do not need winding or may release wind through the rectum.

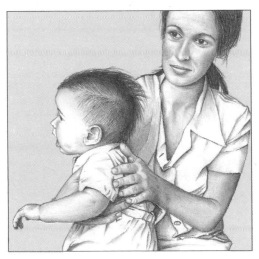

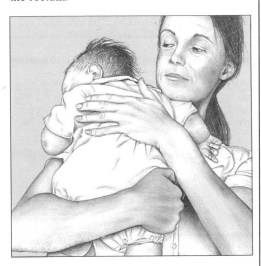

Winding half-way through feeding

Some babies are upset by interrupting feeding in order to wind them half-way through a meal. But winding is necessary in order to stop them getting milk too quickly. If the baby starts crying, turn round in your chair to give the baby a different view, and stroke the baby's back with one hand while supporting the baby's front with the other arm.

The over-the-shoulder position

Another way to wind an infant is to hold the baby against your body, with his or her chin resting on your shoulder, and to apply slight pressure to the middle of the baby's back with the palm of your hand. This position is recommended for a crying baby. Walk round the room carrying the baby and speaking softly, or distracting him or her in some way.

Bathing a baby 1

Have everything ready before undressing the baby.

An infant quickly loses body heat, so it is important that the room is warm and that there are no draughts from open windows and doors. A wall thermometer is useful. Put the baby bath, three-quarters full of warm water, on its stand in front of your chair. Keep a large jug of hot water nearby so that the temperature can be adjusted before putting the baby in the bath.

You will also need: a bottle of liquid bath soap, or baby soap in a dish; cotton wool balls; one large and one small, soft, synthetic make-up sponge; baby oil; talcum powder; cotton buds; baby shampoo; hairbrush and fine comb; ointment for the nappy area; and nail scissors.

Before starting the bath put on a towelling apron with waterproof backing. On a rail, put: a large towel; two muslin nappies for patting the baby dry; a folded nappy with liner, pins and plastic pants; a wrapping blanket and clothes.

Babies dislike having their faces washed, so use cotton wool balls, dipped in warm water, for the first few weeks and then change to the smaller of the two sponges. The larger sponge may be used to rinse off the soap while the baby is in the bath.

Babies often develop nappy rash, usually from prolonged contact with stools and urine; constant use of ointments and petroleum jelly (Vaseline) reduces the likelihood of this occurring.

Dry skin is common among newborn babies. Baby oil, gently massaged into the skin, can relieve the condition. But test the oil first on the baby's ankle to make sure that there is not an allergic reaction.

Cradle cap, a patch of yellowish, greasy material on the baby's head, commonly occurs. It can be removed by rubbing baby oil into the scalp several times a day. Once the area is soft, the material can be carefully removed using a toothcomb. At bath time, shampoo and rinse the hair. Brush the hair in all directions, several times a day to help prevent cradle cap's recurring.

Throughout bath time reassure the infant by speaking softly. A newborn infant is frightened by loud noises and quick, jerky movements, and reacts by crying.

Handle the baby gently when dressing him or her. Babies much prefer staying undressed.

Clothing should be simple to slip on and take off because the baby may be crying and thus stiff and rigid from exertion. Loose clothes with press studs are preferable to clothing that has to be pulled over the head.

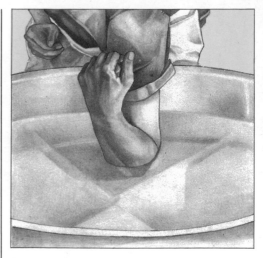

Bath and temperature

Whatever the kind of baby bath, make sure that it is sufficiently deep to contain enough water to cover the baby while bathing. (A tub with slanted sides prevents the baby from being covered with water.)

To test the temperature of the baby's bathwater dip an elbow into it. The water should be just above body temperature, and this temperature should be maintained.

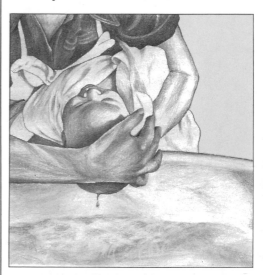

Washing the head

Wrap the baby tightly in a towel. Tuck him or her under one arm, supporting the head with that hand. Using the other hand massage the shampoo into the hair and scalp. Do not be afraid to massage the soft spot on the baby's head. Rinse off all the soap with warm water and dry the hair with a muslin nappy.

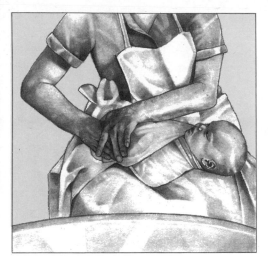

Lap or changing mat

The difference between dressing and undressing a baby on the parent's lap, and
doing so on a changing mat, is largely a
matter of convenience. Most babies prefer
the lap: they enjoy the closeness and security
of being held by the parent.

If a mat is used, it should have padded
edges, and should be covered with a towel
before the baby is put on it.

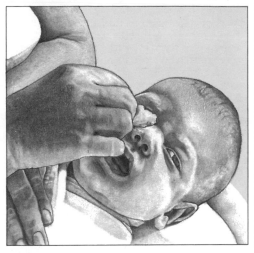

Washing the face

Wrap the baby firmly in a towel that has
been folded into a triangle, before starting
to wash the face. The baby will feel secure
lying on your lap.

Use a fresh cotton wool swab dipped in
water to wipe each eye. The outside of the
mouth should also be washed with a new
cotton wool swab. Then wash the rest of
the face and dry with a soft towel.

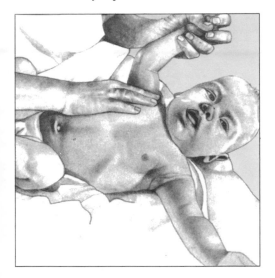

Soaping the baby's front

Soap the front of the baby all over. The skin
creases of the neck, armpits, umbilicus, groin
and buttocks need particular attention:
moisture, peeling skin and milk may often
become trapped. The creases can easily
become inflamed and sore if they are not
washed, carefully rinsed, and equally
carefully dried.

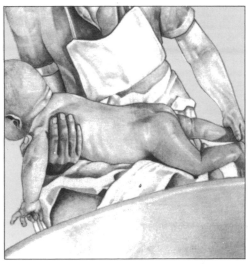

Soaping the baby's back

Soap the baby's back next. Turn the baby
over by supporting him or her from the
front with one arm, the hand round the
baby's armpit. The baby then is face-down
on your lap. You can now use your other
hand to soap and massage the baby's back.
Massaging is good for the baby's skin. The
baby can now go into the bath.

Bathing a baby 2: holding and handling

In the early weeks, bath-time may take longer than anticipated because the parent is often inexperienced and anxious. As soon as the parent is more relaxed, the baby will feel more secure and tolerant of handling.

Make sure in these early days that the room and bath temperatures are kept constant throughout the bath-time. For the first six weeks, the temperature in the room should be 21–24°C (70–75°F). After six weeks it may then be 18–21°C (65–70°F). The bathwater should be kept to 37–40°C (100–104°F), slightly higher than normal body temperature. Keep a jug of warm water near the bath to top up the bathwater should it cool down too much.

Be kind to the baby: handle him or her with warm hands.

Most babies love being in the water, but hate coming out of it and often start to cry and shiver. The baby should then be wrapped immediately in a towel and held tightly for a moment. This helps a baby to relax again. Now slowly start to dry the baby, either on your lap or on a changing mat. Be sure that a soft, absorbent towel covers the plastic mat before you lay the baby on it. Now gently open the towel in which the baby is wrapped and pat dry with a muslin nappy. Always try to keep the parts of the body covered that are not actually being dried.

When the baby is dry, apply ointment to the nappy area, then begin to dress the baby. Put on the vest first to keep the body warm, then the nappy and plastic pants, and finally the nightgown. All this time, the baby is impatient to be fed. But do not let crying distract you from what you are doing.

Finally the baby is ready to be wrapped in a receiving blanket and fed.

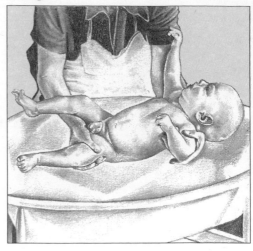

Holding a slippery baby

Hold the baby face-up, supporting the head behind the neck by grasping the arm farthest from you, with your thumb over the baby's shoulder and your fingers wrapped round the baby's arm. Put your other hand under the baby's nearer leg and buttocks, and firmly hold the baby's leg farthest from you.

Lower the baby slowly into the water.

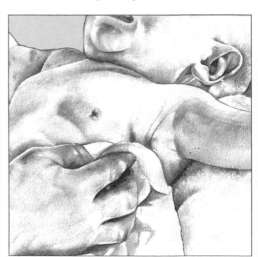

Washing under the arms

Newborn babies, especially chubby ones, sweat a lot. Consequently, in the first few weeks, parents may discover sticky substances in the baby's armpits which may cause a skin irritation. The armpits should be well soaped and then thoroughly rinsed in the bath. Pat dry and apply a little baby powder. Remove excess powder with a cotton wool ball.

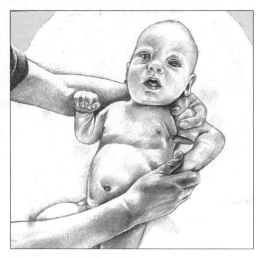

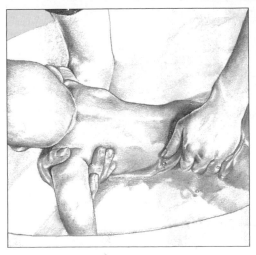

Rinsing off the soap

Release your grip on the baby's leg once
he or she is in the water. With your free
hand take a sponge and rinse off the soap
in the baby's armpits, under the neck, in
the groin, around the buttocks, and between
the fingers. In the warm water the baby's
tightly clenched fist will probably open.

Held in this position, a baby should feel
secure.

Swimming position

Hold the baby over your forearm, your
thumb on the shoulder farthest from you,
fingers encircling the baby's arm. The
baby's head then stays well clear of the
water. Most babies enjoy this position, and
are happy to be sponged.

To lift the baby out of the tub on to your
lap, drop the sponge and place your hand
under the baby's lower abdomen.

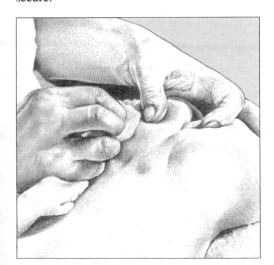

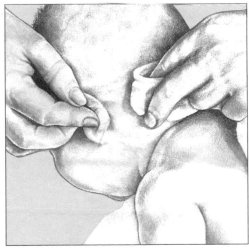

Drying in the creases

It is easy for a new parent to overlook some
of the baby's folds and creases when drying
the baby after a bath. One of the areas
requiring most attention is that of the
buttocks, which are almost always damp or
dirty in the early months. Take great care to
dab dry in the deep crease at the top of the
buttocks, where redness and soreness can
sometimes occur.

Drying behind the ears

Cracked skin behind the ears can be painful
but is not serious. Daily washing behind,
above, and below the ears is important.
Apply petroleum jelly (Vaseline) behind the
ear lobes when they are clean and dry.

Crusts may develop either as an extension
of cradle cap, or as the result of milk trickling
down the cheek and behind the ear when the
baby is lying on one side.

Changing a nappy

Ideally, a baby's nappy should be changed both before and after feeding. Until the age of about six weeks, most babies protest loudly and tearfully against anything that delays feeding time. So, provided that the baby has not had a bowel movement, it is better not to distress the baby before feeding as this allows a peaceful feed. After the baby has been fed, he or she will not mind being changed.

Some parents, especially mothers, like to change a newborn baby on their lap; others prefer to use a waterproof changing mat on a bed or a dresser top. The mat should be covered with a soft towel so that the baby is not placed on a cold plastic surface.

No matter how clean the baby is kept, the skin in the nappy area may become sore and red. When the first signs of nappy rash appear, add extra absorbency by folding a towelling nappy in half and wrapping it round the baby's waist, over a clean ordinary nappy. Secure the extra nappy with a nappy pin, like a skirt. When nappy rash occurs, plastic pants must not be worn.

To prevent a nappy from becoming stained, rinse the stools off the nappy as soon as possible by holding the nappy under running water in the lavatory pan. It should then be put into the soaking bucket containing sterilizing solution and covered with a lid.

Always make sure the baby is left in a safe place, warmly wrapped, while disposing of dirty nappies. Older babies frequently roll over and accidents can occur. The parent's hands must be thoroughly washed after a nappy change and it is advisable to use hand cream to prevent chapping.

The older baby

When a baby sleeps through the night, an extra nappy, either a muslin or disposable one, should be put inside the towelling nappy to provide extra absorbency. A non-absorbent nappy liner ("ever-dry") can be wrapped over the nappy area inside the nappy. This allows urine to pass through into the nappy and helps to keep the skin dry.

At night-time the nappy change is: a muslin nappy, folded lengthways to give three thicknesses, or a disposable pad put inside a towelling nappy which is folded into the kite shape (*see* below). The "ever-dry" liner is put over the nappy area and the muslin and towelling nappies can now be brought up between the legs and firmly secured to the other ends with two nappy pins. Finally, put on a pair of large plastic pants.

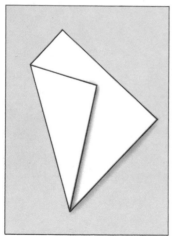 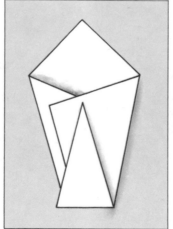 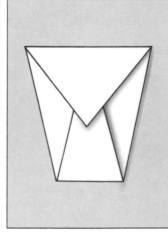

Folding into a kite shape

To fold the kite-shaped nappy, lay the towelling nappy flat in a diamond shape with a point at the top and bottom. Then fold each of the side points towards the centre. Next draw the narrow "tail" end of the nappy up towards the centre, folding it about two-thirds of the way from the bottom. Finally, fold the top flap towards the centre. The size of the nappy can be adjusted to the baby's size by altering both the length and width.

This provides an excellent nappy for day-time use and can be used with a nappy liner or one-way nappy (a special fabric treated so that the urine passes through to the towelling nappy) to keep the baby's skin dry. At night a folded muslin or disposable nappy can be put inside for extra absorbency. Plastic pants can then be put on over the nappy.

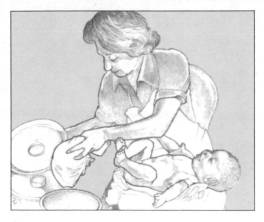

1

Have ready a clean nappy, with nappy liner, folded to shape; nappy pins; plastic pants; cotton wool swabs; a sponge or flannel; warm water in a bowl; baby soap; a bucket with a lid; and petroleum jelly (Vaseline) or ointment against nappy rash. Remove the old nappy and put it in the bucket: a dirty nappy on the floor risks spreading infection. Wipe away any stools with tissue paper or cotton wool. Wash the nappy area with soap and warm water. Rinse off the soap, pat dry, and apply ointment.

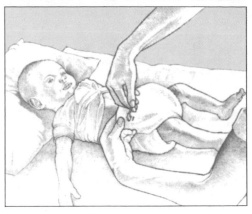

2

For the first few weeks, the average seven-pound (3kg) baby will be more comfortable in a muslin nappy, folded in four and then into a triangle. This can be lined with a disposable liner to prevent staining the nappy fabric.

As the baby grows, use a towelling nappy. The kite-shaped nappy is more absorbent because it is folded in a way that its thickness and size can be adjusted. It also ensures that the baby has less bulk between the legs when he or she begins to walk.

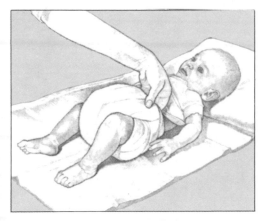

3

Lay the baby on the kite-shaped nappy with the widest end of the nappy at the baby's waist. Draw the narrow "tail" of the nappy up between the baby's legs. Nip in the inside edges of this flap to reduce bulkiness between the baby's legs, and draw the flap up and over the baby's stomach. Bring forward the points from the back of the nappy and tuck them under the front points while keeping two fingers inside as a protection against pricking the baby when inserting the nappy pins.

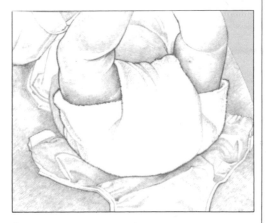

4

Correctly fitting a kite-shaped nappy results in this pair of neat, well-fitting pants. The shape makes for a good fit around the top of the baby's legs, so that leaks are prevented. A pair of soft plastic pants can be worn over the nappy. The pants should not fit too tightly over the stomach or around the thighs. Air should circulate in the nappy area to counteract the ammonia in the urine and stools, which can harm the baby's delicate skin. Discard plastic pants when they become hard and stiff.

Cleanliness

Most parents are nervous at first about handling tiny and apparently fragile newborn babies. As the mother or father becomes more confident, routine baby care is easier.

To maintain the health of a newborn baby, a basic rule is to keep the baby clean. In the early weeks this means daily attention to the following areas.

Care of the genitals

Hospitals and visiting nurses are sometimes reluctant to explain how to clean a baby's genitals, and may recommend not touching them. Such inattention can lead to infections that could otherwise have been prevented.

The genitals of a baby girl must be kept clean. It is not necessary to wash inside the lips of the vulva during the first week after birth, but the parent should thereafter from time to time wipe the genitals, from the front toward the anus, with a cotton wool swab dipped in warm water or baby oil.

It is important to do this. Any stool or vaginal discharge left on this area, which can even happen after a bath, can cause a vaginal or urinary infection if it is not carefully cleaned away.

With a baby boy, never attempt to pull back the foreskin of the penis. The foreskin and the tip of the penis are united at birth and only gradually separate. It is unnecessary to pull back the foreskin in order to wash the penis until the child is about four years old.

Circumcision

Medical opinion is divided about the value of circumcision. If for social or religious reasons a baby is to be circumcised, the operation should be performed before the tenth day after birth. There are two common methods: (1) cutting and then stitching the foreskin (the traditional method), and (2) applying a plastic cone to the penis, inside the foreskin, stitching round it, and then cutting. The foreskin and the cone fall off together within two or three days.

After a baby is circumcised, a gauze bandage is usually applied, which should be carefully soaked off in the bath after twenty-four hours, or when the doctor advises. The gauze bandage must never be pulled or bleeding may start. After the bandage has been soaked free, dry the area with a soft towel. Apply a sterile piece of gauze impregnated with petroleum jelly (Vaseline) to prevent nappies from sticking to the skin. Similar dressings should be used for at least two more days. After that time, the skin should have healed.

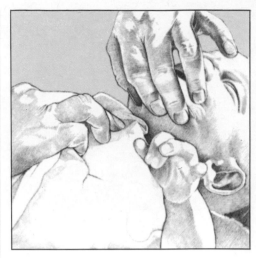

Soreness under the chin

The newborn infant often has a short neck with many creases. These must be carefully washed and thoroughly rinsed.

After taking the baby out of the bath, gently tilt back the head and, ensuring that it still remains supported, carefully dry under the chin to prevent it becoming sore.

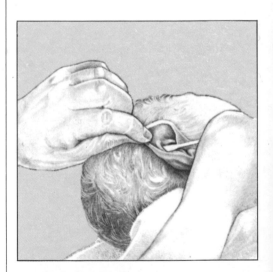

Cleaning the ears

A newborn baby's ears can frequently collect all kinds of extraneous matter: saliva, milk, juice, fluff, in addition to the normal wax.

Clean the ears with a moistened cotton wool swab. Use a fresh one for each ear. Carefully wipe around the shell-like folds of the outer ear. Clean away the wax at the entrance to the ear hole. Never insert the cotton wool swab into the baby's ear passage.

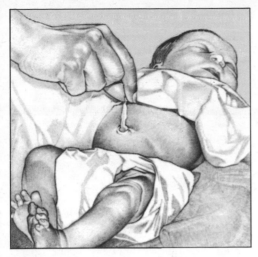

Care of the navel

The umbilical cord usually falls off between the sixth to the tenth day after birth.

A slight discharge under the cord is usual and normal. Lift the stump and carefully clean at the base with a cotton wool bud dipped in surgical spirit. Then apply a medicated powder. The baby must not wear plastic pants over the navel till it is dry.

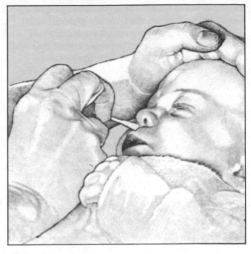

Cleaning the nose

It is important to check daily that there is no blockage in the nose.

If there is an obstruction, such as catarrh or crusts, hold the baby's head gently with one hand, and with a cotton wool bud in the other wipe around the entrance to each nostril. Never insert the cotton wool bud up the baby's delicate nostril.

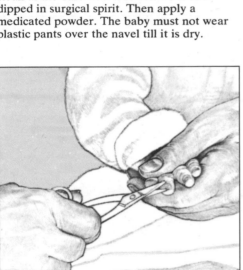

Cutting the nails

A baby's fingernails are soft but sharp. In the early weeks, unless a parent cuts the nails, a baby may scratch his or her own face. The best time for cutting the nails is after a feed. Hold the baby's hand firmly. Cut straight across the nails, and avoid leaving sharp points.

A baby's toenails do not usually require cutting for the first four to six months.

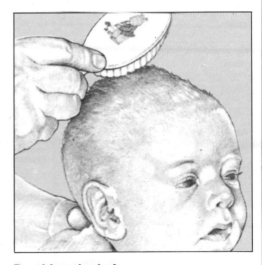

Brushing the hair

The hair should be washed two or three times a week with a baby shampoo and rinsed with warm, clean water. For details of washing, *see* p.784.

Brushing is also excellent for the circulation to the scalp, and helps to prevent the common condition known as cradle cap. Do not be afraid to brush over the fontanelle (or "soft spot").

Feeding solids

There is no set time for introducing solid foods into a baby's diet. Some parents start offering their baby cereal as early as at six weeks, but this may sometimes cause colic or diarrhoea. Generally, a baby thrives on a milk diet for the first three months, or even longer: it depends on the individual baby. But any time between the ages of three and five months is perfectly suitable for the introduction of solids.

Remember that solids given to a baby represent a replacement for milk, and an addition to the baby's previous total consumption. Milk is easy to digest and goes through a baby's system fairly rapidly; solids take longer. The result is that the number of feeds per day can probably be reduced by one, once the baby is on solids. Fortunately, the baby usually sleeps through the 6am feed soon after solids are started, which is convenient for the mother.

There are many signs to tell a parent when a baby needs more than merely milk.

A baby is ready for solids when he or she: wakes during the night demanding to be fed, having for some time previously slept right through every night

gains only 30 or 60 grams (one or two ounces) or nothing at all, during a week

seems restless between feeds during the day and wakes up too soon before each feed, crying

is no longer satisfied by an 240ml (eight-ounce) bottle; or, if breast-fed, interrupts nursing and plucks at the mother's clothing, trying to chew it

shows a readiness to chew by picking up objects and trying to put them in the mouth.

A baby's first solid food should consist of cereal, fruit, or vegetables, depending on temperament and build.

An average-sized (or even plump) baby should be started on fruit or vegetables. An active baby, who may be thinner, can be started on cereal, which should preferably be fed at the 6pm feed.

Begin with only one teaspoonful of the new food at one meal-time, gradually introducing new foods and flavours over a

Suggested Feeding Times	Feeds, with additional solids			
	1st week	2nd week	3rd week	4th week
6am*	Milk			
10am	Milk	Milk 1 teaspoonful strained fruit	Milk 2 teaspoonfuls strained fruit	Milk 3 teaspoonfuls strained fruit
2pm	Milk 1 teaspoonful strained vegetables	Milk 2 teaspoonfuls strained vegetables	Milk 3 teaspoonfuls strained vegetables	Milk 4 teaspoonfuls strained vegetables
3:30-4:30pm	Juice	Juice	Juice	Juice 1 teaspoonful plain yogurt or 1 teaspoonful mashed banana
6pm	Milk	Milk	Milk ½-1 teaspoon unmixed cereal but not wheat	Milk 1-1½ teaspoonful another cereal
10-11pm*	Milk			
* This feeding may have been dropped				

period of weeks. The chart here suggests how to do this.

Any change in feeding pattern may result in the baby's showing no weight gain during that week, or even a weight loss. But such a stasis or loss will be made up for by the baby's increased intake of solids during the following week. A cold, an upset stomach, or cutting teeth may have the same temporary effect.

The method of judging how much food a baby needs is by assessing the total intake of solids, milk and juice, as well as other fluids, and by regular weekly weighing to monitor and ensure a steady weight gain. There is, in addition, the pleasure of seeing a contented baby.

Any increase in the amount of food given to a baby must be gradual. One teaspoonful more at selected times (see the chart) is the suggested amount, especially of fruit and vegetables, for one week at a time. And if the baby is gaining weight too rapidly, cereals should not be increased for at least another week.

When the baby has reached the stage of having five or six teaspoonfuls of pure vegetables at lunchtime, some meat, fish, or cheese may be added. The baby's milk consumption should be decreased at this meal for better overall volume balance.

Having started on solids at age four months (for example), a six- to seven-month old infant generally has three main meal-times, plus an afternoon snack of a teething biscuit and a bottle of fruit juice.

A sample day's menu for a baby at this stage might consist of:

8-9am	8oz (225gm) milk; 3-4oz (90-115gm) fruit, including a little cereal. (On alternative days, a teaspoon of egg yolk, can be given and slowly increased.)
12-1pm	5-6oz (142-170gm) milk; 4-6oz (113-170gm) total of meat, fish, or cheese, plus vegetables.
afternoon	Juice; rusk.
5:30-6pm	8oz (225gm) milk; 4-5oz (113-142gm) total of cereal, fruit, and/or savoury food.

Food should be pureed for a baby up to age seven months; the puree should be of a sufficiently thick consistency for the baby to be able to suck it from a spoon. Mince or grind food for a baby seven to ten months old. After this age, most babies can eat food that has been cut up into small pieces.

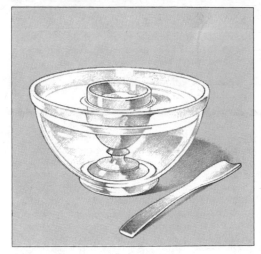

1
Keep small quantities of food warm by serving them from an eggcup that has been placed in a bowl or jug of hot water, kept ready on a nearby tray or table. Babies are puzzled by their first taste of solid foods and some may refuse the first spoonfuls.
Offer a little milk first and then a taste of the new food, before the rest of the milk.

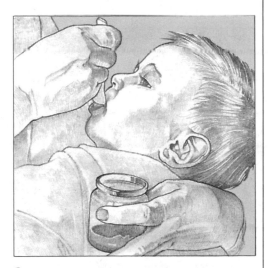

2
Hold the baby firmly in one arm and wrap a muslin nappy under the baby's chin, covering the arms and hands. Use an almost flat, rounded plastic spoon. Place it just inside the baby's mouth, resting it on the lower lip. The baby then sucks the strained food into his or her mouth. Babies may make a face at the taste of a new food but they soon become accustomed to it.

Normal functions: sleeping, crying, teething

Sleeping

The number of hours sleep required each day is not the same for every baby. It depends on the individual baby and on environmental circumstances. Not all babies require the same amount of sleep, and parents should be aware that each baby develops his or her own sleeping pattern.

The chart at the foot of the page shows the average total number of hours of sleep a baby may take, at ages from birth to one year, during any twenty-four hours. It is immediately noticeable that as the baby's age increases, there is also an increasing divergence in the average number of hours of sleep that different babies may require.

Although newborn babies generally sleep for a total of about twenty hours a day, it is usually for three or four hours at a time, with feeds between periods of sleep. By age of six weeks the baby begins to sleep for longer periods at night and for shorter periods during the day. It is at this stage that the baby begins to enjoy, for the very first time, staying awake for a while after being fed. At such a time, lying on a bed, the baby can be encouraged to use his or her eyes. A colourful mobile is useful for this, and may also promote movement and exercise.

It is a mistake to believe a baby can sleep anywhere in any surroundings. Like an adult, a baby prefers quiet and undisturbed rest. A baby who is frequently carried about from one place to another, disturbed by the slamming of car doors, or awakened by loud noises in unfamiliar surroundings, may develop lifelong sleep problems.

Crying

It is important to remember that a baby usually has a reason for crying. Crying is a baby's means of communication, generally indicating a need: a parent or baby sitter soon learns to recognize the sounds and to interpret the reasons.

Among those reasons are: hunger; wind pains; wet or dirty nappy; lack of attention; teething; sudden bright lights; noises; boredom; and others.

Crying patterns vary as much as do sleeping patterns, and some babies cry more than others. Most babies up to the age of two or three months quite normally have a crying period each day. Parents should not become upset. One method which is commonly successful in soothing a baby is to walk around slowly, holding the baby upright looking at you.

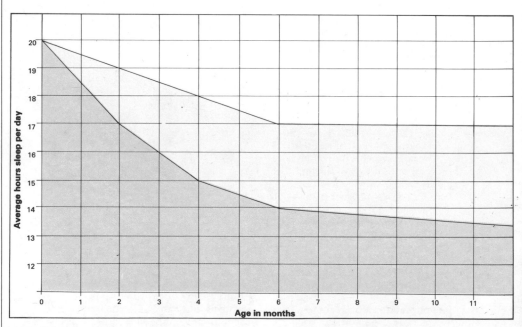

Patterns of sleep

Babies' sleep patterns vary enormously. The amount of sleep a baby needs depends on his or her individual temperament. It is not possible to make a baby sleep if he or she is overtired or not tired at all. It is most important to watch for signs of tiredness, usually irritability and fretting, to give the baby the chance to fall asleep.

Teething

All babies have to go through the process of teething, but some find it less disturbing or painful than others. The twenty milk teeth, or baby teeth, are already present in the jaw at birth and start appearing any time after birth, but usually at about six to eight months.

There are thirty-two permanent teeth, which start to develop when the baby is born. Eventually they begin coming through at age five to six years.

There are many signs by which a parent may know that a baby is teething: the cheeks may become red and blotchy; the gums may swell; the baby may frantically suck the fingers or anything else that comes to hand. Alternatively, the baby may have difficulty sucking; a cough may develop because of the extra saliva swallowed when a tooth is erupting; the baby may pull or rub the ears; and dry or sore patches may appear on the face and body. If the baby sleeps on the stomach, put a nappy under the face to absorb dribbling and prevent skin soreness.

A baby who is teething may wake up crying several times each night, and persist in crying even when soothed. At such a time, offer the baby a drink of cool water or diluted fruit juice. Teething jelly, rubbed into the gums, often gives temporary relief. If this does not help, give a pain-relieving medicine containing paracetamol.

Teething, despite many old wives' tales, does not cause a multitude of symptoms such as: vomiting and diarrhoea, fevers or fits. If any of these occur, consult a doctor.

Care of the teeth

Vitamins A, C, and D, calcium (all in milk) and fluoride are vital for healthy teeth.

To keep the baby teeth healthy, parents should not permit bad eating habits: the baby should never be given undiluted sugary juices, nor a dummy dipped in honey. Sweet drinks and foods are harmful to teeth, destroying the enamel. Once the baby can chew food, meals should be finished off with a piece of apple or some water. When the baby is one year old, clean the teeth after each meal with a soft, small brush, brushing the teeth up and down, and making a game of it so that it becomes a pleasurable part of the daily routine. Use toothpaste containing fluoride. Many babies are given additional protection with fluoride drops from the age of one month if the fluoride content of the local water supply is insufficient.

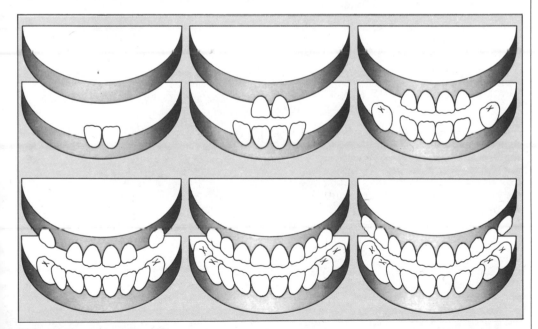

The emergence of teeth

The age at which teeth begin to appear varies from baby to baby. Some are born with a tooth already cut, others do not begin teething until after the age of eighteen months. The plan shows the order in which the twenty milk teeth usually emerge, each taking about three weeks to do so. Again, babies may have individual patterns.

Pot training

Voluntary control over the bladder and the bowels begins at about eighteen months to two years of age. Accordingly, it seems a waste of time to most parents and doctors to start toilet training an infant before that age.

There are, however, younger babies who show definite signs that they do not like a dirty or wet nappy.

Once the baby can sit on his or her own there is no reason why the infant should not sit on a pot after one or two meals. Most babies do not object to this and, on the contrary, may enjoy playing with their toys while sitting there. Many babies will "perform" – and whether this is due to voluntary or reflex action does not at this age really matter.

More important is the parents' attitude, which should remain relaxed. A parent should not mind whether the baby has "performed" or not.

Toilet training method

Start the training programme in the morning. Put a fresh nappy on the baby before he or she has breakfast. At the end of the meal, if the baby is still dry and clean, sit him or her on the pot or potty chair. This should be placed on the floor near to or against the slatted side of the cot or playpen: the baby sits with the back to the cot. To prevent him or her from toppling over or crawling away, slot a large nappy or scarf through two of the slats, bringing the ends forward under the baby's arms to be tied together in the front. The infant seldom objects, especially if he or she is given a toy to play with while this harnessing is carried out. It is a good idea to reserve some favourite toy or toys just for the potty session.

Each potty session should last no longer than five minutes. Stay with the baby during the first few times, but only as company and not playing with him or her. After several days of this routine, the parent should leave the baby but remain within a reassuring distance.

At the end of five minutes, the baby should be unharnessed and lifted from the potty. If there is anything in the potty, the parent should express approval. If not, the parent should merely say something casual like: "We'll try again tomorrow." (Parents must not show anxiety at such a time.)

This routine can gradually be carried out more than once a day, but not so often that the baby gets the impression that he or she is spending a large part of the day on the potty.

If the baby cries and obviously objects to sitting on the potty, abandon the toilet training for about a month, then try again.

Eventually most babies develop a regular potty habit, and defecation occurs after breakfast. The habit usually continues into adult life (and is due to the normal reflex of the large bowel emptying after a meal enters an empty stomach).

At night, a towelling and muslin nappy should still be worn. Some babies in order to remain dry, must be potted in the evening before the parents go to bed.

Choice of pot or potty chair

The pot or potty chair should sit firmly on the floor so that the baby cannot tip over and become frightened. The circumference of the top of the pot should fit the baby's bottom. A toilet seat that can be fitted to the ordinary adult toilet is too high for a baby to relax on. It may be dangerous and is certainly not suitable for a baby starting toilet training: it is much easier for an infant to relax when both feet are firmly and comfortably resting on the floor.

Some doctors and parents recommend that pot training should begin at age eighteen months. By then a baby has control over bowel movements and may be aware of a full bladder in time to indicate it to a parent.

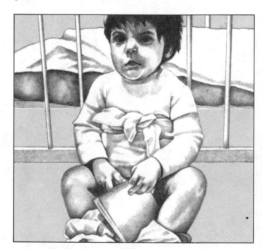

Duration and security

Leave the baby on the potty for not more than five minutes, with some favourite toys. There is no danger of the baby falling off if tied firmly against the cot or playpen. The baby may also be discouraged from wanting to get off the potty.

However, if the baby rejects the potty and struggles to get free, do not insist that he or she remains on the potty for as long as five minutes.

Comfort in the cot

Swaddling the baby

A newborn baby is much happier if he or she is wrapped up firmly. This custom, called swaddling, is considered old-fashioned and even unkind by some people, but modern research has shown that it is a practical way to help a baby to sleep peacefully.

Remember that the infant is not used to unlimited space, having been confined for months to the restricted space of the womb. Swaddling makes the baby feel more secure and helps him or her to adjust little by little to the outside world.

Newborn babies have little or no control over their limbs and they often wake themselves with the jerky movements of their own arms and legs. The well wrapped-up baby does not experience this.

How long a parent continues to swaddle a baby depends on whether the baby is of a calm or restless temperament. But for up to three months it is usually beneficial. At three to six weeks, the baby's hands need not be swaddled so tightly, allowing him or her to reach the mouth.

If the baby is put to sleep on the stomach, leave the arms free but wrap a blanket round the waist and legs to prevent the baby wriggling up the cot and pushing his or her head against the top of the cot.

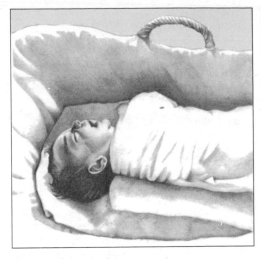

Cot position

Do not let the newborn baby sleep flat on the back. If the baby brings up milk with wind, he or she could choke. Instead, put the swaddled baby on one side in the cot or pram.To prevent the baby from rolling over, place a rolled nappy against the baby's back, just below the head. This is made by first folding a towelling nappy in half and then tightly rolling it.

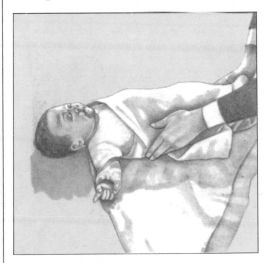

Wrapping the baby

Lay the baby on a wrapping blanket that has been folded to form a triangle. The fold should be under the baby's neck and shoulders. Place one of the baby's arms across his or her chest in a flexed position at a 45° angle. Draw one corner of the blanket over the baby's arm and chest, and tuck it smoothly under the baby. Repeat with the other corner.

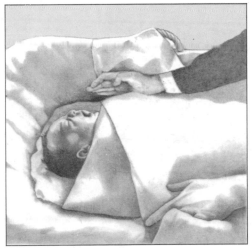

Well tucked in

Once the baby is on his or her side, fold two over-blankets into separate triangles. Criss-cross the folded edges over the baby's uppermost shoulder tucking the remaining loose ends of the blankets firmly under the mattress. This keeps the baby warm and prevents the sudden jerking movements that may occur during sleep and wake the baby up.

Transporting a baby

Choosing a pram

The baby's pram is probably the most expensive piece of equipment parents have to buy, and should be chosen with care.

A pram with large wheels is smoother in motion than one with small wheels. However, a pram with small wheels at the front and large ones at the back is easier to push over the edge of a pavement.

Parents living in an urban flat often find the most convenient kind of pram is one that can be detached from a foldable frame. The only disadvantage with this kind of pram is that the lighter structure becomes unsafe when the baby is about one year old, and is able to rock the pram.

Ensure that the pram has safety straps, or attachment points for straps. When a baby starts to twist or turn, he or she must wear straps at all times. The pram must have good brakes, checked frequently.

The interior of the baby's pram must be easy to clean. There should be an attachable hood and cover, and a firm mattress. If the pram is for use outside, attach a net over the front while the baby sleeps.

For the convenience of the parent a pram should have adjustable handles. A shopping tray under the chassis is useful, or a hanging basket at the end.

The carrycot

The carrycot should have a wipeable interior and exterior. The handles must be strong and positioned towards the head end for even balance when carrying the baby. Most carrycots are light in weight and convenient for travelling. Remember that a baby grows quickly, so that the carrycot cannot be used for infants over the age of nine to twelve months.

If the carrycot is to be used as a pram, a folding chassis should be bought with strong attachments to the carrycot.

The backpack

A backpack is a useful additional item to the pram. The baby must be able to support his or her own head before sitting in a backpack, usually around the age of four months. The pack should have adjustable shoulder straps for the parent. It should also be equipped with safety straps for the baby, or attachment points for a harness.

Some backpacks have a small strut that folds out at the back to support the pack on the ground. This strut is to enable the parent to put the pack on comfortably from a table top when the baby is sitting in the pack, and should never be used to convert the pack into a seat for the baby: this is not safe.

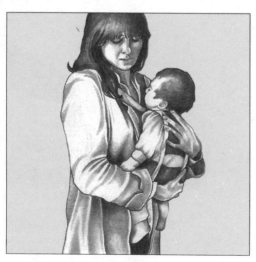

Sling carriers

Many parents use a sling carrier, which makes it possible for the baby to accompany a parent while shopping as it leaves the parents' hands free. Most infants enjoy the closeness and the movement.

The parent should wait until the baby can support the head before using this carrier. And great care must be taken not to trip up.

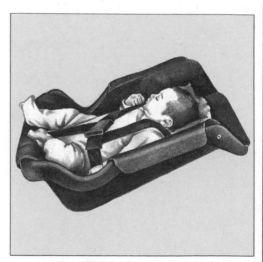

Safety car seat

While the baby is in a carrycot, safety straps must be attached to the back seat of the car to keep the carrycot firmly in position. When the baby has grown out of the carrycot, a child's safety seat must be used – but only on the back seat.

Never sit on the front seat holding a child on your lap; if holding is necessary, sit on the back seat with the child.

The baby's temperature

A newborn baby is unable to control body heat as efficiently as an older child. External changes in temperature can alter a baby's body temperature considerably. Unless a baby is kept well covered, serious chilling (hypothermia) may occur in cold conditions. In the same way, overheating may result from a baby's being left in the sun on a hot day. Parents must be aware of potentially dangerous situations.

Cold

A baby's bedroom must be maintained at a temperature of at least 15.5°C (60°F). A thermostat heater is an efficient method of keeping the room warm throughout the night. During the winter, warm the baby's cot with a hot water bottle before placing him or her in it, but remember to remove the bottle first. Never use an electric blanket on a baby's bed. Make sure that the baby is warmly dressed in cold weather and well covered with blankets, for a tiny baby does not move much during sleep and loses heat.

Heat

During hot summer weather, a baby should wear light, loosely fitting, cool clothing. As long as he or she is protected from direct sun, the baby can lie outside in nothing but a nappy. Overdressing causing overheating is one of the most common reasons for irritable babies during the summer.

Never leave a small baby unattended in a car. This is especially important during the summer, because if the car is in direct sun, the baby can become dangerously over-heated. A baby under the age of three months is unable to lose excess heat.

During car journeys, check frequently to make sure that the sun is not shining directly on to the baby. Always protect the baby's head from the sun.

Illness

When a baby becomes ill, the body temperature is not necessarily above normal. A reading from a thermometer is an inaccurate guide to a baby's state of health. Other warning signs must also be considered.

The most obvious signs that a baby has an infection or illness are: a sudden loss of appetite; the baby is irritable or, alternatively, lethargic; and there may be vomiting or diarrhoea. These signs are a more accurate indication than a temperature reading.

However, during an illness, the doctor may ask the parent to take the baby's temperature. It is dangerous to place a thermometer in a baby's mouth, and difficult to keep one underneath a baby's arm for a sufficient length of time. The best way to take the baby's temperature is in the back passage (rectum).

A rectal thermometer has a rounded, stub end. This type of thermometer can be used for taking oral temperatures as well, so when buying a thermometer buy a rectal one.

Finally, do not keep a feverish baby's room too hot. If the baby has a high temperature, keep him or her covered with light clothes and a sheet only. The doctor may recommend sponging with tepid water to keep the baby's temperature down.

Taking a rectal temperature

Make sure that the mercury line is first shaken below the thermometer's lowest mark. Then take the baby's rectal temperature using the method described below.

It usually takes up to two minutes for a rectal thermometer to register the body temperature. Although the normal body temperature varies from person to person, the average is 37°C (98.6°F) for an oral temperature, and 37.6°C (99.6°F) for a rectal temperature.

Wash the thermometer carefully after use with cool water and soap. Never use hot water, because this will break the bulb.

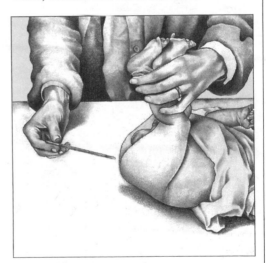

Taking the rectal temperature

Lay the baby on his or her back. Dip the end of the thermometer in petroleum jelly (Vaseline). Hold the baby's legs up with one hand, and gently insert the bulb into the anus. Do not push further if the thermometer meets an obstruction. Slide it in about 2½ cm (1 inch). Talk calmly to the baby throughout the procedure, and do not frighten him or her by gripping the legs too tightly.

The growing child

In a general discussion about the care of your infant and child, only the broadest outlines of what you should do can be given. In some things you need skilled advice, or the reassurance that what you are doing is right. Regular visits to your doctor maintains a relationship with an expert who can help if your baby is ill. The clinic also advises on many things that cause concern, as well as discussing a child's normal development.

Your baby relies on you not only for food and physical safety, such as warm clothing, a comfortable cot and a dry nappy, but also for the help in learning about his or her surroundings and the family and friends who live in them. Your baby feels your emotions when you feel them but may not understand them. If you are unhappy or upset, your baby cries and frets. When you are cheerful and happy your baby gurgles and laughs. Your uncertainty when handling your baby produces tensions and tears as he or she feels momentarily insecure; this is why, by picking up your baby, a nurse can sometimes stop the crying. The nurse's confidence gives reassurance to your baby.

A first baby often reflects the parents' anxieties about progress and development in a way that does not occur with future children. By then the parents know what is normal and have confidence about handling small babies and children built on experience with their first child.

Despite this complete dependence of a newborn baby on the parents, there is a slow and steady progress to independence. At first this is difficult to see and feel, but it is essential that it is recognized. Your baby develops a personality from an early age, and begins to assert an individual way of doing things. At first this is scarcely noticeable, but gradually you realize that your baby's crying has various forms. It may be caused by hunger; discomfort from a wet nappy; wind; pain from colic; boredom; and the desire for attention. Crying for love is normal and healthy, but can easily become a way of maintaining your attention all the time. Do not neglect your baby, but be able to recognize a well-fed but bored baby, crying only for attention, who will usually fall asleep in a few minutes if left alone in a warm cot.

As your baby grows, his or her diet changes, and new foods are introduced. This is a time when your baby may assert himself or herself. It is an excellent chance for your baby to achieve some form of independence. Any of us can have a few dislikes, as well as favourite foods, but usually only a few. A new taste or food is often rejected by a baby, so leave it for a few days before introducing it again, preferably in a different form or texture. At this stage be prepared to be firm and offer the new food early in the meal when the baby is still hungry and may eat it without complaint. It is wise only to offer a little the first time. Be prepared to stop the meal until the baby eats the small amount before continuing. Your resolve to be firm, at the right moment, prevents dislikes developing that could lead to a natural anxiety about your baby's nutrition.

Babies do not need teeth before solids are introduced into the diet. They chew with their gums as well as their teeth. Some babies are born with a tooth and others may not grow them until nearly a year old. Teething usually starts about the age of four to six months. This is the age when drooling and exploring the mouth with the fingers is normal. It occurs whether a tooth is present or not. A tooth that is cutting through the gum may cause restlessness and discomfort for a few hours and, naturally, several teeth appearing within a week or two is a disturbing and unpleasant experience for anyone, adult or baby. However it is not sufficient to produce fever, diarrhoea, convulsions, rashes, and a multitude of other symptoms and signs that are commonly attributed to "teething". If these things happen, it is essential to find out why, and not to blame the normal, natural stage of cutting a tooth. The discomfort of teething may be relieved by allowing your baby to chew on a ring, or by rubbing the gum with special preparations, obtainable from your chemist.

As babies grow and develop, their understanding increases and they become frustrated by finding that they cannot do things like finding toys, crawling, and standing. This not only leads to tears at the failure to achieve what they want, but also moments of rage and anger. It is important that you are aware of this and do not rush to help your child. Let your baby try again, as the achievement is worth the battle. Your pleasure and praise at your child's success gives that additional fulfilment. This helps to build determination and independence, and prevents the child from always relying on outside help in a difficult situation. There are times, however, when you must interfere; moments when danger, like climbing out of the cot or falling down the stairs, far outweigh the possibility of satisfactory success. If your reaction is too swift your baby may be resentful and cross. It is better to distract your baby before a dangerous situation is reached. Warn of the hazards even if the only thing that is understood is a firm "no".

Anger is a frightening thing to a small child. Not only your anger towards him or her, but also your child's anger towards you. You can help by letting him or her know that your temper expresses a dislike at what your child has done, not a dislike of your child. After the violence of the emotion has passed, you are the same loving parent as before. It is important, however, that your child learns that losing his or her temper has not achieved anything, otherwise he or she may start using anger as a weapon to succeed when other methods have failed. The child with temper tantrums eventually learns to control them when he or she finds they are ignored and a waste of energy and time.

A small child gets great pleasure from the rhythm of simple poetry and music. The enjoyment is often greater than the understanding. From an early age, nursery rhymes and songs can be enjoyed by mother, father, and child, and may quickly develop into a bedtime ritual of a series of familiar rhymes and stories. This must be kept flexible. Introduce new stories before ending with the favourite one when the lights are turned off.

An older child may well extend a familiar story with his or her own imagination into a world where characters seem real. One in particular may become a daytime "companion" with whom the child talks and discusses problems and things to do. This is a normal and healthy stage in development and not a cause for concern. It is a form of play and a sign of a secure and intelligent child.

Play

Play is an unsuitable word in many ways. To an adult, play implies relaxation, whereas to a child there is no difference between playing and working. A child at play is not filling up his or her time until the next important "adult" activity, but making the best possible use of time. If a child plays hard, it implies an underlying ability to work hard in the future. Playing is initially a way of learning basic physical skills. The mother or father who plays peekaboo teaches the baby to look around. Later the baby increases hand skills by offering and taking back toys, or pushing trains and cars across the floor. As co-ordination increases the child enjoys the new abilities by building towers with bricks or "drawing" all over sheets of paper.

Toys come in all shapes and sizes. Improvised toys can be just as successful as manufactured ones. Don't be tempted to think an expensive toy will be played with for longer than a cheap one. Some toys are safe and others are dangerous. Some are easy to play with, and others too complicated for your child's age. Your child must be neither overwhelmed by the complex toy, nor bored by the simple one.

The baby needs a toy to look at, feel, and chew, and sometimes listen to. A rattle is a simple and safe toy. In its various forms, even when hidden in a cuddly toy, it makes a successful companion in the cot. As a baby grows, toys must supply a challenge to ingenuity. By the time a child is walking, toys are not only a practical test of ingenuity, but also an aid to imagination. The child soon stops dragging a doll around by the leg, and starts to dress it, change the nappy, and put it to bed. The child also shows enthusiasm for active and physical games.

Playing with toys not only tests skills, but is also a way of learning to play with children of the same age. A young child seldom plays directly with other children, partly because of the lack of skill, but also because of a feeling of possessiveness for toys and belongings. By the age of two, sociability is increasing out of a similarity of interest and friendship. Friendships may be tested by disagreements and quarrels. Similar interests and enthusiasms, and the need for a friend to play games with, helps to resolve most disagreements in the same way that your child has learned to cope with disagreements in your own family. Your child can share and enjoy experiences with other children, and feel the benefit of independence from you.

It is not only against you that your child is going to assert an independence, but also against others who try and prevent him or her from doing what he or she wants to. This rapidly leads to quarrels with brothers and sisters, who are also trying to do what they want.

The conflict is healthy and natural, even if it leads to lost tempers and tears. It is important not to interfere at the onset of every quarrel. Children must learn that fairness and justice can be achieved from a balance of interest. They soon find out that the sole possession of a favourite toy may lead to the loss of a companion in some other game. Giving and taking in the home is an introduction to the outer world where the same balance has to be achieved to maintain friendships that are built without family bonds.

Inevitably a violent and vicious fight must be stopped, as the older child usually wins. Even so, it is important that the parent should not take sides. The parent is there to prevent real harm. At this point the children frequently ask, either directly or indirectly, for parental judgement on the quarrel. An explanation of your judgement must be given. At the same time point out that no matter who was right in the quarrel, violence on either side is the wrong way of resolving a problem and that both children are equally at fault in this, and must be aware of it.

An awareness of others and their reactions is also developed through your child's relationship with animals and family pets. At first your pet is pulled and hugged without concern for its comfort or safety. Gradually the child learns how to handle it without causing pain or harm, more as an individual and less as a living, furry toy.

The death of a favourite pet is often the first introduction to the idea of life and death. As a child is unable to think of abstract ideas, death must be discussed in a matter-of-fact way, and a logical explanation of what happens after death must be given. It is just as difficult for your child to accept that the puppy is dead, and buried in the ground, as it is to accept the death of a grandparent.

Do not be afraid to show grief after the death of a relative. Your child must learn about emotions, and how to express them. This is a way of learning how to cope with his or her own feelings. The child realizes that not only does everyday life continue, but also that grief becomes less acute and gradually fades. It is difficult for a child to cope with personal emotions if the parents seem to have none. Your child may think you callous, or may feel that such feelings are abnormal and wrong, and try to suppress them.

Immunization

The time that this is due is a balance between the probability of your baby catching the natural infection, and the body's ability to cope with immunizations. A newborn baby, particularly when being breast-fed, has a protection (immunity), which is transmitted from the mother, against various infections. This protection lasts for only a few weeks. The baby then has to develop his or her own immunity. This can occur only when the baby's tissues are mature enough to produce the antibodies, substances produced by the body to fight infection. This ability to develop immunity begins at the age of three months and then steadily increases during the succeeding few months. This is why a series of immunizations has to be given to build up a protection. The schedule that your doctor advises you to follow is built on the balance of experience.

Illnesses

Because you know your child in health and sickness, you are probably the first to realize when an illness starts. Your cheerful, enthusiastic child becomes tearful and quiet at the onset of illness. A child on the verge of illness, like an overtired child, may rebel against the idea of giving up a game, or going to bed.

Young children find it difficult to explain

Development of drawing skills

Two-year-old child
The picture on the right shows a two-year-old child's drawing of a person. The head and facial features are the most prominent parts in the drawing. This is because, even at this age, a child learns to associate specific facial expressions with adult approval or disapproval.

Three-year-old child
The picture on the far right shows a three-year-old child's drawing of a man. The head and face are still the major components of the drawing, but the body also appears although in a very rudimentary form and out of proportion with the head.

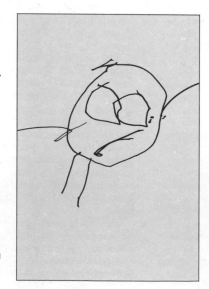

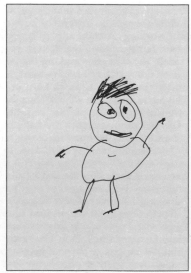

what is the matter with them. Vomiting and diarrhoea are obvious signs of illness, but a child may not mention a headache or sore throat. Symptoms can be misleading, for example, aching limbs or stomach-ache may be caused by tonsillitis or influenza. A child with a high fever may feel hot and seem sleepy, but yet complain of nothing. As a parent you know all the variations of behaviour in your child and can assess most accurately whether something serious is wrong.

When your child is sick, he or she needs your care, and loses the desire for independence. Extra attention often helps in these circumstances. A child is delighted to be tempted with favourite foods and drinks, and to have stories read to him or her. After the illness, life returns to normal. The extra care and affection does not mean the child will expect it in the future. If you are really anxious about your child, you must consult your doctor. Expert help reassures your anxiety, and with the right treatment your child will make a rapid recovery.

Your relationship with your child is an example to him or her of how to make friends with others on an understanding of personal consideration and affection, humour, and shared interest. As the child grows into an adult, his or her increasing independence alters the relationship between you. He or she becomes a close and loving friend, independent, but still able to turn to you for the wisdom and understanding that comes from your age and experience. This is strong evidence that you have been a successful parent.

Becoming sociable

A child acquires an understanding of other people through relationships with family, friends of all ages, and strangers. He or she learns how to fit in with others, how to make friends, and how to show consideration. Your child must be made aware that the noisy enthusiasm of play may not be welcome to family visitors talking to parents. This helps to develop a considerate, kind, and generous adult whose friendship is valued by colleagues and friends.

As a child grows many changes in attitude become apparent. At first the child is wide-eyed with delight when he or she meets a stranger. After the age of six months the child becomes more cautious, and more dependent on the parents. The child must be left to discover whether a given situation is "dangerous" or safe. Leave the child alone to find out, but stay close at hand. This is important at children's parties, where a parent can stay until the child feels secure enough to join in the games.

However, if a child becomes unusually shy, it may be because the parent is overprotective. This can prevent the child from making his or her own assessments. As such a child develops, he or she lacks confidence about the ability to judge a situation, and instead tries to avoid it.

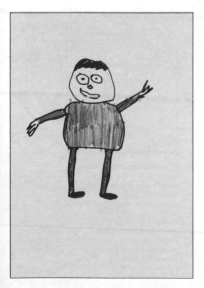

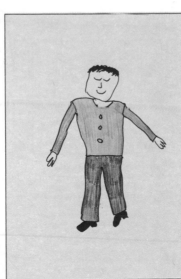

Seven-year-old child
The picture on the far left shows a seven-year-old child's drawing of a man. The child's nervous system has by now developed sufficiently to enable him or her to draw a relatively life-like picture that shows all the main features – the head, body, arms and hands, and legs and feet.

Fourteen-year-old child
The picture on the left shows a fourteen-year-old child's drawing of a man. By this age, the nervous system has matured almost completely and the child has a high degree of coordination between hand and eye. This can be seen in the drawing in which the person's features are in lifelike proportions.

In the older child, shyness may stem from a fear of teasing. Teasing may be aimed at some obvious or imagined defect. A birthmark or deformity may be the focus of comment by other children; or they may pick on some minor problem, such as blushing. Teasing always continues if the child reacts openly to it. The teasing soon stops if the child is able to ignore it, although sometimes a child is called a nickname by which he or she becomes known throughout school life, regardless of the initial reaction.

The parent's attitude should reassure the child that family love is unaltered, and as far as he or she is concerned, the nickname has no significance. The attitude of those the child loves gives him or her the best basis for ignoring teasing.

On a practical basis, it may be possible for any real defect to be improved by medical treatment. This is worth discussing with your doctor if the problem is worrying the family or your child.

A child soon encounters bullying. Why a child becomes a bully is complicated. It may be because he or she is overprotected, because he or she is spoiled, or because there are tensions at home that are not noticeable to strangers. It is difficult for an outsider to take a bully in hand without causing problems between families. Explain to your child that the bully may be a very unhappy child, and that in any case, violence on your child's side is not going to make the situation better.

Sexuality

The pleasure and warmth of sexuality start at birth. The pleasure that both parent and child feel through being cuddled and handled is the warmth of close, loving physical contact. This is your baby's first sex education. All human beings enjoy this warmth, and it is essential for a baby's normal growth and happiness.

A baby's mouth is the most sensitive and appreciative area of the body; it tells the baby about the outside world. As a baby grows and develops he or she discovers face, hands and fingers, feet and toes, and genitals. The exploration of the body is a normal and healthy stage of development. Most babies find pleasure in touching their genitals, but this is only an extension of experiencing a stimulating external world. The pride the child has in the genitals is understandable; the pride is part of the pleasure of being an individual.

The genital phase is accompanied by an interest in the process of excretion. The child notices with interest the curious fact that urine and faeces appear from the body. The child may enjoy feeling the consistency of the faeces. It is important that as a parent you should not make your child feel guilty about this, but explain that faeces and urine are unwanted parts of a working body, and should be thrown away.

Problems with sexuality can occur if a child is bored, or if there is a lack of outside stimulus and interest. This can happen if the child is unhappy, perhaps because there are

Toys for different ages

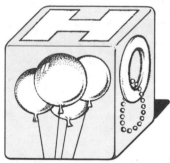

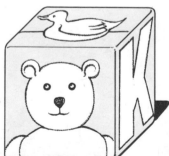

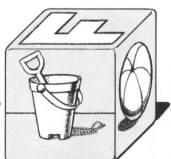

Up to six months
Balloons or streamers for the baby to watch. Toys suspended across the cot or pram within reach of the baby's hands. Rattles that small hands can easily grasp. Teething rings, or interesting things, too large to swallow but satisfying to bite and chew on or to suck.

Six to eighteen months
One or two soft toys to hold and snuggle. Plastic ducks, boats, and fishes for the bath. Jugs and cups for pouring. Toys on wheels to push and pull. Balls to roll and follow. Household objects, like paper, to rattle and tear. Building blocks to pile up and knock down. Hammer and pegs.

Eighteen months to three years
Bucket and spade for the sand box. Swings and slides. Simple jigsaw puzzles. Toy telephone. Thick crayons and large sheets of paper. Paints and big brushes. Blackboard and chalk. Dolls to dress and undress. Miniature cooking utensils. Doll's house.

parental stresses and strains, or for other reasons. Compulsive infantile masturbation may start as a pleasurable distraction from the less pleasant realities of everyday life.

Masturbation occurs almost universally in both sexes. In general, the best policy is for the parents to ignore it. Taking a child's hands away from the genitals, or looking disapproving, makes him or her feel guilty and wicked. If the habit does become compulsive, the parents must talk to the doctor and try to find the root of the anxiety. As the child becomes happier, so the compulsion stops.

Talking about sex

All children ask questions, and sooner or later these include queries about sex. Simple questions need simple answers. There is no need to launch into a lengthy sex lecture at the slightest provocation. Children are not interested. They only want to know the answer to the immediate question in a way that is understandable. If a child wants to know more, he or she can ask. The child may find it difficult to believe the answer, and may ask the same question two or three days later. It is often easier for a child to believe that a newborn baby is bought at the shop than it is to understand that it takes nine months to grow inside the mother's womb after the father has implanted a seed in an egg located there.

If your child does not ask questions, use examples. For instance, if the mother becomes pregnant again, let the child feel the growing baby moving inside, and explain about it at the same time. A description of how the cat has kittens is a help toward understanding childbirth. Watching an animal suckling its young introduces the topic of breast-feeding. Children may see dogs mating. If your child asks about it, he or she is ready to know. You could even mention the fact that it is possible to prevent fertilization occurring by using contraception.

The whole topic should be discussed openly enough to stop your child feeling that questions about sex are different from questions on any other subject. This leaves your child free to ask about sex when he or she is ready to understand.

It is always difficult to know how much a child remembers and whether he or she has linked up apparently isolated questions into a complete understanding. By the time a child goes to school, much of the initial curiosity has died down. There is often an apparent lack of sexual interest until puberty. The child has an increased understanding, but decreased interest.

Children often tell each other fairy stories of their own making about how they arrived in the world. Your child may even be happy with both versions, the fairy tale and the reality. This kind of make-believe is normal. Sometimes the fantasy and mystery is much more exciting than the reality, and is a temporary escape.

A child not only has to learn the mechanics

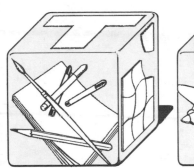

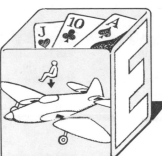

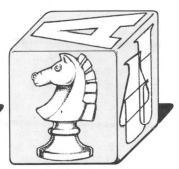

Three to five years
Ready-mixed and powder paint with plenty of paper. Pencils and colouring crayons. Construction sets with large pieces in wood or plastic. Toys to "play house" with. Garage, fort, or farm sets. Round-ended scissors and a scrap book. Dominoes. Cards for simple games. Tricycle.

Five to eight years
Construction sets with small pieces. Modelling kits for careful painting and gluing. Carpentry tools to build up into a set. Dice, board games, and more complicated card games. Glove puppets, and string puppets for the older child. Scooter, bicycle, and stilts for outdoors.

Eight years and over
Practical chemistry sets and realistic scientific equipment. Weaving, raffia, and basketmaking sets. Sewing and mending sets. Board games – draughts, chess, and Monopoly. Toy theatre. Conjuring and magic sets. A box with dressing up clothes and masks.

of sex, but also has to understand morality. This, like other aspects of behaviour, is an important example set by you as parents to your children.

Modesty is not a natural part of a child's life. He or she begins by constantly having a nappy changed, as well as being washed and touched. The child accepts parental nudity, and differences in appearance. Clothing for a child is for warmth, not modesty. The child has to learn that strangers are not seen in the nude, and likewise strangers are unlikely to see him or her in the nude.

Privacy is a concept that gradually develops. A young baby may sleep in the parents' room for convenience at first. As the child grows, a separate room is necessary, not only for the parents' peace and privacy, but also to give the child a feeling of territory. You should respect your child's territory in the same way as you expect your child to respect yours.

Children often share a room. A brother and sister can continue to do this until the onset of puberty when their own developing modesty indicates a need for different rooms. Children of the same sex may continue sharing a room unless they become too incompatible in temperament.

Explaining perversions

A major problem for parents is to warn children of the dangers of strangers, without making them frightened of an outside world that may already be causing stresses and anxieties. A child is more likely to be puzzled rather than frightened by a man who exposes himself. The child cannot see the need to do it, as nudity is part of life at home. If your child is frightened by such an experience, explain that such people are in need of help and seldom do any harm, but be careful in the future not to let your child out alone where it may happen again.

The true child molester is a far more serious problem. Every child must be told never to accept lifts from strangers, or to believe people who say that they have been sent to collect him or her from school.

In this era of sexual discussion and television documentary, every child sooner or later asks a question that you are unable to answer. Admit that you cannot answer. Your child understands that there is a limit to everyone's knowledge. Questions about different forms of sexual practice are less easy to deal with. It is best to give the simplest answer possible, and yet still be truthful. Make sure, however, that your child fully understands the range of normal sexual activity before embarking on any other explanations.

A child enjoys learning about new things. He or she often may ask several people about the same thing, partly to compare answers, and partly as a way of remembering. Any member of the family – grandparents, aunts, uncles, or cousins – may be asked the most intimate questions in a direct and innocent manner. These questions require an equally direct and honest answer, however much embarrassment or amusement it gives to you all. Sex, like eating, drinking, and breathing, is an essential part of life.

Discipline

A newborn baby begins to develop his or her own rhythms of life and needs regular food and the outside influence of day and night. These are partly a biological necessity, and partly the discipline of a natural existence. As parents you learn to blend your own routine with your baby's. Bathtime, playtime, mealtimes, and sleep begin to make a pattern that your baby understands and expects. Your routine changes a lot to fit in with your new baby.

This is the basis upon which all discipline is built: the balance between the individual's desire for complete freedom, and the need to fit into the established routine of the family.

As your baby learns to eat with a spoon, the new skill is enjoyed with great enthusiasm. The accent at this age is on enjoying the food, and this includes squeezing it through the fingers, and dropping it on the floor. An older child learns table manners, and the simplest way is to copy those of the parent. The child must understand that consistently bad table manners are inconvenient and unacceptable. The loss of a privilege could be used to support your point, but is only effective if used occasionally.

The child understands discipline provided it is consistent and fair. Your child then knows which areas of behaviour are acceptable, and which are not.

Bedtime can become a problem, particularly if your child is feeling lively, and when you are feeling tired. Your child sees an opportunity to assert himself or herself. A bedtime ritual that ends with a story produces an atmosphere of relaxation. You can allow your child to look at a book, or play with toys in bed for a few minutes before switching the lights off. Your child may need the security of a night light, or of hearing you moving and talking in another room. If your child is constantly calling or reappearing from the bedroom, he or she may be frightened or anxious. You must show your child that you understand these fears, but be firm.

The rhythms and customs of family life are built round the need for a child to help himself or herself. Encourage your child to dress in the morning whenever possible, and appear tidy and on time for breakfast. Encourage your child to be ready to go out with minimal help from you. Your encouragement and praise helps to establish a habit of self-discipline and self-confidence.

Every child must learn at an early age the dangers of traffic and the rules for crossing a road. Your child can watch you and learn before going out into the street alone.

In the outside world a child learns the rules made by society. He or she comes across the police who try to maintain the laws. Children should realize that the police are friendly and helpful. In fact, the role of the police should be presented as an extension of your role at home.

As your child learns about restrictions on behaviour, he or she can be given responsibilities. These include keeping his or her room tidy, and helping the family with the general running of the house. Each child should be given jobs that are entirely his or her own responsibility, such as feeding a pet, or collecting the post. It shows the child that the family relies on him or her.

Punishment should only be an occasional weapon used in the longer process of discipline. There are rewards for good behaviour, and punishment for bad behaviour. Every child understands this. It is important not to get into a habit of threatening punishment and not carrying it out.

Physical punishments should be used sparingly but if they must be used, should be immediate and directly related to the offence. A sharp smack on the hand of a naughty infant is often salutary and effective. If you have a normal affectionate relationship with one another, it does little harm. An older child may not be so impressed and often perseveres despite the punishment. It is often better to use your skill to avoid a direct conflict.

Your anger makes a strong impression on your child. Too much parental anger and temper soon loses its effect. Anger at the right moment is frequently a sufficient punishment.

Honesty is the basis of all human relationships. Children can understand that stealing is wrong because they do not like their own personal possessions being stolen. More subtle forms of human behaviour are learned from the example of the child's parents.

These include consideration, and courtesy. As your child grows, he or she imitates you in many things, and works out a personal morality from your example.

Acceptance of discipline at an early age establishes a way of life in which your child feels secure. Personal security is based on the emotional and moral structure that is the foundation of acceptable adult behaviour. Throughout your child's early life, he or she challenges and questions discipline. You must be logical and sympathetic to your child's challenges because he or she is only experimenting and trying to find out the full range of acceptable human behaviour.

Schooling

Day nursery or kindergarten introduces a child to children of the same age, new adults, and a new set of disciplines. The child learns from the new equipment and toys available, and from the teacher's ability to instruct new and interesting skills.

By the time a child starts a more formal education, he or she has discovered how to cope with a new environment, and how to compromise the desire for freedom with the minor restrictions of an institution's discipline. The child also learns the enjoyment of making friends. You can help in this adjustment by showing an interest in your child's work and play, and by talking to the teachers about your child's progress. Your involvement is appreciated by teacher and child.

Any child may have anxieties and fears about the first few days at a school. This is normal and most schools let you stay for a little while until your child has met the new classmates and teachers, and has had a look around the school. Most children fit into a pattern of school life and discipline in a few days. The rule structure at a school is usually sensible, and punishments usually fair. Problems may arise from bullying and teasing. Talk to your child and ask how things are going each day. This support is essential, and it is often surprising how, with your reassurance, he or she is able to cope with school problems of this kind. Much of the problem is due to an underlying feeling of insecurity and apprehension. A secure, sociable child is most likely to remember schooldays as being happy ones.

Whether your child is clever or not, and skilful at sport or not, is unimportant compared with his or her ability to make friends, and remain happy in the school. This gives you a greater pleasure than any other form of success as a parent, and is the basic quality essential for a happy life.

Age-by-age charts

Section contents

Introduction

The age-by-age charts are designed to show how an average child may develop, year by year, from birth to adulthood. Similarly the age-by-age charts that concern adults (*see* pp.882–927) outline the normal changes that may be expected to occur at any one age. In addition to this, the age-by-age charts for both children and adults also show the various disorders that may affect people at different ages. Disorders are described in the age group where they are most likely to occur, although this classification is not, of course, exclusive. The alphabetical index of children's disorders (*see* pp.880–881) and the classified index of adult disorders (*see* pp.928–933) provide comprehensive guides to the different disorders described for every age group.

The charts of normal development describe behaviour and achievements that are *usually* found at the age in question, but that do not, by any means, *always* occur. It is very important to realize that slight variations are not signs of abnormality, and parents should not feel anxious if their child appears different from what they suppose a "normal" child should be. If anxieties persist, however, consult a doctor for advice.

The charts of disorders consist of a description of the symptoms of each condition, with an outline of the ways the disorder may be treated. There are also notes that discuss other questions related to the disorder itself, or to its treatment.

A person using the age-by-age charts should consider whether he or she is more interested in what can happen at a particular age, in general terms, or whether he or she is concerned about a specific illness or disorder.

In the former case, turn first to the beginning of the section that relates to the age in question, where information can be found describing events that normally occur at this age. In the case of children, emphasis is placed on health care, physical growth, and the development of speech, hearing, vision, motor skills, and understanding. For adults the information is more general.

If, on the other hand, the reader wants to know about something specific, for example, an illness about which he or she is concerned, then the first step should be to refer to the index that relates to childhood disorders, or the index of adult disorders, and turn to where the subject is described.

At birth: introduction

The table below summarizes the process of childbirth, following the sequence of stages from the onset of labour to the actual delivery of the baby. The first stage of labour begins when there are regular, powerful contractions at intervals of 10 to 30 minutes.

In almost every case a newborn child is healthy, normal, and perfectly formed.

Furthermore, with modern antenatal care, if a baby is not developing normally, this can be detected before the birth so that all necessary precautions can be taken to ensure that the baby survives.

Antenatal check-ups are an important part of health care during pregnancy and can do much to make the birth trouble-free.

STAGE	SYMPTOMS	DURATION
Onset of labour This is usually identified by one of three events. (1) The "show", which is the discharge of a bloodstreaked, jelly-like substance from the vagina, caused by loosening of the plug of mucus from the neck of the womb. (2) "Breaking the waters", which occurs when the strong bag (amniotic sac) surrounding the baby and containing the waters (amniotic fluid) starts to leak. (3) Regular contractions of the uterus.	Dragging pains in the abdomen; slight nausea; lower back pain; aching at the top of the legs.	
Stage one Labour begins with the regular contractions of the uterus. Contractions feel like cramp pains in the abdomen and lower back. The neck (cervix) of the womb dilates gradually with each contraction until it becomes wide enough to allow the baby to emerge. The cervix is about 10cm (4 inches) wide when fully dilated.	Lower abdominal discomfort and pain. Contractions occur at intervals of 10 to 30 minutes. Frequency increases to 2-minute intervals.	3 to 24 hours (10 hours on average) for a first baby; 1 to 24 hours (6 hours on average) for subsequent births.
Stage two The second stage of labour begins when the cervix is fully open. The mother usually feels a strong urge to push or bear down. The baby normally passes head first through the birth canal. When the baby's head has emerged it is seen to rotate. Then further contractions are followed by the emergence of first one shoulder and then the other. When the shoulders are delivered, the rest of the baby follows easily.	Discomfort in lower pelvis; strong urge to press down. Forceful contractions every 1 to 2 minutes, each lasting about 1 minute.	30 to 60 minutes for a first baby; less than 30 minutes for subsequent births.
Stage three The period from the delivery of the child to the delivery of the afterbirth (placenta) after it has separated from the lining of the womb is known as the third stage of labour. An injection is usually given at this stage to make the muscles of the womb contract, so that expulsion of the afterbirth is speeded up.	Usually no discomfort. Some contractions while the afterbirth is being expelled.	15 to 30 minutes in most cases.

SYMPTOMS AND SIGNS	TREATMENT
Absent limbs Whole or part of limb missing at birth; affecting one or more limbs. In some cases, limb present in undeveloped form, or with fingers or toes missing.	Mechanical device attached to undeveloped limb; in many cases no treatment possible.
Achondroplasia Dwarfism; short legs and arms; head and body nearly normal in size.	No treatment.
Angioma *See* **Birthmark: angioma**	
Bat-ear One or both ears sticking out from the head.	If necessary, plastic surgery when the child is about six years old.
Birthmark: angioma Swelling made up of blood vessels or lymph vessels; usually occurring in skin.	None required unless angioma presses on an important structure; usually heals naturally within about five years.
Birthmark: mole Small area of pigmentation of the skin; often slightly raised; occurring anywhere on the body.	No treatment necessary.
Birthmark: mongolian spots Area of pigmentation that may be slate grey to blue in colour; usually on the lower part of the back; sometimes on the thigh; can occur anywhere on the body.	None; usually disappears naturally within a few years.
Birthmark: pigmented Dark brown, pigmented area of skin.	No treatment necessary.
Birthmark: port-wine stain A flat, purple, or deep-red discoloration of an area of skin; caused by abnormalities in blood vessels in the skin.	Surgical removal, if the birthmark is small, so that removal does not cause extensive scarring; camouflage of stain for cosmetic reasons.
Birthmark: strawberry Raised area of dark-red pigmentation; usually small at birth; grows rapidly for about a year; may bleed easily if scratched or injured.	Protect from accidental damage; cover the birthmark if it is likely to be scratched or rubbed; wait for natural disappearance; surgical removal is rarely necessary.
Blindness Not always noticed at birth; sometimes eye lens seems opaque; iris may appear defective; in most cases, lack of response to light noticed when the baby is about a month old.	Special education in a school for the blind; precautions for safety in the home; in all cases, consult a specialist.
Blue baby Blue colour to the skin and lips; rapid breathing after slight exertion; difficulty sucking; often underweight.	Specialist assessment and treatment required immediately.

Use of the drug thalidomide during pregnancy resulted in the birth of children with this abnormality. The best-known non-chemical reason for a child being born without normal limbs is that growth has been disturbed by an intra-uterine device that has remained in the womb during pregnancy.

Achondroplasia is an inherited disorder. Intelligence is not usually affected.

Moles can be removed by plastic surgery, later in life. The most common reason for this is cosmetic.

Mongolian spots are more common in people with dark skin, but can also occur in people with fair skin.

A pigmented birthmark may be disfiguring. Removal by plastic surgery is sometimes unsatisfactory, because a large scar is left.

A port-wine stain remains the same size in proportion to the rest of the body as the child grows.

In most cases, after a strawberry birthmark has stopped growing, it gradually decreases in size, and disappears in a few years.

A defect in the iris is often associated with other deformities, for example a cleft palate. A child may be born with a cataract if the mother was ill with German measles during the early stages of pregnancy.

This condition is usually a result of congenital heart disease. It may also be caused by the respiratory distress syndrome (see p.816), in which the blood is not adequately oxygenated because the lungs do not inflate correctly.

SYMPTOMS AND SIGNS	TREATMENT
Brain haemorrhage Irritability; high-pitched crying; in some cases, convulsions after a few hours of inactivity.	Immediate hospital treatment; surgery (ventriculo-peritoneal shunt), or removal of cerebrospinal fluid from the spinal canal (spinal tap), to relieve pressure on the brain; drug therapy; and further treatment in an oxygen tent.
Breasts, swollen Firm swelling of breasts; occasionally, slight discharge of milk; occurs in babies of either sex.	Treatment not required; swelling disappears naturally after a few days.
Breathing problems *See* **Intermittent breathing,** p.816; **Respiratory distress syndrome,** p.816.	
Bruising Local swelling and discoloration, often showing where instruments, such as forceps, have been used to assist the birth; bruising on the top of the scalp common in a normal delivery.	Treatment not necessary; bruising disappears within a week.
"Caput" Swelling on top of newborn baby's head; disappears after a few hours.	None required
Cerebral palsy (spasticity) Rarely appears until the baby is about one month old.	
Cleft palate and lip (hare-lip) A split in the upper lip; sometimes two splits; sometimes only one side; in some cases extending back through the palate on the roof of the mouth.	Plastic surgery to close the defect; treatment starting in infancy; closure of lip possible, in some cases, soon after birth; severe cases need treatment until about the age of twelve. Generally, cleft lip treated at three months, and cleft palate closed at a later date.
Club-foot Foot bent downwards and inwards; may affect one or both feet; sometimes associated with spina bifida (*see* p.818).	Consultation with an orthopaedic specialist; gentle manipulation and splinting usually sufficient.

Congenital anomalies
Causes

Congenital anomalies are found in about two-and-a-half per cent of all babies. There are many possible causes, some of which are associated with chromosomal abnormalities. Down's syndrome (mongolism) is more common in the children of older parents. Some infections, such as German measles, may cause abnormalities. Certain drugs, if taken by the mother during pregnancy, may also cause abnormalities in the child. Treatment of the mother with X-rays during early pregnancy may harm the foetus. A poor diet is thought to be a significant cause of congenital illness. Physical injuries may occur to a baby that grows in an awkward position in the womb, and damage may also occur if an object, such as an intra-uterine device (IUD), remains in the womb as the foetus is developing. Finally, some anomalies may be inherited. These may be obvious at birth, as in the case of a cleft palate, or appear only later in life, as in the case of haemophilia.

A brain haemorrhage may cause the death of the baby. In some cases it may lead to cerebral palsy (*see* p.812). A haemorrhage may also be associated with damage to the baby's skull. If a haemorrhage occurs, this possibility should be investigated.

The condition is caused by the mother's hormones that remain in the baby's circulation after birth. The swelling disappears as these hormones leave the body. In female babies, the vulva may also be swollen, and vaginal discharge or bleeding may occur.

Bruising is sometimes associated with a wryneck (*see* p.818), if a muscle in the neck has been torn during the delivery. Bleeding around the white of the eye may occur. In a breech delivery there may be bruising on the buttocks. Bruising may also occur on the legs if these have been pulled or stretched during the delivery.

The baby's skull is squeezed as the head is forced through the birth canal. The top of the skull is the softest part and, as the skull is squeezed, the pressure of the fluid within the skull causes this part to bulge.

See p.824.

There may be problems with feeding. In most cases, feeding is accomplished by the use of a special nipple. In some cases, only tube-feeding is possible. A cleft palate and lip may be associated with other congenital anomalies. Ear infections are common. Long term treatment involves orthodontics and speech therapy.

Club-foot may be an inherited deformity, or the result of the baby developing in a cramped position in the womb. The condition is sometimes associated with other congenital anomalies.

Congenital anomalies
Precautions
The chances of giving birth to an abnormal child may be minimized by taking certain precautions before and during pregnancy. Genetic counselling can advise parents about the likelihood of transmitting hereditary disorders, or of bearing a deformed child. The mother can be immunized against German measles before pregnancy. Drugs that are potentially harmful should not be taken during pregnancy. Examination of the mother's blood, to detect the presence of alpha foeto-protein, may indicate deformities such as spina bifida or anencephaly in the foetus. Examination of the fluid that surrounds the foetus during pregnancy (amniocentesis) may be used to check for abnormal cells or chemicals. If abnormalities are detected by medical investigations during early pregnancy, the possibility of terminating the pregnancy may be considered.

SYMPTOMS AND SIGNS	TREATMENT
Congenital dislocation of the hip No obvious symptoms; detected by a specialist after birth.	Hip joint held in place by special splints; splints required for about six months.
Down's syndrome (mongolism) Short, thick hands, often with only a single crease on palm; small, slanting eyes with eye folds; flattened bridge of nose and back of head; general floppiness of body and limbs.	None; special education and home care required; parents need a specialist's advice.
Eyefolds Additional fold on inner side of eyelid, next to the nose; commonly seen at birth; tends to disappear as child grows and as the shape of the face changes.	None required.
Fingers or toes, extra (polydactyly) Additional fingers or toes; usually on the outer side of the hand or foot; often an inherited condition.	Surgical removal in early childhood.
Fingers or toes, webbed (syndactyly) Skin joining two or more fingers or toes; normal opening prevented; often an inherited condition.	Toes usually left untreated; fingers separated by surgery at about the age of four.
Fracture Local swelling; pain; sometimes obvious deformity of skull, collarbone, or limb.	Examination by a doctor; splinting sometimes required; results usually excellent.
Haemolytic disease of the newborn (Rh factor incompatibility) Anaemia; increasing yellow colour to the skin (jaundice); heart failure; brain damage; cerebral palsy; death may occur.	Exchange blood transfusion; treatment with ultraviolet light to destroy yellow pigment (bilirubin); baby's eyes must be protected from the ultraviolet light.
Heart disease, congenital Breathlessness; slight blueness of skin and lips, as in a blue baby (*see* p.810); easily tired; weak sucking; in some cases there are no symptoms.	Urgently required if symptoms are obvious; in other cases, surgical treatment may be required later in life.
Hermaphroditism *See* **Sex uncertainty,** p.816.	
Hernia (rupture) Soft, local swelling, on part of the abdomen; may appear and disappear without obvious cause; usually can be pushed back, temporarily, into the abdomen; most commonly occurs in the groin, on one or both sides (inguinal hernia); may occur at the umbilicus (umbilical hernia).	Surgical treatment needed for an inguinal hernia; in boys, check also for an undescended testicle (*see* p.838); an umbilical hernia usually grows for six months, then diminishes; normally disappears naturally after about four years.

The cause is not known. It may occur because the muscles that relax in the month before birth become too weak to hold the hip joint in place. It is sometimes inherited.

Down's syndrome is due to an abnormal number of chromosomes. This anomaly is more likely to occur in the case of a child born to an older woman. The possibility of a child being born with Down's syndrome can be anticipated if amniocentesis is used to examine the uterine fluid in early pregnancy.

Eyefolds are normal in Oriental races. Sometimes they occur in non-Oriental families as a genetic variation. Eyefolds are also a sign of Down's syndrome (*see* p.814) but they are not significant unless other signs of Down's syndrome are present as well. Consult a doctor if there is any doubt.

Polydactyly may be associated with more serious conditions and other anomalies.

Other anomalies in the shape or function of a child's fingers or toes may be corrected by appropriate treatment.

Fractures occur rarely, but are more common during a breech delivery. In some cases the fracture may damage a nerve, causing temporary paralysis.

A child whose mother's blood is Rh negative and whose father's blood is Rh positive may be born with Rh positive blood that is incompatible with that of the mother. If blood from an Rh positive foetus mixes with the mother's Rh negative blood, as occurs towards the end of pregnancy, the mother forms antibodies against Rh positive blood. These antibodies do not usually appear in time to affect the first Rh positive child but are likely to affect subsequent Rh positive babies. If these antibodies enter the baby's blood they destroy the Rh positive red blood cells. This causes anaemia and heart failure in the foetus, and jaundice in the baby.

All pregnant women should be examined for Rh negative blood. If a woman is found to be Rh negative, anti-Rh serum should be given to prevent her being sensitized at the birth of her Rh positive baby. If necessary, an exchange transfusion can be done while the baby is still in the womb.

Heart disease may be associated with other congenital anomalies, for example, Down's syndrome (*see* p.814).

At birth: disorders 4

Hydrocephalus

Large head; soft areas of the skull (fontanelles) seeming to bulge; whites of eyes showing below upper lids; symptoms not always obvious at birth.	Early diagnosis important; skilled supervision to monitor pressure of cerebrospinal fluid; surgical treatment to relieve pressure inside skull to prevent damage to brain; regular measurement of head size.

Hypoglycaemia (low blood sugar)

Usually appears about twenty-four hours after birth; drowsiness; refusal to suck; pause in breathing for up to half a minute; sometimes convulsions.	Consult a doctor immediately; intravenous glucose for several days.

Intermittent breathing

Temporary stoppages of breathing; brief stoppages, up to ten seconds, are not serious; longer stoppages may be serious.	Consult a doctor; immediate treatment required for stoppages longer than thirty seconds.

Jaundice

Yellow discoloration of whites of eyes; slight yellow discoloration of skin developing a few days after birth and fading slowly. Yellow colour that increases and does not fade is serious.	Not usually needed for mild jaundice; ultraviolet light sometimes used for premature babies. Increasing jaundice needs urgent diagnosis and skilled care.

Mongolism
See **Down's syndrome,** p.814.

Nerve injury

Lack of movement in a limb or part of the body; sometimes affects one side of the face.	Treatment by a specialist; results usually satisfactory in cases of facial paralysis; often less successful if the limbs are affected.

PKU (phenylketonuria)

None at birth; later, pale skin, and urine that smells like mice; mental retardation, convulsions, and abnormal behaviour in later childhood.	Phenylketonuria (PKU) test forty-eight hours after first feeding, and again before discharge of the newborn baby from hospital; following positive blood test, treatment with diet that is low in phenylalanine.

Premature baby

Birth before expected date; small size; skin appearing red; covering of fine hair (lanugo) that disappears soon after birth; short nails; few skin creases on soles of feet.	Skilled care needed; keep baby warm; use incubator; feed frequently, but in small quantities; additional oxygen may be needed; observe progress carefully.

Respiratory distress syndrome

Rapid breathing; grunting; inability to suck; common in premature babies at birth.	Immediate treatment by a doctor; treatment with mechanical ventilation and continuous positive airway pressure (CPAP); intravenous infusions; care in an oxygen tent.

Rh incompatibility
See **Haemolytic disease of the newborn,** p.814.

Sex uncertainty

External sexual organs not properly formed; sex of the baby uncertain.	Assessment by a specialist; chromosome examination; surgical treatment may be required.

The condition is caused by a defect in the drainage of fluid from the brain. Hydrocephalus is often associated with spina bifida (see p.818) in the newborn, and a baby with one abnormality should be examined by a specialist for the other as soon as possible after childbirth.

This condition occurs more commonly in premature babies. Feeding the baby as soon as possible after birth reduces the chances of hypoglycaemia occurring. In some cases it is associated with other disorders of sugar metabolism. The symptoms resemble those of a brain haemorrhage and it is important to exclude this possibility.

A blue colour to the skin and lips, vomiting, and diarrhoea may be associated with this breathing problem. Prolonged breathing stoppages, known as apnoea, may indicate a serious condition, such as brain haemorrhage or meningitis.

Slight yellow discoloration is normal in most babies and is due to the destruction of excess red blood cells. An immature liver is unable to get rid of the yellow pigment (bilirubin) fast enough. Severe jaundice may be a result of Rh factor incompatibility (see **Haemolytic disease of the newborn,** p.814), a blocked bile duct, prematurity, or an infection. The greatest danger of severe jaundice is that it can cause brain damage.

Facial paralysis is most commonly due to pressure on the nerve during a forceps delivery. Limb paralysis is usually caused by pulling on the limb during the delivery.

Treatment should continue for at least five years in order to prevent brain damage. The disease is due to the failure of the body to metabolize the amino acid phenylalanine correctly. The disease is inherited. All children should be tested for phenylketonuria in the period immediately following birth.

Premature babies are more likely to develop breathing problems, infections, hypoglycaemia, and jaundice, so they must be treated with particular care in the days after birth. In most cases, progress is rapid and such babies catch up with the growth of children that are not premature. A premature baby weighs under 5.5lb (2.5kg).

This syndrome occurs because the baby's lungs do not expand normally at birth. If the oxygen content of arterial blood increases, the baby has a good chance of survival.

It is important to determine the sex of the child as early as possible in infancy, and before the baby leaves the hospital. Failure to do so may lead to social as well as medical problems.

SYMPTOMS AND SIGNS	TREATMENT

Skull and brain deformities
Absence of cranium and brain (anencephalus); baby stillborn or dies soon after birth. Small skull (microcephalus); face normal size; leads to severe mental handicap.
   See also **Hydrocephalus,** p.816.

No treatment of anencephalus; mental handicap associated with microcephalus needs special treatment and care.

Sneezing and sniffling
Difficulties in breathing through nose; nose partly blocked; nose running.

None usually required.

Spasticity
See **Cerebral palsy,** p.824.

Spina bifida
Failure of the lower part of the spine to close; abnormality may not be obvious if spinal opening is covered by skin; indications include dimple, lump, tuft of hair, or cyst containing clear fluid like a blister, over lower spine; in serious cases, a raw open area in which spinal nerves can be seen; paralysis of lower body and limbs in severe cases.

No treatment needed if skin is not damaged; form in which there is a cyst can often be treated surgically; serious form, in which spine is uncovered, is difficult to treat; urgent surgical operation to close skin over spinal cord essential; child may live if infection can be prevented; specialist care as the child grows.

Tongue-tie
Tongue unable to stick out of the mouth; ligament (frenum) beneath the tongue unusually short, restricting movement.

Usually unnecessary; if no natural improvement, surgery may be required if advised by the specialist.

Urethra, abnormal opening
Small opening along the underneath of the penis (hypospadias); rarely, along the top (epispadias).

Surgical operation to repair defect; usually done at about the age of five.

Uvula, split
Double-ended uvula; visible when the mouth is open.
   See also **Cleft palate and lip,** p.812.

None required.

Vernix
Oily film (vernix caseosa) covering the baby's skin at birth; collection of this in groin and in armpits.

Wash face and groin; remove excess from creases; skin covering usually left for several days after birth.

Vulva, swollen
Swollen external genitals in a baby girl; sometimes associated with enlarged clitoris and vaginal discharge; genital area inflamed.

None required if swelling disappears within one or two weeks.

Wryneck
Head turned to one side at birth; chin tilted downwards; persistence of this deformity after birth.

Turn head gently in opposite direction to the deformity several times a day for six months; consult doctor; a minor operation may be needed to repair damaged muscle.

In microcephalus, the skull is small because the brain does not grow normally. This may be due to a fault in the genetic make-up of the child, or to damage from an infection such as German measles or toxoplasmosis, contracted by the mother during pregnancy. Microcephalus may also be the result of brain damage caused by asphyxia at birth, or to a disease, such as meningitis, that sometimes prevents the brain from developing correctly.

This is relatively common in the newborn, particularly if the nose is small. A low bridge to the nose and narrow nasal passages are usually the causes of sniffling and as these grow larger the symptoms disappear. Sneezing in the newborn is more commonly the result of sensitive nasal passages than of infection.

Babies with severe spina bifida often have anencephalus or hydrocephalus as well. Severe spina bifida causes the spine and the spinal cord to be deformed and this may lead to paralysis of the legs and the inability to control the muscles of the bladder and anus. Infection of the cerebrospinal fluid, leading to meningitis, is a common cause of death. Genetic counselling is advisable because of the risk of a subsequent child being born with spina bifida. Certain types of spina bifida can be detected early in the pregnancy by methods of prenatal diagnosis.

There are usually no problems with sucking or with the development of speech, unless the frenum is very short. Surgical division is not usually necessary, but, if it is required, it is a minor operation.

The purpose of surgery is to reconstruct the urethra so that the opening is in the normal place. Part of the foreskin is commonly used to cover and close the abnormal opening. For this reason circumcision must not be done.

The vernix is thought to provide protection against infection. It may also protect against excessive heat loss. It is usually washed off during the first day after birth.

This condition is often associated with swollen breasts (*see* **Breasts, swollen,** p.812). It is caused by the presence of maternal hormones in the baby's blood. Slight menstruation can occur.

A wryneck is usually the result of a neck muscle being torn during the delivery. Sometimes a lump can be felt in the affected muscle. Exercising the neck gently in the manner described will usually encourage the muscle to grow correctly. Consult a doctor if there is any doubt or if progress seems slow. Occasionally a wryneck is a symptom of a bone abnormality, in which case this will appear on an X-ray.

Birth to age 1½: normal development 1

Each section of the age-by-age charts begins with an outline of the normal achievements of a child of the age group being considered. The stages of development, in this case of a baby from birth to age eighteen months, are represented in chart form. It should be remembered that these charts can only present an outline of average development, because babies can vary enormously in the rate of their individual progress. Certain babies will be more advanced in some things and slower in others. Sometimes progress is rapid over a wide range of abilities, whereas at other times it may be held back, perhaps by illness or accident. If parents are concerned about their child's lack of progress, they should consult a doctor.

The problems and disorders that can affect a baby at birth, and in the months following birth, are illustrated in charts that emphasize the main symptoms, how to treat them, and also show other problems that can arise.

Vision
Achievements include at:

Birth:	closes eyelids to bright light
Two weeks:	momentarily looks at objects
One month:	briefly follows parent's face and may smile
Two months:	follows moving objects with eyes
Three months:	begins to focus and starts to move head as well as eyes
Four months:	looks at own hands and focuses easily on nearby objects
Five months:	looks at surroundings and searches for lost toy
Six months:	looks at and picks up object
Nine months:	looks at small objects
One year:	interested in simple shapes
Fifteen months:	recognizes simple pictures

Hearing
Achievements include at:

One month:	responds reflexively to loud noise (startle reflex)
Four months:	opens or widens eyelids in response to loud noise
Five months:	turns head to right or left towards sound
Nine months:	locates noises to one side of, or below, head
One year:	turns head towards sounds from any direction

Speech
Achievements include at:

Three months:	laughs
Seven to eight months:	says "Da" and "Ma" "Da-da" and "Ma-ma"
Ten months:	has one word with a particular meaning
One year:	uses a few words correctly (for example, "dog")
One year to eighteen months:	develops own language mixed with many normal words; often understood by family and enjoys experimenting with new sounds; some children speak well (for example, may describe events accurately)

Physical movement
Achievements include at:

Birth:	can just lift head when lying on stomach; head lags behind when pulled to sitting position
One month:	may hold head up for a moment when sitting
Two months:	raises head when

820

Achievements include at:

Two months:	lying on stomach but constantly drops head when in sitting position
Three months:	pushes up with forearms; only slight head lag when pulled to sitting position
Four months:	looks around when in sitting position with only slight head wobble; slight support from legs when held in standing position
Five months:	head steady when looking around; no lag when pulled to sitting position; starts to dribble a great deal
Six months:	holds out hands to be lifted up; able to support most of own weight when standing; sits in chair, if supported; rolls from stomach onto back
Seven months:	supports self on legs while holding onto mother's hands; rolls from back onto stomach; chews
Eight months:	can sit unaided, and can stand up holding a support; begins to crawl
Ten to twelve months:	begins to walk by holding onto a person's hands or onto furniture; drooling stops
Twelve to fifteen months:	stands alone and then takes first few steps with feet spaced widely; often falls over; crawls up stairs
Fifteen to eighteen months:	begins to walk normally and may run;

Achievements include at:

Fifteen to eighteen months:	may begin jumping; able to get onto chair; walks up stairs holding bannister; throws ball without falling over

Use of hands

Achievements include at:

Birth to three months:	holds objects by reflex
Three months:	pulls at clothing; momentarily grasps toy; clasps hands together
Four months:	shakes rattle; plays with hands
Five months:	takes toy that is offered; holds bottle
Six months:	drops one toy when another is offered; puts toes in mouth
Eight months:	picks up small objects using finger and thumb
Nine months:	uses index finger to pull toys and will deliberately let them drop; puts toys into parent's hand
Ten months:	plays games by dropping toy for parent to pick up and then drops it again
Eleven months:	plays games by giving someone a toy and insisting on taking it back; plays with ball
Twelve to fifteen months:	makes marks with crayons; takes off shoes; plays with blocks
Eighteen months:	builds small tower with three or four blocks; manages spoon; scribbles; turns pages of a book

Birth to age 1½: normal development 2

Understanding

Achievements include at:

One month:	looks at parent's face
Two months:	smiles when parent talks
Three months:	laughs when spoken to
Four months:	enjoys toys and is excited when fed; likes to sit up; holds onto toy when it is pulled
Five months:	looks towards sound; smiles at mirror; looks for, and finds, lost toys
Six to seven months:	puts food into mouth; shy with strangers; plays peekaboo with adults; attracts attention by making noise
Eight months:	tries to prevent face being wiped; excited by favourite food; understands "no"
Nine months:	waves goodbye; tugs parent's clothing; helps when being dressed (for example, puts arm out for sleeve)

Achievements include at:

Ten months:	makes deliberate actions (for example, puts toys into a box); understands simple question like "Where is the dog?"
Eleven months:	likes pictures in a book; likes simple nursery rhymes and remembers the way they are told
One year:	enjoys kisses; understands questions like "Where is your sock?"
One year to fifteen months:	manages cup and feeding; asks for things by pointing; kisses pictures of things that are recognized; sometimes refuses to do things
Fifteen to eighteen months:	able to point to ear, eye, or nose, and to pictures of dog, or car; helps with housework; will fetch objects on request; helps when being undressed; shows anger when parent stops playing; starts to take a long time with meals

AVERAGE INCREASE IN WEIGHT DURING FIRST 18 MONTHS

Teeth

Developments include at:

Birth:	in rare cases a child may be born with one or more teeth
Six months:	lower middle incisors
Seven months:	lower outer incisors
Seven to nine months:	four upper incisors
One year:	lower first molars
Twelve to fourteen months:	upper first molars
Fifteen to eighteen months:	upper and lower eye teeth

Disease prevention and health care

Immunization

Suggested schedule:

Five months:	diphtheria, tetanus and whooping cough (triple) injection; oral polio vaccine
Six months:	diphtheria, tetanus and whooping cough (triple) injection; oral polio vaccine
One year:	diphtheria, tetanus and whooping cough (triple) injection; oral polio vaccine
Fifteen months:	measles injection

Immunization programmes must begin soon after birth, as infectious diseases can be more serious in babies than in adults.

Whooping cough vaccination is not recommended if the baby has had a convulsion, if there is any sign of a brain disorder, or if there is a family history of epilepsy. If in doubt, consult a doctor.

Mumps vaccination may be given at any age, but it is not usually recommended by doctors except for adults who have not had the disease.

Health care

Weight, length, and head circumference measured on each visit. Suggested schedule:

At birth:	thorough medical examination; blood test, if required for legal or medical reason, for example blood group, rhesus factor, syphilis, anaemia, jaundice factor; test for hypothyroidism
One to two weeks:	thorough medical examination; Guthrie (PKU) test; circumcision, if required; vision check
One month:	thorough medical examination
Two months:	thorough medical examination; vision check; hearing check
Three months:	thorough medical examination
Four months:	thorough medical examination
Five months:	through medical examination
Six months:	thorough medical examination; vision check; hearing check
Eight months:	thorough medical examination; blood test, if recommended
Ten months:	thorough medical examination
Twelve months:	thorough medical examination
Fifteen months:	thorough medical examination
Eighteen months:	thorough medical examination

Most medical examinations are given at a local health clinic or at a similar clinic run by a G.P.

SYMPTOMS AND SIGNS	TREATMENT
Allergy to cows' milk May include: skin rash; breathing difficulties; running nose; diarrhoea; vomiting after feeding; weight loss.	Consult a doctor; avoid cows' milk in the diet.
Anaemia Pale skin; lethargic behaviour; often breathlessness when crying.	Consult a doctor; diagnosis from blood test; full investigation to detect deficiency of iron salts; small quantities of iron salts added to the diet; vitamin C given, in form of orange juice, to increase iron absorption; iron supplements usually given in liquid or tablet form.
Anal bleeding Blood in the faeces; evidence of pain (screaming) on defecation; constipation.	Consult a doctor; give the child plenty of fluids to prevent constipation; suppositories or lubricants inserted on a gloved finger may be required.
Anal swelling Swelling at anus; red tissue protruding through anus; sometimes colic and vomiting.	Consult a doctor or go to hospital immediately.
Autism Child that shows no signs of affection; lack of response to people, so that deafness may be suspected; lack of interest in cuddling; ignores interruptions; child may show repetitive mannerisms.	Consult a doctor for advice and definite diagnosis; special treatment sometimes helpful.
Bow-legs A gap between knees when feet are placed together; generally a normal occurrence in children when they start walking.	Consult a doctor for an opinion; normally no treatment necessary unless other conditions are present; condition normally corrects itself, from about two years of age.
Bronchitis Cough; fever; rapid breathing.	Consult a doctor for diagnosis; keep child in warm, humid room; hospitalization for serious cases; antibiotics or antispasm cough mixture may be prescribed.
Catarrh Blocked nose; difficulty breathing; cough; thick mucus running from nose; cough worse at night; sometimes vomiting in the morning.	Consult a doctor; antihistamines help to dry nasal mucosa; increase environmental humidity; antibiotics rarely helpful; avoid using irritant nose drops.
Cerebral palsy (spasticity) Lack of movement; differences in movements of each side of the body; child seeming to be too quiet; muscles feel stiff; child failing to suck normally; one hand, or both, remaining closed.	Assessment by a specialist; repeated examinations, over several days or weeks required for complete diagnosis; deformities prevented by moving limbs gently, several times each day; limbs moved through normal range to teach correct position and use, and to relax muscles.

Cows' milk is a common cause of allergy in babies, particularly if this milk is given in the first month of life.

Blood tests should be repeated even when the condition appears to be cured. Iron deficiency anaemia is the most common type of anaemia, particularly in premature babies or in those that have been fed solely on milk for more than six months. In some cases anaemia may be a symptom of a more serious disease. Consult a specialist if there is any doubt.

Anal bleeding is often the result of constipation. Hard faeces sometimes tear the mucosa lining the rectum, causing an anal fissure. Anal bleeding may also be due to an intussusception or a rectal prolapse, both of which are serious, so consult a doctor immediately.

A prolapse of the rectum is the most likely cause of anal swelling (*see* **Rectal prolapse,** p.836), but swelling may also be a symptom of an intussusception (*see* p.834).

Many autistic children are intelligent and some show relatively advanced behaviour in one particular respect. Some autistic children develop a special relationship with one person.

If the condition persists, an orthopaedic specialist should be consulted, particularly if bow-legs are associated with club foot. A child may appear to have bow-legs because of the normal bulge of the outer sides of the calves, when compared to the inner sides. Bow-legs are diagnosed by the separation of the knees.

Bronchitis may develop after a cold and is sometimes accompanied by vomiting or diarrhoea. Bronchiolitis, commonly called wheezy bronchitis, is the most common variety and may be an indication that asthma will develop later in childhood, particularly in a child who has eczema (*see* p.830). The condition may also be associated with cystic fibrosis (*see* p.828).

Recurrent minor respiratory infections cause excess nasal mucus production, leading to blockage of the narrow nasal passages of a young child. This may be troublesome, particularly at night. If the child swallows mucus during the night, vomiting is likely to occur in the morning. As the baby grows, the nasal passages widen and immunity develops.

Cerebral palsy may occur if the baby is premature, if the baby has severe jaundice at birth, if the mother had diabetes during pregnancy, or as the result of a birth injury.

SYMPTOMS AND SIGNS	TREATMENT
Chest deformities Funnel breast, a depression of the breastbone resembling a funnel; pigeon breast, a protruberance of the chest in front; altered shapes of the normal chest.	Surgical treatment seldom needed but may be given for cosmetic reasons. Discuss with a specialist, because operation may be dangerous.
Coeliac disease Starts about age six to twelve months; loss of weight; swollen abdomen; plentiful, frothy, floating diarrhoea; loss of appetite. See also **Cystic fibrosis,** p.828.	Consult a doctor, who may recommend a diet free of gluten, the protein in wheat and rye that causes the symptoms; gluten-free diet may have to be maintained for rest of patient's life.
Cold Fever; running nose with catarrh (see p.824) and cough; sometimes diarrhoea.	Keep in warm room; plenty of fluids; consult a doctor who may give antihistamine drugs to dry nasal secretions; children's nose drops may be used for few days, particularly before feeding, because sucking is difficult with a blocked nose.
Colic Screaming and drawing up of knees in small baby. See also **Colic, infantile,** p.826.	Further burping of child after feeding; sips of sweetened water; cuddling; change of nappy; all these may be necessary.
Colic, infantile (three-month colic) One to two hours of recurring colic; taking place most evenings in babies one to three months old.	If simple measures fail (see **Colic,** p.826), consult a doctor; antispasm medicine before baby's meal.
Conjunctivitis Red eye with sticky discharge.	Keep eye clean by bathing with warm, weak salt solution two or three times a day.
Constipation Occasional passing of hard faeces; may accompany a fever (see p.832); sometimes occurs after diarrhea (see p.830) or vomiting (see p.838).	Increase fluids by mouth; in older babies more fruit and vegetables produce a larger stool; children's suppositories may help restart defecation.
Convulsions Sudden body rigidity and loss of consciousness; sometimes followed by generalized shaking that lasts between fifteen and sixty seconds; convulsion may be followed by continued unconsciousness, for several minutes, before return to normal colour and consciousness.	Hold baby on side with head down to allow any vomit to leave mouth and to prevent inhalation of vomit into lungs; do not try to force anything into mouth; consult a doctor.
Cot death See **Sudden infant death syndrome,** p.838.	

Funnel breast is rarely associated with underlying disorders, but pigeon breast may be associated with congenital heart disease, asthma, or rickets. Funnel breast may be an inherited condition.

The doctor may examine the faeces for excess fat, or carry out tests to determine whether the small intestine is absorbing sugar and iron properly. A diagnosis of coeliac disease is usually confirmed by making a biopsy of the small intestine. In some cases the biopsy is repeated after six months of gluten-free diet.

A young baby may still have some protection against colds because of immunity transferred from the mother. Nevertheless, older children with colds should not go near the baby, and the mother should wear a mask if she is developing a cold.

Serious causes of colic include intestinal obstruction (*see* p.834) and intussusception (*see* p.834). It is also associated with some infections, particularly ear infections.

The colic may be due to abdominal discomfort and pain after crying, because the crying causes air to be swallowed. The baby may cry because it is bored, or because it has been fed in a hurry. Feed the baby slowly with small amounts of solids and keep the baby sitting up in a chair for a short time after feeding.

Conjunctivitis commonly occurs with a cold (*see* p.826), or other virus illness. If the discharge is increasing, discuss the condition with your doctor. Conjunctivitis is often contagious and cloths or towels used for the patient should not be used by other members of the family.

Constipation is commonly due to insufficient fluid in the diet. Constipation and anal bleeding (*see* p.824) may be due to a painful crack in the anal skin, whereas constipation and colic (*see* p.826) may indicate an intestinal obstruction (*see* p.834). Prolonged constipation, from birth, may be due to Hirschsprung's disease (*see* p.834) or cretinism (*see* p.828). Breast-fed babies may have a normal stool only about once or twice a week.

Convulsions are most commonly caused by high fever (*see* p.832), brain damage at birth, or epilepsy (*see* p.856). If the convulsion occurs with a high fever, sponge the baby down at once with tepid water, and keep temperature below 39°C (102°F) with sponging and children's aspirin.

SYMPTOMS AND SIGNS	TREATMENT

Cough
See **Bronchitis,** p.824; **Catarrh,** p.824; **Cold,** p.826; **Croup,** p.844.

"Cradle cap"
Brown, flaking skin on scalp; flakes become thick if not treated; this is a normal and common occurrence.

Rub regularly with baby oil or olive oil; shampoo regularly and carefully; comb and brush flaking skin away. If scalp becomes red or looks sore, consult a doctor.

Cretinism
Child appears normal at birth but develops mentally and physically more slowly than normal; sucks poorly and develops constipation (*see* p.826); thick, pale skin; large tongue; swollen abdomen; crying sounds gruff and hoarse.

Diagnosis made by a specialist after a blood test to detect levels of thyroid hormones; gradually decreasing doses of thyroid hormones are given until baby is normal.

Croup
See **Croup,** p.844.

Crying
Persistent crying without noticeable cause; as babies get older mothers can usually tell one cry from another.

Consult a doctor if anxious; give something to drink; change nappy; cuddle to reassure.

Cystic fibrosis
Intestinal obstruction by thick faeces; usually occurring three to four days after birth; intestinal obstruction is least common but most severe symptom; other symptoms are of varying severity; baby fails to grow normally despite good appetite; frequent foul-smelling diarrhoea; swollen abdomen; recurrent infections.

Doctor makes diagnosis by means of a "sweat test", which measures the salt content of the baby's sweat; X-ray examination of chest and lungs; mother must be taught how to hold baby to encourage drainage of mucus from lungs; nutritious diet; vitamins and pancreatic enzymes are usually prescribed.

Dandruff
Dry, white scales on the scalp.

Shampoo scalp frequently; if condition persists, consult a doctor.

Deafness
Child who is strangely silent; who does not respond to sounds; who appears to lack awareness of surroundings; or whose hearing does not seem to develop normally (*see* **Normal Development: Hearing,** p.820).

Consult a doctor; examination of ears for wax or foreign body; antibiotics to treat middle ear infection. Do not push anything into the ears when trying to clean them.

Dehydration
Glazed appearance in eyes; sunken eyes that feel soft; fontanelle, in the cranium, appears sunken; reduced urine output; dry mouth; flabby skin; weak cry; sometimes slight fever and constipation after a period of diarrhoea that is a common cause of dehydration.

Serious condition; severe dehydration can occur rapidly in a small baby; consult a doctor immediately; if baby unable to drink diluted milk or fruit juice, intravenous fluid replacement may be necessary.

"Cradle cap" improves naturally as the baby grows and usually disappears within twelve months.

Failure to diagnose cretinism produces a mentally deficient child. Umbilical hernia commonly occurs.

The child may be hungry, thirsty, too hot or too cold, have a wet nappy, be lonely or bored, or have pain due to a colic condition (*see* p.826); crying may also be a reaction to the mother's anxiety or a way of attracting the mother. Some babies naturally cry much more than others.

All body secretions of a child with cystic fibrosis are abnormally thick, and this contributes to the child's susceptibility to chronic chest infections, pancreatic failure, and sometimes liver disease. A person with cystic fibrosis requires lifelong specialized care.

Dandruff is a common occurrence at about three to nine months and is associated with "cradle cap" (*see* p.828). The condition may be severe in babies with eczema (*see* p.830) or very dry skin.

Because it is difficult to test the hearing of an infant, and because the symptoms of deafness may resemble the symptoms of other conditions, parents who are in any doubt about their child's hearing should consult a doctor. Generally, deafness and pain in the ear are caused by middle ear infections that need urgent treatment. In some cases a mild, chronic infection may be painless, but in need of treatment nevertheless. Deafness in both ears is usually easier to detect than deafness in one ear. A baby often ignores stimuli without being actually deaf.
   See also "**Glue**" ear, p.844.

Dehydration may occur with fever (*see* p.832), vomiting (*see* p.838), or diarrhoea (*see* p.830). The condition may also be caused by heavy sweating, as a result of the baby's being left in a hot room or having on too many clothes, as well as by any illness in which fluid consumption is reduced.

Birth to age 1½: disorders 4

SYMPTOMS AND SIGNS	TREATMENT
Diarrhoea	
Liquid stools; often occurring without illness; blood in faeces or colic (*see* p.826) are more serious symptoms; severe diarrhoea, or diarrhoea with vomiting may cause dehydration (*see* p.828).	Avoid fruit and vegetables in diet; kaolin mixture, from chemist, may produce more solid stools; give plenty of fluids to avoid dehydration; consult a doctor if severe diarrhoea persists for more than two hours; more than five diarrhoeal stools in a small baby can cause rapid dehydration.
Dry skin	
Dry, scale-like appearance of areas of skin; surface of skin flaking off.	Consult a doctor; use creams to keep skin moist.
Dwarfism	
A baby who does not grow at the normal rate; slow development of a particular part of the body.	Consult specialist; treatment depends on cause; diagnosis from X-rays, blood tests, or associated symptoms.
Ear problems: bat-ear	
See **Bat-ear,** p.810.	
Ear problems: discharging ear	
A flow of waxy secretion or pus from the ear.	Consult a doctor urgently for treatment and antibiotics.
Ear problems: ear pain	
Crying; restlessness; holding ears; other indications that the child has earache.	Earache is a sign of infection or inflammation of the ear; consult a doctor for antibiotic or other appropriate treatment.
Ear problems: ear pulling	
A child constantly pulling on an ear.	Ear pulling is not a sign of infection. Babies like to play with their ears and may pull them when tired or bored.
Eczema	
Red, roughened patches on the skin causing irritation and scratching.	Discuss with a doctor; careful use of hydrocortisone creams; antihistamine drugs; use of specially medicated cleansers in place of common soap when washing; avoidance of wool clothing and, occasionally, certain foods. Gloves worn at night will help prevent scratching.
Eye problems: blindness	
See **Blindness,** p.810.	
Eye problems: blocked tear duct	
Persistent flow of tears from one or both eyes.	Consult a doctor; if condition persists, it can be relieved by passing a small probe down the duct to clear it.

Dehydration (*see* p.828) is dangerous and a doctor must be consulted as soon as possible if signs of dehydration appear. Coeliac disease (*see* p.826) and cystic fibrosis (*see* p.828) are serious causes but diarrhoea may occur with almost any respiratory or other infection, for example cold (*see* p.826), ear infection, or bronchitis (*see* p.824), and may also be caused by antibiotics.

See also **Green faeces,** p.832.

Dry skin, in its most severe form, is a congenital abnormality. In hot climates, sweating may aggravate the problem.

Some babies are small because their parents are small and a premature baby (*see* p.816) is usually a small baby. Feeding problems, or heart disease may also inhibit normal growth. Failure to grow normally may be due to a serious condition such as coeliac disease (*see* p.826), to some disorder such as cretinism (*see* p.828) or to a congenital abnormality such as achondroplasia (*see* p.810).

A discharging ear sometimes occurs after a prolonged period of crying in a child who has a cold (*see* p.826) and this may be a sign of an infected middle ear and of a burst eardrum. Continued discharge may cause soreness on the side of the neck and cheek. Remember to check for deafness (*see* p.828) when the ear seems better.

A baby over ten months old may indicate that an ear is hurting by crying, by holding the ear, or by refusing to allow anyone to touch the ear. Ear pain often occurs with a cold (*see* p.826) or a throat infection. Vomiting (*see* p.838) may occur. Recurrent ear pain may be due to swollen adenoids blocking the Eustachian (auditory) tube. Check for deafness (*see* p.828).

In babies eczema generally starts on the scalp or face, but in older children it develops most commonly in the creases of the elbows, and behind the knees and ears, although it can occur anywhere on the body. Bleeding and infection may occur from scratching. The condition seldom develops before the age of three months and usually improves after three years. Eczema varies greatly in severity from time to time and from one baby to another. There is usually a family history of allergy. In some children, after the natural improvement of eczema, asthma may develop. The use of desensitizing injections against allergies seldom helps eczema. Smallpox vaccinations must never be given to a child with a history of eczema.

A blocked tear duct in a baby is a tear duct that was not fully opened at birth. Sometimes blockage is caused by conjunctivitis (*see* p.826), or by a cold (*see* p.826), if the infection has spread to the tear ducts.

SYMPTOMS AND SIGNS	TREATMENT
Eye problems: cataract Eyes with opaque lens; appearance of a grey spot, seen through the iris; clouding of lens may or may not interfere with vision.	Consult an eye specialist; severely opaque lens should be surgically treated when the child is six months old.
Eye problems: conjunctivitis *See* **Conjunctivitis**, p.826.	
Eye problems: squint Eyes look in different directions; one eye that appears to wander, independently of the other, from object at which child is looking; symptoms may be noticed as early as six or eight weeks of age.	Examination by an eye specialist to ensure both eyes are healthy and that one is not merely nearsighted and "lazy"; treatment required if squint persists or is present at six months of age; cover normal eye to allow weak eye to develop; early surgery, when about one year old, produces good results if squint is due to lack of muscle balance.
Failure to thrive A baby showing slow physical development; slow weight gain; lethargy; a baby that appears weak and seldom cries.	Consult a doctor if the condition persists for more than three weeks.
Fat baby Baby is overweight and lethargic; late walking; appearing to be behind expected physical achievements.	Discuss feeding with a doctor; reduce sugar and carbohydrate intake; avoid sweetened drinks between meals; increase fresh fruit and vegetables in diet.
Feeding problems: food fads Refusal of many different kinds of food; preference for one or two particular foods.	Parents should be firm and produce a normal nutritious meal; end meal by leaving baby hungry if baby will not eat food that has been refused; give all the originally intended foods; repeat at next meal until baby starts eating disliked food.
Feeding problems: food refusal Refusal to feed; particularly when a new food is introduced.	Baby may have eaten enough or may want to drink; try some other item of food before trying the unwanted food again; further refusal may be ignored at the first meal but the next day try again and be prepared to stop meal if baby will not eat it.
Fever Baby who appears hot, fussy, flushed, or lethargic; chill and shivering; baby thirsty but refusing food; feeling cold at onset, but then feeling hot; fever confirmed by taking temperature.	Give plenty to drink; give children's aspirin mixture to reduce fever; if fever over 40°C (104°F), consult a doctor as soon as possible; sponge baby with warm water or put in bath; call a doctor if other symptoms occur or if you are anxious.
Green faeces Green faeces being passed; occurring with diarrhoea.	In young babies, increase amount of milk; give clear fluids if diarrhoea occurs; treat as diarrhoea (*see* p.830); faeces will return to normal colour when diarrhoea stops.

A cataract in a baby is a congenital abnormality that can be caused by the mother's having contracted German measles during pregnancy. *See* **Blindness**, p.810.

There is often a family history of squint. The sudden onset of squint at any age needs thorough investigation.

Failure to thrive is most commonly caused by inadequate nourishment, or by an illness, such as congenital heart disease (*see* p.814). The condition may also be a result of a lack of affection, and this should always be considered as a possibility. Other possible causes include cerebral palsy (*see* p.824), cretinism (*see* p.828), coeliac disease (*see* p.826), cystic fibrosis (*see* p.828), and lack of pituitary growth hormone.

The condition is rarely, if ever, due to disease. Obese parents tend to have obese children. Overweight babies usually grow into overweight adults, partly because of the family eating habits, and partly because parents consider the obese shape to be a healthy one.

In some cases obesity results from too many sweet foods. Food fads are usually associated with feeding problems, such as food refusal, that have not been controlled. In general, there is no harm in selecting foods for which the child has shown a preference, provided that the child does not try to manipulate the parents.

It is normal for a baby's appetite to diminish after about twelve months, because the growth rate also slows down. Refusal of a food that has been previously eaten is usually a sign that the baby wants to assert itself. A gradual approach allows the parent to be sure the baby is not becoming ill, vomiting (*see* p.838), or experiencing diarrhoea (*see* p.830). Once the baby has been able to refuse one food it may refuse more as a way of defeating the parent. Every baby and child should be allowed one or two dislikes.

Fever is often the first symptom of another illness, for example, a cold (*see* p.826), and is sometimes associated with diarrhoea (*see* p.830), or vomiting (*see* p.838). A fever usually disappears in twenty-four hours if treated sensibly. Recurring fevers, with no obvious cause, must be assessed by a doctor.

Green faeces occur with diarrhoea and are caused by unchanged bile salts leaving the intestine. The condition is commonly a sign of underfeeding in young babies. Look for the underlying causes of the diarrhoea. Green faeces may also occur when the baby is given fruit juice for the first time.

SYMPTOMS AND SIGNS	TREATMENT

Haemophilia
Intermittent spontaneous bruising under skin or into joints; continued bleeding from open wounds or tooth sockets.

Medical assessment with blood tests to confirm diagnosis; child needs to be protected against injuries; long trousers with knee pads, gloves, and special helmet for head and face when in situations likely to lead to injury; bleeding episodes or surgery treated with special antihaemophilia globulin injection prepared from normal blood.

Hiatus hernia
Upper abdominal pain, causing crying and extreme discomfort, may occur; vomiting (*see* p.838), particularly when lying down; moderately large amounts of food regurgitated, with mucus.

Diagnosis made by X-ray after swallowing barium; food should be thickened with cereal; keep baby propped upright day and night; antacids given to reduce stomach acidity.

Hiccups
Regular swallowing spasm; sharp intake of breath; common in babies; rarely lasting more than a few minutes; occurring particularly after feeding.

Not usually necessary; holding baby upright may help; give small amount of boiled water to drink.

Hirschsprung's disease
Constipation (*see* p.826) from birth; 90 per cent of babies with this condition fail to pass normal meconium (dark green-brown stool) within twenty-four hours of being born; abdomen becomes swollen and gas is passed; episodes of swelling and severe vomiting (*see* p.838), relieved by passing gas; child usually grows slowly despite eating well.

Once diagnosis is made, a doctor may recommend saline enemas to empty intestine until child is old enough for surgical removal of abnormal section of large intestine.

Hives
See **Urticaria**, p.850.

Intestinal obstruction
Abdominal swelling or distention; colic (*see* p.826); vomiting (*see* p.838); constipation; failure to pass gas.

Consult a doctor as soon as possible.

Intussusception
Vomiting; sudden onset of severe colic (*see* p.826); short periods of normal behaviour and sleep before further colic; diarrhoea (*see* p.830) at onset, with stools that look like red jelly, then constipation (*see* p.826).

Diagnosis by a doctor, who may feel lump in abdomen; barium enema may not only confirm the condition but will usually relieve it; urgent surgical procedure often required.

Jaundice
See **Jaundice**, p.816.

Meningitis
High-pitched cry; fever (*see* p.832); irritability; sometimes vomiting; staring eyes; lethargy; stiff neck.

Urgent examination by a doctor; lumbar puncture in hospital and antibiotic treatment.

Haemophilia is a hereditary disorder of the blood. It is transmitted genetically through women, but women are rarely, if ever, affected. The condition occurs because the person's blood fails to clot normally, and this allows excessive bleeding to occur. Repeated joint bleeding causes damage to the joint, producing a deformity and swelling.

Haemophilia varies in severity from individual to individual but also, sometimes, with the seasons of the year. Sports, except for swimming, are prohibited.

A hiatus hernia is caused by a weakness in the diaphragm at the point where the oesophagus passes through. This allows food to flow back into the oesophagus, particularly when the baby is lying down, rather than to be held in the stomach. Frequent vomiting

may cause loss of weight and failure to thrive (see p.832). The condition usually improves in the first year.

Hiccups do not indicate that there is anything wrong with the baby's feeding. Sometimes a little regurgitation may occur, but this is normal.

The pain is seldom severe during episodes of swelling or distention. Hirschsprung's disease is about four times more common in boys than in girls. It is a congenital abnormality in which a segment of large intestine develops without a nerve supply. This prevents faeces passing through so that the intestine behind becomes distended with faeces and gas.

Removal of the abnormal segment alleviates the condition. Episodes of fever (see p.832), diarrhoea (see p.830), and acute illness may occur due to infection.

Dehydration (see p.828) and fever (see p.832) may develop if the condition is untreated. Intestinal obstruction may be caused by a twisted intestine (volvulus) or a strangulated inguinal hernia (see p.814) that obstructs the passage. Other causes include

intussusception (see p.834) and congenital anomalies (see p.812) of the intestine. Rarely, the condition is caused by appendicitis (see p.842) or intestinal infection.

The intestine squeezes part of its own internal surface, causing it to fold upon itself and so to form a blockage. Rarely, a soft lump sticks out from the anus. The condition may occur in healthy babies, aged three to

twelve months, who have had recent minor infections such as a cold or diarrhoea.

The baby's neck is seldom stiff but the fontanelle, the soft spot on the scalp, may be bulging. Treatment must start as soon as possible, in order to prevent death. The

condition can lead to hydrocephalus (see p.816), deafness (see p.828), nerve paralysis, convulsions (see p.826), or mental handicap.

SYMPTOMS AND SIGNS	TREATMENT
Nappy rash Red, sore buttocks; nappies smell strongly of ammonia.	Wash area gently with soap and water; rinse and dry carefully; leave exposed to the air whenever possible; avoid paper nappies and plastic pants; apply creams or ointments for protection; use soft, clean nappy washed with soap, not detergent.
Nightmares Waking at night screaming; staring into space; usually occurring between nine and eighteen months old, when too young to explain; nightmares may occur more than once.	Seldom necessary to make special visit to a doctor; reassure baby until sleep returns.
Osteomyelitis Acute tenderness, swelling, and redness over a bone; cannot move limb and cries when touched; fever (*see* p.832), vomiting, and general illness.	Consult a doctor urgently; prompt antibiotic treatment will relieve condition quickly; delay may make surgery necessary.
Pyloric stenosis Persistent vomiting (*see* p.838) after food is given; excessive drooling; voracious appetite; from the age of three weeks, vomiting may increase in frequency and force; constipation (*see* p.826) or green faeces (*see* p.832); weight loss, despite good appetite.	A doctor may feel lump in abdomen while baby eats; barium meal may be given to baby (barium sulphate mixture which is X-rayed as it passes through the stomach and intestines) to confirm diagnosis; operation to cut stomach muscle in spasm; normal feeding usually possible days after operation.
Rash: nappy rash *See* **Nappy rash,** p.836.	
Rash: milia Small white pinhead spots on nose and cheeks.	No treatment necessary.
Rash: red skin, diffuse Vague mottled rashes; occurring in many minor illnesses, particularly colds (*see* p.826); also occurring in hot conditions.	Consult a doctor, particularly if other symptoms are present; rash is often a symptom of a more serious illness.
Rash: urticaria (hives) *See* **Urticaria,** p.850.	
Rectal prolapse Red lump protruding from anus in healthy baby; particularly in one who has been constipated; most likely to occur after straining.	Contact a doctor immediately, keep child comfortable; place warm, wet cloth over rectum until a doctor can see child.
Regurgitation Burping up of small amounts of food, usually milk, just after feeding.	None necessary; bib or piece of cloth to protect clothing; sit baby upright after feeding.
Rickets Bony lumps on skull; swelling of wrists and ankles; swollen abdomen; bow-legs (*see* p.824); slow in learning to crawl and walk.	Diagnosis made by doctor; additional vitamin D in diet, and plenty of milk.

"Ammonia rash" may be helped by rinsing nappy in a special preparation or in vinegar. "Thrush" (candidiasis, moniliasis) forms red areas and needs to be treated with special creams from a doctor. Babies with excessive dandruff (*see* p.828) or eczema (*see* p.830) are particularly likely to develop nappy rash.

There should be a natural improvement within a few weeks. Do not be surprised if the baby stands and shakes the bars of the crib. Nightmares may be due to an overactive imagination, or to a temporary feeling of insecurity.

Osteomyelitis is difficult to diagnose in a small baby because the child may appear ill without the bone tenderness being noticed. The child typically becomes extremely irritable, particularly when handled.

The condition is due to a spasm of muscle at the exit of the stomach. The content of the vomit brought up in a case of pyloric stenosis is usually curdled milk without bile. Pyloric stenosis is a congenital abnormality that is much more common in boys than in girls. It seldom starts much before the age of three weeks.

The condition is normal in newborn babies and disappears gradually after a few weeks.

A diffuse rash in a baby usually indicates a raised temperature, and this may be a sign of illness. A rash may also be a sign of an allergic reaction, although this is relatively uncommon in children of this age.
      See also **Eczema,** p.830; **Spotty face,** p.838.

A baby usually recovers from a prolapse of the rectum without treatment, but in some cases an operation is required to fix the tissue in place.

Regurgitation of food is common in many babies, and often accompanies winding after feeding. It is a normal occurrence, and bears no relation to the amount eaten, or to the health of the child.

Rickets is due to a dietary lack of vitamin D, or to lack of sunlight (which encourages vitamin D formation in the skin). It is a condition more common in coloured immigrant children.

SYMPTOMS AND SIGNS	TREATMENT
Skin problems See **Dry skin**, p.830; **Eczema**, p.830; **Rash**, p.836; **Spotty face**, p.838.	
Sleep problems See **Crying**, p.828; **Early morning waking**, p.848; **Fear of the dark**, p.848; **Nightmares**, p.836; **Sleep refusal**, p.848; **Sleep rituals**, p.848; **Sleep walking**, p.866; **Snoring**, p.848.	
"Slow" baby Baby that is unusually quiet and obedient; sleeps well but physically inactive; may not grow fast and may be obese; sometimes constipated.	Discuss with a doctor if concerned about baby's progress.
Spasticity See **Cerebral palsy**, p.824.	
Spotty face Spots on face; particularly around mouth and on cheeks.	A simple baby cream or barrier cream gives some protection.
Squint See **Eye problems: squint**, p.832.	
Sudden infant death syndrome Baby found dead in cot; no warning, or indications of illness.	It is the parents who need treatment for unexpected death of baby; seek help from a doctor; discuss with other mothers who have lost a child in this way.
Teething Increase in drooling; restlessness; rubbing of gums; thumb sucking.	Give baby teething ring to chew; rub gums gently with warm flannel; give comfort and reassurance when baby is miserable; a doctor may prescribe mild painkilling drug, such as paracetamol (children's dose).
Testis, undescended Testicle moves in and out of the scrotum, often not in correct position; in some cases, impossible to push testicle into scrotum.	Consult a doctor; retractile testicles will eventually descend into correct position; treatment required at once if condition is associated with an inguinal hernia (see p.814); otherwise, treatment delayed.
Umbilicus, infected Discharge from umbilicus; inflammation.	Consult a doctor urgently; keep clean with surgical spirit and powder; antibiotics may be required.
Vomiting Small amounts of milk vomited after food common in most babies (see **Regurgitation**, p.836); repeated vomiting of large amounts may be serious.	Discuss with a doctor; repeated vomiting in small baby must be reported within two or three hours, because of danger of dehydration (see p.828).

Normal rates of development vary considerably between children. The baby should be checked for possible cretinism (*see* p.828) or brain damage.

See also **Failure to thrive,** p.832; **Feeding problems,** p.832.

Spotty face is a common occurrence and is often due to inflammation as a result of the baby lying face down and drooling on to a pillow. *See* **Regurgitation,** p.836. The condition is common when there is already some soreness around the lips. Minute yellow or grey spots on the cheeks, without redness of skin, are normal in the first weeks of life.

Sudden infant death may be due to breathing problems (*see* p.812 *and* p.816), prolonged stopping of breathing, catastrophic infection, or accidental smothering by a pillow. It is important that the parents discuss their feelings, which may include a sense of guilt or failure, with a doctor.

If other symptoms, such as fever (*see* p.832), diarrhoea (*see* p.830) or rash (*see* p.836), occur during teething, a separate cause should be looked for. Teething powders and cutting of gums are not necessary in this normal, although uncomfortable, stage of development. Children's aspirin may be used to relieve pain.

It is sometimes difficult to decide on the best treatment for this condition. If both testicles remain undescended after about one year, surgery is usually recommended.

A slight discharge from the umbilicus is normal for about twenty-four hours after the cord falls off, but it should not last longer than this. If untreated, umbilical infection can lead to liver infection.

Vomiting is associated with many conditions, including infections, fever (*see* p.832), intestinal obstruction (*see* p.834), pyloric stenosis (*see* p.836) and hiatus hernia (*see* p.834). It may also occur with diarrhoea (*see* p.830). The combination of vomiting and diarrhoea is particularly serious because of the risk of dehydration.

Age 1½ to age 5: Normal development

This section concerns children between the ages of eighteen months and five years. This age group is considered in terms of normal development and health care, and then in terms of the more common problems and disorders that may occur.

Vision
Achievements include at:

Fifteen to eighteen months:	looks at pictures
Eighteen months:	begins to judge distance; but with difficulty
Two years:	judges distances well
Four years:	able to look at objects near to face and at a distance, and to judge their relationship
Five years:	colour vision fully developed

Speech
Achievements include at:

One year to eighteen months:	develops own language mixed with many normal words; enjoys experimenting with new sounds; some children speak well
Twenty-one months:	joins words together; asks for food or toys
Two years:	uses "I" and "You"
Two-and-a-half years:	uses plurals; forms simple sentences; gives full name; knows simple colours
Three years:	talks all the time; size of vocabulary influenced by parents; may also be a measure of intelligence

Physical movement
Achievements include at:

Fifteen to eighteen months:	begins to walk normally and may run; climbs stairs; able to get into chair; throws ball

Achievements include at:

Fifteen to eighteen months:	without falling over; begins to have dry pants during day
Twenty-one months:	kicks ball; throws overarm; can walk backwards
Two years:	climbs stairs, two feet on each step
Two-and-a-half years:	walks on tiptoe or stands on one leg for a few seconds; pedals tricycle
Three years:	climbs stairs, one foot on each step; stands on one leg
Three-and-a-half years:	skill in more delicate movements; takes off shoes, or coat
Four-and-a-half years:	runs and turns easily; gets completely dressed or undressed but cannot cope with shoelaces

Use of hands
Achievements include at:

Eighteen months:	builds small tower with three or four blocks; manages spoon; scribbles
Two years:	tower of six blocks; opens doors by use of knob; washes hands
Two-and-a-half years:	holds pencil normally; threads large beads; uses both hands equally well
Three years:	able to cope with large buttons when dressing and undressing; feeds self; copies drawn circle
Four to five years:	copies drawn square; shows evidence of left or right-handedness; can catch ball

Sphincter control
Achievements include at:

Fifteen months:	tells parents when pants are wet
Eighteen months:	only the occasional loss of control
Two years:	dry nights when placed on toilet late in evening
Two-and-a-half years:	complete control of all actions except wiping of anus

Understanding
Achievements include at:

Fifteen to eighteen months:	able to point to ear, eye, nose, and pictures of common objects; fetches things
Two years:	most children can identify parts of the body and common objects by name; names simple pictures on cards and can usually identify correct card if asked; shows interest in sexual organs
Three years:	counts to four; asks questions all the time; knows own sex; enjoys playing games with other people; can dress and undress a doll; draws simple pictures
Four years:	able to select one object from a pile of six objects; counts to ten and understands simple abstract questions (for example, "What do you want to do?"); draws pictures of people; knows nursery rhymes
Five years:	knows days of week; may know alphabet and be able to read simple words

Teeth
Development includes at:

Fifteen to eighteen months:	upper and lower eye-teeth
Two years:	second molars, giving a full set of twenty baby teeth; second molars are the last baby teeth to erupt
Five years:	permanent teeth do not usually start to appear until age six or seven, but occasionally may start earlier with appearance of molars in upper jaw or loss of front baby teeth

Disease prevention and health care

Immunization
No immunization is necessary between measles at fifteen months and the age of five, unless the child is travelling abroad. In this case, a BCG (tuberculosis) vaccination may be recommended.

Five years (school entry):	diphtheria and tetanus injection; oral polio vaccine

Health care
Weight and height measured each visit.
Suggested schedule:

Eighteen months:	thorough medical examination
Two years:	thorough medical examination; dental visit
Three years:	thorough medical examination; dental visit; vision test
Four years:	thorough medical examination; dental visit; vision and hearing tests
Five years:	thorough medical examination; dental visit; colour vision, general vision, and hearing tests

SYMPTOMS AND SIGNS	TREATMENT

Abdominal pain
Varies from dull ache to acute colicky pain; located anywhere in abdominal region; may accompany diarrhoea or vomiting, or both.

Consult a doctor if pain continues for more than four hours; never administer laxatives to a young child yourself.

Allergy
Runny nose; wheezing; irritating red patches on face and creases; itching, raised welts; breathing problems.

Assessment by a doctor; removal of cause; possible treatment with antihistamine or desensitizing injections.

Angioneurotic oedema
Large, white, itching swellings on part of face, throat, or genitals.

Immediate medical attention needed if throat is involved or breathing obstructed; mild cases treated with general antihistamine; if itching persists, injections of adrenaline may be used.

Appendicitis
Pain around the navel moving to lower right abdomen; vomiting; fever; usually constipation, but sometimes diarrhoea.

Consult a doctor if symptoms continue for more than two hours; urgent appendicectomy if appendicitis is acute.

Asthma
Wheezing, and difficulty in breathing; dry cough; anxiety due to difficulties in breathing normally; attack sometimes preceded by clear discharge from nose, or sneezing.

Drugs to relax spasm; fluids to prevent dehydration; antibiotics if fever occurs; consult a doctor.

Bed-wetting
Child over four years old shows no signs of being dry at night; or child who has been dry at night suddenly begins to wet the bed.

Discuss problem with a doctor, who can eliminate the possibility of urinary infection or epilepsy as causes of the return of bed-wetting; praise child for dry night; do not punish for wet ones.

Breath-holding
Child takes deep breath as if to give loud yell, but does not breathe out; face goes dark red, then blue; child may fall to ground.

The moment child begins to hold breath, before the teeth are clenched, hook finger in child's mouth and pull tongue forward; this causes child to take reflex breath; consult a doctor if attacks persist.

Bronchitis
Cough; wheezy breathing; fever.

Consult a doctor; deep breathing to clear bronchi of mucus; antispasmodic drugs; antibiotics may be needed; increased intake of fluids; humidifiers and inhalations helpful.

Young children are often unable to describe accurately where a pain is, or what the pain feels like. Abdominal pain may be a symptom of an infection in another part of the body, such as an acute throat infection, or the onset of flu. Acute pain and continued vomiting are serious symptoms. A doctor should investigate the possibility of appendicitis or intestinal obstruction. Recurrent stomach pain may have an emotional origin. If you suspect this to be the case, treat the child with sympathy and understanding. A pain brought on by anxiety is as distressing for a child as a stomach pain from another cause.

A doctor may be able to find the cause of the allergy from skin tests, or the parents may notice that a particular food or environment produces the allergy.

See also **Angioneurotic oedema,** p.842; **Asthma,** p.842; **Eczema,** p.830; **Hay fever,** p.844; **Urticaria,** p.850.

The cause of angioneurotic oedema may not be known. It is an internal allergic reaction, perhaps to a drug or a type of food. The swelling usually subsides within a few hours leaving no after-effects. Rarely, it occurs in families as a non-allergic malady that has a specific chemical cause.

It is often not possible to make a definite diagnosis of appendicitis in a child, but if the doctor advises an appendicectomy, accept the advice. The child usually remains in hospital until the clips or stitches from the operation are removed. He or she can return to school within two or three weeks, and will be back to normal after a month.

Children who have suffered from infantile eczema sometimes also develop asthma. An asthma attack may have a physical cause, for example, an allergy to animals, house mites, or dust. It may be caused by emotional stress. Or it may be the result of an infection, usually one of viral origin. Physiotherapy prevents chest deformities, such as pigeon-chest, from developing as a result of breathing difficulties.

At four years old, 60 per cent of boys are dry, and 90 per cent of girls. At five years old, 75 per cent of boys are dry and nearly 100 per cent of girls. An electric bell that rings when the child urinates may help, as may an incentive chart. Bed-wetting eventually stops. Only two to three per cent of boys wet the bed after the age of twelve. Bed-wetting may be a sign of emotional stress, for example, jealousy about the arrival of a new baby in the family. Indulge the child's need for attention if this is the reason.

Although the child needs an audience for breath-holding, it is a subconscious reaction to frustration, and not necessarily an attention-seeking device. It is impossible to prevent a child meeting some frustrations, but if possible it is better to distract him or her from aggravating situations. Children usually stop having breath-holding attacks by about three years old. Attacks are alarming but not dangerous.

The child may be more comfortable sleeping with the head and shoulders raised. Keep the room warm and humid. A physiotherapist can show the parents how to tip the child's head down and tap the chest to relieve the mucus-congested breathing tubes, but this is seldom necessary except in the case of a child with cystic fibrosis. Bronchitis is more common in families in which someone smokes.

SYMPTOMS AND SIGNS	TREATMENT
Croup High-pitched croaking noise when breathing; shortness of breath; fever; rasping cough; symptoms made worse by crying.	If child shows breathing difficulties, consult a doctor; meanwhile, hot, steamy room produces rapid improvement; sit child up; cuddle and comfort child; hospital admission if croup is severe.
Deafness *See* **Deafness,** p.828; **"Glue" ear,** p.844; **Otitis externa,** p.846; **Otitis media,** p.846; **Waxy ear,** p.850.	
Dirt-eating (pica) Unusual appetite for earth, wood, paper, coal, hair, even faeces.	Parents should give child opportunity of playing with safe things to chew. If child is anaemic, a doctor can treat anaemia with iron supplements.
Discharging ear *See* **Otitis externa,** p.846; **Otitis media,** p.846; **Waxy ear,** p.850.	
Fractures Circumstances of injury; sharp pain in limb, or pain becoming progressively worse; limb obviously misshapen; swelling; child unwilling to use limb.	Medical examination; X-ray photograph; treatment either by splinting, traction, or surgery, according to severity of fracture.
"Glue" ear Increasing evidence that child is partly deaf; continued deafness after attack of otitis media.	Medical examination; decongestant medicines; then insertion into eardrum of small plastic tubes (grommets) to drain out thick mucus.
Hair, pulling out Child pulls and sucks hair; occasionally causes thinning; child anxious or bored.	Entertain and distract child; if symptoms persist, consult a doctor.
Hay fever (seasonal allergic rhinitis) Summer sneezing; runny nose; red eyes; eyes oversensitive to light.	Medical examination; antihistamine tablets; desensitizing injections.
Head banging Child rocks or bangs head rhythmically; usually occurs when going to sleep.	Cuddle and comfort child; discuss problem with a doctor.

Croup usually occurs at night. The parents are often more anxious than the child about the coughing. Hot, dry air, as in a centrally-heated room, aggravates the condition. To increase the humidity of the room, keep an electric kettle on the boil. Do not allow the kettle to boil dry. Do not leave the child alone with the hot kettle because of the danger of scalding. Cool air humidifiers are also available.

The chief danger is the risk of poisoning. A parent should be particularly careful to lock away dangerous household chemicals, and never paint cot or wall with lead-based paints. Perfectly healthy children can develop the habit.

Children's bones are fairly soft. It is common for only one side of a bone to crack while the other side bends. This is called a "green-stick" fracture. The orthopaedic surgeon may need only to splint the limb.

If the fractured bone is out of position, it has to be set straight and held in a plaster of Paris cast. This can be frightening for a young child, who may need to be reassured that the limb is definitely inside the cast, and not missing.

In a compound fracture, part of the broken bone tears the surface of the skin. The risk of infection is very high. Immobilize the limb and take the child to hospital. Do not give the child any food, drink, or medicines because a general anaesthetic may be needed.

A child may seem to be backward or to have a speech problem because of undiscovered deafness. "Glue" ear is caused by a build-up of sticky glue-like mucus in the middle ear. There is often no accompanying earache. While grommets are in place, keep the ear dry. The grommets eventually ease themselves out on their own. Water must not get into the ears of a child wearing grommets; hair must be washed carefully, and swimming avoided.

Hair pulling is sometimes due to scalp irritation, such as eczema, or nits. If a bald patch appears on the child's head, consult a doctor. It may be due to a condition called alopecia areata.

Hay fever may be confused with a similar condition, allergic rhinitis. This may be caused by fur, food, or dust, and the symptoms are present all the year round. Skin tests can often identify the specific causes.

Do not scold or restrain the child. The habit is rarely harmful, but it is wise to pad the head of the cot, and to secure it to the floor to prevent the cot from moving.

Age 1½ to age 5: disorders 3

SYMPTOMS AND SIGNS	TREATMENT

Hives
See **Urticaria,** p.850.

Impetigo
Red watery spots; large brown-yellow scabs that spread around lips, nose, and cheeks.

Visit doctor promptly; antibiotic creams; isolate hair and hand-washing materials used by the sufferers from those used by the rest of the family.

Kidney tumour (Wilm's tumour)
Painless swelling of abdomen; blood in urine; possibly fever.

Consult a doctor promptly; blood tests; kidney X-rays; surgery; chemotherapy; radiotherapy.

Laryngitis
Hoarse voice, commonly occurring after cold; cough.
  See also **Croup,** p.844.

Antibiotics; steam inhalations; throat lozenges; relative silence to rest larynx; keep child in warm, humid atmosphere.

Masturbation
Child rocks backward and forward; possibly handles genitals; looks preoccupied; stares and puffs; finally relaxes.

Do not punish child; distract and entertain him or her, but never appear disapproving.

Nightmares
See **Sleep problems: nightmares,** p.848.

Osteomyelitis
Area of sharp or severe pain over bone; swelling; child refuses to use limb; fever, vomiting, and general illness; loss of appetite.

Immediate assessment by a doctor; evidence from blood cultures and X-rays only apparent after first week; antibiotics; sometimes surgery.

Otitis externa (inflammation of outer tube of ear)
Inflammation of the outer ear; moving ear causes pain; canal may look red; ear may be discharging.

Consult a doctor without delay.

Otitis media (inflammation of middle ear)
Severe earache, particularly following a cold; fever; sometimes vomiting, diarrhoea, and abdominal pain.

Consult a doctor who can see if eardrum is inflamed; antibiotics; painkilling drugs; decongestant drugs.

Paraphimosis
End of penis swollen and painful; tight foreskin rolled back constricting end of penis.

Apply cold compress for a few minutes; gently attempt to roll foreskin forward; if this fails, visit a doctor or hospital quickly.

Pigeon toes
See **Walking problems: pigeon toes,** p.850.

Pneumonia
Rapid breathing; painful cough; coughing brings up sputum with streaks of blood; usually high fever; sometimes stiff neck; slight blue colour to lips (cyanosis); use of shoulder and chest muscles to help breathing.

Immediate medical examination; chest X-ray; treatment of bacterial pneumonia with antibiotics; high fluid intake to prevent dehydration; complete bed rest; oxygen therapy. Hospital admission often necessary.

Impetigo can affect previously healthy skin, but often appears with another skin disease, for example, eczema. It is highly infectious, and can be transmitted to other members of the family. It tends to occur on moist, dirty skin, and can be spread by direct contact. If dirty fingernails are allowed to pick at the scabs, the infection may spread to other parts of the body.

This may be accompanied by other congenital anomalies. It is a form of cancer, and needs urgent medical attention. Many children with this tumour can now be completely cured.

Laryngitis occurs more commonly in children whose parents smoke. With careful attention the condition improves in one or two days. Acute laryngo-tracheo-bronchitis (croup) and acute epiglottitis may be serious complications in young children.

This may occur more frequently with autism, but generally it is a normal stage of development. Compulsive masturbation implies that a child is bored, and the problem needs discussion with a doctor. Masturbation usually continues into early childhood, then ceases for a few years before recurring in adolescence.

Osteomyelitis is an infection of bone tissue. It may be chronic or acute. Antibiotic treatment within the first twenty-four hours is usually successful, but if treatment is delayed, surgery may be necessary.

The disorder may be due to swimming, or from poking a foreign body, such as a bead, into the ear canal. Boils are sometimes associated with otitis externa in which case it may be necessary to surgically drain the boil.

A child may show all the symptoms but still not be able to tell the parents that it is the ear that is causing pain. A child with otitis media may not have a fever, or feel ill. Only a specialist can make an accurate diagnosis by looking at the eardrum.

This may happen if the foreskin has been forced back for washing before the fine fibres attaching it to the end of the penis have separated naturally. A doctor may decide to circumcise the child to prevent paraphimosis recurring.

Pneumonia often attacks a child recovering from another illness such as gastroenteritis, measles, or whooping cough. The child will be more comfortable propped up in bed during the illness.

SYMPTOMS AND SIGNS	TREATMENT
Quinsy (peritonsillar abscess) Acutely sore throat on one side; difficulty in swallowing; purple-red swelling near tonsil; high fever.	Immediate medical attention; antibiotics; painkilling drugs; incision and drainage of abscess under general anaesthetic.
Roseola infantum (exanthema subitum; sixth disease) High fever for two to three days; red, blotchy rash appears on face when temperature falls; recovery begins after three or four days.	Keep temperature down with aspirin; sponging with tepid water if necessary; give plenty of fluids.
Sleep problems: early morning waking Child wakes two or three hours before family; playfulness makes further sleep impossible.	Blinds or heavy curtains over window to reduce morning light; sufficient toys within reach to provide entertainment.
Sleep problems: fear of the dark Child unreasonably frightened at night; unable to sleep; more frightened in strange surroundings or when ill.	Nursery night light; an open bedroom door; normal sounds of family within earshot.
Sleep problems: nightmares Child wakes up at night terrified; screams; cries; sometimes able to relate content of dream.	Reassurance; cuddles; staying until child sleeps; leaving light on.
Sleep problems: sleep refusal Child refuses to go to bed; refuses to go to sleep; stays awake for two or three hours.	Stop afternoon sleep; start bedtime ritual that encourages child to relax.
Sleep problems: sleep rituals Excessive time-wasting rituals before child settles to sleep.	Make sure child is not afraid of the dark; break ritual gradually with something equally enjoyable; stop new rituals from developing.
Sleep problems: sleep walking *See* **Sleep walking**, p.866.	
Sleep problems: snoring Noisy breathing through mouth when asleep.	None necessary, unless there is an obstruction, such as adenoids, or a foreign body in the nose.
Talking, delayed Child over two and a half years old shows no signs of talking.	Assessment by a doctor; spend more time talking to child.
Temper tantrums Two to four year old expresses immense anger; throws toys; screams and yells; goes red in face; usually ends in tears.	Stay calm; leave door open, and go into another room; do not try to stop tantrum by shouting back.
Throat infections *See* **Croup** p.844; **Laryngitis**, p.846; **Quinsy**, p.848; **Tonsillitis**, p.850.	

Quinsy often occurs after a severe attack of tonsillitis. If it recurs, a surgeon may decide to remove the tonsils (tonsillectomy).

Roseola infantum seldom affects children over the age of three. It is only mildly infectious. It has an incubation period of ten to fourteen days. There are no complications associated with this disease, but the child may suffer from convulsions brought on by a high temperature. Immunization is not available.

Unfortunately for the rest of the family, this is normal between the ages of two and six. If you have to get out of bed to change the child's nappy, show by your manner that it is inconvenient.

Night fears are normal and relatively common. Reassure the child that although there is nothing to be afraid of, the fears are not unusual. If you go out for an evening, show the baby sitter the lights that the child prefers to have left on.

A nightmare may be caused by a frightening experience, a television programme, or the onset of illness. Some children feel better the moment they wake up, others need time to recover from the dream. Nightmares seldom occur before the age of four. They are normal, but if they occur as often as two or three times a week, talk to a doctor.

A child who refuses to go to sleep may be afraid of the dark, or may feel insecure. Sleep requirements vary from child to child. Do not insist on a rigid "lights out" discipline if child is afraid. Do not disturb a child who is quiet.

Most children need some kind of ritual, such as stories or lullabies, before going to sleep. Only if the rituals are too long or complicated may they become a problem. Many young children need to hold something, such as a soft toy, when going to sleep, and this is harmless.

Some children snore whenever they sleep. Others develop the habit after a cold, or as a result of enlarged adenoids. If you are worried about the snoring, talk to a doctor.

Many children use their own language, but nevertheless understand all that is being said around them. Such children will speak normally if adults speak with them.
    See also **Autism,** p.824; **Cerebral palsy,** p.824; **Cretinism,** p.828; **Deafness,** p.828.

A child in a tantrum cannot stop, so shouting back does not help. The child needs an audience. He or she is more likely to calm down if left alone. Avoid trouble as much as possible by distracting the child. Children usually grow out of temper tantrums by about age four.
    See also **Breath-holding,** p.842.

SYMPTOMS AND SIGNS	TREATMENT
Tonsillitis Inflamed tonsils; sore throat; sometimes earache; headache; fever; neck stiffness in some cases.	Medical examination; antibiotics; painkilling drugs; bed rest.
Urinary infections Frequent urination; painful urination; blood-stained urine; cloudy urine; possible loss of appetite; vomiting; fever; bed-wetting.	Medical examination; urine tests; investigation by X-ray; appropriate drugs.
Urine, red Painless, red urine.	Medical examination.
Urticaria (hives) Rash of small white hives or welts; reddened skin; severe itching; welts join to make large, raised, white areas; then disappear.	Application of antihistamine; injection of adrenaline sometimes given if symptoms persist.
Walking problems: bow-legs Conspicuous gap between knees when ankles are touching.	None necessary, but avoid bulky nappies.
Walking problems: flat feet Complete undersurface of foot in contact with ground when standing.	None; medical examination if parents are worried; remedial exercises seldom necessary.
Walking problems: knock-knees Knees turn inwards when child stands; when knees touch, feet remain apart.	None; condition usually corrects itself by the age of six or seven.
Walking problems: late walking Child makes no attempt to walk by the age of two.	Medical examination if parents are concerned.
Walking problems: limping *See* **Congenital dislocation of hip,** p.814; **Fracture,** p.844; **Osteomyelitis,** p.846; **Rheumatic fever,** p.864.	
Walking problems: pigeon toes Toes point inwards when child stands; sometimes accompanied by bow-legs.	None necessary.
Walking problems: splay foot Child walks with feet turned outwards.	None necessary.
Waxy ear Yellow, greasy discharge from ear.	Consult a doctor if at all doubtful that discharge is wax; wipe wax from outer ear, not canal.

Repeated attacks of tonsillitis scar and reduce the size of the tonsils. Large tonsils, even if they seem to meet at the back of the throat, hardly ever cause an obstruction to breathing, and are usually functioning well. The decision to remove the tonsils may be made by the surgeon. It is rarely done before the age of four.

Urinary infections are more common in girls because the urethra is shorter than in boys. Occasionally, congenital abnormalities of the kidneys and bladder make urinary infections more likely. X-ray examinations can confirm if there are any congenital abnormalities.

Red dye in sweets, or beetroot, often stain the urine red. Blood makes the urine cloudy. Large quantities of blood in the urine make it red or brown. If it is caused by a urinary infection, nephritis, or a kidney tumor, other symptoms are usually also present.

If urticaria recurs regularly, try to discover the cause. It may be a reaction to a particular food, drug, or insect bite. Urticaria is unpleasant, and can be dangerous if it involves the throat.

Bow-legs are normal in the first two years; a thick layer of nappy between the legs may increase a child's bow-legged appearance. Most children need no treatment. The only disorder that causes bow-legs is vitamin D deficiency (*see* **Rickets,** p.836).

Feet vary from family to family. The fact that a foot works well is more important than the way it looks. In many children, the arch only appears when the foot is being used, for running, walking, or standing on tiptoe. All babies have flat feet at first.

Although knock-knees may be caused by rickets, they are usually a normal part of development and most obvious between the ages of two and three. If you are anxious, discuss the problem with a doctor.

The age at which walking starts varies greatly from child to child. If development is steady and normal in other fields, the parents have no reason to worry.
See also **Congenital dislocation of hip,** p.814; **Rickets,** p.836.

This is a normal condition for children between one-and-a-half and four years old. It improves naturally. Sometimes pigeon toes make a child walk on tiptoe.

It is normal for a toddler to begin walking with toes pointing outwards. As balance improves, the child's feet become more parallel. A child who begins walking with parallel feet often ends up pigeon-toed to balance.

Wax is a natural secretion that keeps the canal of the outer ear clean. Cotton wool sticks tend to pack wax back down the canal. Pushing things into the ear to clean it is dangerous, and encourages the child to do the same. It is also dangerous to use an ear syringe to clear wax from the ears of young children as this may damage the eardrum.

Age 5 to age 11: normal development

This section of the age-by-age charts deals with a time of great physical and intellectual change, beginning with the school age child, and ending with the child who is on the threshold of adolescence.

Intellectual ability varies enormously from one child to another, and is determined by heredity and the home environment as well as by the child's education. Development occurs in spurts so that a child who seems to be doing less well than the rest of the class at one time, may suddenly catch up and, six months later, appear to be in advance of the rest, both physically and intellectually. This variation is seen most clearly in the height of children at this age. A child whose growth starts early may be, for a time, several inches taller than a child of the same age whose growth starts late.

Parents who are anxious about their child's achievements should discuss the situation with a teacher and with a doctor. Their worry may be making the child anxious, and so inhibiting his or her work. Alternatively, a child may be more than usually tired because of the energy spent in a growth spurt.

The first part of this section emphasizes growth characteristics that are considered normal for the age group and so outlines the general patterns of development of children at this age.

Physical development

Achievements include at:

Five years:	runs and turns easily; gets completely dressed and undressed but cannot cope with shoelaces; catches a ball; able to copy a square; helps parents with housework, such as washing dishes, or gardening
Six years:	draws simple pictures with considerable detail; writes own name

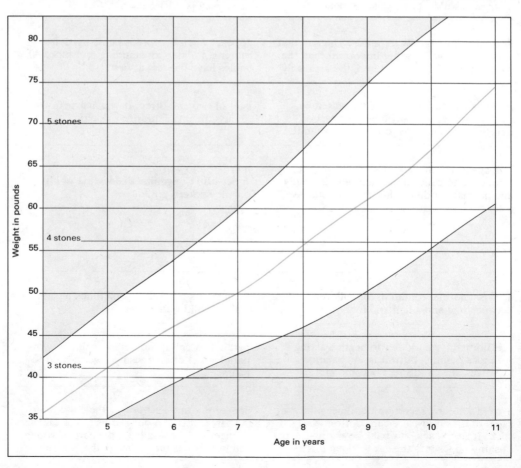

Seven years:	many children can ride a bicycle safely; good coordination in playing with a ball; difficulty with bat or tennis racket
Ten years:	begins to play tennis, or ping-pong successfully
Eleven to thirteen years:	rapid increase in strength and skill; able to compete successfully with adults; onset of puberty with associated physical changes such as menstruation; breast development may be noticed between the ages of ten and eleven, and menstruation between ten and sixteen; pubic hair development may occur between the ages of eleven and fourteen; voice changes occur between twelve and fifteen.

Understanding

Achievements include at:

Five years:	knows days of week; may know alphabet and be able to read simple words; able to answer complicated questions; enjoys singing
Six years:	reads simple messages; recognizes traffic signs; counts and may do simple addition; talks about television programmes; knows left from right hand
Seven years:	begins to learn to tell the time; writes name, age, and address; able to explain words (for

Seven years:	example "A ball is a round toy")
Eight years:	reads simple books; writes simple arithmetic; can explain simple concepts (for example "An apple is a kind of fruit")
Nine years:	reading more complicated sentences; reading alone; writing improving; begins to understand rules of spelling; enjoys pretending to buy and sell; runs errands effectively; shops for mother
Ten years:	understands the idea of historical time; also has a concept of future and has ideas about a career
Ten to thirteen years:	immense differences in achievements due to differences in intelligence, ability to concentrate, parental influences, and schooling

Disease prevention and health care

Immunization

Health steps to be taken at:

Five years (school entry):	diphtheria and tetanus injections; oral polio vaccine; other injections such as cholera or typhoid should be given in advance of going to area of risk
Ten years:	tetanus injection; oral polio vaccine
Eleven years:	German measles vaccine for girls.

Health care

Annual visit to dentist and doctor; annual vision and hearing tests.

SYMPTOMS AND SIGNS	TREATMENT
Anxiety Crying; nail biting; tics; stuttering; frequent nightmares; recurrent unexplained pains; school phobia.	Discover reason for anxiety; discuss problem with a doctor.
Baldness (alopecia) Patchy loss of hair from scalp; or sudden, total loss of hair from scalp; exposed skin clear and smooth; stumps of hair round edge of patch.	Consult a doctor; investigate any possible emotional cause of baldness; otherwise, only treatment is wearing a toupee.
Boil Small, red, painful lump; sometimes fever; boil develops a head within three days; boil bursts, releasing pus; pain subsides.	Local steam heat to bring boil to a head; clean surrounding skin with surgical spirit. If red streaks appear radiating from boil, if a lymph gland becomes tender, or if boils recur, consult a doctor, as antibiotics may be required.
Cerebral palsy (spasticity) *See* **Cerebral palsy**, p.824.	
Chilblains Numb, white area on fingers, toes, ears, or nose; red, burning, swollen, intensely itching area as skin warms up; blistering and ulceration in severe cases; occurring in cold, damp weather.	Loose-fitting, warm hand and footwear; in severe cases, tablets to increase blood flow to skin; cream to reduce itching; dry dressing to prevent chilblain from being rubbed; improve nutrition to treat chilblains, and also to prevent condition recurring.
Chorea, Sydenham's (St Vitus's dance) Involuntary twisting movements of arms and legs; associated with rheumatic fever; grimacing; develops from fidgeting to contorting movements lasting several months; movements cease in sleep.	Hospitalization and assessment; sedative drugs if severe; penicillin to prevent further attacks of rheumatic fever.
Clumsy child Child moves awkwardly; bad at games; bumps into things; drops things; falls over frequently; slow to learn hand skills.	Refrain from constant nagging; allow child to practise hand skills; consult a doctor if concerned.
Colour blindness Inability to tell difference between red and green; or occasionally yellow and blue.	None.

Children, like adults, become anxious. Some children openly express anxiety, and can tell parents their problems. Other children express their anxiety through rebellion, or anger. A child may be anxious because of stress between the parents, or strange behaviour in the family. Another common cause of childhood anxiety is the fear of failure, a reaction against parents who constantly push the child. If a child suffers from a stammer or tic, constant nagging increases the anxiety, and the annoying habit. Once the cause of the child's anxiety is known, the problem should not be too difficult to solve.

If this condition is left untreated, the hair grows back of its own accord, but the child's and the parents' anxiety is increased. Baldness in children is sometimes brought on by a serious emotional shock.
   See also **Lice,** p.862; **Nits,** p.864; **Ringworm,** p.864.

Single boils may occur at any time, but recurring boils appear most commonly on the buttocks and at the back of the neck, especially in boys between eight and ten years old, and in the armpits at puberty. Recurring boils are not caused by poor hygiene, but frequent showers help to clear the skin. A doctor may also recommend antiseptic soaps and creams, and antibiotic lotions. Recurring boils are sometimes associated with the development of diabetes, and a test of the child's urine is advisable to exclude this possibility. In general, boils heal themselves, and immunity to staphylococcus bacteria, the most common cause, develops naturally.

Chilblains occur when the surface blood vessels constrict in cold weather. Tight shoes encourage chilblains. Children with a tendency to develop chilblains must keep warmly wrapped up at the first sign of cold weather. Once a chilblain has formed, it takes time to heal, but usually resolves itself within two weeks.

There is no cure, but this rare condition eventually improves of its own accord. Formal schooling is missed for the duration of the disease, so speak to the doctor about the possibility of arranging education for the child while he or she is being treated.
   See also **Rheumatic fever,** p.864.

Many children are clumsy for no apparent reason, but sometimes clumsiness is caused by "minimal brain damage" at birth, which is thought to be like a mild cerebral palsy. Slow improvement does occur, but the child needs patient and understanding teaching from the parents. Most children eventually become normally co-ordinated.

This is an inherited genetic disorder occurring more often in boys than girls. It often goes undiscovered until the child has an eye test, either by an eye specialist, or during a medical examination. Colour-blind people are unable to take up certain professions, for example, piloting aircraft.

SYMPTOMS AND SIGNS	TREATMENT
Dental problems: decay Pain in tooth or ear; broken tooth; sometimes bad breath.	Immediate dental attention.
Dental problems: loose teeth Milk tooth loose in socket.	None.
Dental problems: overcrowding Permanent teeth emerge cramped and crooked.	Orthodontal care.
Depression Unusually tearful and touchy child; obvious unhappiness; signs of remorse; sometimes anger and rebelliousness; sleep disturbances.	Discover cause of depression; discuss problems with a doctor, if depression persists.
Diabetes Persistent thirst; frequent urination; weight loss; sometimes drowsiness and loss of consciousness.	Admission to hospital for urgent care; intravenous fluids; injections of insulin.
Dyslexia Child has difficulty reading and writing; no comprehension of the written form of even familiar spoken words.	Assessment for any problems with eyes essential first; if no visual defects, consult a doctor, especially for advice on correct teaching method.
Epilepsy: grand mal Unconsciousness; rigid body; jerking movements of arms and legs; clenching of teeth; grunting noises; in many cases incontinence; may be confused and frightened one or two minutes after attack; then gradual recovery, often sleep. Seizures sometimes preceded by characteristic warning sensations known as "aura".	Stay with child and move dangerous objects away; if vomiting starts, turn head to side to avoid choking; do not restrain limbs; do not push anything into mouth; when convulsion is over, get medical assistance. Modern drug therapy allows an epileptic to lead a normal life but, nevertheless, working with dangerous machinery should be avoided.

Prevention is better than cure. Milk teeth need as much care as permanent teeth. Discourage sweet and sugar consumption. Prevent children from eating sweets between meals, but allow sweets at the end of a meal when the mouth is still moist with saliva. Encourage tooth brushing at least twice a day, three times a day if possible. The novelty of an electric toothbrush is often enough to encourage a lazy child. Adults must not assume that the loss of a milk tooth does not matter because it is not meant to be permanent. A child should be taken to the dentist regularly even when there is no obvious sign of tooth decay. The visits accustom the child to the idea of going to the dentist, and the dentist can detect a problem before it becomes severe.

The first teeth of children are known as milk teeth. These are replaced naturally as the second, or permanent, teeth develop. Milk teeth loosen naturally and fall out from the age of six years onward. Sometimes months elapse before the permanent teeth come through. If a toddler falls and knocks out a milk tooth that was not loose before, wash it carefully and hold it firmly in the socket for a few minutes. If this is done quickly, the tooth will "take". It is important to do this because if a milk tooth is lost before time, the surrounding teeth grow incorrectly. The permanent teeth may then emerge out of position.

An orthodontist is a specialist trained to deal with crooked and overcrowded teeth. Occasionally some teeth are removed to make room for the others, but usually braces are fitted and tightened from time to time, to correct the position of the teeth. Braces may be uncomfortable at first.

Depression in children is more common than is often realised. It may follow the death of a much-loved pet or of a close relative; a change of home and loss of friends; or it may occur as a reaction against a tense family atmosphere. Depression in childhood is not an indication that it will recur in adult life.

Diabetes in early childhood is relatively rare, but when it occurs it develops suddenly. Careful control with insulin injections is necessary for the rest of the person's life; nevertheless the outlook is good. Diabetes should not affect the choice of profession in the future. It is important that the child learns to test the urine and administer the injections independently. Parents must try to make the child feel as normal as possible. Infections in a diabetic are often more serious and must be treated as quickly as possible.

The inability to read and write prevents the child from benefiting from normal education. The child may become anxious and frustrated, feeling excluded and a failure. Sympathetic and understanding teaching is required. Special classes are often helpful. Forcing a left-handed child to write with the right hand can cause apparent dyslexia. Dyslexia does not indicate a lack of intelligence.

A doctor assesses the cause of the seizure by observing the electrical activity of the brain with an EEG. Epilepsy may occur as a result of brain damage at birth, or it may occur spontaneously. It is often associated with cerebral palsy. Epileptic children should be encouraged to lead a normal, active life, while taking certain precautions, such as avoiding heights.

SYMPTOMS AND SIGNS	TREATMENT

Epilepsy: petit mal
Momentary loss of awareness; blank look; staring eyes; then return to normal.

Treatment with appropriate drugs prevents attacks; sometimes spontaneous improvement occurs.

Fainting (syncope)
Dry mouth; hot then cold feeling; noises sound distant; vision becomes grey; possible nausea; loss of consciousness; sometimes vomiting during recovery; weakness and lethargy for half an hour after attack.

At onset of symptoms, lie down; or sit down with head between knees; retain position for at least five minutes.

Growing pains
Vague aches and pains in limbs; no obvious cause; sometimes occurring at onset of flu or a cold.

None; aspirin, reassurance, and understanding in severe cases.

Hair ball (trichobezoar)
Habit of eating hair; noticeable hair loss; vomiting; abdominal pain; child often emotionally disturbed.

Consult a doctor; diagnosis by barium meal; surgical removal of hair ball.

Hay fever
See **Hay fever,** p.844.

Headaches, recurrent
Pain, anywhere in head; variable intensity and duration; possibly nausea.

Medical examination; painkilling drugs.

Infectious diseases: chickenpox (varicella)
Two to three days of fever; red spots on trunk; after a few hours, spots turn to clear blisters; new spots appear in first three days on face, inside mouth, and in ears; numerous spots cause severe irritation.

Dab calamine lotion on spots; cut nails to prevent scratching; cool light clothing; antihistamines reduce itching.

Infectious diseases: erythema infectiosum (fifth disease)
Sudden onset of rash; bright red cheeks; faint irregular rash on limbs; rash more obvious when warm or in bath.

Keep patient cool; sponging with tepid water if temperature rises; nourishing fluids when appetite is poor.

Infectious diseases: German measles (rubella)
Mild fever; sore throat for one or two days; fine, pink rash behind ears, spreading over face, then body; rash lasts two or three days; tender, swollen glands at back of head for about ten days; joint pains may last longer.

Keep temperature down; nourishing fluids when appetite is poor.

In some cases a child suffering a petit mal attack may appear to be day-dreaming. But the difference between day-dreaming and a petit mal attack is that nothing can attract the child's attention for the few seconds that the attack lasts. Petit mal can occur very frequently, several times an hour in some cases, and this may interfere with a child's education. Even in mild cases, medical treatment is advisable, because momentary unconsciousness may be dangerous. Most children recover after several years.
See also **Convulsions,** p.826.

Fainting commonly occurs when a child is tired or hungry, or after standing for a long time. It may also be brought on by the shock of seeing something unpleasant, or by pain. Boys sometimes faint when standing up at night to urinate. If this occurs more than once, advise the boy to sit on the toilet when using it at night.

"Growing" pains may occur because of fatigue, or as a result of a minor knock when the child is playing. The pains usually occur in the muscles, not the joints, and are not caused by rheumatic fever. If the child is eager to run out to play, the parents can assume that the pain is not too serious. However, whatever the reason for the pain, it is real to the child, and should not be dismissed as unimportant if it causes worry.

The habit of hair-chewing must be stopped. The cause of the habit must be investigated, and the child usually needs psychiatric help. Sometimes a hair ball is discovered long after the habit of chewing hair has stopped.
See also **Baldness,** p.854.

Headaches, without other symptoms, often affect older children. They are usually caused by tension and stress. The parents and doctor must try to find the cause of the anxiety. The child needs reassurance and understanding. Recurrent headaches are seldom due to eye strain.
See also **Migraine,** p.874.

Chickenpox is one of the most infectious childhood diseases. It has an incubation period of up to twenty-one days, but usually develops in fifteen days. The child is infectious from one day before the outbreak of spots, to six days afterwards. A child who has come in contact with chickenpox should be kept in quarantine for twenty-one days. Complications are rare in chickenpox. Immunization is not available. In some cases chickenpox causes shingles (Herpes zoster) in adults who are only partly immune.

The incubation period of fifth disease is six to fourteen days. The child is infectious from the onset of the illness until about five to seven days after the fever subsides. A child who has come in contact with fifth disease may be kept in quarantine for fourteen days. There are no complications, and immunization is not available.

German measles is a mild childhood disease, but a specific diagnosis is essential in case the child has come into contact with a woman who is in the early stages of pregnancy. If this is the case, the pregnant woman must consult her doctor. German measles has an incubation period of up to twenty-one days after last contact, but usually develops within fourteen days. The child is infectious for seven days before the rash appears until five days after the rash appears. If quarantine is advised it should be maintained for twenty-one days, but most schools do not exclude children exposed to this infection. Immunization is offered to girls at the age of 11 through the school medical service.

SYMPTOMS AND SIGNS	TREATMENT

Infectious diseases: influenza (flu)

Sudden onset of shivering; high fever; sweating; aching muscles; headache; sore throat; cough; symptoms last four to six days; fatigue lasts one to two weeks.

Keep temperature down with aspirin and sponging with tepid water; nourishing fluids when appetite is poor; throat sweets to soothe throat.

Infectious diseases: measles (rubeola; morbilli)

Fever; dry cough; sore throat; runny nose; red eyes; tiny white spots (Koplik's spots) inside mouth; then red spots developing into a pinkish red rash behind ears; rash spreads over face, on to limbs and trunk; lasts three to five days.

Keep temperature down with aspirin; sponging with tepid water if necessary; nourishing fluids until appetite returns; antihistamines to reduce nasal congestion; wash eyes if crusted; nurse in a quiet, darkened room; doctor may give injection of gamma globulin if complications are likely.

Infectious diseases: meningitis

Sometimes cold-like symptoms for two days; then severe headache; vomiting; convulsions; in some cases, red rash on skin and inside mouth; stiff neck; dislike of light.

Urgent medical attention; isolation in hospital; study of cerebrospinal fluid to confirm diagnosis; rapid treatment necessary to prevent development of the disease; antibiotics; nourishing diet with plenty of fluids.

Infectious diseases: mumps

Fever; headache; salivary glands in front of ears and under jaw swell and become painful after two to three days; swelling remains for up to ten days; eating and swallowing may be painful.

Keep temperature down; sponging with tepid water if necessary; give plenty of fluids; nourishing diet with soft food; frequent mouthwashes and drinks; painkilling drugs; ice packs held against glands may give some relief.

Infectious diseases: poliomyelitis

At first an influenza-like illness; fever; aching muscles; then temporary improvement followed by relapse; high fever; headache, dislike of bright light. In about one case in ten this relapse leads to muscle weakness and paralysis and, in rare cases, death.

Urgent medical care; complete bed rest; hospitalization; painkilling drugs; mechanical respiration needed if respiratory muscles paralyzed; paralysis treated by physiotherapy; muscle tendon transplant if paralysis is permanent.

Infectious diseases: scarlet fever

High fever; sore throat; headache; vomiting; stomach ache; fine, red rash beginning around neck and on chest, spreading over body; area around mouth remains pale; skin peels on and after seventh day; tongue is white initially, then bright red spots appear; exhaustion.

Keep temperature down; sponging with tepid water if necessary; nourishing fluids by mouth when appetite is poor; antibiotic drugs to be taken for at least ten days.

Children tend to suffer less than adults during an attack of flu. Complications may develop in the form of bronchitis, otitis, pneumonia, or sinusitis. The child is infectious for twelve hours before the fever starts, until the end of the fever. Vaccination against the specific influenza virus protects most people in a severe epidemic, but is not usually recommended for children.

Measles is highly infectious. It has an incubation period of up to fourteen days, although it usually develops in ten days. The child is infectious from the onset of fever until five days after the rash first appears. A child who has come into contact with measles should be kept in quarantine for fourteen days. Complications, should they occur, may be serious. They include chest infections, sinusitis, middle ear infections, and encephalitis, an inflammation of the brain. The latter needs urgent hospital treatment. Measles vaccination is given at the age of fifteen months, and provides nearly complete protection against the disease. Even the rare cases that are not fully protected suffer only a mild form of the disease. Older children who have not been immunized should be given measles vaccine within two days of contact with case if their health is poor.

Meningitis is spread by meningococcal bacteria. There is a slight chance that other members of the family will catch it. This is prevented if all contacts take appropriate antibiotics or sulphonamides. The child stops being infectious two days after antibiotic treatment begins. A child who has come into contact with meningitis should be kept in quarantine for two weeks (two days if the child takes antibiotics). Complications are not common, but include arthritis, nerve paralysis, deafness, abscess inside the skull that presses on the brain, and collapse culminating in death.

Mumps is usually mild in childhood, and not as infectious as other childhood diseases. It has an incubation period of twelve to twenty-eight days, but usually develops within eighteen days. The child is infectious for two days before the onset of symptoms until ten days later, or until three days after the swelling has subsided, whichever is longer. A child who has come into contact with mumps should be kept in quarantine for twenty-eight days. Complications include deafness, encephalitis, meningitis, and inflammation of the pancreas or thyroid gland. Inflammation of one or both testes is fairly common after puberty. Similar inflammation of ovaries is rare. Vaccination may be carried out during childhood.

Poliomyelitis is a highly infectious disease. Although many children can be affected by it and suffer from flu-like symptoms only, the serious cases result in paralysis, and even death. It has an incubation period of up to twenty-one days, but usually develops within fourteen days. The child is infectious for about three weeks after the onset of illness. A child who has come in contact with polio must be kept in quarantine for twenty-one days. Three doses of oral vaccine in infancy and booster at 5 and 10 years give complete immunity with no side-effects.

Scarlet fever is a streptococcal infection that affects the throat, and also causes a rash. Contacts sometimes get the same throat infection without the rash. Children seldom complain of a sore throat during the illness. It has an incubation period of one to three days. Throat swabs are taken after the illness to ensure the infection has cleared. A child who has come in contact with the disease should be kept in quarantine for three days. Complications include rheumatic fever, acute nephritis, hair loss, and ear infection, but all complications are reduced by early antibiotic treatment. There is no immunization available, but antibiotics are given to the contacts to prevent further spread.

SYMPTOMS AND SIGNS	TREATMENT

Infectious diseases: whooping cough (pertussis)

Mild fever; runny nose; slight cough that becomes severe; bout of coughing ending in a "whoop" as air is inhaled; distress; vomiting; increased weakness; difficulty sleeping; gradual improvement after six weeks.

Antibiotics at early stage; cough suppressants seldom helpful; nourishing fluids, and light food; hold a distressed child firmly and securely during bout of coughing.

Learning problems

See **Cerebral palsy,** p.824; **Clumsy child,** p.854; **Deafness,** p.828; **Depression,** p.854; **Down's syndrome,** p.816; **Dyslexia,** p.854; **Epilepsy: petit mal,** p.858; **Overactive child,** p.864.

Leukaemia

Pallor; fatigue; malaise; fever; bruising of skin; sometimes acute sore throat and illness at onset; often pain in limbs.

Special drug therapy.

Lice (pediculosis)

Itching scalp; itching skin around hair; possible secondary infection; tiny white dots sticking to hairs.

Consult a doctor; shampoo hair with anti-louse preparation; treat all the family; wash clothes and bedding.

Lisping

Inability to pronounce "s" sound correctly.

Assessment by a doctor if severe, or if lisping continues longer than normal.

Lying and cheating

Various mannerisms that imply child is not being truthful; may include blushing, shuffling, staring parent in eye, aggression; signs vary from child to child.

Discover cause; compulsive liar may need professional help.

Meningitis

See **Infectious diseases: meningitis,** p.860.

Mental handicap

See **Cerebral palsy,** p.824; **Clumsy child,** p.854; **Cretinism,** p.828; **Down's syndrome,** p.814; **Hydrocephalus,** p.816.

Nail-biting

Child chews and nibbles nails; nails excessively short; cuticles sometimes ragged and bleeding.

Find underlying reason for nail-biting; discussion with child; habit is not harmful but is unsightly; gloves worn at night may help; bitter-tasting nail polish useful only if child wishes to cooperate.

Whooping cough is one of the most serious of the childhood infectious diseases. It may have an incubation period of up to twenty-one days, but usually develops within ten. The child is infectious from the onset of symptoms, for about three weeks. Complications include middle ear infections, bronchial pneumonia, and sinusitis. Encephalitis may also occur. Children should be immunised against whooping cough at an early age.

Leukaemia used to be fatal within a few months, but with modern treatment the life expectancy is much greater and may be curative. The doctor makes the diagnosis from blood cells taken from the bone marrow. Leukaemia is the commonest form of cancer in children, but it must be remembered that it is still a rare disease. Children with Down's syndrome (*see* p.814) have a greater chance of developing leukaemia.

If the parents discover a child has lice, they must tell the school teacher who can make sure the lice do not spread. They are extremely contagious and can spread to the cleanest heads. They are becoming an increasing problem because insecticide-resistant strains are developing.
See also **Nits,** p.864.

Lisping is a normal part of speech development. It tends to recur when the child loses the milk teeth at the front of the mouth. However, continued lisping and mispronunciation may occasionally be due to partial deafness. If a doctor recommends speech therapy to correct the lisp, it is wise to begin the therapy before the child attends school regularly.

In young children truth and fantasy intermingle. It is normal for a child under seven to tell stories that are transparently untrue. If an older child grossly exaggerates a story, the parents must make it clear that they know the real truth, but should avoid a direct confrontation. Compulsive lying is usually a cry for help. The child has a need to be found out. The parents should seek expert advice. Parents must show children by example that honesty is an important rule in life.

Nail-biting is an extremely common habit in children over the age of five. They find the habit soothing. Painting the nails with bitter-tasting substances only helps a child who has already decided to stop. Drawing attention to the habit usually makes the child defiant. The parents should try to appeal to the child's sense of vanity, and point out that it makes the hands look ugly. Nail varnish often helps girls to stop. Compulsive nail-biting that causes bleeding may require professional assessment.

SYMPTOMS AND SIGNS	TREATMENT
Nephritis, acute About two weeks after throat infection; blood in urine; urine appears dark and cloudy; backache; generally unwell; swelling around eyes and ankles; headaches.	Hospitalization; medical examination; penicillin; restricted fluid intake; diet low in salt and protein, high in carbohydrates.
Nits Tiny white dots along shaft of hair.	Wash hair with anti-louse shampoo following the instructions exactly; treat all the family.
Nosebleed Sudden bleeding from one nostril; usually due to injury; onset of influenza; something pushed up nose.	Sit down; bend head forward to prevent blood running into throat; mouth breathing and pressure over bleeding nostril for at least ten minutes. If bleeding does not stop after twenty minutes, seek medical advice.
Overactive child (hyperkinesis) Restlessness; inability to sit still in class; short concentration time; poor academic and personal performance at school; slow reading and writing; small sleep requirement.	Consult a doctor and the school staff; specialized schooling; sometimes special drugs to aid concentration.
Pneumonia See **Pneumonia,** p.846.	
Psoriasis Small red spots on skin; developing into dry, scaling discs; commonly on knees, behind elbows, or elsewhere on skin.	Consult a doctor; drugs and creams to control condition.
Rheumatic fever About two weeks after throat infection; fever; sweating; joints inflamed and feel hot; swollen and painful joints; pain may move from one joint to another; skin rash; nodules under skin on back of head, elbows, and knees.	Medical examination; hospitalization and complete bed rest; penicillin and aspirin-like drugs in large doses; careful regular assessment and drug control with penicillin for many years to prevent another attack.
Ringworm (tinea capitis) Ring of blisters, growing outwards; bald patches, if scalp affected; skin on patch dry, grey, and scaly; stumps of hair visible on patch.	Antifungal cream prescribed by a doctor; wash brushes, combs, and towels separately; other members of family must not use anything that has come in contact with infected parts of the patient's body.
St Vitus's dance See **Chorea, Sydenham's,** p.854.	
Scabies Red rash; severe itching; small grey burrows under skin may be visible; usually occurs on webs of fingers and toes, in pubic area, and sometimes on buttocks.	Consult a doctor promptly; hot bath; rub body firmly with rough flannel to expose burrows; paint body with prescribed lotion; leave to dry; repaint; repeat for three days; launder all bedding, towels, and clothes at high temperature.

Acute nephritis is caused by a reaction between the kidney tissue and other agents. Streptococcus bacteria were formerly thought to be the main cause. Although there is a possibility that chronic nephritis will develop, most children recover without complications.

See also **Infectious diseases: scarlet fever,** p.860.

Nits are the eggs of the head louse. They are anchored so firmly to shaft of hair that nothing can pull them off. In addition to using special shampoo, the hair can be combed with a nit comb.

See also **Lice,** p.862.

A bloodstained discharge from the nose that smells means that the child has put a bead or some other small object up the nostril. This needs medical attention. Some children have a tendency to have frequent and alarming nosebleeds. This is usually caused by dilated blood vessels inside the nose. A doctor will be able to verify this and give appropriate treatment. Nosebleeds are a symptom of certain blood disorders, but are rarely a symptom of leukaemia. Some children suffer from nosebleeds at the onset of puberty. These are more common in boys than in girls.

This condition is more common in boys than girls. The symptoms are usually noticed in the first few months of life, but seldom cause a problem until the child begins school. On investigation, a doctor may discover minimal brain damage at birth is the cause.

See also **Clumsy child,** p.854.

Psoriasis is a familial skin disease. It is not curable, but can be controlled. Patience and understanding from the rest of the family is needed to help the child to come to terms with the condition. It is seldom itchy, and may suddenly improve, particularly in sunlight.

Heart inflammation commonly occurs with rheumatic fever, and heals to form scar tissue. Complete bed rest reduces the severity of the valve damage, but should heart symptoms occur later in life, cardiac surgery may be required. Rheumatic fever is caused by the body's reaction to the bacteria, streptococci, that cause throat infections.

See also **Chorea, Sydenham's,** p.854; **Nephritis,** p.864; **Scarlet fever,** p.860.

Ringworm is a fungal infection that occurs in various forms, each type affecting a different part of the body. It is highly contagious. Prompt treatment usually clears the child's scalp of the infection within three weeks, but the hair may take a little time to cover the patch. The child must be kept away from school and the family must be careful to prevent the infection spreading.

Scabies is caused by a mite that is just visible to the naked eye. It is highly contagious, although it can live for only twenty-four hours away from the body. All members of the family must be checked for suspected scabies. The itching is worse at night when the mites are active. Additional skin infection, such as impetigo, may be caused by the scratching. The body's allergic reaction to the mite takes about a month to develop. Should the child be infected for a second time, the symptoms start at once.

SYMPTOMS AND SIGNS	TREATMENT

School phobia

Tears; tantrums; headaches; stomach pain; nausea; sometimes vomiting as the time for school approaches; truancy.

Discuss with teacher to exclude possibility of bullying or teasing at school; give child help and reassurance; consult a doctor if concerned.

Sinusitis

Pain below eyes; pain on one side of face or in forehead; general headache; sometimes fever; excess catarrh and post-nasal drip; rare in children under seven years old.

Medical examination; nose drops; decongestant drugs; antihistamine drugs; often antibiotics.

Sleep-walking

Child wandering about at night; unaware of surroundings; seldom knocks into things; may be able to answer questions; has no recollection of incident the next day.

Lead child back to bed; do not wake; but if child is in middle of nightmare, it may be sensible to wake; keep window shut if child is going through a sleep-walking phase.

Sore throat

Pain on swallowing; pain in throat; often fever.

Aspirin; throat lozenges; for severe sore throat, medical examination; throat swabs; prescribed antibiotics.

Stealing

Child steals from family; or steals from pockets and lockers at school; attempts to hide stolen article.

Speak firmly to child; explain that stolen articles must be returned; do not humiliate child.

Stuttering and stammering

Hesitation over words; sometimes contortion of face, mouth, and tongue in effort to get word out.

In minor cases, ignore stutter; persistent stutter needs speech therapy.

Testis, torsion of

Sudden, severe pain and swelling of scrotum; severe abdominal pain; often intermittent pain; sometimes vomiting and fever.

Seek urgent medical assistance; surgery required to prevent permanent damage to testis; testis is untwisted and repositioned during the operation.

Although school phobia may stem from a fear of teasing or bullying, it is often a reaction against parents who constantly push their children to achieve better results. Sometimes school phobia has nothing to do with school at all, and is caused by emotional problems in the family. A child who refuses to eat breakfast, or vomits after breakfast, should not be forced to eat. A fruit drink, toast, or nothing at all, is better than a battle before school. The child makes up for a lost breakfast at lunchtime. A child who has been happy at school before, and suddenly develops a violent phobia may need specialist help.

See also **Depression,** p.864; **Truancy,** p.868.

Sinusitis occurs after a cold, and may be accompanied by fever. The area of the face above the sinus may be tender to touch. Immediate treatment allows the sinus to drain. Repeated untreated infections may damage the natural drainage mechanism and lead to chronic infection.

Sleep-walking is most common between the ages of seven and fifteen. It may be due to anxiety about exams, or some other worry. Once the cause has resolved itself, the sleep-walking usually stops. Although children's natural safeguards still seem to function, it is safer to keep a potential walker's window shut. Consult a doctor if sleep-walking occurs regularly, so that EEG test can exclude the possibility of a more serious problem, such as temporal lobe epilepsy.

A small child often has difficulty in describing exactly where a pain is. Even when the throat is inflamed, or possibly ulcerated, the child may still be complaining of other symptoms, for instance stomach pain, or headache. Sore throats occur with tonsillitis, colds, and influenza, as well as the more serious diseases such as infectious mononucleosis, diphtheria, and scarlet fever. Severe sore throats must be investigated by a doctor because they may be caused by streptococcal bacteria. This can lead to acute nephritis (*see* p.864), rheumatic fever (*see* p.864) or scarlet fever (*see* p.860).

A child under the age of three who steals does not fully understand about possessions, but a child of school age should have grasped this idea. Stealing is usually considered to be a cry for help. If the child takes money, it may be used to buy sweets for the class. Such a child is probably trying to buy affection. The parents should maintain a sympathetic attitude, but must not condone stealing. More pocket-money may be enough to make the child feel more like the others at school. If stealing continues, the parents should seek professional advice. Stealing is sometimes accompanied by compulsive lying.

See also **Lying and cheating,** p.862.

Stuttering is more common in boys than girls. It tends to run in families, but is not genetic. The reason for this is probably that a family with a stutterer over-reacts to the normal stage of hesitant speech that children go through. A child has a lot to say and naturally trips over words. If the family appear worried, or try to correct the hesitant speech, the child is likely to develop a persistent stutter. Speech therapy aims to restore the child's confidence in the ability to produce fluent speech. More than half the children are cured, and the rest improve considerably.

Torsion occurs when the testis twists the spermatic cord, thus obstructing the blood supply. The testis swells. The condition is painful. If the condition is left untreated, the testis will be destroyed in a matter of hours. If one testis is involved the other may be in danger, and so the surgeon often secures the position of the other during the same operation. Torsion of the testis is thought to be caused by a congenital defect.

SYMPTOMS AND SIGNS	TREATMENT
Thumb-sucking Child sucks thumb when tired, when worried, or for comfort.	Appeal to child's sense of vanity; do not use physical restraints.
Tic Rapid, repeated movement of face or body; twitch worse when child concentrates; part of body affected works normally when required; blinking and grimacing commonest forms; twitch disappears during sleep.	None; discover reason for possible anxiety; do not try to stop child twitching; do not mention twitch.
Tonsil and adenoid problems Inflamed tonsils; sore throat; blocked nose; snoring; earache; sometimes deafness.	Acute infections treated with antibiotics; consult a doctor, who may recommend surgical removal.
Truancy Child who sets off for school but does not arrive; sometimes forges parent's note; does not tell parents about absence from school.	Discuss problem with a doctor and teacher; discover whether other children are encouraging child to join them, then talk to parents; treat child with love and understanding; try to find out underlying worry.
Warts Small nodules, usually on hands and fingers. Warts on sole of foot (verrucas) may be painful.	Medical examination; removal by means of liquid nitrogen, dry ice, acid, foot soak or electric cautery (burning); most disappear without treatment.
Worms In many cases symptoms are not apparent; in others, worms may be visible in faeces; sometimes intermittent diarrhoea; flatulence; abdominal distension; anal itching, particularly at night.	Medical examination; treatment with appropriate antiworm medicine.

Thumb-sucking is a harmless habit until it begins to affect the position of the permanent teeth. Explain to the child that the habit is pushing the teeth forward, and that to correct the position, the child may have to wear a brace in the future. Wearing a glove at night, or painting the thumb with a bitter substance, may help to remind a child who has decided to stop the habit anyway. Soreness of the thumb may become painful, because of moisture or because of friction from sucking. In such cases the child usually changes to suck the other thumb.

A tic may result from a habit that used to have a useful purpose, for example, flicking hair out of the eyes. The habit continues even when the hair is cut. If the parents constantly nag the child to stop, another tic of a different nature is likely to develop. They are most common between the ages of eight and twelve, and tend to improve as the child gets older.

Tonsils and adenoids build the body's immunity and are important parts of the body's resistance to respiratory disease. If scarring occurs as a result of repeated infections their usefulness is reduced and it may be necessary to remove them. Children of school age encounter many infections, and at this age the tonsils and adenoids are proportionally at their largest.

The truant child usually has a history of bad behaviour at school, and a poor school record. Helping the child with homework, and involving yourself in the work, may be enough to take the anxiety out of school. Accompany the child to the school in the morning.
See also **School phobia,** p.866.

Warts are thought to be caused by a viral infection. They are not usually uncomfortable unless they appear on the foot, where the pressure of walking on them hurts the foot. Verrucas are mildly infectious, so a child with verrucas should not be permitted to go barefoot, for instance, in a swimming pool. The foot should be covered with a protective slipper, to prevent other children catching the infection. Sometimes "seedling" warts appear around the site of a wart that has been removed. In many cases warts disappear naturally after a few months.

Worms that infest the human intestine include hookworms, roundworms, tapeworms, or threadworms.

Age 11 to age 18: normal development

Normal development of children between the ages of eleven and eighteen is extremely varied. This section of the age-by-age charts gives general indications of the normal changes that parents and their children can expect. A list of the most common problems and disorders encountered at this age follows this outline.

Adolescent development is closely related to situations at home, in school, and in the community. These circumstances affect mental and emotional development particularly. In addition to this, physical growth and sexual development do little to help, and may do much to complicate, the process of growing up. An understanding of this process, from the information given, will help parents to appreciate what their child is going through in the crucial, and sometimes difficult, transition from child to adult.

Physical growth
Developments include at:

Eleven to sixteen years:	in girls most rapid growth occurs between age eleven and fourteen; in boys it occurs between age twelve and sixteen; height increases, on average, by six to twelve inches; weight by between one and five stones; legs grow first; then hips, chest, and shoulders develop; and finally the trunk increases, giving depth to the chest
Sixteen to eighteen years:	growth complete in girls; in boys it usually continues, slowly, for a year or two more; in some cases there is "delayed adolescence", in which a growth spurt occurs at this age

Female sexual development
Developments include at:

Eleven to fourteen years:	development of hips may be noticeable since age nine; early breast development evident from age ten; breast

Developments include at:

Eleven to fourteen years:	swelling rapidly from age twelve, with nipple pigmentation; size of vulva increases; hair grows in pubic region and in armpits; onset of menstruation between age ten and sixteen
Fourteen to sixteen years:	breasts fully grown; slight vaginal secretion is normal; armpit and pubic hair fully developed

Male sexual development
Developments include at:

Twelve to sixteen years:	increase in size of penis and testicles; spontaneous erections; appearance of pubic hair; temporary breast swelling occurs in ten per cent of boys; voice beginning to deepen
Fourteen to sixteen years:	full development of pubic hair; appearance of armpit and facial hair; nocturnal emission of sperm; deep voice
Sixteen to eighteen years:	starts to shave; normal adult sexual interests and abilities

Emotional understanding
Developments include at:

Twelve to fourteen years:	friends tend to be of own sex; interests mainly concern school, sports, and home; particular interest in factual information; no real interest in moral, social, or political questions
Fourteen to sixteen years:	interest in opposite sex with "dating"; tendency to stay in groups; steady friend or companion often changes every

Developments include at:

Fourteen to sixteen years: few weeks; bursts of great enthusiasm often fail to last; admiration of "cult" or public figures, often of same sex; transient homosexual phase; ability for abstract thought now fully developed

Sixteen to eighteen years: deeply involved with opposite sex; rejection often causes considerable sense of hurt; wanting to be accepted as mature and adult; rebellious against authority; sexual anxieties and problems sometimes conflict with other interests and schooling; friends tend to be of similar intelligence and are usually at a similar stage of rebellion against authority; interested in politics, and in anti-establishment ideas

---

Disease prevention and health care

Immunization
Health steps to be taken at:

Eleven years: German measles (rubella) injection for girls

Thirteen years: Skin test for tuberculosis; if negative, followed by BCG immunization; if positive, followed by investigations for tuberculosis

Thirteen to eighteen years: Tetanus injection and oral polio vaccine often given; injections for foreign travel if required (for example, against cholera, typhoid, or other diseases likely to be encountered)

Health care
Health steps to be taken at:

Twelve to fourteen years: medical check-up once; six-monthly dental check-ups; discussion about emotional, physical, and sexual changes that are taking place; importance of personal morality and ethical values must be stressed

Fourteen to eighteen years: medical check-up once; six-monthly dental check-ups; informal discussion of sexual matters; explanation of venereal disease; encourage the child to visit doctor alone; contraception should be explained

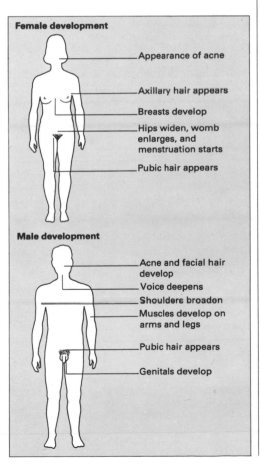

Female development

Appearance of acne

Axillary hair appears

Breasts develop

Hips widen, womb enlarges, and menstruation starts

Pubic hair appears

Male development

Acne and facial hair develop

Voice deepens

Shoulders broaden

Muscles develop on arms and legs

Pubic hair appears

Genitals develop

Age 11 to age 18: disorders 1

SYMPTOMS AND SIGNS	TREATMENT
Acne	
Disfiguring pustules on face and neck; particularly affecting forehead, cheeks and chin; also chest, back, and shoulders; severe cases result in scarring.	Keep hair and skin clean; creams that cause skin to peel sometimes used to expose blocked pores; supervised ultraviolet light treatment helps in some cases; antibiotics in severe cases.
Anorexia nervosa	
Loss of weight; often extreme emaciation; failure to eat; sometimes vomiting after meals; monthly periods cease; skin sometimes becomes covered with fine hair; denial that there is a problem.	Persuade patient to see doctor; psychiatric care; drug therapy; in severe cases, intra-venous feeding is necessary.
Anxiety	
Irritability; agitation; nail-biting; inability to sleep well; inability to concentrate.	Attempt to discover underlying worry; doctor may help.
Appendicitis	
See **Appendicitis,** p.884.	
Bornholm disease (pleurodynia)	
High fever; headache; severe muscle pain in chest; illness lasts between four and seven days.	Aspirin or stronger painkilling drugs; high fluid intake; bed rest; consult doctor.
Chancroid	
Pustule or ulcer on genitals or anus; abscess in groin; ulcer sensitive and inflamed; smelly discharge from ulcer.	Consult doctor; drug therapy; abstinence from sexual intercourse.
Cystitis	
Frequent and painful urination; cloudy urine; sometimes fever; in some cases, blood in urine.	Consult doctor; urine tests; antibiotics.
Delinquency	
Violence; overt aggressiveness; rebellion against parental authority, and against society; stealing; "gang" activities.	Parents should discuss the problem with people who are accustomed to dealing with adolescents, for example, a doctor, youth officer or social worker; constructive group activity; team work.
Depression	
Moodiness; persistent lack of enthusiasm; feelings of failure; sleep difficulties; feelings of isolation and loneliness; drop in standard of school work; overeating; anorexia nervosa; thoughts of suicide.	Keep adolescent involved in family affairs; show friendship and affection; discuss realistic worries; seek the advice of a doctor if condition continues; drug therapy may help.

Acne is a disfiguring complaint occurring at an age when physical appearance is important. In nearly all cases, the problem gradually disappears after about age twenty. Parents should be sympathetic and help to maintain the child's self-confidence. In girls, acne is often worse just before menstruation. Some types of skin are more likely than others to develop acne.

Anorexia nervosa is much more common in girls than boys. The girl usually denies that anything is wrong. She is often convinced that she is obese, despite evidence to the contrary. This is a psychological illness. One interpretation is that the girl is trying to stop herself becoming an adult, thus avoiding social and sexual responsibilities. It is a sign of underlying insecurity and depression. A milder type of anorexia nervosa may occur when the girl alternates between periods of weight loss, and periods of excessive eating and weight gain. Both disorders are different from "crash" dieting and slimming crazes, and should not be confused.

Anxiety is a common problem during adolescence. The child may be worried about examinations, about school activities, or about making friends, particularly with the opposite sex. The parents should try to appear interested and helpful without forcing the child to tell them about the problem. If it is a sexual problem, the child may find difficulty in talking about it. If the symptoms continue, suggest a visit to the doctor. Depression sometimes accompanies the anxiety that stems from a feeling of failure at school.

Bornholm disease is an infection spread by a virus. The pain is so acute that the illness may be confused with pleurisy. A relapse may occur if the patient is too active in the month following the illness. Depression and fatigue frequently occur in the course of recovery from Bornholm disease.

A chancroid is a rare but highly infectious sexually-transmitted (venereal) disease. It is distinct from the syphilitic chancre, which is a painless ulcer. Chancroid often leaves a scar.

Cystitis is an infection of the bladder. It is more common in girls than boys because the female urethra is shorter, and infecting organisms from outside the body can reach the bladder more easily. It may occur for no apparent reason, and is sometimes caused by sexual intercourse, or by the use of internal tampons during periods. Recurring attacks need careful investigation, because they may be associated with a more serious disorder.

Delinquency is a social, rather than medical, problem. It is most likely to occur in adolescents who have a disturbed family background. The liking for "gang" activities can often be successfully redirected into team work. The pressures within the group help to discipline the delinquent. Youth clubs and social work may also help.

Adolescence is a difficult time in which many social and personal adjustments must be made. The adolescent has to cope with increasing responsibility, sexual problems, often important examinations, and the realization that social pressures and conflicts commonly suppress individual interests. Teachers at school often notice a change in the standard of the child's work.
See also **Anxiety**, p.872.

Age 11 to age 18: disorders 2

SYMPTOMS AND SIGNS	TREATMENT

Drug abuse: hard drugs

Abnormal behaviour, including: sudden changes in habits or appearance; extreme lethargy; unusual enthusiasm; extraordinary statements; confusion; moodiness; lack of concern for personal appearance; weight loss; in some cases, scratch marks, or persistent sniffing and nasal irritation.

Seek expert advice; avoid violent confrontations; maintain secure, friendly family situation. Hospital treatment and psychiatric care may be required.

Drug abuse: soft drugs

Lack of enthusiasm; lethargy; sore and red eyes.

Try to discover any underlying anxieties; discuss problem in relaxed manner.

Glandular fever

One to two weeks of lethargy; general ill-health; headaches, followed by fever; other symptoms may include severe sore throat, difficulty in swallowing, swollen neck, enlarged lymph nodes felt in armpits and groin, faint rash, jaundice; doctor may detect enlarged spleen.

Consult doctor; diagnosis from blood tests; painkilling drugs; occasionally antibiotics to reduce risk of secondary infection.

Gonorrhoea

Discharge from penis or vagina; pain on passing urine; painful erection; in girls: symptoms mild or absent, but sometimes low abdominal pain.

Immediate assessment by specialist; antibiotics; abstinence from sexual intercourse.

Granuloma inguinale

Painless nodule in genital area; nodule grows and ulcerates.

Immediate assessment by specialist; antibiotic therapy.

Hepatitis, infectious

Fever for four or five days; often nausea and vomiting; muscle aches; severe headaches; finally yellow colouring of skin and whites of eyes (jaundice); dark urine; often fatigue; depression, and weakness during recovery.

Bed rest at home; hospital admission in severe cases; light, low fat diet, mainly carbohydrates and extra vitamins; no alcohol for six months after the infection.

Jaundice

Yellow colour to skin; yellow whites of eyes.

Assessment by doctor.

Masturbation

Stimulation of external genitals, usually until orgasm is achieved.

None necessary.

If parents think that one child may be using addictive drugs, they should discuss their fears with their other children, who may be better informed than the parents. In cases of addiction to hard drugs it is important that a doctor is consulted. In many cases a teenager finds it easier to talk the problem over with a doctor, who can then advise parents on how to handle the problem.

Adolescents often experiment with drugs, and in some cases, experimentation leads to active rebellion against the authority of their parents. In many cases, however, spying on a teenager's activities only increases the need to rebel. If parents suspect that their child is experimenting with marijuana, they must try to discuss this without obvious criticism. They can then warn the child about the dangers of drug abuse, without having a direct confrontation. Most teenagers come into contact with soft drugs. They may find them discussed, or used, by friends. In most cases, however, a teenager from a happy, stable, and caring family is reasonably well-equipped to get through the difficulties of adolescence, without feeling the need for drugs of any kind.

Symptoms of glandular fever vary considerably in severity, and may appear only as a low grade fever with minimal sore throat. The worst phase of the illness lasts about seven or ten days, and is followed by a gradual but steady improvement over several weeks. During the acute phase the patient may be able to eat only soft foods, such as jelly and ice-cream. It is essential that the fluid intake is kept high. During convalescence extra rest is necessary, because excessive activity can cause a relapse.

Gonorrhoea is a highly contagious sexually transmitted (venereal) disease. By the time a child has reached adolescence, the parents should have discussed the problems and dangers of sexuality and venereal disease in an open and frank manner. If this has been the rule in the family, the teenager is less likely to contract the disease, and will also be able to ask the parents for advice if symptoms of venereal disease appear.

Granuloma inguinale is a relatively rare, sexually transmitted (venereal) disease.

Infectious hepatitis is inflammation of the liver that is caused by a virus infection. There are three main types of the disease: virus A, virus B, and virus non A non B. Virus A is contracted by drinking water or eating food that has been contaminated by the faeces of an infected person. Virus B is usually transmitted either in saliva or in the faeces of an infected person. It is also spread by contaminated hypodermic needles, and is common among drug addicts. Virus non A non B is the commonest cause of post-transfusion hepatitis. Infectious hepatitis can best be prevented by good sanitation. Injections of gamma globulin give protection against virus A hepatitis for about four months.

Jaundice is a symptom that may indicate infectious hepatitis, mononucleosis, gall bladder disease, a form of anaemia, or obstruction of the bile ducts.

Most adolescent boys, and many adolescent girls, find masturbation relieves sexual tension. It is a normal habit, but parental and school attitudes may make the teenager feel guilty. Masturbation does not cause physical or psychological problems, other than those associated with guilt.

SYMPTOMS AND SIGNS	TREATMENT
Migraine	
Vision disturbances that may include flashing lights, abnormal vision, and diminished field of vision; followed by severe headache, often on only one side of head; nausea; vomiting; dislike of bright lights, noise, or movement.	Immediate doses of soluble aspirin; antimigraine (ergotamine) drugs; injections or suppositories needed in rare cases to control vomiting; frequent attacks may require daily treatment with drugs.
Nonspecific urethritis (NSU)	
Slight, milky discharge from urethra; frequent urination; pain on urination; symptoms rare in girls.	Assessment by specialist; drug therapy; abstinence from sexual intercourse.
Obesity	
Excessive fatness of body and face; in severe cases, knock-knees; backache and recurrent respiratory diseases.	Reduce food intake; exercise.
Periods, failure to start	
Girls not menstruating by age fifteen.	Discuss with doctor; gynaecological assessment six months later; sometimes assessment of hormone levels; in rare cases, hormone treatment.
Periods, heavy	
Excessive bleeding; prolonged bleeding; often accompanied by low abdominal pain; loss of clots of blood.	Assessment by gynaecologist; examination to investigate possibility of infection; drugs to control blood flow, pain, and irregularity of periods.
Periods, irregular	
Intervals of up to three months between periods; variable severity of periods.	Usually none necessary; consult doctor if worried.
Periods, painful	
Low abdominal, colicky pain for first day or two of menstruation; low backache; pain down outside of thighs; sometimes vomiting; sometimes fainting.	Assessment by doctor; regular doses of painkilling drugs; antispasmodic drugs and, occasionally, antinauseant drugs may be used; in severe cases, three to four months of hormone treatment.
Premenstrual tension	
Irritability; depression; headache; feeling of "heaviness"; breast tenderness for a few days before the onset of a period; some girls show antisocial behaviour and poor school performance before the onset of menstruation.	Speak to doctor; drugs to reduce excess body fluid; sometimes hormone therapy.

Migraine headaches may occur occasionally, or as often as two to three times a week. It commonly occurs before or during menstruation, at times of mental stress, or just after a period of tension, when the patient finally relaxes. There is often a family history of migraine. Vomiting attacks in childhood may develop into true migraine headaches at the onset of puberty. Occasionally migraine is associated with a certain type of food. *See* **Headaches, recurrent,** p.858.

This is a common sexually-transmitted (venereal) disease, caused by one or more organisms that have not been definitely identified. It is important that both partners are tested and treated, even if one has had no symptoms.

Obesity is a common problem. Overfeeding may have started at birth. Parents who tend to overeat encourage similar eating habits in their children. An increase of weight at puberty is natural, due to the hormone changes occurring at this time. If parents are concerned about their child's weight, they should discuss the problem with a doctor. A child should eat a high-protein diet with plenty of fresh fruit and vegetables. Parents should approach the problem with under-standing and sympathy, because an obese teenager is often eager to cooperate in an effort to lose weight, whereas parental rejection can lead to secret overeating.
See also **Depression,** p.856; 872.

The age that menstruation begins depends on the family, race, and health of the individual. The menarche (onset of menstruation) usually begins between the ages of eleven and fourteen, but is commonly delayed until the age of fifteen or sixteen. Breast and pubic hair development occur first. Rarely, the membrane that partly covers the vaginal entrance (hymen), closes it completely. Menstruation occurs, but the menses cannot escape. This may cause local discomfort.
See also **Anorexia nervosa,** p.872.

Occasionally the first period is heavy and prolonged, and periods tend to be heavy until they become regular. Emotional stress often makes the problem worse. Frequent, heavy periods can cause anaemia, and a doctor should be consulted in case dietary iron supplements are required.

It is normal after the first period for subsequent ones to be irregular. A second period may not occur for three months, but the intervals lessen and regularity is usually achieved within the first year, although some girls never become regular. This may cause problems in the future, particularly when estimating the delivery date of a baby, or if trying to use the rhythm method of contraception. Sometimes irregular periods are caused by anxiety, or nervous disorders such as anorexia nervosa (*see* p.872).

About ten per cent of girls between the ages of fourteen and eighteen have periods that are sufficiently painful to prevent them attending school. This may be due to an infection of the womb or ovaries, and the doctor should assess this possibility. Periods are often more painful during times of anxiety and stress.

Mild premenstrual symptoms are normal, but if they occur frequently and severely, seek the advice of a specialist.

SYMPTOMS AND SIGNS	TREATMENT

Sexual problems

Anxiety about sexual appeal and ability; ignorance about sex; fears of homosexuality.

Parents, counsellors, and a doctor should answer questions frankly and openly; informal talks in small groups, with an adviser who is experienced in dealing with adolescent sexual problems.

Suicidal tendency

Talk or threat of suicide; commonly a result of depression.

Stay near teenager; contact a doctor; try to give reassurance; lock away sleeping pills and potentially dangerous drugs; stay with teenager until assistance arrives.

Syphilis

Firm, painless ulcer (chancre), usually on genitals, sometimes on other parts of body, for example, lip; scar forms after about three months.

Immediate assessment by specialist; drugs; avoidance of all sexual contact.

Tinea

Itching, irritation, and inflamed patches of skin; often with blisters; can affect feet, groin, scalp and nails.

Antifungal preparations from pharmacist; if infection persists, consult doctor; keep area clean and dry; use medication twice daily, or as directed.

Tuberculosis

Gradually increasing fatigue; general feeling of ill-health; slight fever; night sweats; weight loss; swollen lymph glands, particularly in the neck; cough, sometimes with bloodstained sputum.

Diagnosis from chest X-ray; blood and skin tests; specific drug therapy for a minimum of one year; bed rest, with a nutritious diet.

Typhoid and paratyphoid fever

Slowly developing fever; headache; slight cough; constipation; scattered pink spots on body; confusion and restlessness; followed by diarrhoea; dehydration; possibly death.

Hospital admission; blood and urine tests; antibiotics, such as chloramphenicol and trimethoprim; intravenous fluids; convalescence.

Vaginal discharge

Discharge from the vagina; a pale, milky discharge is normal; a coloured, smelly, irritating, or painful discharge is not normal.

Usually none necessary. For irritating or offensive discharge, assessment by a doctor; test for infection; appropriate drug therapy.

Venereal disease

See **Chancroid,** p.872; **Gonorrhoea,** p.874; **Nonspecific urethritis,** p.876; **Syphilis,** p.878.

Anxiety and depression are often a direct result of sexual worries. Parents should answer questions truthfully and respect the adolescent's need for privacy. They should encourage discussion and try not to be disturbed by differences between their children's and their own moral codes and views. Adolescents need to make up their own minds without feeling that they have failed to keep up with their parents' standards. Most anxieties about sex are due to ignorance, and to the stories spread at school about sex. Teenagers commonly feel physically inadequate and they need to know that transient homosexual attractions are normal.

Talk of suicide should always be taken seriously, because talk of suicide or attempted suicide is commonly a cry for help. If the ideas persist, or if an attempt is made, a doctor must be consulted.

Syphilis is usually diagnosed in the primary stage, when the chancre appears. Secondary syphilis may develop, with fever and a rash lasting for about ten days, about two months after the chancre has formed a scar. Syphilis is potentially an extremely serious disease and anyone who is in doubt about it should consult a specialist.

Tinea is commonly referred to as "Athlete's foot" when it affects the feet. It is caused by a fungal infection, which can spread from person to person, by walking barefoot in public places, or by borrowing shoes or clothing.
   See also **Ringworm,** p.864.

Tuberculosis is rare in countries with a high standard of living. Immunity in the form of a vaccination (BCG) is available, and is recommended for children at the age of thirteen. Tuberculosis is usually caught from human carriers, and in these cases the bacteria are inhaled into the lungs. It can also be contracted from the milk of infected cows. This type (bovine tuberculosis) infects the lymph nodes. The bacteria can also infect bone, kidney, and brain tissue.

The fever takes up to three weeks to develop. The patient is considered to be infectious until at least six stool cultures are clear of the infection. Complications include pneumonia, perforation of the intestine wall leading to peritonitis, and chronic infection of the gall bladder. Sterilization of water, and careful cooking of all food are wise safety measures. Immunization greatly reduces the severity of the disease if it is contracted.

Many healthy women have a slight discharge. Overenthusiastic washing and douching only aggravates the condition. It is normal for a girl to have a pale, milky discharge for up to two years before the onset of menstruation. A similar discharge may occur a day or two before and after menstruation, and at the time of ovulation in the middle of the month. However, if the discharge is coloured, or offensive, there may be an infection.

Index of children's disorders

Young adults (age 18–35): introduction

The eighteen to thirty-five age group is at a stage of physical and psychological development that should be full of enthusiasm and vitality, characteristic of young adult life.

It is also a time in which the individual should begin to think in terms of preventive medicine, and of having regular check-ups and discussions with a doctor, especially when symptoms occur, however trivial. If a doctor is fully informed about an individual's general health and previous medical history, then he or she can be alert to signs of impending disorder and disease.

The health of a marriage, or a close sexual and emotional relationship, is an aspect that a doctor has to consider carefully, when assessing the patient's overall health.

Problems in sexual and emotional relationships sometimes give rise to physical, psychosomatic, or psychological symptoms. These underlying problems, as well as the specific disorder about which the patient complains, have to be diagnosed and treated if the patient is to feel and remain basically healthy.

A common cause of marital discord is that the husband, or the wife, or both, have unrealistic expectations of each other. A doctor may suspect this situation in the life of a patient who develops symptoms such as headache, backache or abdominal pain, particularly if these symptoms have no obvious medical cause. It may become clear on investigation that the symptoms are caused by a psychological disorder. In women, the symptoms may also be associated with menstrual disorders.

Psychologically based diseases and disorders are not deliberately made up by the patient, but are unconscious expressions of a need to avoid conflict in situations that may be otherwise impossible. For this reason, such patients require prompt medical diagnosis and careful management. It may be necessary for the doctor to give the patient psychological support until he or she can solve the problem alone. When a solution is achieved, the symptoms usually disappear.

Dental hygiene is an important part of general health care, and this is most easily achieved by annual visits to a dentist, who will check for caries, or decay. Such examinations may also reveal crowding of the teeth, because of a small jaw, or because of the slow emergence of wisdom teeth.

The only neurological problem that may be common in young adults is migraine. Psychological problems that develop may be partly biochemical, such as schizophrenia. More commonly, they are social, for example, drug abuse, alcoholism, and smoking.

Many young adults take part in energetic and sometimes dangerous sports and, as a result, are particularly likely to suffer accidents and sports injuries. Common among these are injuries to the fingers, such as mallet finger, to the knee (torn cartilage), and to the wrist and elbow, for example fracture of the scaphoid bone in the wrist, or the development of tennis elbow. Exercise, such as long-distance running, can result in orthopaedic problems, such as stress fractures or heel pain. The onset of some diseases and disorders that may last for life is sometimes seen at this age. Examples include psoriasis, Raynaud's phenomenon, and vitiligo, as well as excessive sweating (hyperhidrosis) caused by anxiety or stress.

Some people suffer from a persistent backache that may be due to ankylosing spondylitis, but can also be caused by gynaecological problems, such as painful periods.

The development of the early signs of pregnancy, for example an absence of periods, causes all women some concern. If the pregnancy is welcomed, the woman will be pleased, but if a child is not wanted, the mother is more likely to be anxious.

Heart problems, apart from fainting, are rare in this age group. The first signs of chest problems are usually attacks of acute bronchitis. In some cases, the recurrent coughing results in the condition known as pneumothorax. Childhood asthma and hay fever tend to improve between the ages of twenty and thirty.

Sexual intercourse is important to most young adults, and there is some likelihood that psychological problems will arise. Disorders related to sexual activity are also relatively common. Among the disorders that may occur in women are salpingitis and vaginitis, both of which may cause sexual intercourse to be painful. Infections that may be passed on by sexual contact include epididymitis in a man; urinary tract problems, such as cystitis, which usually affects women; and the venereal diseases.

Gastrointestinal problems affecting this age group include appendicitis, Crohn's disease and ulcerative colitis. Usually, only the first symptoms of Crohn's disease and ulcerative colitis occur early in adult life. Infectious hepatitis may develop, and occurs most commonly in local epidemics. Cancer in any form is rare.

Increasing deafness is most likely to be due to otosclerosis, but it may also be due to recurring infections, such as otitis media (secondary to respiratory infection), or otitis externa. Eye problems, other than those requiring glasses, are uncommon.

Recurrent boils on the lower part of the back may occur, and if these develop in the cleft between the buttocks, they may be a symptom of a pilonidal sinus. Such boils are painful, but not serious if correctly treated.

Although regular health care is not usually so important at this age as it is in childhood and later in life, any symptoms of ill health should be discussed with a doctor, particularly if they cause anxiety, or continue for more than a few days. Women should have regular gynaecological examinations and cervical smear tests.

Developing the habits of taking regular exercise, preventing obesity, and avoiding an excessive intake of either alcohol or food, will do much to maintain good health. Even more important is the need to stop smoking, because it is at this age that regular smoking is most likely to become a habit. The first step toward ensuring good health in the years ahead is to stop smoking as young as possible.

Health care checklist

Regular check-ups by a doctor are sensible precautions to take against the development of diseases and disorders. At the same time, the following questions are useful to alert each person to danger signals. Use this checklist to assess your state of health, and try to do this regularly, for instance, at the beginning of each month.

Some of the questions apply only to women and some only to men. If the answer to all of the questions is "No", then almost certainly you are in good health, with no need to worry. But, if the answer to any of the questions is "Yes", then a doctor should be consulted for an expert medical opinion.

Q: Skin of face affected by pimples or blackheads? Skin rash on any other part of body?

Q: Frequent sniffing and sneezing? Cough? If cough, blood in cough? Hoarseness? Chest problems? Shortness of breath?

Q: Persistent pain and stiffness in spine, joints, limbs, or any other part of body?

Q: Weight loss that is not caused by dieting? Vomiting? Appetite loss? Indigestion? Nausea? Sudden weight gain?

Q: Change in bowel habits? Diarrhoea? Constipation? Abdominal and stomach pain? Blood in faeces?

Q: Change in urinary habits? Pain when urinating? Blood in urine? Pain in anal or genital region?

Q: Painful periods? Unusual menstrual blood flow? Pain on intercourse? Vaginal discharge? Unexpected vaginal bleeding? Irritation? Sexual difficulties? Anxiety?

Q: Sore that will not heal on penis? Lump that will not go away?

Q: Excessive use of alcohol, heavy smoking, or habit of taking drugs?

Q: Fainting, hot flushes, or sudden feeling of weakness?

Q: Fever, with or without vomiting?

Q: Recurrent severe headaches?

Q: Hearing problems? Itching and painful discharge from ear? Deafness and earache?

Q: Vision problems? Sore eyes? Pain or irritation around eyes?

Q: Lump that does not disappear in breast or other part of body.

Q: Sore that will not heal?

Q: Change in shape, colour, or size of any skin mark or wart?

Q: Nervousness, irritability or depression?

Q: Apathy or lethargy?

Q: Weeping without obvious reason? Feeling of persecution? Hearing voices?

Q: Overwhelming sadness or despair? Feeling unable to cope? Feeling of being rundown or unduly fatigued? Difficulty sleeping? Insomnia?

Q: Pain and swelling around teeth? Sore, coated tongue and sore gums? Lump or sore on tongue or gums? Bleeding gums?

Q: Persistent cold sores around mouth, or lips?

Q: Scalp irritated and itchy, flaking skin? Sudden loss of hair? Persistent sores on scalp?

SYMPTOMS AND SIGNS	TREATMENT
Abortion *See* **Miscarriage,** p.888.	
Acne *See* **Acne,** p.872.	
Allergy *See* **Allergy,** p.842; **Asthma,** p.906; **Hay fever,** p.844.	
Amenorrhoea No menstrual periods; primary: periods never start at puberty; secondary: periods cease.	Assessment by gynaecologist; pregnancy test; hormone therapy sometimes required if pregnancy test negative.
Ankylosing spondylitis (bamboo spine) Increasing pain and stiffness in lower spine; symptoms worse in the morning; periods without pain; increasing rigidity of spine over several years.	X-ray of spine; blood tests; aspirin-like drugs; antirheumatic drugs; regular physiotherapy; breathing exercises.
Anorexia nervosa *See* **Anorexia nervosa,** p.872.	
Appendicitis Initially slight nausea and vague central abdominal pain; pain gradually increases and moves to right lower abdomen; slight fever, gradually increasing in severity; headache; in most cases, constipation; vomiting; abdomen tender to touch.	After two hours, consult a doctor; urgent hospitalization for surgical removal of appendix (appendicectomy); eat and drink nothing until hospitalized; do not take laxatives for constipation.
Bronchitis, acute Cough; thick sputum; central chest pain during coughing bouts; fever; general feeling of illness.	Steam inhalation; sedative cough mixtures; if necessary, antibiotics prescribed by a doctor.
Crohn's disease Abdominal pain; diarrhoea two or three times a day; loss of appetite; loss of weight; mild fever; weakness or fatigue; severity of symptoms may vary over many years.	Diagnosis from history of illness and from barium meal or enema, and X-ray of gastrointestinal tract; symptoms usually controlled with drugs; sometimes operation is necessary.
Dandruff White, scaling skin from scalp; sometimes with itching; rarely, inflammation.	Wash hair with medicated shampoo two or three times a week; brush hair regularly and vigorously.
Drug abuse *See* **Drug abuse: hard drugs,** p.874; **Drug abuse: soft drugs,** p.874.	

The most common cause of amenorrhoea in this age group is pregnancy. Other causes include ending a regular course of the contraceptive pill, a serious illness, prolonged anxiety, early onset of the menopause, which sometimes affects older women in this age group, and also anorexia nervosa, which is more likely to affect younger women.
See also **Periods, failure to start,** p.876.

In some cases, other joints become swollen and painful, or the eyes become red and sore. Physiotherapy helps to maintain normal back movement and posture.

An appendicectomy is done through a cut in the lower abdomen that leaves only a small scar. The patient stays in hospital for five to seven days. If the appendix is not removed quickly, it is liable to burst, causing peritonitis, a serious infection of the internal abdominal surface. If peritonitis develops, prolonged treatment with antibiotics may be necessary.

The infection often develops after a cold, influenza, or other respiratory illness. It is also associated with asthma. The condition is aggravated by smoking, a dusty atmosphere, or a cold, damp environment, and can develop into pneumonia. Repeated attacks of acute bronchitis damage the bronchi and can lead to chronic bronchitis.

The cause of Crohn's disease is not known. Parts of the gastrointestinal tract become inflamed. In most cases, the end of the small intestine and the beginning of the large intestine, are the places affected. The acute form is often mistaken for appendicitis. The chronic form may lead to intestinal obstruction, or abscesses, that, in rare cases, may involve adjacent organs, for instance, the bladder or the skin.

Dandruff is the normal shedding of dead skin cells from the scalp. Dandruff is more noticeable in people with congenital dry skin, or eczema. Another disorder, seborrhoeic dermatitis of the scalp, produces larger scales that are yellow-brown and greasy.

SYMPTOMS AND SIGNS	TREATMENT
Epididymitis Pain in the groin; swollen, tender testicle; sometimes fever; pain when urinating.	Consult a doctor; antibiotics; bed rest; support for scrotum; painkilling drugs.
Fainting Dry mouth; cold perspiration; nausea; vertigo; disturbed vision; buzzing in ears; loss of consciousness; collapse.	At first signs of fainting, lie down; alternatively, sit with head between knees; avoid standing or sitting upright.
Fracture, scaphoid (wrist) Pain in wrist; stiffness of wrist; after falling on outstretched hand.	Consult a doctor; plaster cast applied, even for a suspected scaphoid fracture.
Fracture, stress Pain, usually in a limb or in a foot; associated with repeated minor injuries; most commonly caused by long-distance running or walking.	Consult a doctor; plaster cast may be required.
Hay fever *See* **Hay fever,** p.844.	
Heel pain Pain in heel, aggravated by walking and running; tenderness deep under heel; sometimes tenderness behind heel.	Consult a doctor; sponge rubber pad in shoe; injection of corticosteroid drug may help; in some cases, plaster cast necessary; rarely, an operation.
Hepatitis *See* **Hepatitis, infectious,** p.874.	
Hodgkin's disease Gradual onset of mild fever; night sweats; weight loss; lethargy; enlarged lymph nodes noticeable in neck; sometimes bone pain after drinking alcohol.	Consult a doctor; blood test; lymph node biopsy; radiotherapy; drugs; sometimes removal of spleen; treatment often successful.
Ingrown toenail Pain on side of affected toenail; infection commonly occurs; inflammation; swelling of toe; thickening of skin.	Cut nail straight across corner; lift and clean carefully under edge with soft brush; wipe with gauze soaked in surgical spirit; if there is repeated infection, consult a doctor; antibiotics, or operation to remove side of nail may be required.
Knee, torn cartilage Inability to straighten knee after twisting injury; swelling; pain for two weeks; followed by recurrent "locking" when knee sticks in one position; or "giving way", when knee fails to support body.	Immediate medical attention; bandaging of knee in straight position; later, operation to remove torn cartilage (meniscectomy) may be necessary.
Mallet finger Inability to extend tip of finger; often caused by violent blow on extended finger, for example, by hard ball.	Immediate splinting, with injured fingertip fully extended and next joint flexed; keep splint on for three weeks.

Epididymitis is an inflammation of the epididymis (beginning of the seminal tube) in the scrotum. It is sometimes associated with prostate problems, and also with venereal diseases, particularly gonorrhoea.

Fainting is caused by a sudden reduction in the blood supply to the brain. It commonly affects pregnant women, but may also occur after standing in a hot room when tired, after a sudden shock, or as a result of a sudden change in posture from lying to standing.

The fracture may not show up on an X-ray for ten days, so a second X-ray is often taken. If a scaphoid fracture is not treated, osteoarthritis of the wrist may result. An operation may then be needed to repair the damaged bone.

Repeated minor strains on any bone may produce a fracture. Runners suffer from stress fractures of the foot (march fracture) or leg; occasionally, javelin throwers or weight lifters suffer stress fractures of the forearm. After treatment, care must be taken not to repeat the injury. Athletes must avoid excessive strain early in training.

Heel pain is most likely to develop in active young adults. X-ray examination may show a "spur" of new bone forming in the ligaments of the sole of the foot. Heel pain can also be caused by the tearing of ligaments in the sole of the foot, or by bursitis on the Achilles' tendon, which is particularly common in women who wear badly-fitting shoes.

Hodgkin's disease is a malignant disease of the lymph nodes. Modern treatment by X-rays and drugs is successful in most cases.

Ingrown toenails occur when pressure on a nail that is more staple-shaped in cross-section than normal causes the sharp edge of the nail to cut into the skin. This cut is easily infected. Any infection is made worse by tight shoes, and by sweaty, dirty feet.

Osteoarthritis may develop if the cartilage is not removed. Even after the operation this condition may develop. A torn cartilage is a common injury among athletes, particularly football players.

If the patient is still unable to extend the finger after three weeks, an operation may be required to repair the tendon that has been torn off the bone of the fingertip by the injury.

SYMPTOMS AND SIGNS	TREATMENT

Miscarriage
Usually in first three months of pregnancy; heavy vaginal bleeding; abdominal pain; loss of foetus.

Contact a doctor or gynaecologist immediately; lie down; painkilling drugs sometimes given; hospitalization for dilation and curettage may be necessary if bleeding persists.

Mononucleosis, infectious
See **Glandular fever,** p.874.

Otitis externa
See **Otitis externa,** p.846.

Otitis media
See **Otitis media,** p.846.

Otosclerosis
Increasing deafness; one ear affected initially; other ear develops symptoms later; patient often able to hear voices more clearly in noisy surroundings; persistent buzzing in the ears (tinnitus).

Consult a doctor; operation on worst ear first requires hospitalization for about one week.

Painful intercourse (dyspareunia)
Pain during sexual intercourse; vaginal discharge; irritation; anxiety.

Consult a doctor; tests for venereal disease; gynaecological examination; counselling.

Pilonidal sinus
Suppurating duct containing hair; recurrent abscess between buttocks or above lower part of sacrum.

Surgical drainage; then operation to remove tissues that cause condition.

Pneumothorax
Sudden chest pain; shortness of breath; pain in shoulder; dry cough; sometimes extreme shock.

Consult a doctor; X-ray of chest; for slight symptoms, no treatment; for severe symptoms, hospitalization; mechanical removal of air from chest.

Psoriasis
Clearly defined patches of red skin; silver-grey scaling; can occur anywhere on body.

Consult a doctor; coal tar; dithranol; corticosteroid cream under plastic dressing; drug therapy followed by ultraviolet light often helpful in severe cases.

Raynaud's phenomenon
White, numb, stiff fingers in cold weather; white colour changing to purple; pain; some swelling of fingers as they warm; sometimes ulceration of finger tip; skin may become smooth and tight.

Consult a doctor; stop smoking; drugs to dilate surface blood vessels; warm clothing; rarely, surgical operation to cut nerves to blood vessels.

Salpingitis
Acute: thick vaginal discharge; lower abdominal pain; fever; pain when urinating. Chronic: menstrual problems; pain during sexual intercourse; painful periods; dull lower abdominal ache; vaginal discharge.

Assessment by gynaecologist; long course of antibiotics; heat treatment; avoid sexual intercourse; sometimes surgical procedure needed.

Sometimes bleeding occurs in early pregnancy without loss of the foetus. This is known as a threatened miscarriage, and the patient should rest in bed for at least two days after the bleeding has stopped.

Hospitalization is sometimes recommended. At least ten per cent of pregnancies miscarry before the fourteenth week. This is usually due to foetal abnormality. Occasionally it is due to hormone imbalance.

People with otosclerosis often find that other members of their family have suffered from deafness. The deafness is aggravated by pregnancy. The condition is caused by a small bone in the ear that sticks to the inner ear

and prevents it vibrating. It is important that the operation is performed before the deafness becomes severe.

Expert medical assessment can exclude possible physical reasons for this common complaint. It is often due to anxiety, but may be caused by poor sexual technique, by

gynaecological problems, such as a tight hymen, vaginitis or salpingitis, or by disorders such as urethritis or venereal disease.

This is more common in dark-haired males than females. The cyst is formed by a hair turning inwards. A draining duct forms and becomes infected. After the abscess has been

drained, and the area has healed, surgical removal of the epithelial tissues prevents recurrence of the condition

A pneumothorax is caused by air entering the chest cavity. This causes part of the lung to collapse. Air enters the cavity either from a chest injury, or from a local emphysema (air-

filled blister) on the internal surface of the lung. An operation is necessary to treat a recurrent mild pneumothorax.

Although psoriasis patches appear and disappear, the condition is usually mild but persistent. One type affects the nails in particular, and another type is associated

with a form of arthritis. The cause of psoriasis is not known. It is more common in women, and usually appears for the first time between age ten and age twenty-five.

The symptoms are caused by a spasm in the blood vessels of the fingers. The cause is not usually known, and is distinct from chilblains or frostbite. The condition may be due to a rare generalized disorder, or an extra

vertebra in the neck that presses on the nerves. In some cases it occurs following an accident.

Salpingitis is an infection of the fallopian tube. The condition can lead to sterility or, in some cases, can cause a subsequent pregnancy to be ectopic (inside the fallopian tube instead of the womb).

SYMPTOMS AND SIGNS	TREATMENT
Schizophrenia Sudden or gradual onset of disorganized and bizarre thinking; feelings of persecution; irrational behaviour; auditory hallucinations.	Consult a doctor; drug therapy; often, hospitalization; antipsychotic drugs, often by injection, to prevent relapse.
Sexual problems *See* **Sexual problems,** p.878.	
Sprain Pain at a joint following injury; swelling; limited movement.	Rest joint; support wrist or arm in sling; support ankle with firm bandage.
Sweating, excessive (hyperhidrosis) Excessive production of sweat; particularly from armpits, palm of hands, and sole of feet.	Consult a doctor if worried; mild tranquillizing drug; special skin preparations; sometimes removal of area of skin from armpit; or operation on nerves in neck.
Tennis elbow Pain and tenderness on outer side of elbow; weakness of forearm muscles.	Rest; antirheumatic drugs; injection of corticosteroid and local anaesthetic drugs sometimes helpful.
Tinea *See* **Tinea,** p.878.	
Ulcerative colitis Recurrent and severe diarrhoea; blood and mucus in stools; frequently fever; weight loss; increasing feeling of ill-health; anaemia.	Consult a doctor; sigmoidoscopy (examination of intestine with lighted tube); barium enema; mild forms treated with antidiarrhoeal drugs; severe forms require hospitalization; blood transfusion; corticosteroid drugs.
Vaginitis Vaginal discharge; irritation; soreness.	Assessment by a doctor; appropriate treatment, depending on the cause.
Venereal disease *See* **Chancroid,** p.872; **Gonorrhoea,** p.874; **Granuloma inguinale,** p.874; **Nonspecific urethritis,** p.876; **Syphilis,** p.878.	
Vitiligo Loss of pigmentation in otherwise normal patches of skin; white hair on patch.	Assessment by a dermatologist; special drugs; increasing amount of sunlight; small patches can be covered by cosmetics.
Wisdom tooth, impacted Pain; swelling at back of jaw; sometimes earache; sore throat.	Dental extraction; sometimes under general anaesthetic.

Schizophrenia is a complicated mental disorder, in which hereditary factors may be significant. A person with a tendency toward schizophrenia may be unable to cope with adolescent anxiety or depression, and is particularly likely to be affected adversely by soft or hard drugs.

A sprained joint is one that has had a ligament damaged by an injury. If only a few fibres of a ligament have been torn, the sprain will heal naturally with rest. Rarely, if a ligament is completely ruptured, surgical repair may be required.

Sweating is the body's normal way of controlling temperature. Sometimes the sweat glands are overactive, and the most common causes of this include anxiety, and stimulating drugs. The condition can produce strong body odour, and may lead to skin problems, such as mild rashes or infection.

Tennis elbow is caused by repeated rotating movements of the forearm, such as in playing tennis or in performing a manual task, such as using a screwdriver, particularly after a long period of muscular inactivity. Rarely, an operation is needed to cure the condition.

The cause of ulcerative colitis is not known. The condition may occur at any age, but is more common between twenty and forty. Haemorrhage and perforation of the intestine are uncommon. The incidence of cancer of the intestine in patients with ulcerative colitis is high. Surgical removal of the colon cures the condition and may be required in some patients with severe forms of this disorder.

Vaginitis may be caused by the organism that causes thrush (moniliasis), or by the parasitic protozoa that causes trichomoniasis. In both these infections, the woman's sexual partner may also be infected. Moniliasis is relatively common during pregnancy, or when taking the contraceptive pill, or after a course of antibiotics.

Ten per cent of persons suffering from vitiligo recover spontaneously. The cause of the disorder is unknown. The patches may be of any size. The disorder may be associated with alopecia areata, pernicious anaemia, diabetes mellitus, or thyroid disorders.

In many persons the jaw is not large enough for the third molar (wisdom) tooth. As it grows, pressure is exerted on the second molars and sometimes on other teeth in the jaw, causing pain and swelling. Dental extraction solves the problem, although post-operative pain and swelling may last for three to five days. Occasionally extraction is followed by pain that appears to be in the ear. The pain begins on the third day after the extraction, and continues for several weeks. This is known as a "dry socket". It is not caused by an infection, but must be treated with frequent anaesthetic dressings.

Mature adults (age 35-50): introduction

Many people in this age group tend to eat and drink too much, and also fail to get enough regular exercise. As a result, many are overweight, if not actually obese. Those who smoke or take other drugs, including alcohol, to excess, usually do so because of psychological stress. Such people commonly persist in these habits, despite their knowledge of the harm being done to their body.

The physical functions and responses of the person in early middle age are gradually slowing down. At this age it is more important than ever to safeguard health if the later years of life are to be enjoyable and not a burden because of illness. A major step toward better health is learning how to control eating and drinking habits.

At this age it is particularly important to understand the relationship between the emotions, the mind, and physical health or illness. This is necessary to help prevent certain diseases and disorders from occurring or, if they do develop, from progressing to more serious conditions. Health care should emphasize preventive medicine. A doctor can help each individual to avoid many of the problems of aging, and to detect others as soon as they occur.

People who have become obese sometimes try to regain their youthful vigour by playing sports too violently or too often. In most cases, such sudden bursts of activity do more harm than good. Strained joints and ligaments are among the least serious problems such violent exercises can cause. Bursitis and frozen shoulder are common in this age group and Achilles' tendon rupture can be the result of a strenuous game of tennis. A slipped disc commonly results from lifting a weight that is too heavy, or from moving awkwardly in some sporting activity that the person is not used to.

Breathing problems may be associated with obesity, but may also be due to a deviated nasal septum, causing a blocked nose and recurrent attacks of sinusitis. Occasionally breathlessness is due to problems such as heart valve disease, which prevents the heart from functioning properly, or to high blood pressure, which may be diagnosed on routine examination by a doctor.

The low-fibre, high carbohydrate diet of many people is a significant factor in some of the gastrointestinal problems that develop. Diet also affects disorders such as colitis and peptic ulcer, which are often associated with stress and anxiety.

Psychological problems that affect this age group are commonly a product of competitiveness, artificially raised expectations (particularly of material achievement), and the related fear of failure. These ambitions are particularly dangerous if they reflect other people's expectations more than the person's own hopes.

A psychological problem that frequently affects people of this age is depression. This may be precipitated by an approaching crisis, or by anxiety about a marriage at the same time as trying to achieve career promotion and social prestige. Depression is particularly likely to affect those who tend to suffer significant changes of mood. The condition is sometimes experienced by those who seem to be the most successful. Typically, such people alternate between an overactive stage, like a mild form of mania, and a depressed state.

Visible signs of aging include problems such as baldness, and the cosmetically unpleasant signs of rosacea. Rosacea may affect women at the time when other gynaecological problems are beginning. Early symptoms of gynaecological or breast cancer may be detected, but these conditions are rare. Other gynaecological problems include premenstrual tension, menstrual disorders, and fibroids, all of which are often associated with menopause. Many of these conditions develop as a result of hormonal changes, with which other endocrine gland problems, such as thyrotoxicosis, may be associated.

The carpal tunnel syndrome is a neurological problem that is associated with fluid retention and premenstrual tension. Bell's palsy is an alarming condition that develops suddenly, for no obvious reason. The variable weakness of myasthenia gravis may also appear at this age and, although this is a rare condition, the transient symptoms may cause concern about the possibility of multiple sclerosis. In multiple sclerosis both alteration of sensation, and loss of muscle power, occur. The gradual spread of weakness, accompanied by loss of sensation, is usually an indication of peripheral neuritis. Fortunately, with the exception of carpal tunnel syndrome and Bell's palsy, neurological problems are rare. Meningitis and encephalitis result from infection but even these are unusual unless there is an epidemic, or the person has recently travelled in areas where these diseases are common.

In this age group, regular dental care is particularly important. Smoking stains the teeth, and can also cause inflammation of the mouth, which may result in gingivitis.

People in this age group are still young enough to correct the effects of physical deterioration due to an inactive, overindulgent, life, and to reverse the process. A balance between work and relaxation reduces the effects of stress in a competitive lifestyle.

Regular exercises, to achieve slight breathlessness, should be done daily for ten to fifteen minutes. Such exercises, combined with a diet that is low in animal fat, high in vegetable fibre, and with only a moderate carbohydrate intake, may do much to prevent heart and circulation problems. In particular, the chances of developing heart disease and arteriosclerosis will be reduced. In addition, gentle exercise will also minimize the dangers of sudden stresses and strains on joints.

Smoking is a major causative factor in heart and lung disease as well as in the development of arteriosclerosis, some forms of urinary cancer, and cancer of the throat. If it can be stopped in middle age, the individual's life will be longer and healthier. In the next stage of life, many of the diseases people suffer are partly the result of lack of care when younger. Sensible health care at age thirty or forty is directly related to a person's comfort and convenience at age fifty or sixty. Regular assessment by a doctor will maintain good health, and the doctor's advice may help you identify potential causes of illness before they become dangerous.

Health care checklist

Regular check-ups by a doctor are sensible precautions to take against the development of diseases and disorders. At the same time, the following questions are useful to alert each person to danger signals. Use this checklist to assess your state of health, and try to do this regularly, for instance, at the beginning of each month.

Q: Skin rash on any part of the body?

Q: Chest pain when taking exercise?

Q: Frequent sniffing and sneezing? Cough? If cough, blood in cough? Hoarseness? Chest problems? Shortness of breath?

Q: Persistent pain and stiffness in spine, joints, limbs, or any other part of body?

Q: Weight loss that is not caused by dieting? Vomiting? Appetite loss? Indigestion? Nausea? Sudden weight gain?

Q: Change in bowel habits? Diarrhoea? Constipation? Abdominal and stomach pain? Blood in faeces?

Q: Change in urinary habits? Pain when urinating? Blood in urine? Pain in anal or genital region?

Q: Painful periods? Unusual menstrual blood flow? Pain on intercourse? Vaginal discharge? Unexpected vaginal bleeding? Irritation? Sexual difficulties? Anxiety?

Q: Sore that will not heal on penis? Lump that will not go away?

Q: Excessive use of alcohol, heavy smoking, or habit of taking drugs?

Q: Fainting, hot flushes, sudden weakness?

Q: Fever? Nausea? Vomiting?

Some of the questions apply only to women and some only to men. You may think of other questions to ask yourself. If the answer to all of the questions is "No", then almost certainly you are in good health. But, if the answer to any of the questions is "Yes", then a doctor should be consulted for an expert medical opinion.

Q: Recurrent severe headaches?

Q: Hearing problems? Itching and painful discharge from ear? Deafness and earache?

Q: Vision problems? Sore eyes? Pain or irritation around eyes?

Q: Lump that does not disappear in breast or other part of body?

Q: Sore that will not heal?

Q: Change in shape, colour, or size of any skin mark or wart?

Q: Nervousness, irritability or depression?

Q: Apathy or lethargy?

Q: Weeping without obvious reason? Feeling of persecution? Hearing voices?

Q: Overwhelming sadness or despair? Feeling unable to cope? Feeling of being rundown or unduly fatigued? Difficulty sleeping? Insomnia?

Q: Pain and swelling around teeth? Sore, coated tongue and sore gums? Lump or sore on tongue or gums? Bleeding gums?

Q: Persistent cold sores around mouth?

Q: Scalp irritated and itchy, flaking skin? Sudden loss of hair? Persistent sores on scalp?

Mature adults (age 35-50): disorders 1

SYMPTOMS AND SIGNS	TREATMENT
Achilles' tendon rupture Sudden severe pain behind calf; inability to stand on toes of affected leg; most likely to occur after jumping or running.	Operation to repair tendon by direct suture; plaster cast for a month; then intensive physiotherapy.
Alcoholism Gradual change in personality; loss of efficiency; forgetfulness; unkempt appearance; vitamin deficiency; cirrhosis of the liver; trembling hands; delirium tremens.	Psychotherapy; tranquillizing drugs; hospitalization; "drying out" in a hospital or clinic; drug Antabuse sometimes helpful.
Anal fissure Severe pain when defecating; bleeding on defecation.	Local anaesthetic ointments and creams; if symptoms continue, surgical stretching of muscle and excision of fissure under general anaesthetic.
Angina pectoris *See* **Angina pectoris,** p.906.	
Arteriosclerosis *See* **Arteriosclerosis,** p.906.	
Arthritis, rheumatoid Painful swelling of joints; most commonly affects finger, wrist, foot, or ankle joints; gradual onset of pain; stiffness, particularly in the morning; general feeling of ill health; fatigue; weakness; increasing deformity of affected parts.	Consult a doctor; drug therapy including aspirin; antirheumatic drugs; gold salts; corticosteroids; physiotherapy; special shoes and splints to prevent deformity; heat treatment for inflamed phase; surgery sometimes necessary.
Baldness Gradual loss of hair; particularly from crown of scalp and sides of temples.	None.
Bell's palsy (facial paralysis) Sudden onset of weakness on one side of face; drooping corner of mouth; inability to close eye; no loss of sensation; no pain.	Consult a doctor immediately; corticosteroid drugs; eye protection until muscles recover; rarely, operation to lift corner of mouth and correct eyelid droop; nerve transplant sometimes helps in severe cases.
Blood pressure, high (hypertension) Often none; occasionally morning headache; slight blurring of vision; breathlessness.	Assessment by a doctor with electro-cardiogram (ECG); blood tests; urine tests; kidney X-ray; drug therapy; diuretics (fluid-removing drugs).
Bronchitis, acute *See* **Bronchitis, acute,** p.884.	

If an operation is delayed for more than two months, the tendon heals, but remains slightly longer than before. This makes it less efficient. The injury is more common in people who are not accustomed to physical exercise. A ruptured Achilles' tendon should not be confused with a strained calf muscle.

An alcoholic often denies excessive drinking, despite being found drinking in secret. This is a complicated addiction. Effective treatment can be given only if the patient co-operates. Attendance at group therapy sessions, such as those organized by Alcoholics Anonymous (AA), is sometimes helpful. Delirium tremens is a serious condition that occurs as a result of a sudden withdrawal from alcohol. Sometimes, heavy drinking is associated with depression or other psychiatric illnesses. That alcoholism may have social origins or causes is suggested by the fact that some professional groups have a particularly high incidence of this condition.

An anal fissure is a tear in the skin lining the anus. Each time a bowel movement is passed, the tear is reopened. It may be a result of chronic constipation, but it may also occur during childbirth, or as a complication of Crohn's disease (*see* p.884).

The word arthritis means inflammation of a joint. Rheumatoid arthritis is a chronic form, the origin of which is unknown, that may lead to crippling deformities. It is more common in women than in men, and often causes depression and considerable social problems.

Baldness is a genetically inherited characteristic that is associated with male hormones. Gradual hair loss also occurs in women after the menopause, but is seldom severe enough to cause concern. However, sudden hair loss in either sex needs medical assessment. It sometimes follows scarlet fever (*see* p.860), or infections of the scalp, for instance, lice (*see* p.862) or ringworm (*see* p.864).

The cause of Bell's palsy is not known. Most cases recover completely within two months. A few cases experience only partial recovery and about ten per cent remain paralyzed.

High blood pressure is usually discovered during a routine medical examination. If the blood pressure is only slightly above normal, the patient is kept under observation, but not treated. High blood pressure increases the risk of a stroke, coronary thrombosis, or heart failure. However, treatment is highly successful, particularly if it is started before the condition becomes too serious. Rarely, hypertension is due to a kidney or hormone disorder. An operation can correct this.

SYMPTOMS AND SIGNS	TREATMENT

Bronchitis, chronic
See **Bronchitis, chronic,** p.906.

Bursitis

Swelling; sharp pain; localized tenderness in elbow, shoulder, hip, knee, heel, or other joint; movement may be limited.

Rest most important; sometimes support in splint or sling; painkilling drugs; injection of corticosteroid drugs or local anaesthetics often helpful.

Cancer, breast

Early symptoms: discovery of painless, firm lump in breast which can be felt with flat of hand.

Immediate examination by a doctor; if necessary, surgical removal of lump and microscopic examination (biopsy) to confirm or disprove diagnosis; in certain cases, biopsy performed with a needle, particularly if the surgeon considers that the lump is a cyst.

Cancer, gynaecological

Early symptoms: vaginal bleeding after menopause; bleeding between periods; bleeding on intercourse; vaginal discharge; all may occur without pain.

Cervical smear test to detect presence of precancerous cells; full gynaecological examination; dilation and curettage of womb to examine tissues lining womb.

Cancer, intestinal
See **Cancer, intestinal,** p.908.

Cancer, lung
See **Cancer, lung,** p.908.

Carpal tunnel syndrome

Waking at night with tingling and pain in thumb, index and middle fingers of one or both hands; symptoms often relieved by shaking hand vigorously.

Consult a doctor; splinting wrist at night or corticosteroid injection into front of wrist gives relief in some cases; if this fails, minor operation to relieve compressed nerve may be effective.

Colitis, mucous (irritable bowel syndrome)

Alternating episodes of constipation and diarrhoea, often with mucus; lower abdominal colicky pain and vague malaise.

Consult a doctor; sigmoidoscopy; barium enema; antispasm drugs; increased fibre and bran in diet.

Coronary thrombosis
See **Thrombosis, coronary,** p.914.

Cystitis
See **Cystitis,** p.872.

Deafness
See **Ear problems: deafness,** p.920.

Depression

Early morning waking; general unhappiness; difficulty in making decisions; loss of sex drive; anxiety (*see* p.864); tendency to avoid people; worse early in day.

Discuss with a doctor; appropriate antidepressant drugs may help; psychotherapy may be needed.

Bursitis may present itself as "miner's elbow", "housemaid's knee", or "typist's shoulder". The condition is due to friction or inflammation of a bursa, a sac of liquid near a joint cavity which cushions and lubricates joint movement.

See also **Bunion,** p.906.

Any lump in the breast must be examined by a doctor as soon as possible, to determine whether it is benign, malignant, or cystic. Additional symptoms may include a puckering of the overlying skin, bleeding from the nipple, or inflammation of the pigmented area around the nipple. Further treatment depends on the extent of spread. Removal of the breast may follow deep X-ray treatment of local glands and cancer-killing drug therapy.

Because some forms of gynaecological cancer may have no symptoms in the early stages, it is important for a woman to have a regular, routine examination, and an annual cervical smear (Pap) test. If cancer is discovered, further treatment may require operative removal of the womb (hysterectomy) and ovaries. Early cancer of the cervix can be treated with local surgical removal, radiotherapy, or laser beam therapy.

Carpal tunnel syndrome is more common in women than in men. It is usually worse during pregnancy or before a period, and is sometimes associated with rheumatoid arthritis (*see* p.894), or with an underactive thyroid gland. The condition is caused by the ligaments in the wrist swelling and compressing the median nerve that passes through them.

The patient is often anxious, tense and at times depressed. He or she may experience diarrhoea early in the day or after meals. The sigmoidoscope examination and the X-ray allow the specialist to observe the state of the internal surface of the bowel, and help to determine whether the bowel is diseased. The cause of the condition is not known but other more serious diseases, such as cancer (*see* **Cancer, intestinal,** p.908), diverticular disease (*see* p.920), and amoebic dysentery must be checked for.

A severe state of depression can lead to suicidal thoughts or to an attempt to commit suicide. If so, there may be a need for hospitalization for further treatment. Depression is particularly likely to follow traumatic events, such as a death, or the birth of a baby. It is also common after prolonged or serious illnesses, or as a result of an injury, although it can occur without apparent cause.

SYMPTOMS AND SIGNS	TREATMENT

Deviated nasal septum
Difficulty breathing through one nostril; recurrent attacks of sinusitis (*see* p.866); snoring; catarrh (*see* p.824).

Diagnosis made by a doctor; operation to break and straighten septum between nasal cavities, with partial removal of septum.

Diabetes mellitus
See **Diabetes mellitus,** p.910.

Encephalitis
Confusion; fever (*see* p.832); severe headache (*see* p.858); stiff neck; dislike of bright light; vomiting (*see* p.838).

Doctor will have patient admitted to hospital to confirm diagnosis and for treatment; lumbar puncture made to examine cerebrospinal fluid.

Epididymitis
See **Epididymitis,** p.886.

Fibroids
Often no symptoms; heavy periods, which may cause anaemia (iron deficiency in blood); sometimes frequent but painless urination; infertility.

No need for treatment unless symptoms severe; fibroids may be removed in order to treat infertility, but this can be difficult; rarely, removal of womb.

Frozen shoulder
Painful limitation of movement of shoulder that gradually increases in severity; pain then ceases, leaving joint stiff; slow improvement over six to twelve months.

Consult a doctor; rest arm in sling; pain-killing and antirheumatic drugs; gentle exercises and heat treatment; sometimes injection of corticosteroid drugs may help.

Gingivitis
Soreness and bleeding from gums, which may lead to loosening of teeth.

Regular brushing of teeth; use of dental floss to remove bacterial formation (plaque) from teeth; regular visits to dentist; consult a doctor if condition persists.

Haemorrhoids (piles)
Irritation, soreness, and sometimes pain in anal region with bleeding on defecation; often a small lump can be felt; symptoms vary in intensity; in some cases no symptoms.

Anaesthetic creams and suppositories under direction of a doctor; if symptoms persist consult doctor again; injection or operation may be needed; include bulk such as bran and vegetable fibre in diet; avoid constipation.

Heart valve disease
Gradually increasing breathlessness when taking exercise; sometimes palpitations (abnormally rapid heart beat); "heart murmur"; ankle swelling; fainting.

Doctor's assessment with X-rays and specialized heart investigation; treatment with diuretics, digoxin, and rhythm-controlling drugs; heart valve replacement surgery if medical treatment ineffective.

Kidney stone
See **Kidney stone,** p.912.

Mania
Extreme, often unwarranted enthusiasm; increased sex drive; physical overactivity; finally, supreme feeling of self-righteousness and power; delusion of grandeur; inability to maintain any single course of action, leading to exhaustion and incoherence.

Consult a doctor; hospital treatment with sedative drugs and skilled psychiatric care.

The symptoms of deviated nasal septum are usually at their worst during a cold (*see* p.826) or during an attack of hay fever (*see* p.844). The deviated nasal septum may have been bent since birth, or it may be the result of a nose injury.

Encephalitis is usually a result of a virus infection. It may be a complication of mumps or measles and sometimes develops because of poisoning with a metal such as lead. Encephalitis lethargica may be associated with the development of Parkinson's disease (*see* p.924) about twenty or thirty years later.

Fibroids are benign swellings of the normal uterine muscle. They slowly increase in size until menopause (*see* p.900) because of hormonal stimulus. After the menopause, fibroids usually shrink, and rarely become malignant. The condition is more common in women who have never been pregnant.

Often, an X-ray of the shoulder does not reveal anything abnormal. The patient may not have a history of injury and the pain may start spontaneously for no obvious reason. Frozen shoulder sometimes develops following coronary thrombosis (*see* p.914).

A lack of dental care allows infection to reach the bone under the teeth. Gingivitis is relatively common in diabetes (*see* p.910), pregnancy, or during drug treatment for epilepsy (*see* p.910), and often develops as a result of a lack of vitamin C. The condition is most commonly seen in the elderly.

Haemorrhoids, which can be external to the anus, or internal, are masses of swollen, inflamed veins in the rectum. The characteristic irritation is due to inflammation of the overlying skin. Haemorrhoids are commonly caused by constipation or pregnancy. Sometimes haemorrhoids can be very painful, and may swell, because of a thrombosis. Relief may be gained by applying an ice bag to the affected area, taking painkilling drugs, and resting in bed. The condition may take several days to disappear.

Sometimes, more than one heart valve is diseased, and heart failure (*see* p.912) may develop with atrial fibrillation (*see* p.906). Most patients know that they have a "heart murmur", and from this a specialist can detect which valve is involved. The disorder may be due to a congenital abnormality, or it may be due to damage following rheumatic fever.

Mania can develop as a result of the use of stimulant drugs, but usually occurs as a relatively rare form of depression (*see* p.896), known as manic-depressive illness.

SYMPTOMS AND SIGNS	TREATMENT

Ménière's disease
See **Ear problems: Ménière's disease,** p.910.

Meningitis

Severe headache; vomiting; neck stiffness; dislike of bright light or sound; moderate, irregular fever; irritability; loss of appetite.

Consult a doctor urgently; hospitalization for bed rest and skilled care; lumbar puncture for examination of spinal fluid; liquid diet needed; possibly intravenous feeding; corticosteroid drugs and antibiotics, if appropriate.

Menopause (climacteric)

Irregular periods of varying length; hot flushes, sweats and mild depression (*see* p.896); premenstrual tension (*see* p.902); periods sometimes cease, although these other symptoms continue; may last several months or years; may be no symptoms.

Consult a doctor; gynaecological examination necessary; drugs or hormones may stop flushes and regulate periods.

Menstrual disorders

Irregular periods with heavy clots; periods that occur too frequently, or infrequently; painful periods (*see* p.876).

Consult a doctor; investigations of cause and then appropriate treatment; sometimes curettage of lining of womb.

Migraine
See **Migraine,** p.874.

Multiple sclerosis

Double vision; weakness or tingling in limbs; dizziness or bladder problems; blindness; symptoms likely to disappear, then return, leading to increasingly abnormal gait, muscle weakness, and finally paralysis.

Consult a doctor; diagnosis made from history of recurring symptoms; physical examination and lumbar puncture to examine spinal fluid; sometimes corticosteroid drugs help during an acute attack; physiotherapy and rehabilitation may also help.

Myasthenia gravis

Muscle weakness after use; commonly affecting eyes, resulting in drooping lid and double vision; but any muscle group may be involved.

Consult a doctor; special tests to confirm diagnosis; treatment with drugs usually controls disease; muscle fatigue improves with rest; surgical removal of thymus gland said to be effective in some cases.

Obesity

Weight twenty per cent above normal average for height, age, and sex; breathlessness; sweating; painful joints; increased fatigue; sometimes anxiety (*see* p.872) or depression (*see* p.896).

Consult a doctor; appetite-reducing drugs may be prescribed in early stages; increase exercise gradually; reduce alcohol and carbohydrate intake; develop healthy diet.

Peripheral neuritis (polyneuritis)

Pain, weakness and tingling in peripheral nerves connecting brain and spinal cord with muscles, skin, organs and other parts of the body; may include loss of sensation and numbness of extremities.
See **Carpal tunnel syndrome,** p.896.

Consult a doctor; may need diet with vitamin supplements; physiotherapy; possibly surgical decompression of nerve; acute condition may need hospital treatment.

Meningitis is an inflammation of the membranes (meninges) which cover the brain and spinal cord. It is caused by bacteria, such as meningococci, or viruses, that infect the meninges directly from the surrounding tissue, or indirectly through the blood.

Menopause is the end of menstruation, and of the female reproductive life. The climacteric is the period of time when hormonal changes cause the symptoms of flushes, palpitations, and sometimes depression, which may be accompanied by a loss of interest in sex. Hormone replacement therapy is a temporary help for the years during which the body adjusts to the new hormone levels.

Menstrual disorders are a complex problem that may require hormones to regulate menstruation if the trouble is hormonal in origin. The condition may also be a result of fibroids (*see* p.898), menopause (*see* p.900), or salpingitis (*see* p.888). It is also sometimes caused by thyroid disorders.

Multiple sclerosis is more common in women than in men and rarely starts after age forty-five. In many patients it does not develop as far as paralysis. The cause is not known but it may be due to a chronic virus infection of the nervous system.

The severity of myasthenia gravis varies greatly from time to time and in different people. In some people, the onset of the disease is acute and is accompanied by severe respiratory problems and difficulty in swallowing. The speech may be slurred and the gait staggering. It rarely occurs in infants.

Obesity increases the chances of developing diabetes mellitus (*see* p.910), osteoarthritis (*see* p.924), high blood pressure (*see* p.894), arteriosclerosis (*see* p.906), heart disease, and bronchitis (*see* p.906). Obesity rarely develops because of hormone problems such as Cushing's disease or myxoedema (*see* p.924). Some people have an inherited tendency to obesity but the condition is usually the result of family dietary customs, particularly excessive carbohydrate and alcohol intake, as well as lack of exercise.

Patients usually recover if the cause is discovered. Causes include: pressure from the spine on a nerve in the neck; arterial disorders such as arteriosclerosis (*see* p.906); some virus infections; poisoning by some metals and chemicals; diabetes; alcoholism; only rarely is the condition associated with cancer. Complications may include lack of control over the bladder and bowels, as well as impotence. In severe cases the skin becomes pale and dry.

SYMPTOMS AND SIGNS	TREATMENT

Premenstrual tension

Irritability; depression (*see* p.896); headaches; constipation; breast tenderness; increase in weight in the ten days before menstruation.

Consult a doctor; fluid removing drugs (diuretics), mild antidepressants, or hormones may help to relieve symptoms if taken during the ten days before menstruation.

Rosacea

Patchy, red thickening of skin on face, nose and sometimes neck; accentuated by flushing; severity varies greatly from time to time.

Consult a doctor; avoid things that cause flushing, such as hot drinks, alcohol, hot fires; small doses of antibiotics by mouth; sulphur and corticosteroid creams applied to face.

Sinusitis

Catarrh (*see* p.824); face pain; pain in teeth or jaw; often fever in an acute attack; headaches; frequently associated with a cold contracted after flying or swimming.

Consult a doctor; X-rays may be needed to confirm diagnosis; drugs, nose drops and inhalations increase sinus drainage; antibiotics often needed; painkilling drugs when required; repeated attacks may need local heat treatment or surgery.

Slipped disc

Acute pain in lower back spreading to leg (sciatica); or at back of neck spreading along arms to fingers; usually occurs after strain of lifting heavy object; weakness and loss of sensation in area supplied by the nerve; may be very painful to walk.

Consult a doctor immediately; X-rays to confirm diagnosis; painkilling and antirheumatic drugs; immobilization of neck or back in collar or corset; physiotherapy and manipulation sometimes relieve symptoms; surgical removal of disc necessary in some cases.

Thrombosis, venous
See **Thrombosis, venous,** p.912.

Thyrotoxicosis

May include: irritability; anxiety; sweating; restlessness; weight loss despite increased appetite; protruding eyes; palpitations (rapid throbbing or fluttering of heart); trembling hands; sometimes diarrhoea; swelling in neck may be noticed.

Consult a doctor; diagnosis confirmed by examination and blood tests; treatment with antithyroid drugs, radioactive iodine or surgery (thyroidectomy).

Ulcer, peptic

Pain often occurs before eating, and is reduced by ingestion of antacids; symptoms aggravated by alcohol and fried food; sometimes, patients wake in middle of night because of pain.

Consult a doctor; barium meal and gastroscopy confirm diagnosis; medical treatment with milk and alkali mixtures to relieve pain; bed rest; stopping alcohol intake and smoking; various drugs may be effective.

Varicose veins
See **Varicose veins,** p.914.

Venereal disease
See **Chancroid,** p.872; **Gonorrhoea,** p.874; **Granuloma inguinale,** p.876; **Syphilis,** p.878.

Vertigo
See **Vertigo,** p.914.

Premenstrual tension is sometimes associated with menstrual disorders (*see* p.900) and painful periods (*see* p.876). Some patients also suffer from migraine (*see* p.874). The condition usually develops because of hormonal imbalance, and this is why the administration of hormones is often beneficial.

This skin condition is more common in men than in women, and may be associated with anxiety (*see* p.872), particularly in people who have an inherited tendency to develop sebaceous gland disorders. Rhinophyma (swollen red nose) may occasionally occur, and this can be treated by cosmetic surgery.

The discomfort is mainly felt in the cheek bone and sometimes above the eyes, rarely in the interior sinuses. Sinusitis may produce a toothache, a constant cough from postnasal "drip," and a husky voice. The condition is aggravated by smoking and dusty work. Repeated infections of the air spaces or sinuses in the skull prevent normal drainage.

A slipped disc develops because of a rupture of one of the pads of cartilage that act as shock absorbers between the spinal vertebrae. The soft centre of the ruptured disc slips out of place and presses on a nerve. The condition has a tendency to improve, then to relapse after a new strain, so the best method to prevent recurrence is to learn how to lift or carry heavy objects, or not to lift them at all.

In most cases, thyrotoxicosis is caused by the presence of an antibody that overstimulates the activity of the thyroid gland. Heart problems, such as heart failure and atrial fibrillation (*see* p.906), are often associated with thyrotoxicosis in the elderly. Treatment, particularly with radioactive iodine, is sometimes followed by myxoedema (*see* p.924). Thyroid nodules may be found and these require surgery.

The pain after food usually lasts for one or two hours. There may be long periods of freedom from pain, followed by several more weeks of symptoms. Recurrent ulceration may cause perforation, haemorrhage, or obstruction. Ulceration may also continue because of the failure of drug treatment and will then require surgery. Peptic ulcers are aggravated by stress, anxiety, alcohol, tobacco, and some drugs, such as aspirin and antirheumatics. If the patient wakes in the night it is more likely to be because of a duodenal ulcer, whereas pain on eating is more typically a symptom of a gastric ulcer.

The middle-aged (age 50-65): introduction

Men and women between the ages of fifty and sixty-five go through a series of changes in their lifestyle as they prepare for retirement. The changes may be major, but given good health care, these should be pleasant years. But no one at this age can expect to have the same healthy body he or she had as a young adult.

A person of fifty or sixty will usually have a slower reaction time and may take longer to make decisions. He or she will probably function as usual during normal conditions, but may find it harder to respond quickly to changes, or to physical or emotional stress. Unfortunately, as the individual ages, minor disorders become more serious, and the body is unable to compensate for some of the physical changes that may occur.

Foot problems, such as pain from bunions or metatarsalgia, are common, and orthopaedic difficulties, such as arthritis, rheumatism, gout, or the deformity of Dupuytren's contracture, may develop. A major problem is, of course, the loss of some or all of the teeth. Most people adjust to the use of false teeth (dentures). If dentures are fitted correctly, they should allow food to be chewed as thoroughly as with natural teeth.

Diet is probably the commonest cause of gastrointestinal problems. A diet that has too much animal fat can lead to cholecystitis; drinking too much alcohol can cause cirrhosis; and overeating leads to obesity, with an associated weakening of the abdominal muscles, which makes the development of hiatus hernia (or other hernia) more likely.

An incorrect diet, especially in someone who is overweight, can precipitate diabetes mellitus. Diet is also associated with heart and circulation problems, such as arteriosclerosis, which is aggravated by smoking. This arterial disease may cause angina pectoris, coronary thrombosis, and disorders of the heart rate (atrial fibrillation), and may cause heart failure. Heart failure may also occur as a result of heart valve disease, coronary thrombosis, or endocrine gland disorders such as thyrotoxicosis or myxoedema. Heart failure may also be associated with emphysema or severe lung disease. All heart and circulation problems are aggravated by obesity and smoking. The development of varicose veins or venous thrombosis is partly due to an inherited tendency. But it may also be associated with any condition, such as obesity, fibroids, or an abdominal tumour, that increases abdominal pressure.

At this age, a person's vitality may diminish, and in most people the problems of sexuality are less evident because of a reduced sex drive. The gynaecological problems of menopause pass, but the reduced level of hormone production may cause weakening of the pelvic tissue, as a result of which prolapse of the womb can occur. Male problems are usually minor. Apart from an increasingly frequent need to urinate, caused by the increasing size of the prostate gland, the most likely disorder to occur is swelling of one side of the scrotum (hernia). Other urinary problems occur in some cases. These include kidney stone, and pyelonephritis.

Recurrent attacks of acute bronchitis may develop into chronic bronchitis. This is also likely to develop as a result of smoking, or of years of work in a dusty atmosphere. The late onset of asthma is distressing and, unlike asthma in the young, it is rarely caused by an allergy. Pleurisy is not only painful but is more serious in those who smoke.

At this stage of life psychological problems associated with divorce, business worries, or elderly parents, may cause insomnia as well as anxiety and mild depression.

Fortunately, neurological disorders are rare. The severe, unexpected face pain of trigeminal neuralgia is alarming and may be difficult to treat. Epilepsy may develop at this age and, if it does, unlike epilepsy in a younger age group, it often has a cause which can be identified by appropriate tests.

Eye problems may be caused by the altering elasticity of the lens, causing longsightedness, and making it necessary to wear glasses. A detached retina may also occur. Regular eye testing is needed to ensure that the first signs of glaucoma are not missed, because this causes a gradual loss of vision, and may lead to blindness if not treated. Retinitis can also produce a painless, gradual deterioration in vision. Ear problems may arise because of variable fluid pressure in the inner ear. Ménière's disease, causing severe attacks of nausea, variable deafness, and vertigo, is an example.

The main causes of anxiety about health in this age group are heart problems, which have been mentioned, and cancer. Any swelling, change in normal bowel habit, or persistent cough may be suspected as an early symptom of cancer. All such fears must be discussed with a doctor, but only rarely is the fear justified. Blood in the faeces is as likely to be due to diverticulitis as to cancer of the intestine; blood in the urine may indicate an infection, although it may also indicate cancer of the urinary tract.

Any alteration in size, shape, or colour, of a skin mole or marking is more alarming, and must be discussed with a doctor immediately, because of the possibility of cancer of the skin. Other causes of lumps in the skin include the very slow, painless swelling of a sebaceous cyst, and the small nodule of a rodent ulcer.

Prevention of arteriosclerosis can begin in childhood, by avoiding animal fats in the diet. In early adult life smoking can be avoided, not only to prevent lung cancer, arteriosclerosis, and cancer of the urinary tract, but also to protect the lungs from chronic bronchitis, emphysema, and other disorders of the respiratory system. Equally important is

regular exercise. This should be more than a weekly game of golf, or a swim. Daily exercise improves the condition of the heart, and exercises the lungs. In this way, full use is made of the heart and lungs for a few minutes each day. A side effect of this is a sense of mental well-being.

Regular assessment by a doctor will help the individual to maintain good health, and may detect early signs of disease. But even if such check-ups are routine, it is essential not to ignore any symptoms that last longer than a few days, without consulting a doctor.

Health care checklist

Regular check-ups by a doctor are sensible precautions to take against the development of diseases and disorders. At the same time, the following questions are useful to alert each person to danger signals. Use this checklist to assess your state of health, and try to do this regularly, for instance at the beginning of each month.

Q: Skin rash on any part of body?

Q: Chest pain when taking exercise?

Q: Frequent sniffing and sneezing? Cough? If cough, blood in cough? Hoarseness? Chest problems? Shortness of breath?

Q: Persistent pain and stiffness in spine, joints, limbs, or any other part of body?

Q: Weight loss that is not caused by dieting? Vomiting? Appetite loss? Indigestion? Nausea? Sudden weight gain?

Q: Change in bowel habits? Diarrhoea? Constipation? Abdominal and stomach pain? Blood in faeces?

Q: Change in urinary habits? Pain when urinating? Blood in urine? Pain in anal or genital region?

Q: Vaginal discharge? Unexpected vaginal bleeding? Irritation?

Q: Sore that will not heal on penis? Lump that will not go away?

Q: Excessive use of alcohol, heavy smoking, or habit of taking drugs?

Q: Fainting, hot flushes, or sudden feeling of weakness?

Q: Fever, with or without nausea and vomiting? Recurrent severe headaches?

Some of the questions apply only to women and some only to men. If the answer to all of the questions is "No", then almost certainly you are in good health, with no need to worry. But, if the answer to any of the questions is "Yes", then a doctor should be consulted for an expert medical opinion.

Q: Hearing problems? Itching and painful discharge from ear? Deafness and earache?

Q: Vision problems? Sore eyes? Pain or irritation around eyes?

Q: Lump that does not disappear in breast or other part of body?

Q: Sore that will not heal?

Q: Change in shape, colour, or size of any skin mark or wart?

Q: Nervousness, irritability, or depression?

Q: Apathy or lethargy?

Q: Weeping without obvious reason? Feeling of persecution? Hearing voices?

Q: Overwhelming sadness or despair? Feeling unable to cope? Feeling of being rundown or unduly fatigued? Difficulty sleeping? Insomnia?

Q: Pain and swelling around teeth? Sore, coated tongue and sore gums? Lump or sore on tongue or gums? Bleeding gums? Uncomfortable dentures?

Q: Persistent cold sores around mouth?

Q: Scalp irritated and itchy, flaking skin? Sudden loss of hair? Persistent sores on scalp?

905

SYMPTOMS AND SIGNS	TREATMENT

Angina pectoris

Mid-chest pain often extending into one or both arms, also to neck, jaw, and sometimes abdomen; pain occurring after exercise; may also occur in cold weather, after large meals, or following extreme emotion; slight breathlessness occurs frequently; condition improves after a few minutes.

Consult a doctor; examination using electrocardiograph; general treatment resembles that for arteriosclerosis (*see* p.906), and includes weight loss, giving up smoking, low cholesterol diet, medical treatment to reduce blood pressure; use of drugs to prevent attacks and to relieve pain.

Arteriosclerosis

Symptoms caused by narrowing of arteries; if affecting heart arteries, may lead to angina pectoris (*see* p.906), coronary thrombosis or heart failure; if affecting arteries that supply nervous system, may cause episodes of momentary weakness, difficulty in speaking, blindness, or stroke; if affecting other arteries, may cause limping when walking, due to calf pain, or gangrene of the toes.

Discuss with a doctor; stop smoking; reduce blood pressure; lose weight; eat low cholesterol diet; check for diabetes (*see* p.910) and myxoedema (*see* p.924); in some cases, cholesterol-reducing drugs and anticoagulants are prescribed.

Arthritis, osteo-
See **Osteoarthritis**, p.924.

Arthritis, rheumatoid
See **Arthritis, rheumatoid**, p.894.

Asthma

Episodes of wheezing and breathlessness; sometimes associated with coughing; often started by contact with allergic substance or by infection; late-onset asthma, after age fifty, seldom due to allergy; main symptoms include dry, persistent cough, and breathlessness without wheezing.

Discuss with a doctor; treatment with antispasmodic drugs and sprays to relieve attack; regular use of a corticosteroid or disodium cromoglycate (Intal) spray may prevent further attacks; if infection is present, causing acute bronchitis (*see* p.884), immediate use of antibiotics needed; breathing exercises help prevent attacks.

Atrial fibrillation

Rapid heartbeat; irregularities in rhythm and in rate; usually occurring periodically, but may be permanent; feeling of vague chest discomfort; slight breathlessness.

Consult a doctor; electrocardiogram confirms diagnosis; treatment with digoxin to regulate heart rhythm; rarely, electric shock (cardioversion) may be done in hospital.

Blood pressure, high (hypertension)
See **Blood pressure, high (hypertension)**, p.894.

Bronchitis, acute
See **Bronchitis, acute**, p.884.

Bronchitis, chronic

Cough, particularly in the morning, producing clear sputum; sometimes shortness of breath; tendency to suffer attacks of acute bronchitis (*see* p.884); coughing during day.

Any worsening of symptoms must be treated immediately; antibiotics; daily breathing exercises; stopping smoking; if necessary, moving to cleaner, warmer climate.

Bunion

Painful swelling on side of joint behind big toe; usually accompanied by deformity of toe (hallux valgus), in which toe points toward the other toes on foot.

Relieve pressure on bunion with pads and by cutting an opening in shoe; wear low-heeled shoes; consult a specialist; in severe cases, an operation to remove bunion.

The pain is caused by the narrowing of the coronary arteries that supply heart muscle, so that there is an oxygen deficiency in the muscles. Hiatus hernia (*see* p.834), peptic ulcer (*see* p.902) and cholecystitis (*see* p.908) may all cause similar pain. Surgery is considered only if other treatment fails.

Arteriosclerosis is often associated with an increase of cholesterol and other fatty substances in the blood. Early discovery of this, and early treatment may prevent the development of arteriosclerosis.

Arteriosclerosis is also associated with high blood pressure (*see* p.894), diabetes (*see* p.910), smoking and lack of exercise.

If a person has suffered from asthma since early childhood, the symptoms usually improve as the person grows older. However, recurrence of asthma in a severe form may lead to complications that include dehydration, exhaustion, and respiratory distress. Recurrent asthma may cause lung damage and emphysema (*see* p.920), and an acute attack can rupture a lung (*see* **Pneumothorax,** p.888). Patients with asthma become anxious and fearful of further attacks. Tranquillizing drugs may help. Desensitizing injections seldom help late-onset asthma, but a skin test should be done to exclude allergy as a cause.

Atrial fibrillation is more commonly caused by heart valve disease (*see* p.898) in younger patients, and by arteriosclerosis (*see* p.906) or thyrotoxicosis in older patients.

Chronic bronchitis causes lung damage (scarring), emphysema (*see* p.920), and may eventually lead to heart failure. The chronic condition often develops in people working in a dusty environment, for example, in mining and in other industries where the atmosphere is dusty, cold and damp.

Bunions are more common in women than in men, primarily because women tend to wear tight-fitting or high-heeled shoes. The bunion may become infected if the friction of the shoe causes inflammation of the sac of fluid over the joint.

See also **Bursitis** p.896

SYMPTOMS AND SIGNS	TREATMENT

Cancer, breast
See **Cancer, breast,** p.896.

Cancer, gynaecological
See **Cancer, gynaecological,** p.896.

Cancer, intestinal
Early symptoms: alteration of normal bowel habit; alternating constipation and diarrhoea, with mucus and blood; pain; haemorrhoids (*see* p.898) may also occur.

Consult a doctor; investigation with barium meal, sigmoidoscopy, and fibroscopy; blood and cancer cells may be found in faeces; surgery to remove affected part; drug therapy.

Cancer, lung
Early symptoms: cough, with blood-stained sputum, occurring without obvious cause; symptoms resemble acute bronchitis (*see* p.824; 842).

Consult a doctor; chest X-ray; sputum examination for cancer cells and bronchoscopy (a tube passed down the trachea under a general anaesthetic) to confirm diagnosis.

Cancer, oesophagus
See **Cancer, oesophagus,** p.918.

Cancer, prostate
See **Cancer, prostate,** p.918.

Cancer, skin
Early symptoms: any mole or pigmented area of skin that grows larger, changes colour, ulcerates, or bleeds.

Consult a doctor; removal of part of area (biopsy), for microscopic examination to confirm diagnosis; surgery, drug therapy, or radiotherapy may be successful.

Cancer, stomach
Early symptoms: loss of appetite; loss of weight; vomiting; black stools (melaena); sometimes vague indigestion.

Consult a doctor; investigation with barium meal and gastroscopy; biopsy of part of ulcerated area will confirm diagnosis; difficult to treat as diagnosis is usually made late in course of disease; drug therapy effective in some cases; complete removal of stomach (total gastrectomy) may be required; this may also be done to reduce later symptoms of bleeding and pain.

Cancer, urinary tract
Early symptoms of cancer of bladder or ureter: painless bleeding into urine; pain may occur when clots of blood are passed; frequent urination may or may not be a symptom; if kidney swelling can be felt, this is a sign of kidney involvement.

Consult a doctor; investigation of kidneys by intravenous pyelogram; examination of bladder; examination of urine for cancer cells; cancer of the kidney treated by surgical removal of kidney; cancer of bladder treated by local removal or by radiotherapy.

Cholecystitis, acute
Fever; vomiting; severe pain in upper right abdomen; sometimes jaundice (*see* p.816; 874); dark urine.

Consult a doctor; hospitalization; diagnosis with X-ray and cholecystogram; antibiotics; painkilling drugs; intravenous fluids; occasionally, immediate operation to remove gall bladder (cholecystectomy).

In some cases, obstruction of the intestine is the first symptom of cancer and this may be accompanied by abdominal pain and distension as well as vomiting (*see* p.838) and constipation (*see* p.826).

If cancer appears operable, the surgeon may remove part or all of the lung (pneumonectomy). Radiotherapy and cancer-killing drugs are often effective in prolonging the lives of those who cannot be treated surgically. Lung cancer is twenty times more common in cigarette smokers than in non-smokers, and also occurs more frequently in those who have inhaled asbestos, radioactive materials or some other industrial pollutants regularly in the course of their occupations.

Rodent ulcers (*see* p.926), a locally invasive cancer, and squamous cell cancer, commonly occur in fair-skinned people who have been exposed to intensive sunlight for long periods of time. Local removal usually cures the lesion. A dark mole (melanoma) may be malignant and need to be treated by the removal of a large area of skin, and by skin grafting. Melanomas occur most commonly on the legs (particularly of women), and on the trunk (particularly of men), and spread rapidly if not treated.

Several other disorders have symptoms that resemble those of stomach cancer. The commonest disorder with such symptoms is peptic ulcer (*see* p.902). Gallstones (cholelithiasis), pancreatitis, and coronary artery disease also produce similar symptoms.

Renal, ureter and bladder cancer can all occur independently. Each may arise spontaneously. The incidence of cancer of the bladder is increased in some industrial occupations. Cancer of the bladder is most likely to be caused by industrial dyes, or by tars that pass through the kidneys of smokers.

When the acute attack has settled and the patient has recovered, a gall bladder X-ray is performed and then, if necessary, the gall bladder may be removed. The condition is often associated with gallstones.

SYMPTOMS AND SIGNS	TREATMENT

Cholecystitis, chronic
Recurrent indigestion; heartburn; flatulence; discomfort after fatty meals.

Consult a doctor; diagnosis confirmed by gall bladder X-ray; operation usually advised; in some cases gallstones can be dissolved with special drugs.

Cirrhosis
Often no symptoms until late in course of disease; loss of appetite; vague malaise; loss of sex drive; abdominal swelling may occur because of retention of fluid in abdominal cavity.

Stop all alcohol; protein diet with extra vitamins; these measures may halt progress of disease; treatment with corticosteroids, and sometimes a dietary supplement of multivitamins may be helpful.

Diabetes mellitus
Often no symptoms; condition commonly discovered at routine examination of urine; weight loss, despite increased appetite; in some cases, diabetes is indicated by recurrent boils, infection, lethargy, thirst, and genital moniliasis (*see* p.924).

Diagnosis confirmed by test of urine for sugar, blood test, and glucose tolerance test; treatment with special diet to reduce weight and to control intake of sugar; in some cases, pills to stimulate insulin production; less frequently, insulin injections.

Dupuytren's contracture
Nodule in palm of hand; painless, rigid flexion of ring or little fingers that develops gradually; both hands may be affected. Rarely, feet also affected.

Consult a doctor; injection of corticosteroids may be helpful in early stages; gradual contraction can be treated only by surgical means.

Ear problems: Ménière's disease
Buzzing in ear; may last months or years before sudden onset of dizziness, nausea, and vomiting; temporary deafness; several attacks close together, followed by long period without attacks; increasing deafness.

Consult a doctor; antinausea drugs during an attack; various drugs may help between attacks; surgery is effective, but may cause deafness.

Epilepsy
Periodic, recurrent seizures; symptoms of the various forms of epilepsy include: brief periods of impaired awareness; fainting; jerky spasms of one muscle group; generalized severe convulsions; and loss of consciousness; in some cases attacks are proceeded by disturbances of smell or hearing (aura).

Consult a doctor: diagnosis based on the person's medical history and on electroencephalogram (EEG) studies of the brain's electrical activity; special drug therapy is used to control the symptoms of each particular type of epilepsy.

Eye problems: detached retina
Flashes of light; dark spots; a "veil" across vision; partial loss of sight.

Special techniques, using laser beam surgery or freezing, to reattach retina.

Eye problems: glaucoma
Intermittent attacks of dimness of vision, and the appearance of halos around lights; sometimes very severe eye and face pain; partial loss of vision; white of eye becomes inflamed; in some cases, no symptoms.

Examination by ophthalmologist, to detect raised pressure in eyeball; mild cases can be treated successfully with eye drops prescribed by a doctor; in severe cases, operation with careful follow-up.

Eye problems: longsightedness (presbyopia)
Difficulty in reading print, or in seeing near objects.

Vision corrected by wearing bifocal or multifocal spectacles, which help correct both near and distant vision.

Chronic cholecystitis is particularly common in middle-aged women and in diabetics. Severe colic (*see* p.826) and jaundice (*see* p.816; 874) may occur if a gallstone moves into the bile duct, and acute cholecystitis may also develop. Gallstones are usually made from cholesterol, but may consist of only bile salts, or a mixture of cholesterol and bile salts.

Cirrhosis is most commonly due to excessive alcohol intake and is only rarely due to an infection of the bile ducts or to infectious hepatitis (*see* p.874). Complications include jaundice (*see* p.816; 874), which may occur late in the disease, and rupture of a vein in the oesophagus, which will cause massive haemorrhage.

The complications of diabetes mellitus may include arteriosclerosis (*see* p.906), gangrene (*see* p.922), retinitis (*see* p.912), polyneuritis (*see* p.900), recurrent infections, kidney disease, and coma due to excess insulin or excess sugar in the blood. A sudden onset of diabetes is more common in young people and this usually needs urgent treatment with insulin. The likelihood of developing diabetes is increased by alcoholism, obesity, pregnancy, and some thyroid gland disorders. Diabetes is also a condition that tends to run in families.

Dupuytren's contracture affects men more commonly than women. The right hand is affected more than the left. About fifty per cent of the cases have relatives who have the disorder. The condition is caused by thickening and contraction of the tough membrane in the palm that surrounds finger tendons.

The condition is due to an intermittent increase of fluid pressure in the organ of balance of the inner ear. The cause is unknown. The second ear becomes involved in fifteen per cent of patients, and the distortion of hearing is often very unpleasant. A feeling of pressure is often noticed in the ear before an attack starts.

There are several forms of epilepsy, some of them mild. The form known traditionally as petit mal is a brief lapse of consciousness that may last between 5 and 10 seconds. After a more serious attack, involving fainting or convulsions, the person may have a headache or want to sleep. Epilepsy may develop at any age but most cases are diagnosed in people younger than eighteen. In most cases epilepsy cannot be cured, although the symptoms can be controlled; epilepsy is therefore a life-long disorder. Late onset of epilepsy often has a cause such as a brain tumour, a stroke, or following injury.

The condition is more common in those who are shortsighted or have a family history of retinal detachment. It may also develop following an injury to the eye. The sooner treatment is given the better the result.

There are two main forms of glaucoma. The first causes symptoms in one eye only and is usually cured by an operation. The second form causes gradual loss of vision, which is usually not noticed at first, and involves both eyes. Untreated glaucoma causes blindness (*see* p.920). People who are longsighted, and who have a family history of glaucoma, need to be checked annually.

Longsightedness is due to the loss of the elasticity of the lens. Hyperopia, which is longsightedness in a younger age group, is a condition that develops because of the shape of the eye.

The middle-aged (age 50-65): disorders 4

SYMPTOMS AND SIGNS	TREATMENT
Eye problems: retinitis	
Gradual loss of vision; sometimes intolerance of light.	Examination of eye by ophthalmologist; protect eyes from light; consult a doctor for diagnosis and treatment of underlying cause.
Foot problems: metatarsalgia	
Pain in sole of foot at front; thickening of skin and tenderness in this part.	Consult a doctor; muscle strengthening exercises; arch supports not recommended; operation rarely required.
Gout	
Attacks of acute pain in joints; often lasting several days; usually beginning in the big toe and also affecting knee but any joint can be affected; joint becomes swollen and red.	Consult a doctor; diagnosis from appearance of joint and blood test; immediate treatment with antirheumatics, painkilling drugs, or colchichine; long-term treatment with drugs to reduce uric acid in body.
Heart failure	
Ankle swelling; shortness of breath on exercise; often slight cough; breathlessness at night, or when lying down.	Consult a doctor immediately in order that the underlying cause can be discovered and correct treatment given; diagnosis by means of chest X-ray and electrocardiograph; treatment with diuretics; digoxin used to strengthen heartbeat; bed rest, in sitting position; light, low-salt diet; adequate sedation at night until recovery.
Hernia (rupture)	
Swelling, usually in groin or at umbilicus; may be painful if it occurs suddenly, as a result of a strain; swelling often obvious only when standing or when coughing or straining; swelling can usually be pushed flat with gentle pressure, unless strangulation occurs.	Consult a doctor; surgery is only way of curing the condition; hernias in groin can be held in place with a special rupture belt (truss); surgical repair requires hospitalization for one week, then caution for about two months; avoid lifting heavy objects.
Hiatus hernia	
Heartburn; acid taste in mouth; chest pain particularly when lying down, bending forward or kneeling; pain made worse by alcohol, or large meals; mild cases may have no symptoms.	Consult a doctor; barium meal and X-ray, with head tilted down confirms diagnosis; sleep propped up on pillows; antacid mixtures also help.
Kidney stone	
Often no symptoms until stone moves out of kidney; then, severe pain in back, radiating to groin (renal colic); vomiting; blood in urine.	Consult a doctor; diagnosis from examination of urine for blood; strong painkilling drugs; rarely, surgery.
Leukaemia	
See **Leukaemia**, p.924.	
Neuralgia, trigeminal	
Brief attacks of severe pain on one side of face, usually affecting cheek and jaw; episodes sometimes triggered by pain in one area, by eating, touching skin, shaving, or by changes in temperature.	Consult a doctor; some drugs very effective but their use must be carefully controlled; occasionally operation required to cut nerve.

Retinitis may be associated with arteriosclerosis (*see* p.906), high blood pressure (*see* p.894), diabetes (*see* p.910), kidney disease (*see* **Pyelonephritis,** p.914), or infection.

Metatarsalgia may be associated with flatfoot, with wearing high heels, or with rheumatoid arthritis (*see* p.894). The condition develops when the heads of the metatarsal bones lose their arch and touch the ground. As a result, there is greater pressure on the heads of the metatarsals, and this causes pain.

Gout is caused by an increase in the level of uric acid in the blood, which is a result of an inability to excrete uric acid from the body. It is often an inherited disease. Prolonged gout can cause arthritis (*see* p.894) and kidney failure. Sometimes, nodules (tophi) of uric acid are found on the ears or the hands.

Heart failure is the inability of the heart to pump adequate amounts of blood through the body. Because of this, fluid retention occurs. The onset of acute heart failure with severe breathlessness (pulmonary oedema) needs urgent treatment and hospitalization. Sometimes the patient has bluish lips and hands (cyanosis) caused by an excess of carbon dioxide in the blood. In the elderly, confusion and restlessness commonly occur because of poor brain circulation. The condition may be caused by atrial fibrillation (*see* p.906), coronary thrombosis (*see* p.914), heart valve disease (*see* p.898), high blood pressure (*see* p.894), scarring in the lungs due to emphysema (*see* p.920), chronic bronchitis (*see* p.906), or other chest infections.

A rupture is due to local weakness in the muscle wall, allowing abdominal contents, intestine and fat, to push through under the skin. The disorder is more common in obese patients. Sometimes it is impossible to push back the swelling, or the intestines twist inside causing an intestinal obstruction, which leads to local pain and vomiting, and requires immediate treatment.

Hiatus hernia is due to part of the stomach being pushed through a weak point in the diaphragm muscle. It may be congenital and frequently occurs without symptoms. The disorder often occurs with obesity (*see* p.900) and usually improves with dieting. Major surgery is occasionally required to repair the hernia if symptoms are severe.

Kidney stones are caused by calcium abnormalities, sometimes due to parathyroid gland overactivity, as well as to deposits of uric acid in gout (*see* p.912), or to congenital abnormalities of cystine and oxalic acid metabolism. Further stones can be prevented from forming by increasing the intake of fluid and by adapting the diet. A kidney stone may cause inflammation, and ultimately lead to infection, at the point of blockage.

In trigeminal neuralgia there is no evidence of abnormality between periods of pain. The loss of sensation suggests some cause, such as tumour, rheumatoid arthritis (*see* p.894), or multiple sclerosis (*see* p.900), although the actual cause of this disorder is not known. Other similar facial pains, such as the pain after an attack of shingles (*see* p.926), usually last longer.

The middle-aged (age 50-65): disorders 5

SYMPTOMS AND SIGNS	TREATMENT
Pleurisy	
Severe pain in side of chest; pain made worse by breathing and coughing; usually fever.	Consult a doctor; chest X-ray; blood and sputum tests; treatment of underlying condition; painkilling drugs.
Prolapse of womb	
Often no symptoms; sometimes incontinence of urine, particularly when laughing, coughing or straining; feeling of weight or discomfort in vagina.	Consult a doctor; operation to tighten ligaments and muscles that support the womb; usually requires ten days in hospital; as a temporary measure, the prolapse can also be held in place with a pessary.
Prostate problems *See* **Prostate problems,** p.926.	
Pyelonephritis (kidney disease)	
Frequent urination; back pain; fever, sometimes shivering attacks and vomiting.	Consult a doctor; urine specimen for culture of bacteria; antibiotics for two weeks; further urological investigations may be necessary.
Stroke *See* **Stroke,** p.926.	
Teeth, loss of	
Loss of some or all teeth through dental disease.	Consult a dentist for advice about kinds of dentures available; regular check-ups help to reduce decay and loss of teeth.
Thrombosis, coronary	
Onset of severe mid-chest pain, often with distribution like angina pectoris (*see* p.906); sweating; shortness of breath and anxiety; sometimes symptoms are only slight.	Call a doctor immediately; lie quietly and still; immediate, strong painkilling drugs, such as morphine, may be helpful; hospitalization in coronary care unit for three to four days and then mainly bed rest for four more days before gradual movement; discharge after two weeks; regular use of anticoagulants may be required.
Thrombosis, venous	
Superficial venous thrombosis: pain, tenderness and slight swelling over line of superficial vein in one area of leg. Deep venous thrombosis may produce only calf pain and ankle swelling.	Consult a doctor; firm bandaging; painkilling and antirheumatic drugs; exercise; anticoagulant drugs may be necessary for a deep venous thrombosis.
Varicose veins	
Irregular, swollen veins visible in one or both legs; often slight ankle swelling; aching pain in lower part of leg.	Consult a doctor; elastic stockings prevent swelling and aching in legs; large veins can be removed surgically; smaller veins treated by cutting, or by injections; legs bandaged for six weeks.
Vertigo	
Spinning sensation; may be accompanied by nausea and vomiting; unsteady gait brought on by moving head; no deafness.	Consult a doctor; antinausea drugs may help; avoid any movement that is known to cause vertigo.

Pleurisy is caused by inflammation of the membranes between the lungs and the chest wall. It can be caused by bronchial pneumonia (*see* p.918), lung cancer (*see* p.908), a blood clot (embolus), or tuberculosis (*see* p.926).

With a prolapsed womb, if the patient is too old or weak, a plastic ring can be inserted into the vagina, to hold the womb in place. This ring has to be changed at regular intervals, recommended by the doctor. The disorder is usually the result of the ligaments and muscles supporting the womb being stretched during childbirth or because of excessive obesity (*see* p.900).

Inadequate treatment causes damage to the kidneys, which may lead to kidney failure. Infection is more common in patients whose kidneys have congenital abnormalities, or a kidney stone (*see* p.912), and in patients with prostate problems. Infection usually enters through the urinary tract, in women, but is carried by the blood in men.

Great care should be taken in choosing artificial teeth, because dentures that are fitted badly are not only painful but may also damage the mouth. Take care of dentures by regular cleaning. Rest the gums by taking the dentures out of the mouth each night.

A coronary thrombosis may follow angina pectoris, but can occur without a history of heart problems or chest pain. The patient usually feels overtired, in a state of stress, and feeling vaguely unwell for a few weeks before the attack. About fifty per cent of deaths take place before the patient has reached the hospital. Other heart conditions, such as atrial fibrillation (*see* p.906) and heart failure (*see* p.912) may occur at the same time. On recovery, diet and mild, careful exercise are essential parts of a regimen to prevent recurrence of the condition. Obesity (*see* p.900), smoking and arteriosclerosis (*see* p.906) are contributing factors to coronary thrombosis.

A superficial venous thrombosis is not serious and usually improves without complications. A deep venous thrombosis may cause problems if the blood clot (embolus) is released. If an embolus reaches the lungs it may cause the death of lung tissue, leading to pleurisy (*see* p.914) and, in severe cases, death. A superficial venous thrombosis can occur as a result of an injury, varicose veins, or ulceration of the leg.

Varicose veins develop because of weakness or absence of valves in the veins of the leg. This may occur after a venous thrombosis (*see* p.914), after valves are damaged by back pressure, as may occur during pregnancy, or as a result of a congenital defect. Varicose veins are cosmetically disfiguring in the early stages, and there is a tendency for varicose veins to recur. Eczema of the lower legs, haemorrhage or ulceration may also occur, particularly in the elderly.

Benign positional vertigo is of unknown cause, but seldom improves. Vertigo may be caused by vestibular neuronitis, an infection of the nerve of balance that is severe at first, but usually improves. The condition may also occur because of wax in the ear (*see* p.920), or arteriosclerosis (*see* p.906).
    See also **Ménière's disease,** p.910.

The elderly (age 65+): introduction

The gradual changes of late middle age can cause a rigidity of mental attitude, despite a minimal deterioration in intellectual function. The physical alterations in the body are partly due to the wear and tear of a lifetime of activity, or to disease, and partly because of a natural slowing in the nervous and muscular reactions.

Elderly people who remain in good physical and psychological health have active and useful lives. They may have accidents of any kind, but falls are most common, and fractures of the wrist and hip occur.

Such fractures may be complicated by the orthopaedic problems of osteoarthritis, and by loss of calcium from the bones, osteoporosis, which may lead to curvature of the spine and difficulty in standing straight. Fingers may become deformed by Heberden's nodes.

Prostate enlargement is a common male problem in this age group and is characterized by an urgency to urinate. This condition may be complicated by other ailments of the elderly, such as difficulty in walking because of an arthritic hip, which can make going to the toilet a problem.

Social isolation, particularly as experienced by those living alone, can be intensified by ear problems that cause deafness, even if this is only due to wax, as well as by eye problems, such as blindness and cataract. The cycle of events following minor illness may result in skin problems. Reduced resistance may allow shingles to develop, and the use of antibiotics may lead to the development of moniliasis in moist areas of skin, or in the vagina. The gradual onset of chronic forms of leukaemia may cause fatigue, weakness, and malaise, and may reduce a person's resistance to infections.

In those who smoke, or who have chronic bronchitis, chest problems that arise from emphysema will be intensified. In such people, pneumonia may follow any respiratory infection.

An active, elderly person who eats well should have few problems with constipation, but the condition is a common complaint in those who are inactive and who eat foods that are high in carbohydrates and low in fibre. Constipation may lead to a partial blockage of the intestine, and a type of diarrhoea in which liquid faeces bypass the harder mass. These symptoms may also indicate cancer or diverticular disease. Constipation may be a symptom of the glandular disorder myxoedema (hypothyroidism). It is also common in immobile arthritic patients who are being treated with painkilling drugs.

The combination of myxoedema, arteriosclerosis, and diabetes commonly results in arterial damage, which may cause a coronary thrombosis, gangrene or a stroke.

It is essential for the elderly person to maintain an active routine, to stimulate both body and mind. The diet of a person aged sixty-five or over must contain adequate protein, as well as fresh fruit and vegetables to provide bulk and vitamin C, particularly during the winter months. Vitamin deficiency is a common result of a bland diet of cheap, processed foods, which are easy to prepare, but are of only poor nutritional value. A combination of poor diet, inadequate heating of the home and poor health, may cause confusion and death due to lowered body temperature (hypothermia).

Hypothermia is a particular hazard for elderly people who live alone and who do not receive many visits from relatives or friends. Left alone for days during the winter, elderly people may simply sit, become confused, and eventually die. Neighbours should check on the well-being of such people.

Psychological problems of the elderly are made worse by a sense of loneliness and isolation, by the onset of depression following the deaths of close relatives or friends, and by loss of memory, leading to confusion. This confusion may be intensified by any disorder, such as deafness or blindness, by diseases such as pneumonia or leukaemia, as well as by the common problem of failing to understand the correct dosage of drugs, which may cause the elderly to take an excessive number of tranquillizers. Sleep may be disturbed by prostate problems, the discomfort of arthritis, pain from cramp in the leg, breathlessness from heart failure, or coughing from bronchitis and emphysema.

These are only some of the problems of the elderly. Such problems can be overcome by encouraging a healthy attitude towards the years of retirement, before psychological problems present difficulties. A strong interest in life and the world in general can make the difference between a long life of health and happiness, and a short life plagued by physical and psychological problems. Planning for retirement is particularly important. The person who does community work, or who has an absorbing hobby, is usually healthier than the person who does very little or nothing with his or her time.

For those who are less active there are, in most cities and small towns, social clubs for the elderly as well as special centres for their use during the day. Those who have lost relatives or friends through death, and those who live alone, can find companionship in such centres, which often have a visiting nurse; this is particularly valuable for people who are ill or crippled.

A common fear of people as they grow older is that they will succumb to senile dementia, lose their independence, and become confused and baby-like. The major cause of senile dementia is arteriosclerosis, a hardening of the arteries that supply blood and nourishment to the brain. This condition may be avoided by a sensible health care programme through earlier years. This can be started as early as age twenty-five. If senility develops, early medical care is necessary. Seeing that this medical care is given is the responsibility of relatives and friends.

If a person's physical or mental deterioration is accelerating, there may be no choice but to put him or her into a nursing home, hospital, or institution, where there are special facilities. The emphasis must be on early diagnosis and treatment. Because a person suffering from senile dementia usually has no awareness or insight into his or her condition, it is up to an alert observer to notice the onset of the disease.

Health care checklist

Regular check-ups by a doctor are sensible precautions to take against the development of diseases and disorders. At the same time, the following questions are useful to alert each person to danger signals. Use this checklist to assess your state of health, and try to do this regularly, for instance, at the beginning of each month.

Q: Skin rash on any part of body?

Q: Chest pain when taking exercise?

Q: Running nose? Frequent sniffing and sneezing? Cough? If cough, blood in cough? Hoarseness? Chest problems? Shortness of breath?

Q: Persistent pain and stiffness in spine, joints, limbs, or any other part of body?

Q: Weight loss that is not caused by dieting? Vomiting? Appetite loss? Indigestion? Nausea? Sudden weight gain?

Q: Change in bowel habits? Diarrhoea? Constipation? Abdominal and stomach pain? Blood in faeces?

Q: Change in urinary habits? Pain when urinating? Blood in urine? Pain in anal or genital region?

Q: Sore that will not heal on penis? Lump that will not go away?

Q: Excessive use of alcohol, heavy smoking, or habit of taking drugs?

Q: Fainting, hot flushes, or sudden feeling of weakness?

Q: Fever, with or without nausea and vomiting?

Q: Recurrent severe headaches?

Some of the questions apply only to women and some only to men. If the answer to all of the questions is "No", then almost certainly you are in good health, with no need to worry. But, if the answer to any of the questions is "Yes", then a doctor should be consulted for an expert medical opinion.

Q: Hearing problems? Itching and painful discharge from ear? Deafness and earache?

Q: Vision problems? Sore eyes? Pain or irritation around eyes?

Q: Lump that does not disappear in breast or other part of body?

Q: Sore that will not heal?

Q: Change in shape, colour, or size of any skin mark or wart?

Q: Nervousness, irritability or depression?

Q: Apathy or lethargy?

Q: Weeping without obvious reason? Feeling of persecution? Hearing voices?

Q: Overwhelming sadness or despair? Feeling unable to cope? Feeling of being rundown or unduly fatigued? Difficulty sleeping? Insomnia?

Q: Pain and swelling around teeth? Sore, coated tongue and sore gums? Lump or sore on tongue or gums? Bleeding gums? Uncomfortable dentures?

Q: Persistent cold sores around mouth?

Q: Scalp irritated and itchy, flaking skin? Sudden loss of hair? Persistent sores on scalp?

The elderly (age 65+): disorders 1

SYMPTOMS AND SIGNS	TREATMENT

Arthritis, osteo-
See **Osteoarthritis**, p.924.

Blood pressure (hypertension)
See **Blood pressure, high (hypertension)**, p.894.

Bronchial pneumonia

High fever; cough with sputum; shortness of breath; chest pain.

Consult a doctor; treatment with antibiotics, breathing exercises and steam inhalations; X-ray confirms diagnosis.

Cancer, oesophagus

Early symptoms: feeling that food sticks in throat or behind breastbone when swallowing; heartburn, in some cases.

Consult a doctor; investigation with barium meal and oesophagoscopy; difficult to treat but removal of tumour may be possible; otherwise, surgical operation to shorten oesophagus after removing affected part; radiotherapy; in some cases, a plastic or metal tube is inserted to prevent tumour from blocking oesophagus.

Cancer, prostate

Early symptoms: frequent and difficult urination; blood in urine; in some cases, the first symptoms, caused by secondary deposits, are bone pain that may be associated with backache or with spontaneous fracture of lower leg or thigh.

Consult a doctor; examination of prostate may detect irregular, hard enlargement; biopsy of prostate confirms presence of cancer on test; treatment with hormones frequently causes prostate cancer to decrease in size, and may prevent growth for many years; if cancer has not spread, removal of prostate gland may be curative; X-ray confirms presence of cancer in bones; radiotherapy to bone stops local pain.

Cataract
See **Eye problems: cataract**, p.920.

Corns

Tender, thickened skin over or between toes, due to friction from rubbing of shoes.

Consult a chiropodist; protection with special pads; removal of thickened skin with softening solutions or plasters.

Cramp in calf and foot

Severe, spontaneous muscle cramps; usually occurring during night; occasionally when resting during day.

Consult a doctor; massage muscle and pull foot so as to stretch calf muscle; recurring cramps may be prevented with pills prescribed by a doctor; exercises before patient goes to bed, to move limb through full range of movement, may also help; cradle over feet in bed to relieve leg from weight of bed clothes.

Curvature of spine (kyphoscoliosis)
See **Spinal curvature**, p.926.

Deafness
See **Ear problems: deafness**, p.920.

Bronchial pneumonia is an infection of the air passages (bronchi) in the lung. It usually occurs as a complication of bronchitis (*see* p.906), influenza, or lung cancer (*see* p.908). Sometimes it develops after an operation, and is a potential danger in any illness that affects an old person.

Cancer of the oesophagus is most commonly associated with excessive intake of alcohol. A muscular disorder (achalasia) that affects the junction between the oesophagus and the stomach may also lead to the development of cancer.

Cancer of the prostate is often discovered only when the patient undergoes surgery for prostate problems (*see* p.926). Although prostate cancer is the commonest form of cancer in men over sixty-five, in many cases it has no effect on life expectancy, because it is relatively easy to control.

Corns may be sufficiently painful to prevent normal walking. It is important that the feet of the elderly should have regular attention, so that the person is not prevented from getting enough exercise. Wearing comfortable, well-fitting shoes is also important.

The cause of this type of cramp is not known, so treatment is difficult. Cramp that affects the calf and foot at rest is not due to a poor arterial blood supply, and does not cause pain in the calf muscle when the person is walking. Pain in the calf when walking (intermittent claudication) is usually a symptom of arteriosclerosis (*see* p.906).

The elderly (age 65+): disorders 2

SYMPTOMS AND SIGNS	TREATMENT
Diverticular disease Diarrhoea or constipation; lower abdominal pain; rectal bleeding; in severe cases, fever; in chronic cases, symptoms occur intermittently.	Consult a doctor; antispasm pills; high-fibre diet; antibiotics if necessary; diagnosis made with barium enema and sigmoidoscopy; thorough examination necessary to exclude possibility of cancer.
Ear problems: deafness Gradual or sudden loss of hearing.	Assessment by a doctor; special hearing tests to diagnose type of deafness; hearing aid may be suggested before deafness becomes extreme.
Ear problems: wax Deafness and sometimes irritation in ear.	Examination of ear by a doctor; softening of wax with warm oil; syringing ear with warm water removes softened wax.
Emphysema Gradual and increasing breathlessness; difficulty expanding chest; often slight cough; recurrent attacks of bronchitis (*see* p.884), frequently accompanied by wheezing.	Condition confirmed by special breathing tests and chest X-rays; stop smoking; bronchitis treated with antibiotics; lose weight if obese (*see* p.900); breathing exercises and drainage of secretions from lungs are helpful.
Encephalitis *See* **Encephalitis,** p.898.	
Epilepsy *See* **Epilepsy,** p.910.	
Eye problems: blindness Sudden or momentary blindness in one or both eyes or gradual loss of vision.	Consult a doctor and ophthalmologist; eye problems must be assessed by specialist, with correct equipment; treatment depends on the cause of blindness.
Eye problems: cataract Gradually increasing mistiness of vision; cloudy appearance in the pupil; distortion or loss of vision; no pain.	Surgical removal of lens; this is usually done when useful vision is lost in worst eye.
Eye problems: lid disorders Inflammation of lids; irritation; redness; thickening of eyelid.	Consult a doctor; blepharitis is treated with antibiotics and corticosteroids; a cyst may be treated by incision under local anaesthetic; if the edge of the lid is turned inward (entropion) or outward (ectropion), or if the lid appears to droop (ptosis), a minor operation may be required.

Diverticular disease is infection of the blind pouches (diverticulae) that form in the wall of the large intestine. It is relatively common in the elderly. Severe attacks of diverticulitis may lead to an abscess formation, infection of the abdominal cavity, or intestinal obstruction. These disorders may need surgery.

In the elderly, deafness may be due not only to wax in the ear but also to Ménière's disease (*see* p.910), or to a condition affecting the bones in the middle ear (*see* **Otosclerosis**, p.888). The gradual deafness of old age may be accelerated by working with noisy machinery. Sudden deafness may be due to wax (*see* p.920) in the outer ear, or to a haemorrhage into the inner ear. Deafness is also a social problem, because it can cause the deaf person to feel isolated. Speak slowly and clearly.

The problem of wax in the ear is more common in people with ear infections. Some people form wax more easily than others, and should have regular ear examinations to prevent hard wax causing irritation.

Emphysema is caused by a breakdown of lung tissue that leads to a reduction of the surface area and the elasticity of the lungs. The condition is more common in people with chronic bronchitis (*see* p.906), and those who smoke. Heart failure (*see* p.912) may occur because of lung damage, which prevents a normal flow of blood.

Sudden blindness in both eyes is very rare, but may be caused by a stroke (*see* p.926). Sudden blindness in one eye is usually caused by a disorder such as a detached retina (*see* p.910), arteriosclerosis (*see* p.906), or multiple sclerosis (*see* p.900). Gradual loss of vision is most commonly caused by cataract (*see* p.920), glaucoma (*see* p.910), or retinitis (*see* p.912). Gradual blindness may also be a result of chronic infections of the conjunctiva, such as trachoma or pressure on the optic nerve from a tumour in the brain. Momentary blindness may occur with migraine (*see* p.874) and some forms of arterial disease. Gradual loss of vision in one eye may not be noticed for some time if the other eye is healthy. The apparent suddenness of the condition may be caused by the discovery, rather than the onset, of the disease. Deterioration in vision is common with increasing age.

Cataract, a gradual loss of lens transparency, may be associated with diabetes (*see* p.910), but it may also occur following eye injury or infection. The condition is usually due to deterioration with age, although it also occurs as a congenital defect in some infants.

Blepharitis, an inflammation of the eyelid margins, is often associated with seborrhoea or irritation from dust or tobacco smoke. A cyst on the eyelid is due to a blockage of a gland. Entropion and ectropion are usually due to ageing or scar formation. Drooping of the eyelid is usually a result of muscle weakness.

The elderly (age 65+): disorders 3

False teeth
See **Teeth, loss of,** p.914.

Fissure-in-ano
See **Anal fissure,** p.894.

Fracture, Colles' (wrist)

Painful, swollen wrist; wrist twisted backward and outward; occurring after a fall on an outstretched hand.	Consult a doctor or go to hospital immediately; injury repaired under general anaesthetic; plaster cast for six weeks; recovery aided by physiotherapy.

Fracture, hip

Inability to stand; pain in hip; one foot turned outward; occurring most commonly after a fall.	Call an ambulance immediately; treatment depends on point of fracture; operation to pin broken parts of bone together; sometimes necessary to replace head of femur; recovery is usually rapid, and most patients leave the hospital after two weeks.

Frozen shoulder
See **Frozen shoulder,** p.898.

Gangrene

Gradual darkening of tissue; fingers or toes particularly affected by "dry" gangrene, in which skin appears to shrivel; if area swells, becomes painful, and discharges, this indicates infection ("moist" gangrene).	Consult a doctor immediately; keep area cool; cover with light, dry dressing; "moist" gangrene treated with antibiotics; amputation of foot or leg may be necessary.

Glaucoma
See **Eye problems: glaucoma,** p.910.

Haemorrhoids (piles)
See **Haemorrhoids (piles),** p.898.

Heart failure
See **Heart failure,** p.912.

Heberden's nodes

Swellings, sometimes tender and slightly reddened, on the end joint of the fingers; occurring particularly in elderly people.	Consult a doctor; injections of corticosteroids; wax baths may reduce tenderness; no treatment required in most cases.

Hernia (rupture)
See **Hernia (rupture),** p.912.

Hiatus hernia
See **Hiatus hernia,** p.912.

Hypothermia

Mild confusion; slurred speech; staggering when moving; lethargy; may lead to coma and death; occurring when the body is too cold.	Cover with blankets; give warm drinks, but not alcohol; hospitalize as soon as possible.

Hypothyroidism
See **Myxoedema** p.924.

Colles' fracture is the commonest kind of fracture in people over age fifty. Complete repair of the fracture may be difficult and, in some cases, weakness, stiffness, and slight deformity of the wrist persists. Occasionally the tendon that controls the thumb is damaged after the plaster cast is removed. This requires a surgical procedure to repair it.

Hip fractures are common in the elderly. Successful treatment depends on the patient's swift return to normal activity. Encouraging the patient's confidence, which may have been shaken by the accident, is particularly important, because the muscles of an older person weaken rapidly if they are not exercised.

Gangrene occurs because the blood supply to the affected tissue is inadequate or lacking altogether, causing the tissue to die. Gangrene is more common in people with diabetes (*see* p.910), or with arteriosclerosis (*see* p.906), but may also occur with frostbite, or following an accident. The elderly must take great care with foot hygiene and the treatment of corns.

Heberden's nodes are associated with minor underlying osteoarthritis of the joint. The disorder is a result of an inherited tendency to produce a thickening of fibrous tissue, usually from repeated movement, over the roughened edge of the joint cartilage.

Hypothermia occurs because the body is unable to produce sufficient heat to maintain the correct body temperature. This may occur either because of excessive loss of heat, or because of failure of the body to produce it. It is a particular hazard in the elderly, in whom it may be associated with heart failure (*see* p.912) or malnutrition, and in the newborn, particularly in cold weather.

SYMPTOMS AND SIGNS	TREATMENT

Leukaemia

Gradually increasing fatigue and weight loss; bleeding from gums; spontaneous bruising; malaise; liable to recurrent infections; in some cases, sudden onset of high fever; bronchial pneumonia (*see* p.918).

Consult a doctor; diagnosis made from examination of blood and bone marrow; various treatments with drugs and radiotherapy; results often excellent; sometimes blood transfusion required if anaemia is severe.

Memory, loss of

Inability to remember names, and recent events; tends to increase in severity in the elderly; sometimes accompanied by loss of physical skills.

Consult a doctor; treatment depends on whether cause of it can be found; additional vitamins and certain drugs may help.

Moniliasis (candidiasis, thrush)

Sore, slightly irritating skin infection; occurring in moist skin folds; mouth, armpit, groin, vagina, and skin under breasts most commonly affected.

Consult a doctor; keep area clean, dry and powdered; treatment with antifungal preparations.

Myxoedema (hypothyroidism)

Gradual development of lethargy and drowsiness; thickening of skin of face; slight loss of hair; deepening voice; constipation; feeling the cold.

Consult a doctor; condition hard to detect in early stages; blood test confirms diagnosis; treatment with thyroid hormone effective, but must be continued for life.

Osteoarthritis

Stiffness, pain and swelling of joints; usually affecting joints in legs, where use has damaged joint surfaces; also common in hands; pain and swelling aggravated by movement and improved by rest.

Discuss with a doctor; X-ray to confirm diagnosis; use of aspirin and antirheumatic drugs helps; weight loss if obese; exercises to strengthen surrounding muscles; sometimes injections of corticosteroid drugs produce improvement; in severe cases, surgical treatment with joint fixation (arthrodesis) or joint replacement, particularly in hips and knees, may stop pain and allow normal movement.

Osteoporosis

Gradual loss in height with curvature of spine; in elderly, often occurs without pain; sometimes backache which may become severe after a slight accident.

Consult a doctor; occasionally cause can be found; X-ray of spine necessary to exclude other causes of back pain; treatment with painkilling drugs; orthopaedic corset and exercises prevent immobility.

Parkinson's disease

Slowly progressive trembling; usually starting in one hand and then spreading through both arms; walking with shuffling gait; expressionless, immobile face; staring eyes.

Treatment may control, but does not cure; atropine-like drugs may be used at first; then levodopa or amantadine, often with great success.

Pleurisy
See **Pleurisy**, p.914.

Leukaemia is cancer of white blood cells (leucocytes). The disease affects bone marrow, and may cause swelling of the spleen and lymph nodes. There are various forms of leukaemia. The acute condition is more common in childhood and a chronic one is more common in older adults.

In some cases, the memory of an individual is excellent, except for certain information, such as names of people and objects. Loss of memory may be due to the gradual death of brain cells as an individual ages. The condition can occur prematurely, however, and may be aggravated by arteriosclerosis (*see* p.906), hypothyroidism, stroke (*see* p.924), brain tumour, alcoholism (*see* p.894), or drug abuse (*see* p.874).

Moniliasis is caused by a fungal organism that normally lives in the intestine. The fungus can spread to the skin in certain circumstances. A warm and moist environment, such as the interior of the body, is favourable if other organisms have been killed through antibiotic treatment. Other factors favouring development of moniliasis include lowered resistance due to diabetes mellitus (*see* p.910), and the effects of cortisone treatment. The fungus occasionally invades the lungs and intestines of people who are seriously ill and taking antibiotics. This complication requires hospital treatment.

Deafness (*see* p.920) sometimes occurs, but it is a rare complication. Increasing vulnerability to cold may lead to hypothermia (*see* p.922). In myxoedema, some circulation problems may result from a raised cholesterol level. Myxoedema can cause menstrual disorders (*see* p.900) if it develops in people of a younger age group. Myxoedema also develops, in some cases, as a result of the treatment of thyrotoxicosis (*see* p.902).

Osteoarthritis is most likely to occur in joints that have been damaged or overused, for example, in a knee that has had its cartilage removed, in the hips of athletes, and in the hands of manual workers. Early treatment, with physiotherapy, prevents stiffness and deformity, and also helps to maintain mobility in an elderly patient.

Osteoporosis is more common in women than in men, and often occurs after menopause. A course of treatment with hormones, calcium, and vitamin D may prevent the condition getting worse.

In Parkinson's disease, trembling is often increased by anxiety (*see* p.872) or by the desire to pick something up (intention tremor). Mild dementia and depression (*see* p.896) are common. In patients who have had encephalitis (*see* p.898), the neck sometimes twists and the eyes roll upwards. The condition is commonly associated with ageing, and with arteriosclerosis (*see* p.906).

SYMPTOMS AND SIGNS	TREATMENT

Prolapse of womb
See **Prolapse of womb**, p.914.

Prostate problems

Poor stream when urinating, and difficulty starting and stopping; hesitation and dribbling when urinating; need to urinate during night; frequency of urination during day gradually increases.	Consult a doctor; examination of urine; kidney X-ray; may require operation to remove prostate gland; cancer of prostate (*see* p.918) treated with hormones; infection treated with antibiotics.

Rodent ulcer

Small, firm pearl-like nodule on skin; nodule grows slowly; centre may ulcerate.	Doctor must be consulted; diagnosis made from microscopic examination; radiotherapy or surgical removal are usually effective.

Shingles (herpes zoster)

Dull ache in one area of body followed in few days by mild fever and red rash that forms blisters, pustules and then scabs.	Consult a doctor; painkilling drugs; calamine lotion and vitamin injections may help; antiviral skin solution may lead to rapid improvement, if condition is treated early.

Spinal curvature

Back bent sideways and forwards; onset may be gradual and painless, or fairly rapid and accompanied by pain.	Consult a doctor; X-rays and blood tests confirm diagnosis; physiotherapy; anti-rheumatic drugs; occasionally spinal support may be needed.

Stroke

Sudden onset of weakness or paralysis of one side of face and body; may be followed by slow recovery, with some weakness remaining for a few months; or may lead to coma and death.	In early stages, hospitalization; nursing and medical care; physiotherapy; in some cases, use of anticoagulants; rarely, operation needed.

Thrombosis, coronary
See **Thrombosis, coronary**, p.914.

Thrombosis, venous
See **Thrombosis, venous**, p.914.

Tuberculosis

Usually lung infection with cough; sometimes with blood-stained sputum; loss of weight; night sweats.	Consult a doctor; chest X-ray and sputum tests confirm infection; treatment with at least two antituberculin drugs for at least eighteen months; may need bed rest; nutritious diet; isolation to prevent spread of infection.

Varicose veins
See **Varicose veins**, p.914.

Vertigo
See **Vertigo**, p.914.

In some cases, infection of the prostate (prostatitis) causes the painful frequent urination. Blood may be found in urine. A sudden blockage of urine flow rarely occurs. The size of the prostate gland (prostatic hypertrophy) normally increases with age, but this size increase may also occur because of cancer of the prostate.

About seventy-five per cent of rodent ulcers occur on the face, neck or ears. If untreated, ulceration of the skin may spread into local structures, such as the ear cartilage and the nose. The condition is a locally malignant skin tumour that develops most commonly in fair-skinned people. It may occur as a reaction to exposure to prolonged, intense sunlight.

Shingles is caused by the same virus that causes chickenpox. The shingles virus infects the nerve endings in the body. A face infection of shingles needs special care to avoid eye damage. Pain (postherpetic neuralgia) may continue for months or, rarely, years after the infection.

Spinal curvature is usually due to the gradual compression of a vertebra as a result of osteoporosis (*see* p.924) but sometimes it develops because of a slipped disc (*see* p.902) or a sudden collapse of a vertebra from bone disease. The condition may be associated with nerve pain in the arms and in the legs, causing sciatica.

Incontinence is a problem in the early days after a stroke. There may also be speech problems if the right side of the body is involved in a right-handed person. In some cases, a major stroke is preceded by a series of "warning" strokes, from which the patient recovers completely. This indicates that a narrowed artery is the cause. Often, minor strokes are followed by excellent recovery. Strokes are caused most commonly by arteriosclerosis (*see* p.906), which leads to a clot or a haemorrhage in a brain artery. In younger people, strokes are due to haemorrhage of a weak part of an artery. Strokes may also be caused by narrowing of a neck artery, or by circulation problems that cause a clot formation.

Tuberculosis may spread to involve bone, kidneys, or lymph nodes. Rarely, it may cause a form of meningitis (*see* p.900). In many cases, the patient is reasonably fit. Vaccination with BCG, a mild form of tuberculosis, gives protection against the disease. People who have come into contact with tuberculosis patients need careful follow-up examinations, as well as skin tests to assess their immunity.

Index of adult disorders 1

Accidents and sports injuries	18–35	35–50	50–65	65+
Achilles' tendon rupture		p.894		
Bursitis		p.896		
Fracture, Colles' (wrist)				p.920
Fracture, hip				p.920
Fracture, scaphoid (wrist)	p.886			
Fracture, stress	p.886			
Frozen shoulder		p.898		
Knee, torn cartilage	p.886			
Mallet finger	p.886			
Sprain	p.890			
Tennis elbow	p.890			
Cancer				
Breast		p.896		
Gynaecological		p.896		
Hodgkin's disease	p.886			
Intestinal			p.908	
Leukaemia				p.924
Lung			p.908	
Prostate				p.918
Skin			p.908	
Stomach			p.908	
Urinary tract			p.908	

Chest problems	18–35	35–50	50–65	65+
Asthma			p.906	
Bronchial pneumonia				p.918
Bronchitis, acute	p.884			
Bronchitis, chronic			p.906	
Emphysema				p.920
Pleurisy			p.914	
Pneumothorax	p.888			
Tuberculosis				p.926
Dental problems				
Gingivitis		p.898		
Teeth, loss of			p.914	
Wisdom tooth, impacted	p.890			
Ear problems				
Deafness				p.920
Ménière's disease			p.910	
Otosclerosis	p.888			
Vertigo			p.914	
Wax				p.920
Eye problems				
Blindness				p.920
Cataract				p.920
Detached retina			p.910	
Glaucoma			p.902	
Lid disorders				p.920
Longsightedness (presbyopia)			p.910	
Retinitis			p.912	

Index of adult disorders 2

Foot problems	18–35	35–50	50–65	65+
Bunion			p.906	
Corns				p.918
Cramp in calf and foot				p.918
Heel pain	p.886			
Ingrown toenail	p.886			
Metatarsalgia			p.912	
Gastrointestinal problems				
Anal fissure		p.894		
Appendicitis	p.884			
Cholecystitis, acute			p.908	
Cholecystitis, chronic			p.910	
Cirrhosis			p.910	
Colitis, mucous		p.896		
Colitis, ulcerative	p.890			
Crohn's disease	p.884			
Diverticulitis				p.920
Haemorrhoids (piles)		p.898		
Hernia (rupture)			p.912	
Hiatus hernia			p.912	
Obesity		p.900		
Ulcer, peptic		p.894		
Gland problems				
Diabetes mellitus			p.910	
Myxoedema (hypothyroidism)				p.924
Thyrotoxicosis		p.902		

Gynaecological problems	18–35	35–50	50–65	65+
Amenorrhoea	p.884			
Fibroids		p.898		
Menopause		p.900		
Menstrual disorders		p.900		
Miscarriage	p.888			
Painful intercourse (dyspareunia)	p.888			
Premenstrual tension		p.902		
Prolapse of uterus			p.914	
Salpingitis	p.888			
Vaginitis	p.890			
Heart and circulation problems				
Angina pectoris			p.906	
Arteriosclerosis			p.906	
Atrial fibrillation			p.906	
Blood pressure, high (hypertension)		p.894		
Fainting	p.886			
Gangrene				p.922
Heart failure			p.912	
Heart valve disease		p.898		
Hypothermia				p.922
Thrombosis, coronary			p.914	
Thrombosis, venous			p.914	
Varicose veins			p.914	
Male problems				
Epididymitis	p.886			
Prostate problems				p.926

Index of adult disorders 3

Neurological problems	18–35	35–50	50–65	65+
Bell's palsy (facial paralysis)		p.894		
Carpal tunnel syndrome		p.896		
Encephalitis		p.898		
Epilepsy			p.910	
Meningitis		p.900		
Multiple sclerosis		p.900		
Myasthenia gravis		p.900		
Neuralgia, trigeminal			p.912	
Parkinson's disease				p.924
Peripheral neuritis (polyneuritis)		p.900		
Stroke				p.926
Nose problems				
Deviated nasal septum		p.898		
Sinusitis		p.902		
Orthopaedic problems				
Ankylosing spondylitis (bamboo spine)	p.884			
Arthritis, osteo-				p.924
Arthritis, rheumatoid		p.894		
Dupuytren's contracture			p.910	
Gout			p.912	
Heberden's nodes				p.922
Osteoporosis				p.924
Slipped disc		p.902		
Spinal curvature				p.926

Psychological problems	18–35	35–50	50–65	65+
Alcoholism		p.894		
Depression		p.896		
Mania		p.898		
Memory, loss of				p.924
Schizophrenia	p.890			
Skin problems				
Baldness		p.894		
Dandruff	p.884			
Moniliasis (candidiasis; thrush)				p.924
Pilonidal sinus	p.888			
Psoriasis	p.888			
Raynaud's phenomenon	p.888			
Rodent ulcer				p.926
Rosacea		p.902		
Shingles				p.926
Sweating, excessive (hyperhidrosis)	p.890			
Vitiligo	p.890			
Urinary problems				
Kidney stone			p.912	
Pyelonephritis (kidney disease)			p.914	

Taking care of your body

Section contents

Introduction

In almost every culture in human history, men and women have taught their children how to keep themselves clean, perhaps sometimes merely as a social necessity, but much more commonly as a protection to their children's health. To most people, hygiene implies washing and keeping clean more than anything else.

This section would be very short if the need for cleanliness was all that hygiene implied. After all, most people wash at least once a day, and some bathe just as often. Many people enjoy their daily rituals and do not regard them as tedious duties. But in this book, hygiene is more specifically the avoidance of illnesses and disorders. To this end, this section gives not only instructions for maintaining full health through hygiene, but also a list of the illnesses and conditions that are the penalties for ignoring hygiene.

Another aim of this section is to discredit some of the popular (but mistaken) myths about health that have generally arisen from an incomplete understanding of how the body works.

A daily hygiene routine is essential for good health. It should include general cleanliness, care of the skin, hair, nails, hands and feet, eyes and ears, and teeth. Each part of the body is dealt with separately on the following pages, and the consequences of neglect are explained from a medical point of view. The section does not deal with cosmetic beauty. Care should always be taken when using cosmetics as explained in the section **The skin.**

Some people need to take more care with their personal hygiene than others. A pregnant woman is particularly susceptible to fungal infections of the vagina such as thrush. This is because of hormonal changes in the body during pregnancy. The hormones also affect the ligaments and muscles in the back and pelvis. A pregnant woman must concentrate on good posture at all times as explained in **Looking after your back.** This not only reduces the likelihood of backache, but also makes pregnancy less tiring.

A person who suffers from diabetes mellitus must pay particular attention to daily cleanliness. The smallest abrasion, caused for example by a long toenail digging into another toe, can become infected.

In addition to personal hygiene routine, it

is important to have regular health tests. A doctor can advise a person on how often the tests should be carried out, but as the section on **Routine health tests** explains, disorders such as glaucoma, short- and longsightedness, dental decay, and cervical cancer can be detected and treated before they have advanced to a serious degree.

Many myths surround sex, and the section on **Sex and health** sets out to allay all the anxieties and fears that doctors are continually encountering. A healthy sex life is discussed, and warnings are given (where appropriate) about some sexual practices.

Diet plays an important part in the maintenance of good health. Vitamin deficiency diseases are rare in Western society, but the rich and varied foods available have brought problems of their own. Most experts agree that there is a strong link between heart disease and a diet high in animal fats. The richness of diet also eliminates the need for a person to add bulk to a meal in order to feel satisfied. Low bulk diets cause constipation, and disorders such as diverticular disease. A low fibre diet is also thought to be associated with cancer of the large intestine. The section **Food and health: nutrition** explains that a balanced diet supplies all the vitamins and minerals a body needs, and dispenses with the necessity to take additional vitamin tablets.

Obesity is another threat to good health. A fat bouncing baby used to be regarded as healthy, but it is now understood that a fat baby often develops into a fat child, and a fat child may grow up to be a fat adult. A fat person runs a high risk of coronary heart disease in middle age, and is more likely to suffer from conditions like high blood pressure, diabetes mellitus, intertrigo, haemorrhoids, and varicose veins. The nutrition section includes advice on the types of food that can be included in a controlled diet.

Adequate relaxation is as essential to healthy living as a balanced diet and looking after the physical body. Without a good night's rest the individual is less able to cope with the stresses and strains of modern society. Without the opportunity to take a rest when under great physical strain the individual can damage the normal functioning of the body by putting it under too much stress.

Mental and physical breakdown can occur under conditions that push us to our limits. Types of breakdown such as battle fatigue, or breakdown caused by stress in people who are involved in a catastrophe such as an earthquake, are extreme examples.

The section that deals with **Rest and health** looks closely at how we overcome stress and strain with relaxation exercises and explains why adequate sleep is essential when taking care of your body.

While the human body can survive reasonable environmental fluctuations of climate and season, modern technology has produced pollution which is especially damaging to the quality of life. Mankind may gradually adapt to the environmental hazard that has been created, or may develop some form of control over the hostile environment but, at present, we must learn to live with it as a factor in our health.

The section **The environment and health** points to the various hazards that encroach on our daily lives. Air pollution, the major health hazard in our cities, is caused through factory smoke and car exhaust. Ways are being developed to control or filter out the harmful elements. Pollution of our water supplies by chemicals used in insect and disease control, and soil fertilization can affect the water we drink, the food we eat, and indeed, all aspects of the natural food chain. Waste disposal by burying, dumping, and releasing harmful products in the sea or the earth must, inevitably, cause problems for mankind in the future.

Staying healthy while travelling offers advice about ensuring your mental and physical well-being before the journey so that the journey itself will be as comfortable and incident-free as possible. The section is concerned with all aspects of planning in advance, from making sure that your passport is up to date with the correct visas, to ensuring that travel and insurance documents will not cause mental anguish if last minute delays are encountered. It points out the need for a health check by your doctor before you travel, and mentions the various immunizations that might be needed for international travel.

Hygiene: general cleanliness

Personal cleanliness is important for three main reasons: (1) to remove odour-producing waste and sweat that accumulates on the skin; (2) to prevent skin irritation; and (3) to prevent the spread of infection, either on one's own body, or to other people.

Sanitary awareness in modern society and progress in medical understanding have together reduced the incidence of many diseases, some of which had previously reached the proportions of epidemics. Although cleanliness might no longer be considered next to godliness, it is ordinarily taught in homes and schools as part of daily life and the social requirements.

The routine of cleanliness

From the earliest practicable age, children should be taught a routine of cleanliness. Such a routine, continued from then on, commonly develops into a personal habit in which each individual can take pride in the improvement of his or her own appearance and health. This is particularly important in adolescence.

Girls can use their cleanliness routine as a reassurance in the time of their first menstrual period, and as they become aware of the wish to be attractive. Both boys and girls may be able to avoid some of the unpleasantness of acne through personal cleanliness. Adults may be more casual about maintaining their routine, but it is no less important to them.

Because such a cleanliness routine is a personal matter, what it actually consists of differs from person to person. But careful washing is essential, preferably for the whole body, once a day. It is particularly necessary to wash the hands after visiting the toilet and before touching food. The activities of the day may also make special care necessary in washing: a bath or shower that includes washing the hair, for example, is advisable after most sports. In addition, children should be taught not to put their fingers into their ears, nose, or any other orifice, especially if they are natural finger suckers. They may need encouragement to use soap, and to get dirt off in the bath rather than on the towels afterwards. Most children enjoy baths, and it should not be difficult to accustom them to a washing routine.

For adults, there are times when personal cleanliness is particularly important, especially in working conditions where hygiene is necessary. A person who works in the preparation or serving of food, for example, should be medically checked for infection, even if suffering only a mild stomach upset. If a food handler develops an infection such as a boil or a nail infection, he or she should stop working until the infection clears. Any person with a boil should avoid preparing food if possible, and take extra care in the cleaning of hands and nails. Cuts on the hands and fingers may also harbour harmful bacteria although these cuts may not appear to be visibly infected. As a general precaution, extra cleanliness is also necessary following a bout of diarrhoea or vomiting, in case the cause is bacterial.

Hazards

There are many more serious conditions and disorders that may result from poor personal hygiene, and that are therefore potentially avoidable without much difficulty. But there is one disorder that may actually be caused by the efforts made to maintain personal hygiene. This condition is contact dermatitis, an inflammation of the skin where it has been irritated by a substance with which it has been in contact. The result may be just a slight redness at the site – or it may be an acutely itching area covered with blisters. Common causes of contact dermatitis are household detergents, deodorants, face creams, and the dye in some cosmetics. Once the condition has appeared, the symptoms may remain for a long time. Until the symptoms clear up, the commonest site, the hands, should be protected by wearing cotton-lined rubber gloves.

Another common condition is body odour. The odour is produced by bacteria on the skin surface that break down glandular secretions. The areas that produce the odour, generally the feet, groin, and armpits, should be washed daily with mild soap and water; a deodorant can then be applied. The more sweat the body exudes, the more odour there is likely to be; active jobs and pastimes may demand two, or even three, baths per day. But overactive sweat glands in non-active periods is a medical condition known as hyperhidrosis. This condition may occur during menopause or as a result of anxiety. If the affected areas are not kept clean, fungal infections (such as moniliasis) may invade the damp skin, and cause further problems.

Another hazard of poor cleanliness is skin irritation. Between baths, and especially if the individual is very active physically, the skin becomes covered with the normal debris of dead skin cells, oil (called sebum), and dirt particles. If the debris is not washed off, the number of potentially dangerous bacteria increases, and substances that cause irritation accumulate. Because of the active glands in the area, and because exposure to the air is infrequent, the genitals are usually areas of greatest build-up of debris. As a result, they are most likely to be affected by skin irritation. In severe cases, vulvovaginitis (in a female) or balanitis (in a male) may result.

Serious conditions

General standards of personal hygiene are good in the United Kingdom; most people have their own cleanliness routine that also assures social acceptability. But of course there are individuals who are different, and who usually are not aware of the risks they run. There are a number of unpleasant disorders that are the sole result of failure to care about hygiene, and are therefore totally avoidable with little effort.

Many of these concern either (1) the transmission of bacteria by the hands, and particularly the nails; or (2) irritation and inflammation of the vulva, the penis, or the anus. The nails, for example, are usually implicated in the spread of threadworms (*see below*) and of food poisoning. Care of the hands and nails is hygienically extremely significant; for further information, *see* p.942.

Irritation and inflammation of the vulva and the vagina may be caused by various factors. But if the area is not kept sufficiently clean, the build-up of natural secretions may irritate the skin and cause intense itching.

However, similar itching can be caused by too much cleaning of the vagina. Douching is seldom, if ever, necessary: the vagina's natural secretions keep it clean. Frequent douching can cause serious gynaecological infections, occasionally resulting in sterility.

Inflammation of the end of the penis is known as balanitis. Many factors may be responsible for the condition, but a lack of personal cleanliness, particularly in uncircumcised men, can cause irritation. The penis should be washed daily with mild soap and water—including the foreskin, which should be rolled back gently for the purpose. (But note that in baby boys, the foreskin is attached to the tip of the penis. If the foreskin is rolled back before the age of about two years, the tissue may tear.)

Itching around the anus can be a symptom of many conditions, including threadworms (*see below*). But insufficient cleaning of the anal area after defecation can be a major cause of irritation, especially in combination with too infrequent washing. Although the chief remedy is the obvious one, of improved hygiene and a regular washing routine, there are also forms of medical treatment for the condition. If the itching continues for more than two weeks, medical advice should be sought.

Threadworms
One of the commonest results of a lack of personal hygiene, especially in children, is infestation by threadworms. It is all too easy to become infested with, but very difficult to get rid of, this parasite. The eggs of the threadworm are swallowed in contaminated water, and travel to the small intestine where they develop into adult worms. The female worms move down the intestine and lay eggs in the skin around the anus at night, causing anal itching. The eggs become embedded under the nails during scratching, and are transported back to the mouth to restart the cycle. The eggs can also stick to the lavatory seat, or be transferred to towels, bed linen, curtains, books, and clothing. As a precaution, children must be taught never to scratch around the anus, and to carefully wash their hands each morning, after using the lavatory, and before handling food. Many doctors treat all members of a family when one member is found to have threadworms.

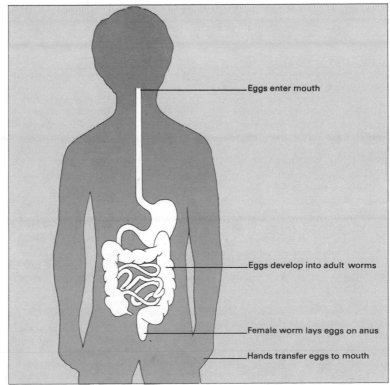

Eggs enter mouth

Eggs develop into adult worms

Female worm lays eggs on anus

Hands transfer eggs to mouth

The skin

The skin is the largest organ of the body. It has three main functions: (1) to protect the tissues beneath from injury, invasion from bacteria, drying out, and damage from ultraviolet light; (2) to inform the body of changes in environment through a network of specialized nerve sense organs; and (3) to keep the temperature of the body constant. Some areas of the body are covered with specialized skin, for example, the palms of the hands, and the soles of the feet.

The skin contains specialized glands. There are three main types. (1) Eccrine glands secrete a salty sweat containing some of the body's waste products. The secretions have a mild antiseptic quality. (2) Sebaceous glands secrete sebum, an oily substance that stops the skin drying out. (3) Apocrine glands, another kind of sweat gland, develop only in hairy areas at puberty, and produce a pungent odour caused by bacterial activity on the glands' secretions.

The skin is vulnerable to many different kinds of disorders, but misuse or inadequate care of the skin can encourage or aggravate problems. Skin conditions can be classified as: (1) those arising from outside invasion of micro-organisms; (2) those caused by bacteria already present on the skin; and (3) self-inflicted injury.

Preventing invasion from outside

The skin can be infected by a virus or a fungus. Infections, such as pityriasis rosea, are difficult to avoid. But an adult is unlikely to suffer a second attack, and provided the skin is not broken down by scratching, the disease disappears spontaneously within a few weeks leaving a clear skin.

A fungal infection can be contracted easily if an area of skin is too moist. For example, fungal infections of the nail bed are common among people who constantly have their hands submerged in water.

Attention must be paid to creases and folds in the skin, especially in hot weather. It is essential to wash and thoroughly dry creases beneath the arms, in the groin, or under the breasts each day. A light dusting of talcum powder helps to keep the area smooth and dry. If this is not done regularly, a condition known as intertrigo may develop. This produces red, inflamed areas of skin that are susceptible to fungal infections, particularly in obese people.

Maintaining the bacterial balance

The skin is covered with bacteria. Most of them are harmless, and some benefit the body in its fight against infection. However, if the balance of bacteria is altered, infection can set in. This commonly occurs following interference with the body's natural defence system. For example, vaginal douching can change the bacterial balance in the vagina, and encourage moniliasis (thrush).

Boils

Another example of harmful interference with the body's natural defences often occurs during home treatment of boils. A boil is a deep infection of a hair follicle. It is caused by staphylococci. Redness and swelling developing around the site of infection is the body's defence mechanism working to isolate and kill the infection. If the boil is squeezed, the staphylococci may spread to another follicle and start a crop of boils. It should be covered with a dressing and left alone.

Similarly, a stye developing on an eyelid should not be rubbed or scratched, however irritating it is. The infection could be carried on the fingers to the other eye. A doctor may prescribe antibiotic treatment.

Impetigo

Impetigo is caused by either a streptococcal or staphylococcal infection. Impetigo can occur as a complication of another skin disorder. It enters through abrasions caused by scratching. To prevent it occurring, a person must never scratch skin made vulnerable by an irritating skin condition. If a member of a group catches impetigo, that person's towels and clothing must be isolated and washed separately to prevent it spreading around the group, and medical treatment must be sought immediately.

Avoiding misuse of the skin

A limited amount of sun is beneficial to the skin. Acne vulgaris often improves when exposed to ultraviolet rays, and the skin manufactures vitamin D from sunlight. Overexposure, however, can lead to serious burning, and prolonged exposure reduces the skin elasticity, resulting in premature ageing of the skin. Prolonged sunshine over many years may produce skin cancer.

Specialized cells in the skin produce a protective pigment, known as melanin. The pigment protects the skin's underlying tissues from ultraviolet rays, and also determines the skin's colour. The amount of damage done to the skin by exposure to sunlight depends on skin type, and intensity and duration of exposure.

Fair-skinned persons with a tendency to freckles are more vulnerable to sunburn because their skin contains less melanin. Dark skin contains more pigment, and is usually thicker than fair skin.

At the beginning of the summer months, fair-skinned people should limit sunbathing to a few minutes a day according to the strength of the sun. The sun is at its hottest at midday, therefore it is safer to sunbathe in the morning or evening. As the skin tans, the length of time in the sun can be increased. Each person achieves an individual amount of suntan that is related to genetic factors as well as to the degree of exposure. Lying in the sun for hours after the maximum tan has been achieved is harmful and unnecessary.

Protection against the sun is essential for fair-skinned people even if they are not sunbathing. Areas such as the back of the neck are particularly vulnerable. A person who burns easily must apply barrier cream to any exposed areas, including the tops of the ears, the backs of the hands, and the soles of the feet, before lying in the sun. If a person is walking on sand, or snow in bright sunshine, barrier creams must be applied beneath the eyebrows, under the nose and chin, and beneath the ear lobes to protect the skin from reflected sun. Cream must be reapplied, particularly after swimming.

Sebum is secreted on to the skin to prevent moisture loss from the underlying tissues. Sebum production varies from person to person, but over-enthusiastic washing with soaps or detergents can dry out the skin, and leave it rough and flaking. The skin on the hands is particularly susceptible to damage. Protective gloves should be worn when using any kind of chemical, or soap powder. Continual use of even a mild household cleaner may suddenly produce an acute allergy. Irritation can cause itching, and scratching can open the skin to infection.

The skin has an abundant blood supply. In fact, almost a third of the blood pumped from the heart reaches the skin. If the blood supply is cut off for more than a few hours through pressure, the tissue dies. This can occur in elderly, bedridden people, resulting in bedsores. People suffering from disorders such as diabetes are particularly susceptible to this kind of skin damage, and must take special care.

Scab formation is a normal part of healing. A scab is formed from blood, serum, and clotting factors such as platelets and fibrin. Scabs must never be picked off because the healing process may be delayed, infection may be introduced into the open wound and scarring is more likely to occur.

Diet has some influence on the condition of the skin. In extreme cases, vitamin deficiency leads to skin disorders. A deficiency of vitamin C causes scurvy.

Total skin area
Skin covers a total area of 1.7 sq. metres (18 sq. ft) in an average sized person, and weighs about three kilograms (7 lb). It is elastic, but gradually loses the ability to return to its original tension with increasing age. Some parts of the body are covered with specialized skin. For example, the palm of the hands, and the sole of the feet are thickened (the darker area in the diagram). This skin contains no hair follicles, and hardly any skin pigment (melanin).

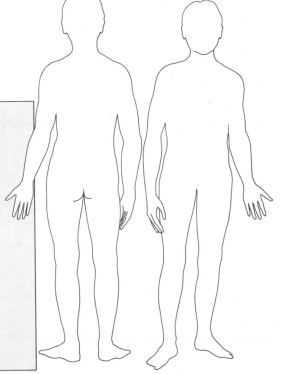

Eyes and ears

The eyes and ears are highly sensitive organs and, although they have a defence system of their own, their delicate structure makes them susceptible to injury and disease. If you want to retain good sight and hearing, you must take care of your eyes and ears.

The eyes

The eyes must be protected from accidents. Blindness can result from injuries inflicted with sharp sticks, fireworks, toy guns, and other objects that children may use as missiles during play. Parents must be firm with their children and explain the possible consequences of careless play. Spectacle lenses should be made of an unbreakable substance, particularly for children.

Foreign bodies

The lid of the eye can shut in a fifteenth of a second. This is a reflex action that responds to the smallest stimulus. However, foreign bodies do become lodged in the eye, and there is a correct way to remove them without causing damage.

If a soft object, such as an eyelash, becomes lodged between the lid and the eyeball, instruct the victim to close the eye. Lead the victim to a good light source, and gently open the eye. If the foreign body is not visible, instruct the victim to look up, down, then to either side as you gently deflect the eyelid in the opposite direction. When the particle is located, lift it from the eye with the dampened corner of a clean handkerchief.

Never try to remove a particle that is stuck to the white of the eye or lying over the centre of the eye. Also never attempt to remove a hard foreign body from the eye unless watering has moved the particle to the inner corner. In both cases, the eye should be covered with a raised eye pad that does not touch the lid or the eyeball, and the victim taken to a doctor.

Eyestrain

A good deal of eyestrain can be avoided by using your common sense to develop good habits for reading and close work.

Always read in good light, but ensure that the light does not reflect directly off the page. Too much glare makes reading uncomfortable. When reading, hold the book at least a foot away from your eyes, and relax the muscles that control the lens by looking at a distant object about once an hour. Do not sit too close to a television screen, or watch television in a dark room. You need extra light for close work.

Adults should have their eyes tested every two years. Children should have their eyes tested once a year. Poor vision can harm a child's social and educational development, and may be mistaken for low intelligence. Early detection of any serious vision defect enables correction that will permit the child to make maximum use of remaining vision.

Every adult over the age of forty should have his or her eyes examined as well as tested every two years, in order to diagnose and treat any disorders before vision suffers irreparable damage.

Spectacles are prescribed to correct longsightedness (hypermetropia) and shortsightedness (myopia), and some other visual disorders. The lenses must be prescribed by an ophthalmologist or optician. Longsightedness may develop with increasing age (presbyopia) because the lens of the eye becomes less elastic. Any disturbance of clear vision strains the eyes and needs correction as soon as possible, or the person may suffer from headaches.

Misuse of cosmetics

Eye cosmetics can produce a violent allergic reaction, particularly the kind containing particles of "glitter". A contact dermatitis may develop after years of use, producing swelling (oedema) and itching around the eyelids, and sometimes involving the whole face. It is a sensible precaution to use hypo-allergenic cosmetics that are now on the market.

Clean all traces of make-up off the eyes each night. Use a mild soap and water, or a mild cleansing oil. If particles of make-up are left on overnight, there is a higher risk of irritation. Mascara tends to make the eyelashes brittle, and they can be damaged on the sheets at night.

A cosmetic that should never be used regularly, if at all, is false eyelash glue. If misapplied it can block the natural flow of tears from the lacrimal glands.

Eye infections

Blepharitis is an inflammation of the edges of the eyelids. The condition can give rise to infected eyelash follicles. If the membrane covering the eye becomes infected, the patient develops "pink eye" (conjunctivitis). The condition may be accompanied by a discharge of pus, pain, and sensitivity to bright light. If the infection is confined to one eye, it can be easily spread to the other eye during the early stages when the patient is unaware of the infection. For this reason, always clean the eyes separately by wiping with cotton wool from the inner to the outer corner. Discard it immediately afterwards and use a fresh one for the other eye.

Levels of perceived sound		
Jet taking off 27 metres (30 yards) away		140dB
Permanent deafness likely		
Pneumatic drill 2 metres (2 yards) away		100dB
Inside underground train	90dB	
Temporary deafness likely		
Busy restaurant	65dB	
Rustling leaves	20dB	

The ears

Part of your daily cleanliness routine should be careful cleaning of the outer part of the ear (auricle) to remove wax secreted by glands in the ear canal. Wipe a clean, damp flannel around the outside contours of the ear as well as behind it. Never try to reach the wax in the invisible, deeper part of the ear with a fingernail, or a twist of cotton wool, because you will push the wax deeper into the ear canal. Once this has happened, the wax – that moves naturally along the canal to the outside and flakes off – hardens to a dark orange lump that irritates the wall of the ear canal and encourages the skin to peel. The build up can completely cover the eardrum and cause temporary deafness. The plug then has to be removed by a doctor.

Wax also tends to trap water in the canal after swimming or washing the hair. This may cause temporary deafness. To relieve it, tip your head to one side and gently pull the external ear up and down. The water can then flow out of the ear.

Protection from injury

The eardrum is vulnerable to many kinds of injury that can result in partial or even total deafness. Never strike an adult, or child, across the ear, because this can force air down the canal and burst the drum.

The ear can also be injured by high levels of noise. Loudness is measured in decibels. Exposure to noise at a level of more than 85 decibels causes temporary impairment of hearing. Continued exposure causes increasing, irreversible deafness. The first symptom of noise damage is a buzzing or ringing in the ears when the noise stops. The buzzing may take days to subside. This can happen in discotheques, if you are part of a band, or if you work in noisy surroundings.

Because of these dangers, if you work in high level noise you must protect your hearing with plugs or ear protectors.

Ear infections

Ear infections need prompt medical treatment. Whenever you have an earache consult your doctor.

Infection can enter the ear when you are swimming or diving, particularly in hot climates. It is a sensible precaution to wear earplugs when swimming. A boil in the ear canal is extremely painful because the surrounding tissues are tight. Never squeeze the boil, but see a doctor immediately.

Foreign bodies

It is not uncommon for a child to push a bead, or any other small toy into the ear. It is most important that parents never try to remove the foreign body. This must be done by an expert. Similarly, should an insect get lodged in the ear, see a doctor.

Nose blowing

An infection of either the nose or the throat can easily reach the ear and cause a painful infection of the middle ear (otitis media). The chance of the infection spreading can be reduced by carefully blowing the nose. If the nose is blown violently mucus can move up the Eustachian tube to the middle ear. Blow your nose gently, and make sure the nostrils are open before you begin to blow.

The Eustachian tube

The purpose of the Eustachian tube is to maintain an equal pressure on each side of the eardrum. Blockage of the tube, which runs from the back of the nose to the middle ear, can lead to deafness and middle ear infection.

A blocked Eustachian tube can usually be cleared by swallowing and gritting the back teeth at the same time. If the block lasts for more than a few hours, medical attention should be sought. The situation is potentially dangerous because any sudden change in pressure can rupture the eardrum.

Hands, feet, and nails

The hands

The hands contain twenty-seven bones and a complex network of tendons and muscles. The palm is protected by a thick, tough layer of hairless skin. The hand is a mechanically complex and highly sensitive structure. Misuse can easily damage it.

Most parents teach their children to wash their hands before meals and after visiting the lavatory. Fewer parents, however, are equally careful to teach exactly how the hands should be washed properly.

To rinse, soap, and rinse again is not enough. Attention should be paid, also to cleaning the finger tips, between the fingers, and the top of the wrist. Dirt under the nails must be removed with a nailbrush designed for the purpose, as soon as is convenient, and certainly before the next meal. The backs of the hands should also be washed.

It should also be made clear to children that there are other times when washing is important: after a game in the park, for example, especially on a dirty surface.

A routine for washing the hands is of extreme importance, not merely as a matter of normal cleanliness or social acceptability, but also as a protective measure. Failure to keep the hands clean can lead to impairment of the sense of touch. A surface coating of dirt or of chemicals found in the home or at work can damage the skin.

Many hand problems are a result of overexposure to harsh detergents, which remove the natural oils and leave the skin leathery, dry, and flaky. You should protect your hands by wearing rubber gloves when doing housework. Applying hand cream may also help.

Injury accounts for the majority of hand problems. But many forms of damage can be avoided, and adequate care can lessen the possibility or effect of injury. Many of these injuries occur during a normal day's work, and may have disabling consequences.

The thick skin that covers the palm helps to prevent minor cuts and abrasions, and usually heals quickly and cleanly. However, a puncture wound may introduce infection into the deeper tissues of the hand. Any deep puncture wound of the hand should be seen by a doctor.

Rings that are complete bands of metal can cause various injuries. Rings should be removed for any manual work, including housework. If the ring catches on a projection, it can cut into the skin. Occasionally, as the hand pulls away, the ring can completely strip the flesh off the finger or, in very severe cases, amputate the finger.

During the last three months of pregnancy the hands swell slightly, and a ring can become too tight. A tight ring constricts the blood flow out of, but not into the finger, resulting in sudden swelling. Once this occurs, the finger needs emergency medical attention, and the ring must be cut off to restore a free blood flow.

Tenosynovitis is inflammation of the sheath surrounding a tendon. Normally, each tendon moves easily within the tendon sheath. Overuse can inflame the tendon and cause grating and pain. The condition can become so serious that the patient can hear the tendon grating. This is known as tenosynovitis crepitans. A doctor should be consulted at the first sign of pain.

One particular form of tenosynovitis is caused by continual overuse of the thumb in occupations that involve a pincer movement of the hand, for example, haircutting. The patient experiences pain in the thumb. Minor surgery is usually necessary to relieve the condition. It can be avoided if a person heeds the warning signs of discomfort and stiffness in the thumb and wrist after a day's work. The thumb should be rested for several days and work resumed slowly during the following months.

Trigger finger is another type of mechanical disorder of a tendon. A lump develops on the tendon of a finger through overuse. The patient develops a flexed and painful finger which straightens with an audible and visible snap. Surgery is the only treatment for the condition, but it can be avoided by not repeatedly misusing a certain tendon.

The feet

The foot contains twenty-six bones and a complex network of tendons and muscles. The two feet support the total weight of the body, balance it when it is stationary, and propel it forwards for walking or running. The sole of the foot is protected by a tough layer of hairless skin that thickens into natural calluses over pressure points.

Routine foot care

Good foot care from infancy, particularly with regard to properly fitting shoes, can prevent many foot problems from developing.

You should wash your feet at least once a day and dry thoroughly between the toes. You should change stockings or socks daily. It is also advisable to change the type of shoes worn at least once a day.

Badly fitting footwear is the major cause of foot problems in modern society. It is important to choose footwear carefully, particularly when buying shoes for children.

Good shoes give support under the instep and heel, and give enough room for the toes to spread inside the shoe. When trying on shoes, wear your normal socks or stockings. Try on both shoes and walk around in them. If there is any discomfort, do not buy them.

Children's feet should be measured regularly since their feet grow quickly and also change shape. The soft bones can easily be deformed by badly fitting shoes. Shoes should be discarded when they become too small. Shoes mould themselves to the first wearer's feet, and therefore should not be handed down from one child to another.

The choice of materials for footwear is important. Shoes should be made of a natural material, such as leather, suede, canvas, or rope. Socks should be made of wool or cotton. Synthetic materials do not absorb sweat nor allow it to evaporate. A damp foot is vulnerable to infection.

Foot disorders
Athlete's foot is a type of fungal infection in which soft, itching blisters develop between the toes. The blisters may spread to the sole of the foot. Fungicidal powders may help to control the infection. But, once acquired, athlete's foot tends to recur and is difficult to eliminate. If the infection persists or recurs, consult a doctor.

Blisters are caused by continual rubbing from badly fitting shoes. Stop wearing the shoes that caused the blister. You should not break a blister. Apply a mild antiseptic and cover it with a dry adhesive dressing. If a blister becomes inflamed, consult a doctor.

Chilblains are caused by an inadequate blood supply to the superficial tissues of the foot and toes in cold conditions. It is a mild form of frostbite. Wearing tight shoes or socks increases the likelihood of chilblains developing.

Claw toes occur when the first joint of the toes points upwards, and the second and third are bent downwards. A badly fitting shoe, or tight sock increases the deformity, and produces corns on the toes.

In **hallux valgus** the big toe is forced outwards. A shoe that crowds the toes together also pushes the top of the toe inwards, and increases the pressure on the first joint, causing a bunion.

High heels throw the weight on to the front of the foot and toes. This encourages the growth of hard skin over pressure points. In extreme cases, a large corn may form on any of the toes. The muscles in the arch of the foot tire easily, and ache by the end of the day.

Metatarsalgia is also a common problem in the elderly, because the arch between the base of the big and small toes is lost.

A badly designed heel can throw the weight of the body on to the outer edge of the foot. Pain occurs in the ball of the foot and, in acute cases, the patient can bear weight only on the heel.

All weight distribution problems are increased by obesity. Careful dieting can prevent, or help many foot disorders.

The nails
Fingernails and toenails are made of a special form of tough skin called keratin. They are formed from layers of this horny material fused tightly together. The growing part of the nail lies beneath the cuticle. A fingernail takes about six months to grow from the nail-bed to the top of the finger, and a toenail takes about a year.

Nails can be affected by any changes in the body, for example, diet or an illness, which may cause cracks or ridges, visible only weeks later as the nail grows. However, some disorders can often be avoided with proper care of the nails.

Routine nail care
The nails should be cut every two to three weeks. The correct way to cut a nail is with small snips along the contour. Toenails should be cut straight across. After cutting, the nails should be shaped with an emery board. File in one direction only, to prevent the nails from splitting.

Nail polish encourages the layers of keratin to split. People who use polish regularly should leave a small area at the base of the nail free, remove the polish completely every six days, and leave the nail bare on the seventh.

Nail disorders
Paronychia is an infection of the nail-bed. A red, painful swelling begins around the side and base of the nail. The cuticle thickens because of accumulating pus, which eventually oozes out around the nail. The condition needs immediate medical attention. To avoid the condition, carefully dry the hands after immersion in water.

Ingrowing toenail causes the nail of the toe to curve under and inwards in the shape of a staple. Tight shoes aggravate the condition. Damp, dirty feet are likely to become infected where the nail digs in. To avoid the condition, the feet must be washed daily. The corner of the nails should be lifted, and accumulated debris removed from beneath the edge.

Teeth

Your permanent, or adult, teeth begin to emerge when you are six years old, and they are bigger and stronger than the first set. Permanent teeth produce a highly effective and efficient bite because they are rooted in solid bone – false teeth can produce only a small proportion of the power of permanent teeth. To keep your teeth and gums healthy you should eat a nourishing and varied diet, follow a strict routine of oral hygiene, and visit the dentist every six months. Children should be encouraged to adopt the same routine from the age of two, and visit the dentist when they are three.

The teeth cut and grind the food in the first part of digestion. The more use the teeth have, the stronger and healthier they remain. A varied diet gives teeth tough and crisp food to chew as well as soft food, and the gums are stimulated at the same time.

Deficiency diseases are comparatively rare in modern society but when they occur, the teeth are one of the areas to be affected first. If local drinking water is low in fluoride, a mineral that is essential for the formation of healthy teeth, your teeth and your children's teeth will be more susceptible to decay. If you know your local water is low in fluoride, your dentist can prescribe fluoride tablets or fluoride toothpaste.

A diet low in vitamin D also makes the teeth less resistant to decay. The condition is common in young children, or dark-skinned people living in northern climates, where the exposure to sunlight is not sufficient for the skin to manufacture the usual amount of vitamin D. A pregnant woman may also suffer from lack of the vitamin. Vitamin D is abundant in sea fish, and is added to most margarines.

Daily routine

Teeth should be brushed twice a day, or better still, after each meal. Choose a toothbrush with a small head to reach well back into the mouth. The bristles should be firm and long to ensure that the gum and tooth can be cleaned with one flicking sweep of the brush, as shown in the illustrations. When your child first starts to clean the teeth, let him or her choose the brush, and provide a stable chair or stool so that the child can reach the basin.

Tooth decay

Poor tooth cleaning habits encourage tooth decay for a number of reasons. Bacteria are always present in the mouth, but when food becomes trapped between the teeth, the bacteria break it down, and form a harmful

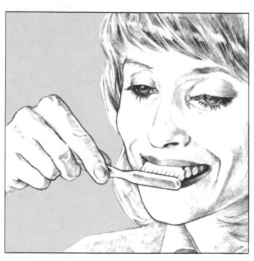

Correct brushing

Lay the side of the bristles flat against the teeth and, by turning the wrist, flick the brush away from the gums towards the tongue. Brush carefully behind the teeth as well. The brushing routine should take at least five minutes a session, with preferably three sessions a day, although two are regarded as adequate. Change the brush every two months.

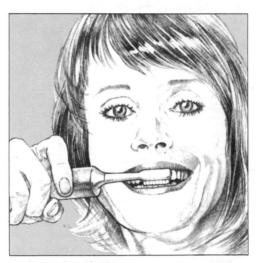

Electric toothbrush

An electric toothbrush is an efficient tooth cleaner. It brushes the teeth up and down in the correct way, and massages the gums if laid gently on them. Children enjoy the novelty of electric toothbrushes, and introducing one into the family often encourages children to brush their teeth more often. The brush attachments should be changed every two months.

acid capable of softening the enamel, and eroding the teeth. The film of saliva, bacteria, and food particles is known as plaque, and if this remains on the teeth, calcium salts begin to form, and build up a hard, chalky deposit around the teeth known as tartar. Although careful cleaning and flossing can remove the particles of food that encourage plaque, no amount of cleaning can remove tartar. Once it is there, the dentist has to scale the teeth to get rid of it.

The gums
The gums also suffer from poor cleaning habits. A healthy gum should come to a fine point between each tooth, and look moist and pink, but if the gum margin is rounded, red, and slightly puffy it means that the early stages of gum disease (gingivitis) have begun. You are not cleaning your teeth correctly, and the gums are reacting to the build-up of plaque and tartar.

Puffy gum margins also occur during pregnancy because of hormonal changes in the mother's body. Pay more attention to oral hygiene during pregnancy, and see your dentist as often as every three months.

Gingivitis can lead to acute infection of the gum and produce a painful boil or abscess. This can even cause the gum to recede

permanently. Once the root is exposed, infection can enter and penetrate into the bony tooth socket, loosening the teeth. This can eventually lead to tooth loss.

The dentist
When you visit the dentist, he or she can detect signs of decay or gum disease before any permanent damage is done. The dentist may routinely X-ray the teeth because decay among the back teeth can be seen more easily on an X-ray. The dentist also checks that existing fillings are not leaking, or damaged in any way. If a filling needs replacing, the dentist drills away the old filling and any infected tooth material, and refills the tooth.

The orthodontist
During the pre-teen years, a child's permanent teeth are emerging and settling down into position. Irregularities are common – there may be gaps between the teeth, or the teeth may be overcrowded and overlapping. The dentist may refer a child to an orthodontist, who takes a series of X-rays before correcting the irregularities with a brace or similar equipment. A brace should not be uncomfortable, but the child must be especially careful about cleaning the teeth.

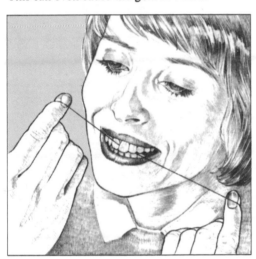

Dental floss
Dental floss is made of a strong thread that is either waxed or unwaxed. Use it every day, preferably at night. Cut off a long piece of floss, wrap each end several times around the middle fingers, and run the centre portion over the tip of the index fingers. With a gentle sawing action, move the floss down between each tooth in turn, and stroke the floss along the gum at the base of the tooth.

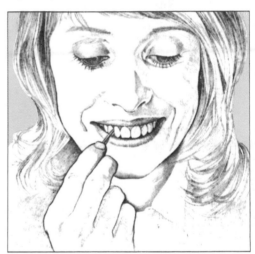

Toothpick
A toothpick is useful for removing large pieces of debris from the teeth, but is not as efficient as floss for cleaning between each tooth. It is, however, more convenient for use in the daytime. Do not force the toothpick down between the teeth, because this can damage the gum. Work the pick downwards with a gentle massaging or rubbing motion. The pick can be made of wood or plastic.

Hair

Hair grows out of small pockets in the skin called hair follicles. The cells in the base of the follicle multiply and gradually push the older, dead cells up the follicle. These dead cells form the hair shaft. The number of follicles on the scalp is determined while the foetus is developing in the womb.

Each hair has a definite period of growth, after which it is shed, and the follicle begins pushing up a new hair. The lifespan of a hair varies according to where on the body it is situated. Eyebrow hairs last for three to five months; hairs on the head last for two to five years. Human hair grows at an average rate of about 1cm ($\frac{1}{2}$ inch) a month.

Hair colour is produced by special cells at the base of the follicle that form coloured pigments in each cell. It is a hereditary factor. Dark hair usually dominates over light-coloured hair: for example, if a child has one parent with black or brown hair and one parent with red or blonde hair, the child's hair is likely to be dark-coloured.

Routine hair care

You should brush the hair daily to remove dirt and dead cells. Do not brush too vigorously, because you may uproot hairs and leave small ridges on the scalp that are vulnerable to infection. The best type of brush to use is made from natural bristle. The best type of comb is one that is saw-cut. Clean the brush and comb every time you wash your hair.

Hair can be washed twice a week without disturbing the natural balance of the oils. Greasy hair may need more frequent washing. After shampooing, a vigorous massage of the scalp stimulates the local circulation and frees small particles that may be adhering to the skin. The hair should be rinsed thoroughly in clean water, and should be brushed gently as it dries.

The basis of all shampoos is a soluble grease-removing agent. Other constituents include scents, colourants, and chemicals to make the shampoo thicker. These additional components may irritate the scalp. Commercial shampoos that claim to cure dandruff or seborrhoea are unlikely to be better than standard varieties. However, shampoos that contain selenium compounds can help these conditions. But prolonged use of such shampoos may be dangerous.

Cosmetic hair preparations

Many commercial hair treatments, particularly hair dyes, can produce an acute allergy, or contact dermatitis. For this reason, hair dyeing should be carried out only by a trained beautician. A person who is susceptible to allergy should ask for a patch test before any new dye is used on the scalp.

You should not attempt bleaching with hydrogen peroxide, dye stripping, or permanent waving at home. These methods can seriously damage the hair. Continual dyeing and bleaching tends to make the hair brittle. Regular use of other preparations, such as hair oils and hair sprays, may encourage dandruff.

Disorders of the hair

There are three main groups of disorders that are commonly regarded as disorders of the hair: (1) those that affect the follicle; (2) those that affect the surrounding skin; and (3) those that affect the hair shaft. Many of these disorders can be avoided or controlled with sensible hair hygiene.

Follicle disorders

Alopecia (baldness) caused by changes in a person's hormones cannot be cured. The condition occurs in men, in whom the pattern of hair loss tends to be inherited. Partial hair loss may affect women after menopause. Sometimes hair loss occurs after a severe emotional shock, a severe illness, or childbirth. Occasionally the body reacts against the hair substance. Sudden alopecia

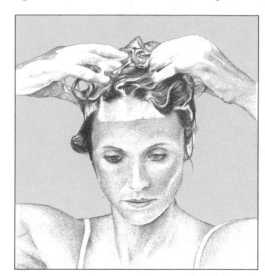

1

Massage shampoo into the hair and scalp with your fingertips, then rinse the hair thoroughly with warm water.

Use two applications of shampoo and carefully rinse the hair with clean water after each application to make sure that all of the lather is removed.

may occur for no apparent reason.

In some cases, a hair transplant may disguise baldness. Non-productive hair follicles are replaced with follicles from another area of the scalp. This procedure is expensive and the results vary. It does not arrest hair loss, which may continue behind the patch of transplanted hair.

Barber's rash is a chronic infection of the hair follicles by staphylococcus bacteria. Small, recurrent boils appear around each hair on the shaved area. It is most common in men, but women who shave axillary hair can also suffer from the condition. A person with barber's rash should stop shaving, and sterilize all shaving equipment after use. A mild antiseptic applied to the area after shaving may also help.

Hirsutism is an abnormal growth of hair. It is more common in women than men, and among some races. It is usually caused by hormonal changes in the body.

Surrounding skin disorders

Ringworm (tinea capitus) is a fungal infection of the scalp. It produces bald patches on the head that are covered with scaling skin and stumps of hair. Ringworm must be treated swiftly by a doctor, because it is highly infectious. Anyone contracting ringworm must use a separate brush and comb, which must be sterilized daily.

Seborrhoea is overactivity of the sebaceous glands of the skin. If this occurs on the scalp, the hair becomes greasy soon after it has been washed. The activity of the glands cannot be altered. The hair should be washed daily. Frequent washing does not encourage greasy hair. Selenium-based shampoos may also help.

Disorders of the hair shaft

Grey hair is due to an increasing number of air bubbles in the hair shaft. The only remedy for grey hair is to dye it. Nothing can stop the follicle producing the hair, but the dead cells can be dyed.

A person with suspected head lice must see a doctor. Towels, brushes, and combs must be sterilized after use, and must not be used by other members of the family.

The crab louse infests the pubic hair, eyelashes, and eyebrows. It may be transmitted during sexual intercourse, or caught from bedclothes or towels.

It is essential to have both varieties of lice treated swiftly, because lice can cause crusting, oozing skin similar to impetigo, and, in the tropics, carry relapsing fever and typhus.

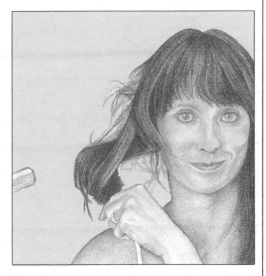

2
Washing removes not only grease and dirt from the hair, but also the natural oils.

A special soft plastic massager may be used to massage hair that is naturally dry. Conditioners, which coat the hair with a layer of wax, can be used after shampooing to counteract dryness.

3
Dry your hair by gently rubbing it with a soft towel. Hard rubbing with a rough towel may split the ends of the hairs.

Drying can also be done with an electric hair dryer. Do not hold the dryer too close to the head because you may burn the hair or even the skin of the scalp.

Looking after your back 1

The spinal column consists of twenty-four vertebrae, the sacrum, and the coccyx. The vertebrae differ in size according to position. Between each vertebra is a cushioned pad of cartilage called an intervertebral disc. The vertebrae and discs are strongest in the lumbar region, which supports most of the weight when a person is standing. The column of vertebrae protects the spinal cord running through the centre of each bone. The spine is further protected by a network of strong ligaments and muscles.

Because the spinal column is such a complex structure, many disorders can affect it. Backache accounts for a large number of working days lost to industry each year. Temporary backache can occur at the onset of a general illness, for example influenza, but many disorders that produce acute or chronic backache are avoidable if a person is careful with his or her back.

Coccydynia

Coccydynia is persistent, severe pain in the lowest area of the spine, the coccyx. The pain increases during defecation, and when sitting, but is reduced, or absent, when the person stands. The condition may last for many months following an injury to the coccyx. The commonest way to injure the coccyx is by falling heavily backwards in a sitting position.

Lordosis and kyphosis

Lordosis refers to the forward or inward curvature of the spine. Abnormal or excessive lordosis usually affects the lumbar region of the spine, and can cause backache. It is common among obese people, and during pregnancy, but may also be caused by incorrect posture.

Abnormal kyphosis is an excessive curvature of the spine in the thoracic region. It may result in the condition popularly known as hunchback. It is frequently associated with scoliosis, a lateral curvature of the spine that is usually caused by incorrect posture. It may also be caused by an injury to the back, by congenital mal-formation, or by various disorders that affect the spine.

Lumbago (low back pain)

Low back pain is one of the most common physical complaints, and often affects young adults or people in early middle age. The symptoms vary from morning back stiffness and difficulty in getting up out of chairs to sudden pain in the sides and an inability to stand upright or move.

Lumbago is usually caused by strained

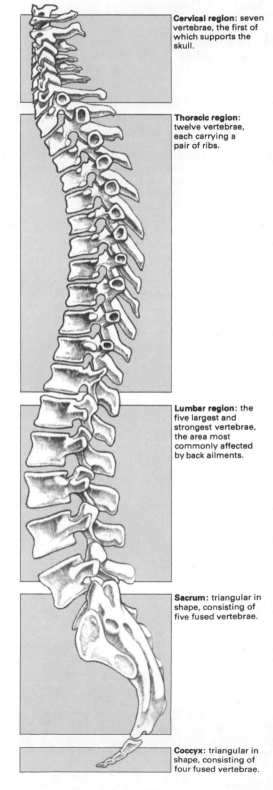

Cervical region: seven vertebrae, the first of which supports the skull.

Thoracic region: twelve vertebrae, each carrying a pair of ribs.

Lumbar region: the five largest and strongest vertebrae, the area most commonly affected by back ailments.

Sacrum: triangular in shape, consisting of five fused vertebrae.

Coccyx: triangular in shape, consisting of four fused vertebrae.

ligaments and muscles in the area surrounding the spine, or an intervertebral disc that has partly slipped. The injury can occur while taking unaccustomed back exercise.

The treatment of lumbago varies according to the severity of the pain or the disability. Good posture, and care taken while bending and lifting, can reduce the possibility of lumbago occurring.

Osteoarthritis

Osteoarthritis is a degenerative disorder of the joints. The onset is gradual after the age of forty-five and is more likely to affect the spine if a person has a previous history of back injury, or has done hard, manual labour for most of his or her life.

Slipped disc

An intervertebral disc consists of fibro-cartilage. The outer part is called the annulus fibrosus and the soft inner core is known as the nucleus pulposus. As the spine bends, pressure is exerted on the discs. If the pressure is too great, the soft centre can rupture through the outer ring and press on a nerve running from the spinal cord to another part of the body. The pain of the injury is felt in the area that the nerve supplies. The injury most commonly affects the lumbar intervertebral discs, because they take the most strain. If this occurs the pain is felt in the buttock and down the leg to the foot (sciatica).

A person can slip a disc by lifting a heavy object, or by taking some form of vigorous exercise that the body is not accustomed to. As with lumbago, treatment varies according to the severity of the injury. Slipped discs are more common in young men than women, and are unusual after the age of fifty.

Whiplash injury of the neck

A whiplash injury occurs when an accident jerks the head backwards and forwards like a whiplash. The sudden powerful force that causes the injury is often the result of a road accident. The ligaments in the neck are stretched or torn, internal bleeding may occur around the site of the injury, and sometimes an intervertebral disc in the neck may tear, causing pain down the shoulder and arm, and tingling in the hand.

A whiplash injury may not at first be apparent, but a few days after the accident the person experiences dizziness, severe headaches, and an inability to turn the head. Treatment depends on the severity. Whiplash injuries can be prevented by the use of headrest attachments on the seats.

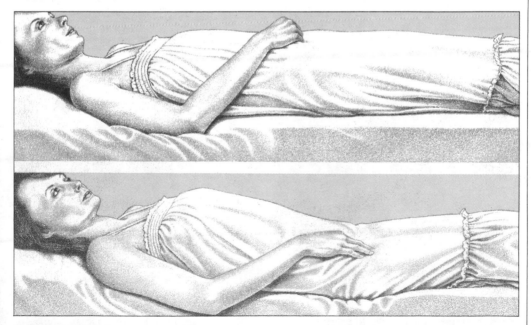

A firm mattress

A sagging bed that allows the spine to curve excessively (bottom) can cause severe back-ache. The mattress should follow the body contours without allowing it to sag (top).

The pillows should support the neck in line with the spinal column. If the base of the bed does not provide firm support, insert wooden boards beneath the mattress.

Looking after your back 2

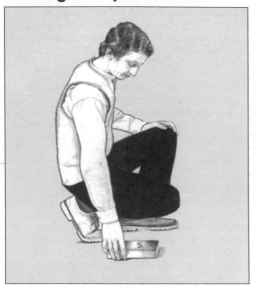

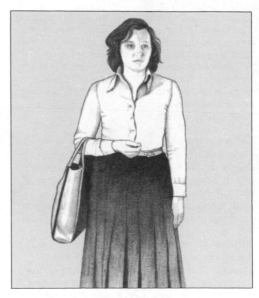

Lifting
To lift a small object from floor level, keep your back straight, and bend your knees. As you retrieve the object with one hand, steady yourself by placing the other hand on your raised knee. Use the leg muscles as you stand, keeping the back straight.

Carrying a handbag
Carry a handbag on the arm. This ensures that the weight of the bag is over the hip. The body is therefore balanced, with the trunk and spine upright. Divide a heavy load into two bags, and carry one in each hand with your arms by your side.

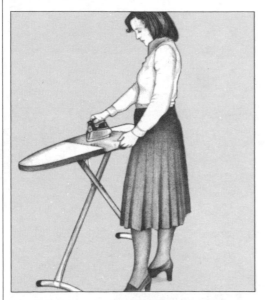

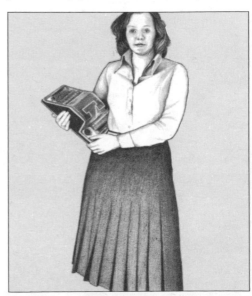

Standing and working
Ideally all work surfaces should be at waist level. If a surface is too low, transfer the weight of the body to one leg. This brings the shoulders nearer to the surface and enables you to keep the back straight. Transfer the weight from one leg to the other as you work.

Carrying an object
Instead of carrying a heavy object in front of you, carry it on your hip. The weight is then taken through the pelvis, and transmitted down each leg, and the back remains straight. The weight of the object can be counteracted by leaning the body in the opposite direction.

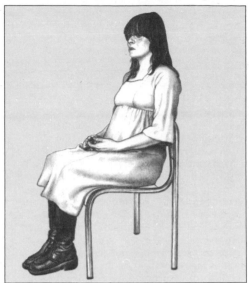

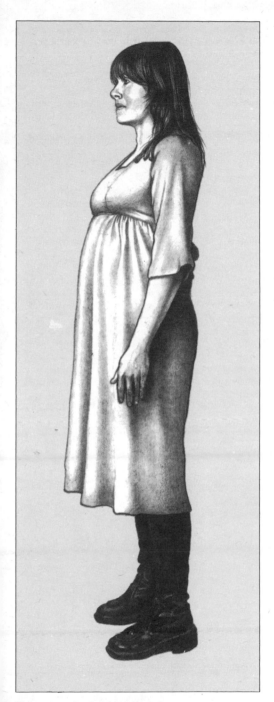

Sitting

During pregnancy it is essential to support the back while sitting. An upright chair with a high back is more comfortable than a low chair or sofa. To reduce pressure in the veins of the leg, place both feet flat on the floor. Do not sit with the legs crossed.

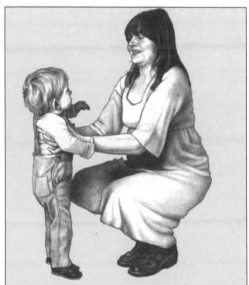

Posture during pregnancy

During pregnancy the small of the back supports much of the weight of the foetus. The back becomes hollow and can cause pain, so good posture is important. Stand with the feet slightly apart, the hips swung forwards, and the back straight.

Lifting

A pregnant woman with a small child can find pregnancy very tiring. It is essential to lift correctly. Bend at the knees instead of at the waist, lift the child with both hands, and keep the back straight as you lift. Let the leg muscles take the strain, not your back.

Routine health tests

A person's main need for a doctor occurs when symptoms of some disorder become apparent or are felt. But many disorders do not produce obvious symptoms until the disease is well advanced. This type of disease can usually be effectively treated if it is identified at an early stage. Routine health screening tests are now a recognized and important part of preventive medicine. Many health tests can be carried out annually by your doctor, but some can be carried out daily, weekly, or on a regular basis by you.

Many individuals decide to have a regular physical check-up by their own doctor, or to have one as part of the health programme recommended by the employer. The tests are often carried out at health centres containing all the facilities and equipment needed for such assessments.

Patients who have a particular problem, such as high blood pressure, diabetes mellitus, or glaucoma, should have regular examinations to ensure that the condition is under control. Some patients are now taught how to take their own blood pressure, and all diabetics must know how to test their own urine for sugar.

Routine testing helps to ensure a healthy pregnancy, because many potentially serious disorders, such as pre-eclampsia, can be identified and treated at an early stage. The development of the foetus can be monitored, and possible problems that may arise during labour can be detected, such as a breech presentation. The obstetrician's examination includes blood pressure recordings, urinanalysis, and weight assessment during antenatal examinations. A pregnant woman is advised to see her obstetrician every four weeks during the first six months, every two weeks for the next two months, and every week during the final month.

Personal health tests

It is important to establish a daily routine of health care, including general cleanliness (p.936), care of the nails (p.942), and the teeth (p.944). Check your eyes in the mirror each morning to make sure that the whites look healthy, and not coloured.

Monitor bowel and urinary habits, but do not become obsessed with regularity, because this differs from person to person. However, if bowel movements cause minor discomfort, increase your intake of roughage.

Each month a woman should examine her breasts for any unusual lumps or other changes. The examination should be carried out a few days after menstruation when the breasts are at their smallest. It is important to examine the breasts at the same time each month, because a woman's cycle produces

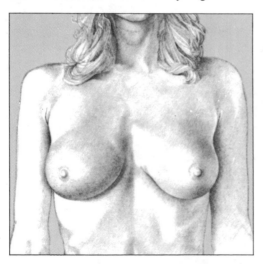

1
Examine your breasts each month at the end of your menstrual period. Firstly, look carefully at the breasts in a mirror with your arms by your side. Raise your arms above your head and turn from side to side. Look for any unusual puckering of the skin, or a change in the normal shape of the breast. Make sure that the nipples look normal.

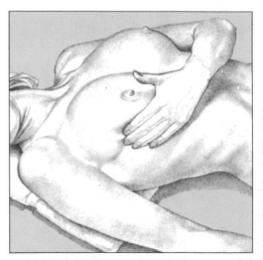

2
Lie down and put a folded towel beneath one shoulder. Keep your arm by your side and examine the breast with the fingertips of the other hand. Press firmly, but gently. Feel the outer edges of the breast, then work in a circular motion towards and around the nipple, gently pinching with finger and thumb feeling for lumps or thickened tissue.

natural changes in the breast tissue that may be confusing. A woman who detects a lump should see her doctor immediately. It must be remembered, however, that the majority of breast lumps are not caused by cancer. There are many other reasons for breast lumps, but it does need investigation.

Six-monthly tests
Every six months you should visit the dentist, who checks the teeth and fillings for any early signs of decay. He or she also checks that you are cleaning your teeth correctly, and not habitually missing an area at the back of the teeth.

Annual tests
A yearly visit to an optician enables him or her to test your eyes for early signs of vision deterioration. The optician also tests the intra-ocular pressure of the eye to detect early signs of glaucoma, a treatable disease that can cause permanent blindness if neglected. This test is particularly important after the age of forty.

During a regular check-up with your doctor, you will be given a full physical examination, including inspection of eyes, ears, nose, skin, glands, and reproductive organs. The doctor may also arrange for chest X-rays, and an electrocardiogram. The doctor takes your weight, your blood pressure, and sends a sample of urine for analysis. Women should have a breast and pelvic examination, and a Pap smear test. Men over the age of forty may have a rectal and prostate examination. The doctor may also advise you to have a blood screening test and a hearing test. The doctor may give you any necessary immunization injections.

Routine health tests at various ages
Infancy and early childhood is a time of rapid growth and development, and regular testing and examination is important. The tests can be carried out by your general practitioner, or at the baby clinic.

Certain tests, such as hearing tests, are carried out at specific ages, because before that age a baby may hear well, but not have sufficiently well-developed co-ordination to react to the noise. The doctor also follows a careful immunization schedule, and inspects the baby's emerging teeth. The baby will not have to visit the dentist until after the age of two and a half to three years.

During later childhood and adolescence, children should have their growth and development checked regularly. Six-monthly visits to the dentist are imperative during these years, because treatment may be necessary to correct malocclusion.

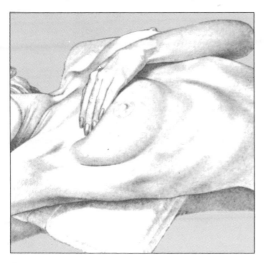

3
Place your hand behind your head and repeat the examination. You are feeling for any lumps or thickening of the tissues. You will soon learn to detect any unusual variations. Even in a small-breasted woman the breast tissue extends to within a few inches of the collarbone and examination must include this often flat area.

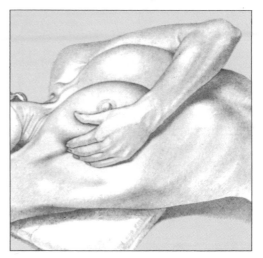

4
Keep your arm raised above your head, and examine the tissue underneath the arm. To do this, begin above the nipple, and work the fingers along towards the armpit. Press your fingers deep into the armpit to feel the lymph gland. You will soon learn what the glands normally feel like. Repeat the examination on the other breast.

Rest and Health

Fatigue

Fatigue is a signal for rest and relaxation. The changes in the body that produce fatigue are not fully understood. A person naturally feels tired at the end of a stressful day, or after heavy physical exercise. But a violently stressful situation, a car crash for instance, produces severe fatigue a few minutes after the event, even if the person is not injured by the accident. If a person does not rest and sleep properly, important faculties such as concentration and reflexes are impaired.

Fatigue also changes a person's ability to cope with stress. In some people, stress produces disorders like diarrhoea, migraine, skin eruptions, and even asthma. Also, many authorities believe that stress may have a direct link with high blood pressure and coronary heart disease. If you push yourself to the limits of fatigue, you will be unable to deal adequately with stress, and your health will suffer.

Rest and relaxation

If you are relaxed you are better equipped to cope with the pressures of everyday living. Many people find it difficult to relax and need to be taught how to, in order to stop wasting energy on needless activity.

Relaxing is a skill. Physical relaxation is best obtained after a period of intense activity, such as a sports game or jogging. This principle applies to relaxation exercises that help you to become aware of the tone of the muscles. It is easy to feel when a muscle is tensed for activity, but difficult to feel when it is fully relaxed. Relaxation exercises systematically tense the muscles throughout the body, starting at the toes and working upwards, then "let go". You can then feel the muscle relaxing.

Deep breathing is also a good way to help relaxation. Lie or sit down comfortably. Place your hands on the abdomen just below the rib-cage. Slowly inhale through the nostrils, and feel the diaphragm filling and pulling the fingers open. Feel the chest expansion spread upwards to the shoulders. Hold your breath for a few seconds, and then slowly exhale through the nostrils. At the end of the exhalation, concentrate on the rib and shoulder muscles in their relaxed state. Many people find that four or five deep breaths prepare them for any stressful situation.

Some people find that meditation and yoga are two successful methods of deep relaxation. Meditation teaches a person to concentrate on a word, symbol, or object (known as a mantra). This enables the person to dismiss all other thoughts from the mind.

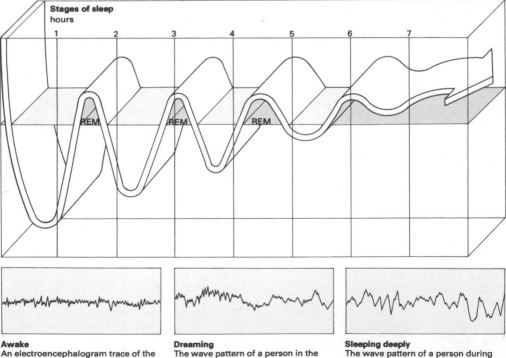

Stages of sleep
hours
1 2 3 4 5 6 7

REM REM REM

Awake
An electroencephalogram trace of the electrical impulses of the brain. The wave pattern is shallow and sharp when a person is alert.

Dreaming
The wave pattern of a person in the rapid eye movement (REM) stage of sleep. It is during this stage that a person dreams.

Sleeping deeply
The wave pattern of a person during deep sleep. The eyes are still, and the person moves less. The pattern is relaxed and free.

Yoga combines mental relaxation with physical harmony. It is a popular pastime, and many classes are now available.

Relaxation is often taught in antenatal classes. In the early months of pregnancy, fatigue may increase feelings of nausea. Most obstetricians recommend a rest period of two hours a day, preferably after lunch.

The aim of relaxation and deep breathing during childbirth is to preserve the woman's energy for effective muscle control throughout labour. Many women continue relaxation and breathing exercises after the baby is born. A new mother should take every opportunity during the daytime to rest and relax while the baby sleeps. This enables her to make up for some of the sleep that may have been lost earlier.

Chronic fatigue produced by the monotony of many kinds of work can be cured only by a long period of rest. A holiday should be at least two weeks long, because it takes two to three days for a person to recover from acute fatigue, aggravated by travelling and organizing the holiday, and another week to overcome chronic fatigue. It is only after about ten days that the benefits of a holiday take effect.

Intercontinental travellers often suffer from jet lag because of the change of time zone. They should have a period of rest on arrival, and should postpone all important decisions until after a night's sleep.

It is also important to rest after a meal. Digestion requires additional blood flow through the intestine after a meal. Physical activity disrupts digestion because the blood is concentrated in the muscles for exercise. The main meals of each day should be followed by a period of half an hour of physical relaxation.

Sleep

Although most people spend a third of each twenty-four hour day asleep, no one fully understands why the body has to sleep. Without sleep a person begins to hallucinate, and mental faculties quickly deteriorate.

When you are asleep, body metabolism is slower, and breathing rate and heart rate both drop. Body temperature also drops, and there is a reduction in muscle tone.

Sleep occurs in two stages. About three-quarters of sleep time is spent in deep sleep. An electroencephalogram during this period indicates slow waves of brain activity. However, there are several periods throughout the night when the waves of brain activity become very active. The eyes move from side to side beneath the eyelids. This is known as rapid eye movement, or REM.

During these periods you are dreaming.

Sleep requirements vary from person to person and from age to age. A newborn baby may need as much as twenty-one hours sleep a day. A growing child needs more sleep than an adult, and parents should try to establish a pattern of regular bedtimes for children. Many young children wake up early in the morning. Although this is annoying for the rest of the family, it is normal. Make sure that the child has plenty of toys within easy reach to play with until the rest of the household is awake. Children often need a nap during the day. Most young children sleep during the afternoon, but some prefer to go back to sleep after breakfast. Allow the child to set his or her own time for a nap.

A major problem for the parent of an adolescent is trying to encourage the adolescent to get enough sleep. Periods of intense physical and emotional activity are interspersed with periods of extreme lethargy which are often due to physical and mental fatigue. Sleep rhythms are also broken by the adolescent's need to maintain an active social life. Parents should encourage an adolescent to sleep at least seven hours a night.

Elderly people tend to require less sleep than an active adult but they make up for sleep lost during the night by napping during the day.

Insomnia

Insomnia is a much misused word. Throughout a full night's sleep you are drifting from deep to shallow sleep, and often wake up. Most people cannot remember how many times they have awakened during the night. But if you think you are suffering from insomnia, a short period of wakefulness may be prolonged with worry.

Sleeping difficulties are often a sign of stress, worry, and depression. You should not resort to sleeping pills to solve the problem. Other ways of promoting sleep include taking exercise before bed, for example, a short walk; drinking a warm milky drink (tea and coffee should be avoided); and relaxing the mind with light reading. If you do wake in the night and are unable to get back to sleep, it is preferable to read a book rather than lie in the dark and worry. Often the distraction of going to the kitchen to get a drink helps you fall asleep fairly quickly when you return to bed.

Chronic insomnia may have a physical or psychological cause, and in such cases medical advice should be sought. A sympathetic doctor can usually find the underlying reason for the insomnia, and prescribe appropriate treatment.

Sex and health

Sexuality is part of everyone's life. Good health helps to maintain libido (sexual drive), and a satisfactory sex life is good for mental and physical health.

Common sexual problems

Ignorance about sexual intercourse is surprisingly common. Some "infertile" couples find that an explicit explanation about sex from their doctor is all that is necessary to overcome problems.

Premature ejaculation is upsetting for a man, and unsatisfying for a woman. Foreplay, and lubricating the vagina before intercourse helps. Because minor penetration difficulties may encourage the man to reach a climax too soon, there are some preparations available on the market that numb the penis, and prolong the time before ejaculation. If premature ejaculation continues, it is often helpful to discuss the problem with a sex therapist who can offer some practical advice.

A woman who is over-anxious about intercourse may involuntarily tighten the muscles around the vagina. This is known as vaginismus. Penetration problems may also be caused by a tougher than usual hymen (the ridge of skin around the vagina). The hymen may tear during intercourse, causing some bleeding and pain. If such problems continue, a doctor may recommend a minor operation to widen the hymen.

During adolescence some teenagers are briefly but strongly attracted to people of the same sex. The attachment may become physical, and include mutual masturbation. It is normal for many adolescents to go through such a phase of homosexuality.

Pregnancy

Intercourse can usually take place quite safely up to the last month of pregnancy. By this time the woman may be disinterested, and frontal intercourse becomes physically more difficult. Intercourse from behind may be easier. Intercourse should, however, not take place if there is any pain, vaginal bleeding, or if fluid is leaking from the amniotic sac, because of the risk of infection. A fluid leakage is cause for immediate medical attention.

After the baby is born, intercourse may be resumed as soon as any tear has healed, but many obstetricians recommend a wait of six weeks and some form of contraception.

Menstruation

No harm will come either to the woman or the man if sexual intercourse takes place during menstruation. However, it is prohibited by some religions, and may be aesthetically disagreeable to many couples.

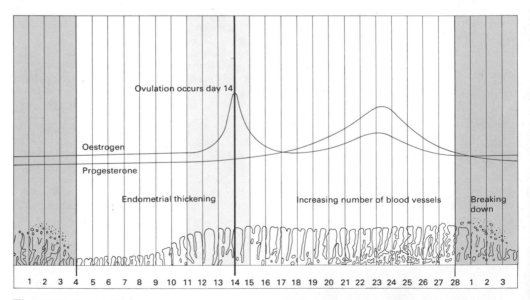

The menstrual cycle

About 500 eggs are produced by a woman in her lifetime but it is unlikely that more than 12 eggs will be fertilized. Each month the lining of the uterus thickens, and then breaks down if the egg is not fertilized. The dark-coloured band indicates the five days of menstruation when blood and mucus flow from the vagina. The light-coloured band indicates the time when sexual intercourse could result in fertilization.

Drugs

The drug treatment of some disorders may reduce libido. Such drugs include those for high blood pressure and hormone disorders, as well as some tranquillizing drugs. Other drugs can have a profound effect on libido; for example, marijuana smoking over a prolonged period of time gradually reduces libido in both sexes.

Social drugs, such as alcohol, reduce the many inhibitions on sexual behaviour, but frequently destroy a man's ability to achieve satisfactory intercourse.

Obesity

Anyone who is overweight may find that libido is reduced. A loss of weight eliminates many physical difficulties during intercourse, and increases the person's sex drive and stamina.

Illness

Most illnesses are accompanied by a reduction in libido. This recovers when the person returns to normal health. In most illnesses, a patient's common sense is the best guide to follow as to when intercourse is safe. After a coronary thrombosis, a return to normal sexual intercourse is encouraged, but the timing should be discussed with a doctor. If angina (heart pain) occurs during intercourse, the patient is sometimes advised to take a drug before intercourse.

Venereal disease

The commonest risk associated with sexual intercourse is venereal disease. Some sexually transmitted diseases can be contracted without sexual contact, although this is uncommon.

Nonspecific urethritis (or NSU) is an inflammation of the urethra, often by an unidentified micro-organism. It is often difficult to cure, and relapses are common. Symptoms usually appear only in the man, and include a watery discharge from the penis and pain during urination. Symptoms in a woman are rare, but a female partner should never assume that her partner alone has contracted the infection.

Gonorrhoea produces symptoms similar to, but more severe than NSU. The symptoms are evident in the man, and may also be present in the woman. A woman may experience pain during urination and have a vaginal discharge. It is a serious disease if left untreated, and can lead to sterility. Treatment is usually with antibiotic drugs. The completion of the full course of treatment is essential.

Trichomoniasis usually produces symptoms in women only. The organism infects the vagina and is most commonly, but not always, transmitted sexually. The symptoms include an irritating vaginal discharge. Men occasionally suffer from a similar irritation in the penis. Treatment is effective, if both partners are treated.

Syphilis is a venereal disease, the final stages of which are now hardly ever seen. It has recently become more common, particularly among homosexuals. The first symptoms of syphilis are painless ulcers on the genitals, around the anus, or sometimes on the lips. The ulcers heal in two or three weeks. About six weeks later, fever and a rash appear. A person who detects any of these symptoms should seek medical help immediately. Although syphilis is easily cured with antibiotics, it is still serious.

Moniliasis (candidiasis), or thrush, is a very common fungal infection that may be transmitted through sexual intercourse. As an infection of the vagina, thrush appears when some other agent upsets the normal bacterial balance in the intestine, from where the infection spreads. Thrush is also common after taking broad-spectrum antibiotics, the contraceptive pill, and during pregnancy, because of the associated hormonal changes. Symptoms include vaginal itching, and a thick greenish-yellow discharge. The infection can be treated with fungicidal suppositories or cream. A man may get a similar irritation on the penis.

Cystitis is inflammation of the bladder. It is much more common in women than men. One form that affects women ("honeymoon" cystitis) can be caused by sexual intercourse. The symptoms include a burning sensation during urination, increasing frequency of urination, and sometimes incontinence. Although the condition is uncomfortable and distressing, antibiotic treatment is usually swift and successful.

If a person detects any symptoms of a urinogenital disorder, it is extremely important that three rules are followed: (1) consult a doctor as soon as possible; (2) complete any course of treatment; and (3) tell the partner if advised to do so by the doctor.

Unwanted pregnancy

For most women, pregnancy is a healthy and happy state to be in. But, for others, a pregnancy may be unwanted, physically dangerous, and damaging to mental health. The consequences of such a pregnancy may be extremely serious. Yet, many people still find the subject of contraception impossible to mention to a partner until too late. Some

Methods of contraception

Oral contraceptive
Contains synthetic oestrogens and progesterones that stop ovulation. A pill is taken daily for 21 days of a 28-day cycle. Virtually 100 per cent reliable.

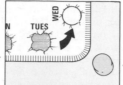

Condom
Thin rubber sheath placed over erect penis before intercourse. Reliable if used correctly with a spermicide jelly. Helps to prevent transmission of venereal disease.

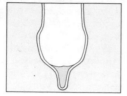

Intra-uterine device (IUCD)
A coil or loop inserted into the womb by a gynaecologist to prevent a fertilized egg from implanting in the womb. Very reliable method after first year of use.

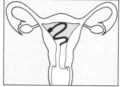

Diaphragm and chemical
Thin rubber cap filled with spermicidal jelly and inserted over the neck of the womb before intercourse. Left in place for eight hours afterwards. Very reliable if used correctly.

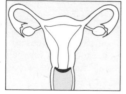

Spermicides
Jelly, cream, or foam introduced into the vagina before intercourse. Unreliable and messy unless used in conjunction with a diaphragm or condom.

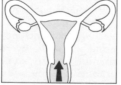

Rhythm method
Abstinence from sexual intercourse for a 10-day period in the middle of the 28-day cycle. Unreliable because monthly cycles are variable.

1	2	3	4
5	6	7	8	9
10	11	12	13	14
15	16	17	18	19

Vasectomy or sterilization
Tube carrying germ cells (vas deferens in the male, fallopian tube in the female) cut surgically. Almost 100 per cent safe. Should be considered permanent.

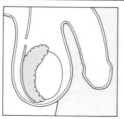

fall back on amateurish alternatives, such as douching after intercourse, or using the withdrawal method. (Douching does not work because, however soon after intercourse it is done, the man's sperm ejaculated deep inside the cervix has already entered the womb. And not only is withdrawal emotionally unsatisfactory, but sperm can escape from the penis before ejaculation.) Family planning clinics and personal doctors offer helpful and confidential advice about contraception.

Unwanted pregnancies may also occur following the birth of a first baby, and during menopause. A woman who has just had a baby should never assume that breast-feeding, or the absence of menstruation means she is infertile. If the couple do not want another pregnancy immediately, they should arrange some form of contraception. (If the woman had been using a diaphragm before, she should have it refitted, because the shape of the vagina and cervix may change following labour). A woman going through menopause must wait at least one year after the last menstruation until she can forget about methods of contraception.

Cancer

Any woman who has started to have regular sexual intercourse should have cervical smear tests when advised to by her doctor. A smear test can detect signs of cancer as early as ten years before serious symptoms appear, thereby enabling treatment to be started during the initial stages of the disease.

Uterine cancer may be associated with prolonged hormone replacement therapy (HRT), which may be prescribed for a woman during menopause if she experiences unpleasant symptoms, such as hot flushes, night sweats, and depression. HRT should be used with care, and a gynaecologist can advise whether HRT is better with a withdrawal period every year or two, or continually with six-monthly or yearly examinations of cells from the uterus.

Libido

Libido is sex drive. It varies among different people, and at different ages. Opportunity to indulge in sexual intercourse also affects libido. A couple who can have intercourse whenever they feel like it experience less urgency than a couple who must take advantage of a chance the moment it is presented.

A woman's libido varies during her menstrual cycle and often reaches its height at mid-cycle, at the time of ovulation, and again during menstruation, possibly because the flow of menstrual blood slightly stimulates the vagina. If a couple's sexual arousal and satisfaction seem persistently incompatible, they should discuss the subject with a marriage guidance counsellor.

The frequency of intercourse varies greatly from couple to couple, within a stable relationship. Some partners may have intercourse two or three times a day, while others may be satisfied with two or three times a month. Similarly, a practice that one couple find natural (for example, oral-genital sex) may repel another couple. But the important thing is that both partners respect each other's needs, and are able to set their own level of activity accordingly.

Sexuality at different ages

A newborn baby boy can have an erection. When a baby reaches the age of about one year, he or she begins to explore the genitals. Once out of nappies, some babies may begin massaging the genitals and occasionally seem to reach some kind of climax. It is important that parents do not stop the child from doing this; babies usually stop handling the genitals after a few months. Only at the onset of puberty might a child start masturbating again.

Parents should answer any questions the child asks on the subject during childhood. Few children are interested in more than a few details at a time. Such questions represent the child's natural need for factual knowledge, and parents should approach the subject unemotionally and informatively. A parent's answer to such questions should be direct and in simple terms that the child can easily understand.

Puberty is a time of rapid physical change when a child's sexual interest awakens. By the time the child has reached this age, subjects such as menstruation, ovulation, fertilization, and nocturnal emission of semen should have been discussed. Contraception also should have been mentioned by the age of puberty.

A year or two before the onset of menstruation it is normal for the vagina to produce a slight discharge. As long as the discharge causes no irritation, and does not smell, it is nothing to worry about. When a girl first begins to menstruate, the periods may be irregular, and occur once every two or three months before settling into a regular rhythm.

If a boy knows about nocturnal emission he will not feel guilty and ashamed about it when it happens. There is normally a long interval between the first "wet dream" and the second. The dreams that cause nocturnal emission of semen are usually symbolic rather than obviously sexual.

Masturbation is a way of releasing a build-up of sexual tension in the adolescent who does not have regular sexual intercourse. Whether an adolescent masturbates several times a night, or not at all, may depend on the individual's upbringing, or temperament, or perhaps only on the way in which emotional and physical energy has been used during the day.

Libido is at its height during a person's early twenties. Many factors can interfere with a person's libido, however, such as fatigue and stress. Some women find that premenstrual tension also disrupts their libido. If such disruption causes problems, the woman should discuss the situation with a doctor who may prescribe drugs to relieve some of the premenstrual symptoms.

Other women find that the contraceptive pill can also reduce libido. The reduction may happen very gradually, but as soon as it becomes a problem, the situation should be discussed with a doctor or gynaecologist, who may suggest a different type of contraceptive pill or contraceptive device.

By middle age, the rhythm of sexual activity has usually settled into a pattern for the couple concerned. Although there is still a great range of variations, the immediate urgency and frequency has usually gone. Some men may find that prostate gland problems stimulate their sex drive, but reduce their performance.

Menopause does not mean the end of a woman's sexual life. Many women find instead that once released from the burden of contraception, they can indulge in sex with renewed vigour. But without the regular stimulation of the hormonal cycle, the vagina can shrivel in size and become dry. Intercourse is beneficial because it keeps the vagina moist and supple. If dryness is causing concern, a doctor may recommend ointments or suppositories.

A woman's partner should be understanding and helpful during the menopause. Some women find that the night sweats make sharing a double bed impossible. If sex life has not been very good before the menopause, a woman may use it as an excuse to stop intercourse altogether. But a satisfactory sex life in early adulthood usually continues into old age.

Although sexual intercourse continues for some people until they are well into their eighties, there is usually a great reduction in frequency. However, the close physical contact of another loving person is a warm and satisfying compensation.

The environment and health

Health and environment are intricately inter-related. Our environment is not only dependent on fluctuations of climate and variations from season to season, but is also affected by factors that are under our own control. This is especially true in the twentieth century when technology has, while improving the lives of millions, also proved to be a danger to human life itself, as the many different types of environmental pollution testify.

Few would argue with this statement, and especially not people who have been the victims of industrial accidents that released harmful products into the environment, permanently damaging health if not actually causing death. Industrial pollution accidents have become commonplace events in the modern world and more and more people have become aware that technology can kill as well as improve life.

Environmental pollution is not only a national health problem today, it is a world problem with grave implications for the survival of mankind. It is the concern of everyone in every kind of environment, and governments are having to plan and implement action to reduce pollution and to make threatening environments less of a health hazard.

It would, however, be an error to consider pollution simply as a physical problem and to assume that all that is needed is legislation for cleaner air, cleaner water, a reduction in noise levels, and the elimination of dirty or toxic products.

Man's distinctive characteristic is adaptability and, rather than becoming extinct, people will probably learn to live in environments that are hazardous. But, now that people are becoming increasingly aware that human interference with nature can reduce the quality of life and health, something can be done to change attitudes. Just as the environment has been changed for the worse in some places, so it can be changed for the better.

Our ability to control the natural environment has made it possible for people to live in areas that were previously considered uninhabitable or at least hazardous. Thus, thanks to the advancement of science and modern technology, communities and towns have sprung up in such extreme environments as the desert of Arizona and the frozen tundra of Siberia. In many ways the natural environment has been modified to suit our own needs. This modification has often produced new dangers, some of which may be anticipated and others which have come to light

accidentally. For example, in some situations rare diseases have developed, possibly as a result of these changes: Legionnaire's disease, which was previously unknown, is able to spread through ventilating systems.

Urban air pollution is a major health hazard, as anyone who lives in a large city knows. For example, air pollution in Tokyo is only surpassed by that of New York. In 1952, fog over London, most of it containing sulphur dioxide, caused thousands of deaths, particularly among those who were already suffering from heart and lung diseases or other respiratory ailments.

Carbon monoxide and other pollutants from car exhaust fumes, especially in large cities, are now recognized as an important factor affecting health. These pollutants have an effect on the central nervous system in a healthy person and evidence has been published suggesting that they can affect the intelligence of children brought up in areas in which the air is constantly polluted by the fumes. Carbon monoxide reduces the oxygen-carrying capacity of the blood and in this way inhibits the normal growth of body tissues. More serious poisoning by car exhaust fumes has been eliminated to some extent by reducing the lead content of petrol.

There are numerous other pollutants that cause ailments ranging from minor respiratory complaints to death from cancer. They may also cause genetic alterations. For example, pollutants like aldehydes, that come from the thermal decomposition of fats, oil, or glycerol, irritate nasal and respiratory tracts, while ammonia from chemical processes such as dye-making and explosive manufacture inflames the upper respiratory passage.

Chlorine from many chemical processes attacks the mucous membranes of the entire respiratory tract and also the eyes. Sulphur dioxide, from coal and oil combustion, causes chest constriction, headache, vomiting, and aggravates respiratory ailments. Suspended particles, such as ash, soot and smoke, from incinerators and manufacturing processes, cause emphysema, eye irritations, and possibly cancer.

Water pollution is a good example of how man has upset nature's balance. Purifying agents are added to the water supply of most cities in an attempt to eliminate the danger of infection from bacteria and viruses. For instance, chlorine has been widely used to neutralize sewage contamination, but there is now some concern that large amounts of chlorine may cause some genetic harm. So, too, is there a controversy about the addition of fluoride to drinking water to decrease dental decay in children. While fluoride has been given widespread medical approval many people still claim that it has some dangers not yet apparent.

Some experts contend that the natural variations in the chemical content of water (that is, the amount of calcium, making the water "hard" or "soft") may have an effect on the incidence of arteriosclerosis and coronary heart disease. Increasingly, public health experts are investigating the correlation between geographical location and the incidence of various ailments.

In the meantime, dumping of industrial waste into rivers, lakes, and the oceans has killed a significant proportion of the life in the waters and has sometimes also destroyed the vegetation as well as bird and animal life surrounding the waters.

Another major cause for concern is the burying or dumping in the oceans of radio-active wastes. Such waste takes many years to decay into a harmless, inactive form. There is also considerable anxiety about the dangers of accidents in nuclear power stations, particularly to those living near them. This anxiety has recently been accentuated by accidents in which some part of the plant has failed and radiation has leaked into the surrounding environment. The safety of the nuclear industry in comparison with other environmental hazards is difficult to assess because the potential danger of a nuclear accident is far greater than the danger in other industries.

Water pollution is seen by many people to be one of the most serious forms of pollution because it also affects the quality of the food that people eat. Years of dumping industrial waste into rivers have produced alterations in the types of food animals that reach people's tables. Pollution is absorbed by the tiny organisms that are the food of the fish eaten by people and, in this way, human pollution is returned by nature to man. For instance, at one time tuna fish consumption was banned by public health authorities because it contained dangerously high levels of mercury. The mercury had been absorbed by the fish from contaminated parts of the sea which had been polluted by the dumping of industrial wastes.

Noise is also now recognized as a pollutant, both at home and at work. People who have to work in a noisy environment have to contend with the occupational hazard of deafness. Not only is physical health affected in this way, but also emotional and psychological health may be affected by the stress caused by a noisy environment. Some industries require workers to wear earplugs, but the incidence of hearing disorders from industrial conditions is high.

It is not only those working in industry who are likely to be affected adversely by noise. People are surrounded by machinery that makes noise and, at least, this can make it difficult to sleep and so lead to other damage to the health. At worst, a high level of exposure to constant noise has been associated with diseases caused by stress, such as colitis, hypertension, and peptic ulcer, as well as some nervous disorders. People who live near large airports in particular often complain that the noise affects their health.

Most of the discussion so far has been about the environment of city dwellers and those working in an industrial environment. This is because such people are more seriously at risk than others. However the environment in the country can also be dangerous and hostile, although in different ways from that in a city. The countryside is less easily controlled, generally speaking, except, of course, for the hazards of chemical pollution from crop spraying and farm poisons. The extremes of temperature may cause frostbite and hypothermia by exposure to unusually cold conditions, while prolonged exposure to sunlight, particularly in fair-skinned people, can cause skin cancer. Skin inflammation or contact dermatitis may result from hypersensitivity to many plants, such as primulas. And the misery of hay fever from the seasonal variations in pollen concentration is very often far greater in the country than in the town.

Most serious of all, however, is the danger of chemical pollution, in all its forms. There is a need to develop new ways to meet the physical and biological threats of this kind of pollution. Aspects of technology are largely responsible for the pollution of the environment, and now methods must be found to clear up the damage. It is reasonable to think that other forms of technology may provide the answers. Such a change in thinking produces many problems, and one of them is economic, the cost of such a clean-up being in terms of millions of pounds. It also necessitates a radical change in industrial practices, and in the general trend towards increasing consumption of goods and hence increasing production of waste. Perhaps what is more important for our future is that people learn to work together to a common end that will be beneficial to us all. The end in question must be the elimination of the worst – if not all – environmental hazards, and a greater understanding of the technology we create.

Food and health: nutrition 1

Plants obtain energy to grow, respire, and reproduce from sunlight and from simple elements in the earth and the air, such as carbon dioxide, water, minerals, and salts. The simple elements are converted into complex food materials which can subsequently be broken down for energy. Humans cannot convert these simple elements into energy, so they have to eat complex food materials either from plants, or from other animals that have previously eaten plants.

The complex materials are broken down during the process of digestion, then absorbed for use in three main ways. The food components can be oxidized and used as energy, the components may be used to rebuild tissue, or they may be used to make new body cells for growth. A well-balanced diet must provide carbohydrates, fats, and proteins in the correct proportions; trace elements such as vitamins and mineral salts; and water and roughage. These must be consumed in adequate quantities to provide energy and must be adjusted to suit each individual's requirements, which vary with such factors as age, sex, physical build, and occupation. An intake of less than 1500 calories a day for a working person will result in weight loss and starvation because the body has to oxidize food stores in the tissues to provide energy. If such a situation persists, death results, often from an infection before complete starvation has occurred. However, if a person eats more than he or she requires for energy, the body stores the excess, initially as glycogen in the liver, and then as fat in the fat cells beneath the skin. A person who weighs 20 per cent or more above the norm for his or her height, age, and occupation is termed obese and health may suffer.

Obesity

About 20 per cent of adults in Britain are obese; many more are overweight. It is easy to change from being overweight to being obese. The chance of dying before the age of sixty is greatly increased if a person is overweight. Obese people run a high risk of developing heart diseases, diabetes, varicose veins, haemorrhoids and, by putting an unnatural load on the joints, may develop arthritis at an early age. An obese person may suffer from skin irritation in the folds of fat, and is likely to develop breathing difficulties in later life.

Obesity is seldom caused by a glandular disorder. The reason is usually that the person is eating more than is being used up in energy. An obese person must reduce the daily calorie intake to a level below that needed by the body, forcing it to use the excess stored in the tissues. Since obesity is a medical condition, it is wise to consult a doctor who can recommend a carefully

MEN'S MEDICAL WEIGHT CHART

| Height | | Average Weight | | Obese | |
cm	(ft in)	stone lb	(kg)	stone lb	(kg)
155	(5 1)	8 12	(56)	10 8	(67)
158	(5 2)	9 1	(58)	10 13	(69)
160	(5 3)	9 4	(59)	11 2	(71)
163	(5 4)	9 7	(60)	11 5	(72)
165	(5 5)	9 11	(62)	11 11	(75)
168	(5 6)	10 1	(64)	12 1	(77)
170	(5 7)	10 5	(66)	12 7	(79)
173	(5 8)	10 9	(68)	12 11	(81)
175	(5 9)	10 13	(69)	13 1	(83)
178	(5 10)	11 4	(72)	13 8	(86)
180	(5 11)	11 8	(74)	13 12	(88)
183	(6 0)	11 13	(76)	14 5	(91)
185	(6 1)	12 3	(78)	14 9	(93)
188	(6 2)	12 8	(80)	15 2	(96)
191	(6 3)	12 13	(82)	15 7	(98)

WOMEN'S MEDICAL WEIGHT CHART

| Height | | Average Weight | | Obese | |
cm	(ft in)	stone lb	(kg)	stone lb	(kg)
142	(4 8)	7 4	(46)	8 10	(55)
145	(4 9)	7 6	(47)	8 12	(56)
147	(4 10)	7 9	(49)	9 3	(59)
150	(4 11)	7 12	(50)	9 6	(60)
152	(5 0)	8 1	(51)	9 6	(61)
155	(5 1)	8 4	(53)	10 0	(64)
158	(5 2)	8 8	(54)	10 4	(65)
160	(5 3)	8 11	(56)	10 7	(67)
163	(5 4)	9 2	(58)	11 0	(70)
165	(5 5)	9 6	(60)	11 4	(72)
168	(5 6)	9 10	(62)	11 10	(74)
170	(5 7)	10 0	(64)	12 0	(76)
173	(5 8)	10 4	(65)	12 4	(78)
175	(5 9)	10 8	(67)	12 10	(81)
178	(5 10)	10 12	(69)	13 0	(83)

controlled diet that maintains all the essential nutrients. Without carbohydrates, for example, the body has to metabolize proteins. An obese person cannot eat large amounts of protein foods and expect to lose weight, because the body is able to convert excess amino acids (broken-down protein) into carbohydrates for storage. So the only way an obese person can lose weight quickly is to eat less. If he or she wants to keep below the danger weight, the new low level of calorie intake must be maintained.

Roughage

Roughage (or fibre) is the indigestible remains of the food that passes through the large bowel. In humans this consists mostly of cellulose, the substance that makes the cell walls of plants. If a person is not eating enough roughage, the large intestine is not stimulated to move the contents along. As the faeces remain in the intestine, more water is absorbed from them, and the faeces become hard.

Unfortunately, Western society now favours foods such as bread made from refined flour, and eats a greater proportion of meat in comparison with vegetables. This low fibre diet leads to constipation, which can cause straining and lead to haemorrhoids. It may also lead to a diverticular disease, in which small pouches on the bowel wall develop and become inflamed. A low fibre diet may also be a factor in the development of cancer of the large bowel and rectum.

It is therefore important to supplement diet with extra roughage. Apart from eating plenty of fresh vegetables, a person who suffers from constipation should take extra bran as cereals, eat wholemeal bread, and drink a minimum of 2½ litres (5 pints) of fluid a day. Regular doses of laxatives must not be taken. If the condition persists, a doctor should be consulted.

Fluids

Body function depends on fluids. Cell protoplasm is fluid, and all essential chemical reactions and exchanges occur within it. Fluid lubricates the food while it is chewed, and also during the digestive process, bringing digestive juices and enzymes with it. Fluids make up most of the blood volume in the form of plasma, and through this medium oxygen, foods, and wastes such as carbon dioxide are carried around the body. In fact, an average human body contains up to 9 gallons (34 litres) of fluid. The kidneys keep the body's fluid level constant, but during the summer, or at times when a person sweats a lot (for example, after physical exercise) it is important to drink an adequate amount of fluid in any form to replace the loss. The only exception is alcohol, because this tends to act as a diuretic and encourage the kidneys to excrete more fluid than normal, dehydrating the body further. If you do want to drink alcohol when you are thirsty, you should also drink at least a litre (2 pints) of non-alcoholic liquid. Mild dehydration over a long period can result in constipation and even the development of kidney stones. Without any fluid at all, death occurs within a few days.

Alcoholic drinks

Alcohol is produced from the action of yeasts on sugar. Alcohol is very high in calories – one fluid ounce (30ml.) of alcohol contains about 75 calories, so it is pointless drinking a low-calorie beer instead of ordinary beer unless you prefer the taste. Spirits have little nutritional value apart from calories but beers and wines contain vitamins and minerals.

Sugar

Sugar is instant energy, but apart from that it contains no other nutritional properties. Sugar occurs naturally in many foods, so added sugars are unnecessary and only serve to encourage obesity. They raise the level of triglycerides (forms of fat) in the blood and this has been associated with coronary heart disease.

Brown sugars contain some minerals; honey is made by bees and consists of fructose and glucose that the human body can use without digesting further. Syrup and molasses contain less calories because they contain more water, but if they are used as sugar substitutes, more is needed to obtain the same amount of sweetness. There has been much controversy about the safety of synthetic sweeteners, so it is sensible to reduce sugar intake rather than use artificial substitutes. In most cases, the palate quickly adjusts to a less sweet diet.

Carbohydrates and fats

Carbohydrates and fats are principally energy providers. This energy can be measured in calories, and every activity that a person takes can be analysed as calories spent. If the balance between calories consumed and calories expended is unequal, a person either stores the excess as fat beneath the skin and puts on weight, or begins to use up existing stores for energy, and loses weight.

Carbohydrates include sugars and starches. Foods such as potatoes, bread, pastas, jams, cereals, and honey are rich in carbohydrates. About half of a person's usual diet consists of

Food and health: nutrition 2

carbohydrates – a third of this is actually sugar itself. Sugar is pure carbohydrate, but other foods in the carbohydrate group, the starchy foods, contain other important nutrients. Potatoes for instance are high in vitamin C, and contain proteins – a quarter of these are in the skin, so an unpeeled boiled potato or a baked potato is more nutritious than a roasted or mashed potato. Bread is also rich in carbohydrates, but brown bread also contains proteins, iron, fat, and vitamins. Even white bread often has added calcium, iron, and vitamins.

Fats and oils

Fats and oils are a more concentrated form of energy than carbohydrates. Animal fats consist mainly of saturated fat and are hard at room temperature, whereas vegetable and fish oils consist mainly of unsaturated fats and are liquid at room temperature. Saturated fats have been associated with heart disease and certain cancers. Many authorities believe that an affluent diet contains a higher proportion of meat and dairy products than the body can cope with. It is sensible, therefore, to reduce the amount of animal fats eaten.

Cholesterol

Cholesterol resembles fat, but most of the cholesterol in the body is manufactured in the tissues. Cholesterol can build up on the inside of blood vessels, causing arteriosclerosis and coronary heart disease, but exactly why it accumulates is not understood. Cholesterol occurs in animal fats, dairy products, and eggs. Even though the causes of arteriosclerosis are not understood, it is sensible to restrict cholesterol intake.

Proteins

Every living cell contains proteins, complex chemical compounds that are broken down into amino acids during digestion. These are absorbed into the bloodstream and transported to different parts of the body, where they are rebuilt into different types of protein. The body can make some amino acids but others have to be made from proteins in the diet. Only eight have to be in the diet; the others can be synthesized. Essential amino acids include lysine that is found in bread, and methoinine that is found in beans. Young babies need two extra essential amino acids, arginine and histidine.

Importance of protein

Proteins are essential for the constant repair and replacement of the body tissues. For instance the skin cells rapidly multiply in the lower layer of the epidermis; hair and nails continue to grow throughout life; and even the bones need gradual replacement of cells that have degenerated, although the process is very much slower.

The proteins responsible for digestion are known as enzymes. Some of the body's hormones are proteins, and antibodies are proteins that group in response to foreign proteins (antigens) that are the cause of a wide range of diseases.

Extra proteins are particularly important during times of growth in childhood, or for pregnant women who are building the bodies of their new babies. Similarly, a woman who is breast-feeding her baby needs extra protein to make milk. Adults who have stopped growing also need protein to replace body tissues that have degenerated.

After a serious illness a person must eat a high protein diet to regain the protein lost during fever – up to a pound of body protein a day when the temperature is raised above 38°C (100°F). Similarly, a person who has been involved in a surgical operation or an accident needs extra protein.

Protein in food

Proteins are present in small quantities in many types of food, although in Western society most of the protein eaten comes from meat, fish, and dairy products. In fact, to achieve the correct adult intake of protein for one week a person would have to eat about four pounds of meat.

However, since protein is present in all foods, other sources help make up the total intake. For example, about twenty per cent of the protein in the diet comes from bread, and about five per cent from potatoes. Even foods such as lettuce and mushrooms contain protein.

A good diet should consist of between five and ten per cent protein.

If a person eats more protein than the body needs for growth and repair, some of it can be converted into carbohydrates and glycogen for storage. But most of it is broken down into its simple chemical compounds and excreted by the kidneys as urea.

The percentage of protein contained in different foods is not an indication of the quality of that protein. A protein source such as cheese, which contains all the essential amino acids, is said to be complete. Incomplete proteins lack one or more of the essential amino acids. Therefore, it is important to eat a balanced diet that contains different protein foods to obtain all of the essential amino acids.

Food	Contents and energy value					
	Water %	Protein %	Fibre %	Carbohydrate %	Fat %	Calories per 30g (1 oz)
Meat						
Beef	64	18	0	0	17	55
Liver	64	19	0	0	16	50
Pork	64	17	0	0	18	75
Chicken	63	20	0	0	16	35
Duck	53	16	0	0	30	120
Turkey	63	20	0	0	16	30
Cod	81	17.5	0	0	0.5	20
Mackerel	68	17.5	0	0	13.5	65
Dairy Produce						
Butter	16	0.5	0	0.5	83	210
Cheese	40	25	0	2	29	110
Egg	74	12	0	1	12	40
Milk	87	3.5	0	4.5	4	20
Vegetables						
Broccoli	90	3.5	1	5	0.5	7
Cabbage	90	3.5	1	5	0.5	6
Carrot	89	1.5	1	8	0	7
Celery	93	2.5	1	3	0.5	2
Kidney bean	12	24	4.5	55	2	15
Lettuce	94	1.5	1	3	0.5	3
Mushroom	92	2	5.5	0	0.5	4
Onion	90	1.5	1	7	0	7
Pea	81	6	1.5	11	0.5	20
Potato	80	2	0.5	17	0	25
Tomato	95	0.5	1	3	0	4
Nuts and Cereals						
Almond	5	16	2	16	59	160
Barley	12	8	1.5	75	1.5	100
Corn	12	22	4	55	7	36
Peanut	5	16	2	16	59	160
Rice	12	7	1	77	1	100
Wheat	10	13.5	1.5	70	3	100
Fruit						
Apple	84	0.5	2	13	0.5	10
Banana	80	0.5	1	18	0.5	12
Grape	81	0.5	0.5	17.5	0.5	15
Grapefruit	88	1	0.5	10	0.5	3
Melon	93	0.5	0.5	5.5	0.5	4
Orange	85	1	0.5	10	0.5	8
Pear	84	0.5	2	13	0.5	8
Plum	85	1	0.5	13	0.5	10
Raisin	23	3	3	68	1	70
Strawberry	87	1	3	8	1	7

Food and health: nutrition 3

Minerals and vitamins

Minerals and vitamins are vital to health – a diet rich in carbohydrates and proteins may lead to illness and death if it is deficient in vitamins and minerals.

Minerals

Calcium and phosphorus are known as the major minerals because the body needs these in fairly large quantities. Both elements are essential for the formation of teeth and bone. Milk and cheese are rich in calcium, and people who live in hard water areas consume as much calcium as they need. A pregnant woman should drink an extra pint of milk a day to provide herself and her baby with sufficient calcium and phosphorus for developing bones. The body does, however, need vitamin D in order to absorb the calcium. Unfortunately, the milling of white flour removes much calcium, but many countries fortify white bread to bring the level up to normal again during manufacture. Phosphorus occurs in nearly all food.

Many other minerals are needed by the body, and these are known as the trace elements because they are needed only in tiny amounts. If a person is eating a well-balanced diet, he or she is consuming enough of the trace elements. Liver is rich in iron, eggs are rich in sulphur and iron, and salt contains sodium and chlorine. Fish also provides sulphur, as does cabbage and poultry – fish also provides iodine. Other minerals such as fluorine, zinc, copper, chromium, manganese, and magnesium are present in all diets.

Vitamins

Vitamins, unlike minerals, are chemical compounds that have no energy value, but seem to act as catalysts. That is, they are responsible for the start and completion of certain essential chemical processes in the body. But like some trace minerals, the body needs only the smallest amount of them; anything over that amount is excreted by the kidneys or stored. It is therefore not usually necessary to take multivitamin tablets or fortified tonics. In some cases it may even be dangerous, because overdoses of vitamins A and D can cause illness and even death.

The importance of essential vitamins was only discovered this century and it was assumed that there were four varieties – A, B, C, and D. Since then research has shown that there are many other varieties.

The vitamin A group includes retinol and carotene. These vitamins are present in fresh green vegetables, milk and butter, liver, and cod-liver oil. Animals obtain most of their vitamin A from the carotene (yellow pigment in vegetables such as carrots). A diet that is deficient in vitamin A reduces a person's resistance to diseases, particularly ones that infect the body through the skin. The linings of the throat and bronchial tubes deteriorate, the skin becomes dry and scaly, and the cornea of the eye may also become affected, causing chronic conjunctivitis. A person's ability to see in the dark rapidly deteriorates.

There are at present seven known varieties of vitamin B. This group plays an important part in the release of energy from carbohydrates, fats, and proteins. Thiamin (B_1) occurs in yeast, liver, pork, and wholemeal cereal; riboflavin (B_2) also appears in liver and yeast, but meat and milk contain it as well; pyridoxine (B_6) is present in almost all foods; and cyanocobalamin (B_{12}) occurs in nearly all animal food. Folic acid, important for development of red blood cells, is present in fresh green vegetables, fruit, dried yeast, and liver. Vitamin B deficiency diseases include beri-beri, and other disturbances. A victim will also suffer from loss of appetite, wasting, and swelling of the hands and feet. Pellagra is a deficiency of one of the B vitamins known as nicotinic acid or niacin, and the victim suffers from diarrhoea and vomiting, skin disorders, and mental disorders. The disorder is sometimes a complication of chronic alcoholism.

Vitamin C (ascorbic acid) is present in citrus fruits such as oranges and lemons, but it also occurs in nuts and fresh vegetables. It is easily destroyed during cooking. A diet without vitamin C results in the disorder called scurvy, characterized by weakness, bleeding under the skin and around the gums, slow wound healing, and various skin disorders. If scurvy is not treated with vitamin C, death may occur from infections.

Vitamin D is also called calciferol, and can be made by the body when ultraviolet rays are absorbed through the skin. Other sources of vitamin D are cream, egg yolk, and cod-liver oil. A lack of it results in rickets in children, and osteomalacia in adults. The bones weaken and soften, and the ends swell.

Vitamin E, or tocopherol, is present in vegetable oils. Experiments on laboratory animals have shown it has an effect on the reproductive system of animals, but this has not been proved to apply to humans.

Vitamin K, known as menadione, is present in green vegetables, particularly spinach and cabbage. A deficiency of this vitamin produces bleeding.

There are a few other vitamins, such as biotin and pantothenic acid, that occur in every type of diet.

Vitamins and minerals

Food	Vitamin A	Thiamin	Riboflavin	Niacin	Vitamin C	Vitamin D	Iron	Calcium
Meat								
Beef			●	●			●	
Liver	●	●	●	●	●	●	●	
Pork		●	●	●				
Chicken				●				
Duck				●			●	
Turkey		●		●			●	
Cod				●				
Mackerel	●		●	●		●	●	
Dairy produce								
Butter	●					●		
Cheese	●			●	●			●
Egg	●	●	●	●		●	●	●
Milk	●		●					●
Vegetables								
Broccoli	●		●		●		●	●
Cabbage	●				●			
Carrot	●				●			
Celery					●			
Kidney bean				●	●			
Lettuce	●				●			
Mushroom			●	●				
Onion					●			
Pea		●		●	●		●	
Potato		●			●			
Tomato	●				●			
Nuts and cereals								
Almond		●	●	●			●	●
Barley				●				
Corn								
Peanut		●	●				●	●
Rice				●				
Wheat		●		●			●	●
Fruit								
Apple					●			
Banana					●			
Grape					●			
Grapefruit					●			
Melon	●				●			
Orange		●			●			
Pear					●			
Plum					●			
Raisin							●	●
Strawberry					●			

Staying healthy while travelling

Preparing for a journey

Any form of travel needs much forethought in planning and preparation. Pack clothing appropriate to the expected climate and type of vacation. Find out as much about the region to be visited as possible. Organize adequate insurance for the medical care of each member of the family, and for the luggage. If you are travelling by air, make sure that the insurance covers an increased air fare you may have to pay if you are to return on a scheduled flight. Make sure that all immunizations are up to date: children must have received protection against measles and whooping cough (prevalent in many countries), and poliomyelitis. Travel documents should include passports and visas, and international health certificates. Drugs to travel with should include a bottle of aspirin, a bottle of anti-histamine tablets, a packet of travel sickness tablets, mild sleeping pills, antidiarrhoeal mixture or pills, insect repellent cream, antiseptic cream, sunscreen cream or lotion, adhesive bandage for minor abrasions, a clinical thermometer, and water sterilizing tablets. Your doctor may recommend antimalarial tablets and antibiotics, and may also provide a prescription for a sufficient supply of any drugs taken regularly for an existing disorder, with a medical report for any concerned authority.

Fitness to travel

Modern transport makes travelling simple and relaxing even for individuals who suffer from serious disorders, or have recently undergone major surgery. If there is any doubt about a person's ability to travel, he or she should consult a doctor before organizing a long journey. People suffering from the following disorders need detailed advice: arthritic problems; cancer; colostomy; diabetes mellitus; ear troubles; heart conditions, such as angina, or a recent coronary thrombosis; neurological problems, such as epilepsy, a stroke, or myasthenia gravis; psychiatric problems still requiring treatment; respiratory problems, such as asthma, bronchitis, or emphysema; sinus problems; urological problems, such as a prostate disorder; and following any major surgery.

Anyone recovering from a cold should also consult a doctor before flying. A minor respiratory tract infection could lead to acute sinusitis or middle ear infection following the changes in air pressure during the flight.

If any member of the family intends to undertake an unusually strenuous activity, such as scuba diving, mountaineering, or hiking, it is important that a doctor checks that he or she is physically capable of that activity. Many schools insist on a medical examination before a pupil is allowed to travel.

Air travel

Always wear comfortable, loose-fitting clothing. If possible, loosen the shoes during the flight to prevent constriction of the feet, which tend to swell slightly. Any swelling can be reduced by simple ankle exercises.

Jet lag is a common problem associated with long flights. Jet lag causes fatigue and slight disorientation during the time that the body's basic biological rhythms are un-accustomed to new sleeping and eating times. The symptoms of jet lag are often aggravated by overeating during the flight,

Table of recommended immunizations for travellers

All immunizations should be at the discretion of your own doctor

IMMUNIZATION	SCHEDULE AND PROTECTION	AREAS RECOMMENDED FOR
Cholera	International certificate valid for six months beginning 6 days after one injection.	All Asian countries; Australasia; many African countries.
Gamma globulin (immune serum globulin)	One injection just prior to departure. Gives three to four months' partial protection against infectious hepatitis.	Countries outside north-western Europe and Australasia where sanitation is of a low standard.
Poliomyelitis	Three doses of oral vaccine at four- to six-week intervals. Valid for five years.	All countries.
Tetanus	Three injections: the second, one month after the first; the third, six months later. Valid for five years, and often combined with the typhoid immunization.	All countries.
Typhoid	Two injections one to two weeks apart. Gives up to two years' partial protection.	All countries except north-western Europe.
Typhus	Two injections seven to ten days apart. Valid for one year.	South-eastern Asia; India; Ethiopia.
Yellow fever	International certificate valid for ten years beginning 10 days after one injection.	Some central African countries; some South American countries.

and a high alcohol consumption that leaves the traveller dehydrated. It is important to drink an adequate amount of fluid, such as water or fruit juice. Small amounts of food should be eaten every few hours. It is often wise to take a mild sedative, prescribed by a doctor, for a few nights after arrival to ensure proper sleep.

People taking regular medication, such as drugs for blood pressure or diabetes, must remember to take the drugs at the prescribed time interval, and not at the local time.

Sea voyages
Motion sickness commonly occurs during sea voyages. Anyone who suffers from motion sickness should take antinauseant drugs the night before a voyage, and again on the morning of the voyage. Antinauseant drugs tend to cause drowsiness, and should not be taken if a person intends to drive a car immediately after a short voyage.

A person taking regular medication should inform the ship's doctor if suffering from motion sickness. The doctor can ensure that treatment is given before the person becomes dehydrated as a result of vomiting.

In rough weather always hold on to a handrail when moving about the deck.

Car, bus, and rail travel
Children frequently suffer from motion sickness during journeys in a car, bus, or train. The condition is aggravated by excitement and apprehension. Children should have a light meal half an hour before the journey, because an empty stomach can increase the feeling of nausea.

Slight dehydration may occur when travelling in a hot climate. Make sure that there is an adequate supply of fruit juice or water for the journey. Elderly people in particular should be encouraged to get out and walk around during stops. This prevents excessive stiffness.

The driver of a car or bus should not remain at the wheel for more than two hours without a stop.

During the holiday
Some precautions can be taken to avoid illness during a holiday.

Sunburn can be avoided by careful attention to a slow tanning programme, as described in **The skin**, p.938. Children are especially sensitive to sunlight, and may remove their clothing when a parent is not looking. Even adults may not be aware that burning can occur on cloudy days as easily as on sunny ones.

Sunglasses prevent headaches caused by glare. Generally, the more they cost, the more protection they offer.

It is essential in a hot climate to drink plenty of fluids and take additional salt to compensate for salt lost in sweat.

Diarrhoea is a distressing but common problem for travellers. Changes in diet introduce new micro-organisms into the digestive system, and cause diarrhoea even though there is no infection. Fluid consumption must be increased to compensate for fluid loss. Antidiarrhoeal drugs and mixtures can control the condition. If the diarrhoea is bloody, or accompanied by a high fever, medical advice must be sought.

Bites and stings are also common in the tropics. Insect repellent creams are helpful, and antihistamines taken at night reduce skin irritation.

To avoid prickly heat rash in the tropics, a person should take frequent showers, and wear cotton clothing. If the rash becomes established, the symptoms can be controlled by cool baths, antiseptic creams and, if necessary, vitamin C tablets.

Swimming can cause infections of the ear; the ears must therefore be carefully dried afterwards. If a person has suffered from otitis externa before, a doctor may recommend the use of ear drops or ear plugs.

Visitors to countries where malaria is common must take antimalarial drugs throughout the visit, and continue taking them for one month after returning home.

Food poisoning
Serious diseases can be caught from infected food. Water can also carry dangerous infections. A traveller should avoid cold, cooked food; salads and fruit, unless peeled or washed personally; tap water; shellfish, unless it is possible to choose them (live) before they are cooked; milk and cream; ice cream and other food from street vendors; and any food that has been open to flies. Water bottled by a reputable firm is usually safe for drinking and tooth brushing. If in any doubt about water, use sterilizing tablets. Hot cooked food is safe as long as it has not been kept warm for more than fifteen minutes.

Personal cleanliness is extremely important when travelling, and the hands must be carefully washed before food is handled.

Returning home
Ensure a proper sleep on returning home to compensate for a tiring journey.

Some tropical diseases have long incubation periods, so it is important to inform your doctor immediately if you become ill shortly after returning home.

Physical fitness and exercises

Section contents

Introduction

This section provides information about getting fit and keeping fit. The first pages explain the importance of physical fitness and show you how you can evaluate your own physical condition. They also contain general advice about health, diet, and recreation. The greater part of the section consists of a series of progressive exercises designed for men and women between the ages of eighteen and fifty. The final pages include supplementary information for anyone who wishes to extend his or her fitness programme beyond the range of the exercises described.

The exercises were planned in consultation with a professional gymnast who has trained many dancers and athletes at his own gymnasium. They are designed for the ordinary person who wishes to get fit and then to keep fit, rather than for people who wish to train for a particular sport, and they conform to the necessary principles of simplicity and safety. All the exercises can be done in your own home, and only the advanced exercises require any form of special equipment.

The warming-up and beginner's exercises (pp.978-985) can be done by anyone, at any stage of fitness. They are designed to prepare the whole body for physical exercise, and then to develop the mobility and suppleness of particular joints and muscles. For people who have not taken regular exercise for some time, the beginner's exercises given here will build up a general level of fitness that can be further developed by the succeeding exercises. For people who are already fairly fit, they will provide the necessary warming-up that must always be done before more demanding exercises are attempted.

The cardiovascular exercises (pp.986-989) are designed to improve the condition of the heart and lungs, and are of special benefit to your general health. If you are unfit when starting this course of exercises, you will attain a good general level of physical fitness by regularly performing these and the succeeding general exercises over a period of about six months. This level of fitness can then be maintained by repeating the exercises at least three times a week. If you wish to develop your strength and fitness further, you can then proceed to the advanced exercises.

The rate of progress for different individuals will vary according to such factors as age, natural ability, and determination.

To obtain the maximum benefit from the exercises, regular practice is vitally important. While developing your fitness (rather than maintaining a level of fitness already attained) you should exercise daily. Each period of exercise builds up from the previous period and leads on to the next. If you exercise less than every second day, you will lose the cumulative benefit.

It is far more beneficial to do small amounts of exercise at frequent intervals than to do large amounts occasionally. If you can only exercise for very short periods of time, you should do as many exercises as you can thoroughly, rather than trying to complete all the exercises in the schedule as quickly as possible. When you next have time to exercise, perhaps later in the same day, do the warming-up exercises and then continue the schedule from where you left off.

The instructions for the exercises have been written as clearly and precisely as possible. Follow these instructions carefully: if you perform an exercise other than in the manner described and illustrated, you will gain less benefit from it, and you may also cause yourself unnecessary strain. All your movements while exercising should be smooth and rhythmical. Sudden or violent movements are less effective in developing strength and suppleness, and can cause strains. Your breathing should be relaxed, and should conform to the rhythm of the physical movements.

The number of repetitions suggested for each exercise is intended as a guide only. If you feel any pain, you should not strain yourself to complete the given number. On the other hand, if you feel that you are able to exceed this number, you may increase your fitness by doing so.

If you follow carefully all the advice given in this section, you should be able to improve your physical fitness with complete safety. There are three necessary precautions, however, which must be emphasized before you start. Firstly, if you are aged over forty, are overweight, are a heavy smoker, or suffer from any form of heart disorder, you should check with your doctor before starting any fitness programme. Secondly, it is always necessary to do warming-up exercises before attempting any form of strenuous exercise, however fit you may be. And thirdly, you should know what your pulse rate while exercising should be, and if it rises too fast or exceeds the proper rate, you should stop exercising. You should also stop exercising if you feel any pain in the chest. Instructions about how to measure your exercising pulse rate are given in the introduction to the cardiovascular and general exercises on p.986. There are reminders about all these precautions at various stages throughout this section.

The general advantages of physical fitness are emphasized in the opening pages of the section. They include improved health, protection against disease, and an increased ability to cope with both physical and mental strain. Many of the rewards of fitness are undoubtedly psychological: a physically fit person is often more calm, cheerful, and self-confident than an unfit person. When starting any fitness programme, you should think carefully about the purpose of exercise, and about the specific results you hope to attain. This will help to sustain your motivation if you are tempted to relax your programme, or to exercise less regularly than you should.

How fit are you? 1

Most people know when they are unfit. The signs of unfitness are obvious: you get tired easily; you find that you can't do all the things you used to do; you feel out of breath after climbing a flight of stairs; you catch colds and other minor infections easily. However, many people are unwilling to acknowledge to themselves how unfit they are.

Fear of the work involved in getting fit, however, is both unnecessary and dangerous. It is unnecessary, because the effort involved in getting fit need not be great, especially since it is largely a matter of self-discipline. And it is dangerous, because if you allow your physical condition to deteriorate, you increase the risk of suffering from heart disease or some other physical disorder.

Finding out how unfit you really are is not a cause for despair, but the first step in improving the whole quality of your life. If you are aged between fifteen and sixty, you can find out initially how fit you are by five simple tests of your physical condition:

(1) Stand in front of the mirror. Look for areas of loose or flabby skin. Are you completely satisfied with what you see? This evaluates general physical appearance and muscle tone.
(2) Pinch your body at the waist, or at a point at the back of your arm between the shoulder and the elbow. Is the fold of skin less than 2.5 cm (an inch) thick? This tests for the first signs of obesity.
(3) Can you hold your breath for more than 45 seconds? This tests the condition of the lungs.
(4) Stand up straight, with your eyes closed and your arms at your sides, and raise one knee. Can you stand like this for 15 seconds without losing your balance? This tests balance and muscular co-ordination.
(5) Find out the pulse rate of your heart. (Feel your wrist and count the beats for 15 seconds, then multiply by four.) Then run on the spot for three minutes. Is your pulse rate now under 120 beats per minute? And does it take less than one minute to return to its original rate? This evaluates the condition of the heart and the circulation.

If your answer to any of these questions is no, your physical condition is not as good as it could be.

Fitness day by day

The process of getting fit and keeping fit is more a matter of common sense and self-discipline than hard work. The exercises described on pp.978-995 are designed to improve your respiration and blood circulation, strengthen your muscles, and improve the strength and suppleness of your joints, neck, and back. They are also designed to increase your powers of physical endurance, reduce fatigue, and help you stay slim.

The rewards of fitness can be attained by any reasonably healthy person who is committed to improving his or her physical condition. For some people, this commitment may involve regular programmes of physical exercises, slimming diets, and taking up sports. For others, less willing or able to alter their daily routine, many less disruptive ways of taking exercise can be equally important and beneficial.

Keep active as much as possible, whatever your occupation. The less active you are, the less your body is exercised and the weaker it gets. Anyone who has been ill in bed for even as little as a week knows how difficult it is to get straight back into working life. This is because there has been little demand on the muscles, heart, lungs, and circulation during the period spent in bed, and their efficiency has correspondingly decreased. Research has shown that people who have desk jobs or who do only light physical work are far more likely to suffer from coronary heart disease than people who's job involves constant physical activity.

Keeping active for long periods may not be easy, especially for an office worker who rides to work each day by car or bus, goes up to his or her office in the lift, sits at a desk most of the working day, and returns home at night to sit in front of the television before finally going to bed. But even a person with this life style can adapt his or her daily routine so that it has a more beneficial effect on physical health: park the car or leave the bus a short distance from the office and walk; use the stairs not the lift; walk around as much as possible in the office; and try to pursue some more active form of entertainment in the evening.

Common sense and self-discipline

Whatever form of physical exercise you decide on, go gently at the beginning. Exercise for short periods and at a slow pace at first, and build up gradually as your muscles become stronger. Do not attempt vigorous or demanding exercises until your body is strong enough to perform them without suffering undue strain. If you are a heavy smoker, are seriously overweight, or are suffering from any form of physical disorder, you should consult your doctor before starting any exercises.

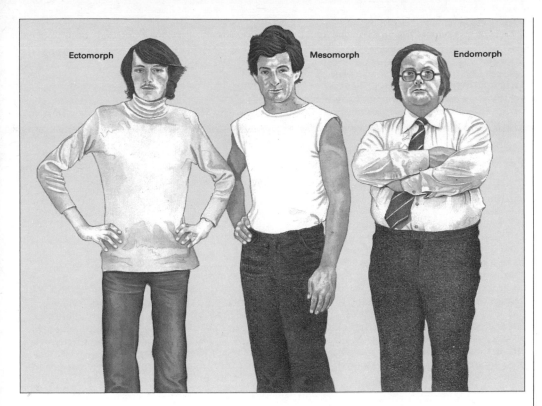

Ectomorph   Mesomorph   Endomorph

To get the full benefit from any fitness programme you should perform the exercises as regularly and as often as directed. The same degree of commitment is also necessary if you decide to give up smoking or go on a slimming diet.

Body types

No one should assume that by following a programme of fitness exercises he or she will naturally acquire the looks and physique of a film star. Human beings are infinitely more variable in size and shape than the stereotype figures preferred by fashion designers and advertisers. One of the things you will discover in the course of improving your physical fitness is the specific type and capabilities of your own body.

A system of categorization for the different body types was established by the American psychologist W.H. Sheldon during the 1940s. According to this system, there are three main physical types, known as endomorph, mesomorph, and ectomorph, each of which represents an extreme. Most of us have bodies with shapes that fall somewhere between these extremes, having attributes from two or more of the classical types.

The endomorph has a rounded body shape.

The endomorph's body is characterized by a round head, a round and large abdomen, large internal organs, rather short arms and legs with slender wrists and ankles, and a large proportion of body fat.

The mesomorph has the body of a classical athlete. It is characterized by a square head, a large heart, broad and muscular chest and shoulders, arms and legs with powerful muscles, and little body fat.

The ectomorph's body is essentially linear in shape. It is characterized by a thin face with a high forehead, a narrow chest and abdomen, long and thin arms and legs, little muscle, and a minimal amount of body fat.

These three shapes rarely occur in their classical forms. Most people can be very roughly described in terms of these types as endo-mesomorphs, or meso-ectomorphs, or some other combination of the extremes. However your own body type may be described, it is important to realize that it cannot be changed. An endomorph will not become a mesomorph by going on a diet, he or she will become a thinner endomorph. Similarly, a mesomorph who sits in the office all day and takes no exercise will become a flabby mesomorph, not an endomorph.

Clearly, certain kinds of work and exercise are more appropriate for each body type.

How fit are you? 2
Flexibility

Exercises to develop flexibility and suppleness are an important factor in maintaining
your body in good physical condition.
Muscular strength and stamina are particularly important for people whose work or
recreation makes heavy demands on the
body. Flexibility, however, is important for
everyone.

Flexibility can be defined as the degree to
which a joint is free to move through its
possible range of motion. The exercises on
these pages are designed to maintain
suppleness of the muscles and tendons
surrounding your joints, and so to maintain
the maximum flexibility of the joints. Each
exercise should be repeated about ten times.

These exercises require only a few minutes
each day but will, if performed regularly,
have long-lasting effects. By developing the
maximum range of movement of your neck,
spine, and joints, you can avoid spraining
ligaments and pulling muscles and tendons,
and also avoid many of the aches and pains
associated with stiffness. Flexibility exercises
are also good for your respiration and
circulation; they help you to avoid developing rounded shoulders and a stooped back,
which can constrict the lungs.

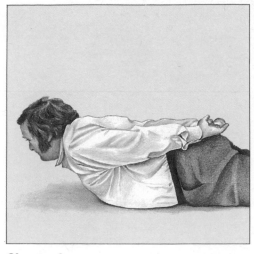

Chest raise

Lie face-down on the floor, with the feet
together and the hands clasped behind the
back. Raise up the head, shoulders, and chest
as far as possible, keeping the legs straight on
the floor. Hold this position for a moment,
and then lower. A friend can help you to do
this exercise by holding your legs in position
as you raise the shoulders and chest.

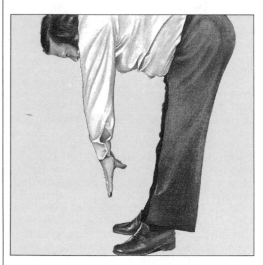

Toe touching

Stand with the feet together, and raise the
arms straight above the head. Keeping the
arms and legs straight, bend forward from the
hips and bring the arms down until the
fingers touch the toes. Then stand upright
again, raising the arms to their original
position. If you are able, try to touch the toes
with the palm of the hands instead of the
fingers, but do NOT strain to do this.

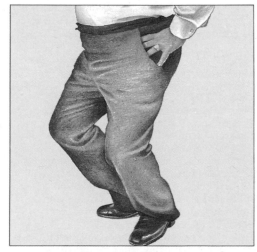

Deep knee-bends

Stand with your feet about 60cm (2ft) apart
and the toes turned outwards. This posture is
necessary because it prevents the body from
swaying or falling over. Hold the arms out
sideways for balance. Keeping the heels on
the floor and the back straight, lower the
trunk of the body by bending the knees as far
as you can. Then return to the original
position.

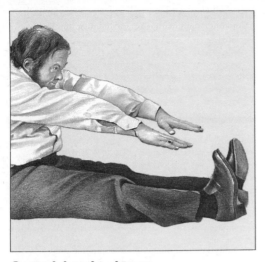

Seated, head to knees

Sit on the floor with legs straight out in front and feet vertical. Raise the arms straight above the head, and breathe in. Lean forwards, keeping the arms straight, and touch the toes with the fingers. Bring the head down as far as you can, and try to touch the knees with the forehead. Then return to the original sitting position.

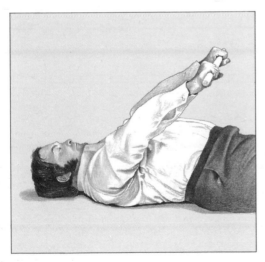

Straight arm pull-over

Lie face-up on the floor, with the legs straight and the hands holding a bar on the thighs with the back of the hands upwards. Keeping the arms straight, raise them from the thighs and bring them back over the head until the back of the wrists touch the floor. Then return them to the original position. Your wrists may not touch the floor at first, but this gets easier with practice.

Fitness for the elderly

In old age, a certain amount of physical decline is inevitable. As the body ages, the arteries gradually harden, the capacity of the lungs diminishes, the muscles deteriorate, the bones become thinner and more brittle, and there is a reduction in both height and weight. Specialized cells in certain organs of the body die and are not replaced, thus reducing the efficiency of these organs. None of these changes, however, need reduce an older person's capacity to enjoy life, and physical exercise remains important.

Many of the advantages of regular exercise taken early in life become apparent only as you grow older. However, it is never too late to start.

Simple flexibility exercises are especially suitable for elderly people. Many of these exercises can be performed while you are sitting in a chair. For neck flexibility, let the neck fall gently forwards or to one side, and then lift it up. For flexibility of the spine and trunk, sit with your arms outstretched and move the whole of your upper body from side to side. For flexibility of the hip joints, sit with the legs outstretched and raise one knee, bending your head gently down towards it as you do so. For flexibility of the ankle joints, cross one leg over the other and move your foot round in a circle, stretching the toes up, down, and outwards as you do so. All these movements can be repeated a number of times, but never strain yourself or force your body to make a movement that causes pain. Remember that the aim of these exercises is flexibility, not muscular strength or endurance.

Other factors related to physical fitness in old age are diet and recreational interests. Many aches and pains, as well as anaemia and other ailments, are caused by diets lacking in essential vitamins, proteins, and nutrients, especially calcium and iron. The diet of elderly people should contain plenty of milk, as well as fruit and fresh vegetables. It is dangerous to assume that older people need less nutritious food than younger people.

Although elderly people should avoid exercise that demands sudden or prolonged effort, physical activity of some kind can be very beneficial. Short but regular walks will exercise the joints and stimulate the circulation. Gardening also provides good exercise, and by planning a garden carefully and using the appropriate tools you can eliminate most of the heavy work. Once you have attained a certain degree of physical fitness, you may even be able to take up swimming, running, or cycling.

Sport and recreation

Many people, especially those who take part in a sport or some other active recreation in their spare time, believe that they get enough exercise during their ordinary daily routine to keep themselves in good physical condition. Whether this is true or not depends very much on the type of sport or exercise, and the regularity with which it is practised. Some of the more popular recreational activities are listed on this page, together with information concerning their real value in promoting physical fitness. It will be noted that even the more active sports have widely differing effects in conditioning your body and keeping you fit.

The information given here is useful for people who already practise these activities, and also for those who wish to choose a recreational activity to supplement their existing exercise programme.

Before you start

The first three exercises listed (jogging, bicycling, and swimming) are known as aerobic exercises: that is, they increase a person's aerobic capacity, which is the amount of oxygen the body can use. The continuous sustained activity demanded by these exercises causes the muscles of the legs and the upper body to contract and relax in a steady rhythm, and causes the heart rate and the breathing rate to increase. Aerobic exercises therefore provide excellent exercise for not only the body muscles, but also for the heart, the lungs, and the cardiovascular system. They increase the efficiency of the heart in pumping oxygen through the body, and of the body tissues in extracting that oxygen. Aerobic exercises are therefore especially beneficial in helping to prevent some forms of heart disease.

Do not, however, believe that you will do yourself any good by setting off on a long run or bicycle ride without any previous preparation. As with other forms of physical exercise, when you start an aerobic exercise you must begin with short periods of relatively undemanding exercise, and build up gradually to more demanding exercise as your body becomes stronger. If you have not taken any regular exercise for some time, or if you are over 40 years old, or if you suffer from any form of physical disorder or ill health, you should consult your doctor before starting.

The same advice also applies to anyone who is about to take up any of the other active sports. Go carefully to start with: if you are unfit, the consequences of sudden strains can be very serious. Even when you are in good physical condition, you should always prepare your body for the heavy demands of a vigorous sport or game by doing warming-up exercises before starting. These exercises stimulate the circulation, strengthen the major joints by thickening the ligaments and increase the power and flexibility of the muscles. They will increase the general efficiency of your body, and reduce the danger of cramp. They should not be so strenuous that you waste any valuable energy before actually starting your main activity, but should gently increase your pulse rate to about 110 beats a minute. For sports such as tennis or squash, the simplest way of warming up is to practise non-competitively for about five minutes before starting your actual game.

Jogging

Jogging requires no special equipment and can be easily fitted in to anyone's daily routine. Because of these advantages the general value of jogging has perhaps been over-rated, but it can certainly be good for the heart, the lungs, and the leg muscles. You should work out a programme, beginning gently and gradually increasing your pace and the distance you cover. Wear warm, loose clothing and thick-soled running shoes. Where possible, run on soft surfaces rather than on streets or pavements.

Bicycling

Like jogging, bicycling consists of regular, rhythmic exercise and is especially good for the heart, the lungs, and the leg muscles. Changes of gradient and weather vary the demands on your body. Continuous periods of bicycling on country roads or special bicycle paths are more beneficial than bicycling in towns.

Swimming

Swimming helps to develop your stamina, suppleness, and general muscular strength, as well as being good for the heart and lungs. Because your body is supported in the water, your spine and joints can move freely and there is no weight on your back, hips, and feet. This makes swimming especially suitable for people suffering from back complaints, arthritis, or rheumatism. To get the maximum benefit from this sport you should practise all the strokes: breaststroke is good for the hips and knees, butterfly stroke improves back and shoulder muscles, and backstroke and crawl are good for the shoulders and trunk. Butterfly is the most demanding stroke, followed by the crawl, backstroke, and then breaststroke.

Continuous periods of swimming are more beneficial than short, fast lengths followed by pauses for rest. You will need to learn how to breathe properly in order to swim for a worthwhile period of time. Do not let yourself get too cold; this can cause cramp.

Skiing

For all-round fitness, cross-country skiing is much more valuable than downhill skiing. It promotes balance, flexibility, and general endurance. Pre-ski training and exercises are especially recommended: they prepare the muscles for the very special demands of this sport, and reduce the danger of falls and injuries.

Tennis and squash

A lazy game of doubles is of little value in promoting physical fitness, but a fast game of singles, played at a pace that demands constant and vigorous activity, can be very valuable. It strengthens the arm muscles and promotes flexibility and balance. Squash is even more beneficial, but you should not attempt to play this game unless you are already fairly fit.

Golf

Golf is chiefly valuable as an aid to mental relaxation. The only real physical benefit comes from the walking involved in progressing round the course, and to get as much benefit as possible you should walk at a brisk pace and carry your clubs on your shoulders, not in a trolley.

Team games

Games such as football and cricket demand a wide variety of skills, and so usually promote all-round fitness. However, the amount of time during which an individual player is actively involved in the game is usually short. The pattern of sudden bursts of effort alternating with longer periods of relative inactivity makes heavy demands on the heart and lungs. The first priority in training for any team game should therefore be the development of general fitness.

Gardening and do-it-yourself

Both these common recreational activities are more forms of relaxation than of physical strengthening. Where vigorous or prolonged activity is demanded, they can have a beneficial effect in developing particular muscles. Generally, however, the effort involved is not sufficient to be of any real value in promoting physical fitness, especially when labour-saving implements or electrical appliances are being used.

Smoking, eating, and fitness

Physical fitness depends not just on exercise, but on the whole way in which you care for your body. The benefits gained from physical exercise will be wasted if you do not pay careful attention to your eating, drinking, and smoking habits.

The dangers of tobacco have been well-publicised. People who smoke a packet of cigarettes every day are twenty times more likely to get lung cancer than non-smokers. Cigarette smoking causes four times as many deaths as road accidents; it damages the lungs and blood vessels, and causes indirect damage to the heart and other organs. It is clear that smoking and physical fitness are incompatible. If you are already a heavy smoker and find it difficult to give up, you should at least cut down the number of cigarettes you smoke each day and smoke only brands with a low content of nicotine and tar. Do not smoke a cigarette right down to the filter, and remove it from your mouth between puffs to reduce the amount of smoke inhaled. If you can stop completely, you will very soon notice the benefits.

Your body can also be harmed by your choice of food and drink. If obesity is defined as weighing 20 per cent more than the norm for one's height, age, and occupation, then a quarter of the population of Britain can be defined as obese. Obesity is associated with backache, foot disorders, arthritis, gallstones, varicose veins, high blood pressure, diabetes, kidney failure, heart attacks, and many other disorders. Incorrect diet is associated with tooth decay, cardiovascular disease, and probably also with some forms of cancer. Again, anyone who is seriously concerned with physical fitness must pay careful attention both to what, and to how much, he or she consumes.

Your body's nutritional requirements are discussed in the section on **Nutrition** (pp.962-967). If you are overweight and decide to go on a slimming diet to improve your physical fitness, you must take care that your diet contains a proper balance of nutrients, dietary fibre, and calories. There are two main types of slimming diet: calorie-controlled, and low carbohydrate. On average, each person consumes about 2,500 calories each day. If you go on a calorie-controlled diet, set yourself a daily target and make sure that the food you consume does not contain more than that amount of calories each day. If you decide on a low carbohydrate diet, you should reduce the amounts of carbohydrate-rich foods you eat. For further information concerning slimming diets, see **Special diets** (pp.684-691).

Warming-up exercises

The exercises in this section are designed to be suitable for anyone, at any age, with or without previous regular exercise. Before starting any physical activity, it is advisable to assess your physical condition (*see* **How fit are you?** pp.972–977) in order to avoid overstraining.

If you are overweight, have any symptoms of a heart condition or circulation disorder, or are older than 40, you should also consult a doctor before you start.

The purpose of these exercises is to help you to improve your physical condition. To achieve this, you should do each exercise daily. Once you are fit, condition can be maintained by going through the exercises about three times a week. The recommended number of repetitions of each exercise should be taken only as a guide; as you become used to the exercises you will be able to increase this number.

It is important to remember while doing these exercises that each stretching movement should be made to the maximum extent that suppleness allows. Also, sudden movements are less valuable than smooth, controlled movements for developing suppleness and strength. Breathing should be relaxed, and should fit in comfortably with the natural rhythms of the movements.

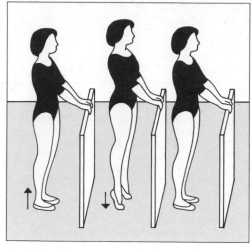

Heels raise

Stand with the heels together and the toes parallel. Hold a firm horizontal support, such as the back of a chair, with both hands for balance. Keep the body and legs straight, and the head up. Stand up as high as possible on the toes, hold this position for a moment, then lower the heels to the floor.
Repeat thirty times.
Purpose: to exercise feet, calves, and ankles.

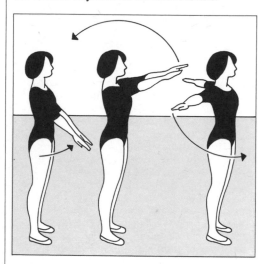

Arms circle

Stand with the feet apart. Start with the hands crossed in front of the body, then raise both arms forwards and upwards in a circular movement past the shoulders. Do not move the torso, hips, or legs, and keep the arms straight. Try to achieve the maximum sweep of the arms, and do not swing the arms too fast. Repeat thirty times.
Purpose: to exercise the shoulders.

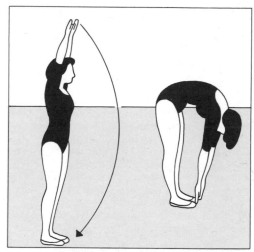

Toe touching

Stand with the feet together. Stretch the arms upwards, draw the chest up and the stomach in, and keep the legs straight. Lean forward from the waist, then down to touch the toes. Do not breathe out until you are standing upright again.
Repeat twenty times.
Purpose: to exercise the backs of the legs and the lower spine.

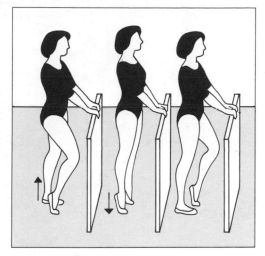

Alternate heel raise

Stand with the heels together and the toes turned out. Hold a firm horizontal support with both hands for balance. Bend the right leg over the line of the foot, keep the toes on the ground, and raise the heel as high as possible. Return to the original position, then repeat with the left leg.
Repeat thirty times with each leg.
Purpose: to exercise feet, calves, and ankles.

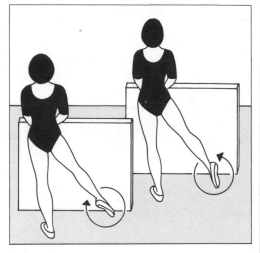

Foot circles

Stand with the heels together and the toes turned out. Hold a firm horizontal support with both hands for balance. Raise the right foot forward, keeping the leg straight. The leg should be at 45° to the midline. Circle the foot slowly, stretching the ankle as much as possible. Rotate the foot fifteen times in each direction, then repeat with the other foot.
Purpose: to exercise feet, calves, and ankles.

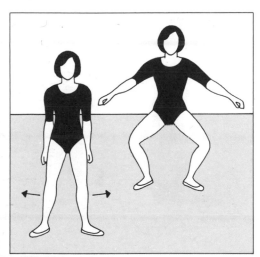

Wide knee-bends

Stand with the heels about 60cm (2ft) apart, and with the toes turned out. Bend the legs over the lines of the feet, keeping the heels on the ground. Keep the back straight and upright, and hold the arms out at the sides for balance. Bend the legs only as far as suppleness and strength allow.
Repeat twenty times.
Purpose: to exercise the hips and thighs.

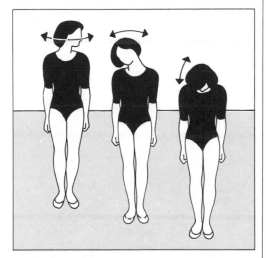

Neck exercises

Sit or stand, with the back straight and the legs together. Turn the head slowly to the right, then to the left, keeping the neck upright. Repeat ten times. Then incline the head sideways, to the right, then to the left, with the eyes looking forwards. Repeat ten times. Finally, bend the head forwards, then backwards. Repeat ten times.
Purpose: to exercise the neck muscles.

Back and chest exercises

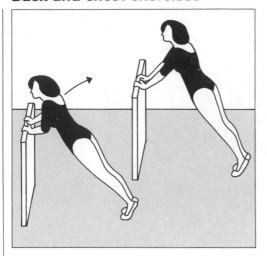

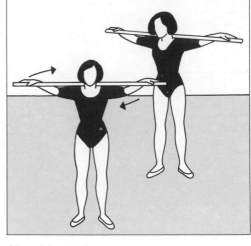

Push-ups
Stand about a metre (3-4ft) away from a firm, horizontal ledge that is about one metre above the ground. Place the hands about a shoulder-width apart on the ledge. While breathing in, bend the arms so that your chest touches the ledge. While breathing out, push up until the arms are straight.
Repeat ten times.
Purpose: to exercise the chest and shoulders.

Shoulder turns
Place a two-metre long stick across the shoulders, so that it can support the out-stretched arms. Stand with the feet apart. Do not move the hips and legs. Turn the upper body as far as possible to the right, then to the left. Keep the back straight, and the arms parallel to the ground.
Repeat thirty times.
Purpose: to exercise the waist.

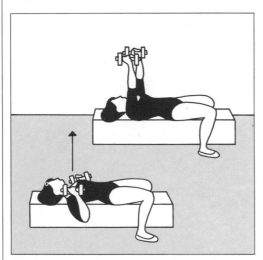

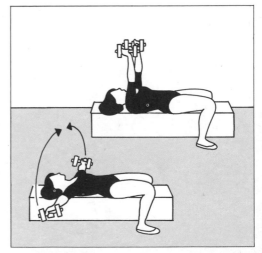

Bench press
Lie face-up on a low bench, with the feet on the floor at each side of the bench. Hold a light weight, such as a plastic bottle filled with water, in each hand. Start with the two weights at the sides of the chest, keeping the forearms vertical, then lift them vertically upwards until the arms are straight.
Repeat twenty times.
Purpose: to exercise arm and chest muscles.

Flying exercise
Lie face-up on a low bench, with the feet on the floor at each side of the bench. Hold a light weight in each hand. Start with the arms vertically above the chest. Swing both arms outwards as far as possible, keeping the arms curved. Keep the arms at right angles to the shoulders.
Repeat twenty times.
Purpose: to strengthen arm and chest muscles.

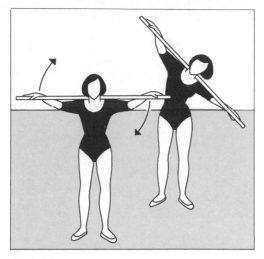

Side bends
Place a two-metre long stick across the shoulders, so that it can support the outstretched arms. Stand with the feet apart. Bend the body at the waist to the right, then to the left, without bending forwards or backwards. Do not allow the hips to sway. Repeat thirty times.
Purpose: to exercise muscles at the sides of the chest and at the waist.

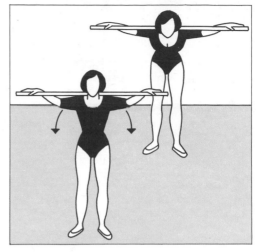

Forward bends
Place a two-metre long stick across the shoulders, so that it can support the outstretched arms. Stand with the feet apart. Keep the legs straight and bend forwards from the hips until the back is horizontal. Keep the back straight and the head up. Repeat twenty times.
Purpose: to exercise the hips and the muscles of the lower spine.

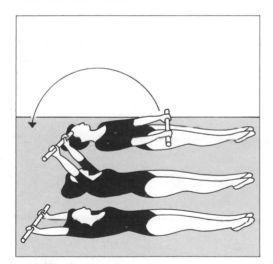

Straight arm pull-over
Lie face-up on the floor. Hold a stick across the thighs, so that the backs of the hands are upwards, and the arms parallel. Swing the stick up and over the head, keeping the arms straight, until the backs of the wrists touch the floor. Breathe in as the arms stretch upwards, and out as the arms return. Repeat twenty times.
Purpose: a breathing and chest exercise.

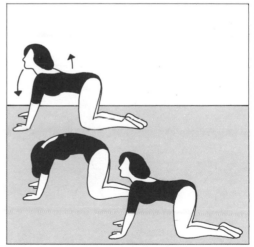

Back exercise (arch and hollow)
Rest on hands and knees, with the thighs upright, and the back horizontal. The fingers should be pointing forwards. Raise the head and hollow the back as far as possible. Then arch the back and lower the head so that the spine is flexed. The movement should be controlled and rhythmical, not violent. Repeat twenty times.
Purpose: to exercise muscles of the back.

Leg exercises

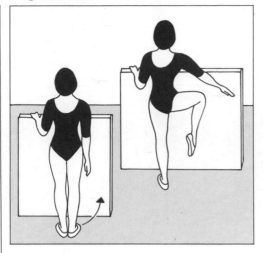

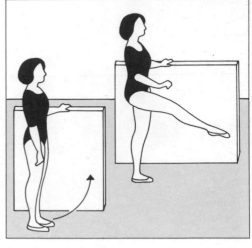

Knee side raise

Stand with the heels together and the toes turned out. Hold a firm horizontal support with one hand for balance. Raise the right knee sideways, keeping the toes pointed. Keep the body upright and move only from the hips. Return the right leg to the original position and repeat with the left leg. Repeat fifteen times with each leg.

Purpose: to exercise the hips.

Leg forward raise

Stand with the heels together and the toes turned out. Hold a firm horizontal support with the left hand for balance. Hold the right arm out sideways. Raise the right leg backwards, then swing it forwards from the hips as far as possible, with the toes pointed outwards. Repeat fifteen times, then repeat fifteen times with the left leg.

Purpose: to exercise the hips and thighs.

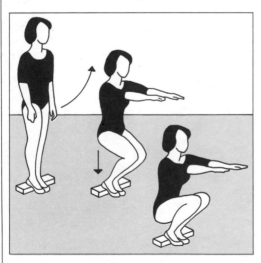

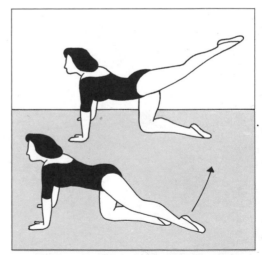

Deep knee-bends

Stand with the heels raised on a block, such as a book or a small step, that is about 5cm thick. Keep the feet together, the back straight, the head up, and hold the arms forwards for balance. Bend the knees, keeping them together, so that you sit on your heels. Then straighten to the standing position. Repeat twenty times.

Purpose: to exercise the hips and thighs.

Kneeling, leg backward raise

Rest on hands and knees, with the thighs upright, and the back horizontal. The fingers should be pointing forwards. Raise the head. Straighten the left leg, then lift it as high as possible without moving the body. Do not bend the knee. Keep the leg straight until all repetitions have been completed. Repeat fifteen times with each leg.

Purpose: to exercise the buttocks and back.

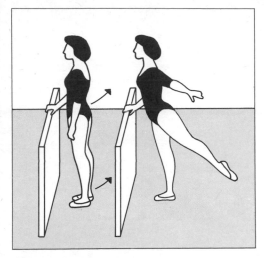

Leg backward raise

Stand with the heels together and the toes turned out. Hold a firm horizontal support with one hand for balance. Lift the left leg forwards, with the toes outwards. Then swing the leg backwards, as far as possible, keeping the legs straight, the body upright, and the toes outwards. Do not allow the body to sway. Repeat fifteen times with each leg.
Purpose: to exercise the buttocks and the hips.

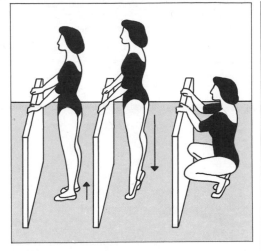

Knee-bends on the toes

Stand with the heels about one foot apart, and with the toes turned out. Hold a firm horizontal support with both hands for balance. Rise up on tiptoe, then squat down, keeping the back vertical. Stand up, and lower the heels to the floor.
Repeat twenty times.
Purpose: to exercise the hips, the thighs, and the calves.

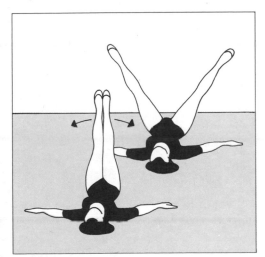

Leg parting

Lie on the back, with the arms stretched out at right angles to the body. Raise both legs so that they are vertical, and point the toes upwards. Spread the legs as wide as possible, so that they make a V-shape, then bring them together again. Do not lower the legs to the floor until the end of the exercise.
Repeat twenty times.
Purpose: to exercise inner thigh muscles.

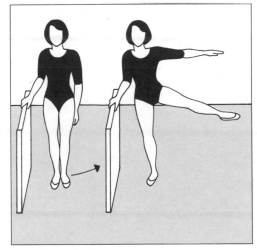

Leg side raise

Stand with the heels together and the toes turned out. Hold a firm horizontal support with the right hand for balance. Keeping the body upright and still, raise the left leg sideways as far as possible, then return it to the original position. Do not allow the leg to veer forwards or backwards. Repeat fifteen times, then repeat with the right leg.
Purpose: to exercise the hip and the thigh.

Abdominal exercises

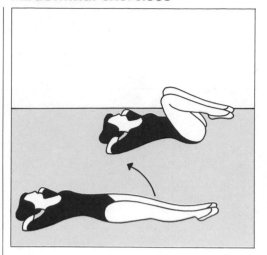

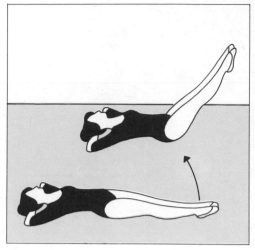

Knees raise

Lie on the back, with the hands under the head, the legs stretched out, the toes pointed, and the feet together. Bend the knees and draw the heels up to the buttocks. Then breathe in, and lift the knees up to the chest, without raising the hips. Return the feet to the floor, then straighten the legs.
Repeat twenty times.
Purpose: to exercise abdominal muscles.

Legs raise

Lie on the back, with the hands under the head, the legs stretched out, the toes pointed, and the feet together. Raise both legs together, without bending the knees, from the floor to a vertical position. Lower the legs to the original position. Keep the legs straight throughout this exercise.
Repeat fifteen times.
Purpose: to exercise abdominal muscles.

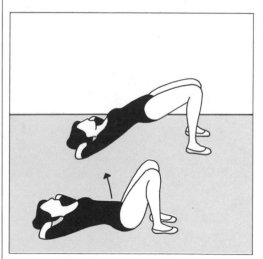

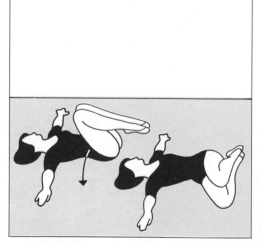

Hip arching

Lie on the back, with the hands under the head. Bend the knees so that the heels are as close as possible to the buttocks. Keep the feet close together. Slowly raise the hips as high as possible, bearing the weight on the shoulders rather than the neck, then lower the hips gently to the floor.
Repeat twenty times.
Purpose: to exercise the buttocks and back.

Hip rolling

Lie on the back, with the arms stretched out at right angles to the body. Bend the knees so that only the toes touch the floor and the heels rest against the buttocks. Roll the legs to the right, then to the left, touching the floor on each side. Keep both shoulders on the floor throughout the exercise.
Repeat ten times each side.
Purpose: to exercise the waist.

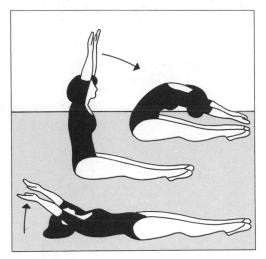

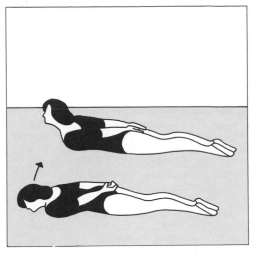

Sit-ups

Lie on the back, with the arms stretched above the head, legs stretched out, toes pointed and the feet together. Swing the arms up, over, and forwards to touch the toes, at the same time as you sit up. As the arms stretch forwards, bend the head towards the knees. Return to the original position. Repeat twenty times.

Purpose: to exercise abdominal muscles.

Chest raise

Lie face-down on the floor, with the feet together either with the toes beneath a bar just above floor level, or with the calves held down by another person. Clasp the hands behind the back. Raise the head and chest as high as possible, then lower to the floor. Repeat twenty times.

Purpose: to exercise muscles of the lower spine, and to stretch the abdominal muscles.

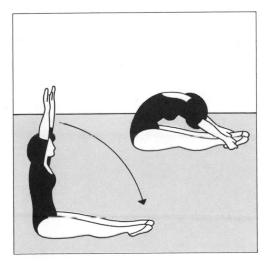

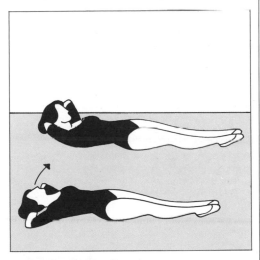

Seated, head to knees

Sit on the floor, with the legs straight and together, and the toes pointed. Hold the body upright and stretch the arms above the head. Draw the chest up and stomach in. Lean forwards, and touch the toes with the hands. Try to touch the knees with the forehead. Then sit upright again. Repeat twenty times.

Purpose: to stretch and exercise the back.

Shoulder raise

Lie on the back, with the hands under the head, the legs stretched out, the toes pointed, and the feet together. Raise the shoulders, arms, and chest at least 30cm (one foot) from the floor. Hold the position for a moment, then lower the head and shoulders gently to the floor. Repeat twenty times.

Purpose: to exercise abdominal muscles.

Cardiovascular and general exercises 1

Cardiovascular exercises improve the condition of the heart and the blood vessels in the body. They do this by making the heart work at a pace that is faster than the normal resting rate, yet not so fast that the heart is strained. In this way the efficiency and the strength of the heart and the cardiovascular system can be increased.

Although these exercises may help to prevent cardiovascular illness, they should not be done by anyone who has had a heart attack. Coronary patients, and anyone who is overweight or who smokes heavily, should consult a doctor before starting these, or any other, vigorous exercises.

The pace at which the heart beats can be measured most conveniently by feeling the pulse of the arteries in the wrist. To do this, turn the right hand so that the palm faces upwards. Place the three central fingers of the left hand on the upper side of the right wrist, close to the base of the thumb. Feel for the pulse with the fingertips on the thumb side of the tendons that are found in the middle of the wrist. Press gently, and count the number of pulses that can be felt in fifteen seconds. Multiply this number by four to calculate the number of pulses, or heartbeats, per minute.

It is important that everyone who exercises knows what his or her own exercising pulse rate should be. If this rate is exceeded, be careful, because strain rather than fitness may result. If you find your pulse rising too rapidly, or going above your calculated exercising rate, you should consult your doctor before taking further strenuous exercise.

The importance of the exercising pulse rate is that it shows each individual, at any time, how vigorously he or she can exercise. If the pulse exceeds the calculated limit, you should slow down; if the pulse does not reach the exercising rate, then the exercise is not vigorous enough.

To calculate the exercising pulse rate, add an "unfitness handicap" of 40 to your age, and subtract this total from 200. Thus an unfit person of twenty should aim to raise his or her pulse rate when exercising to 140; an unfit person of thirty should aim for an exercising pulse rate of 130; an unfit person of forty should aim for an exercising pulse rate of 120; and so on.

Go through the first four exercises to warm up in order to avoid strains during the other exercises. Then do the remaining ten as a sequence that must be completed twice. It is important to do the exercises in the order specified. The whole sequence of exercises should take no more than half an hour.

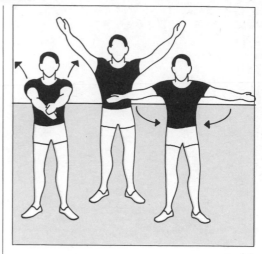

1 Arms circle
With the feet apart, raise both arms forwards, in front of the body. Keep the arms straight, and rotate them from the shoulder. Make the sweep of the arms as large as possible, to achieve most benefit from this exercise. Do not move the rest of the body, or the head, as the arms swing round.
Repeat thirty times.
Purpose: a warming-up exercise.

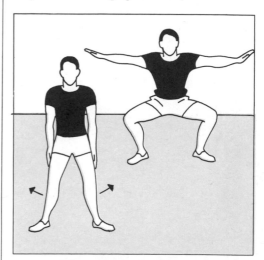

4 Wide knee-bends
With the heels about 60cm (2ft) apart, and with the toes turned out, bend the knees so that they remain in line with the feet. Keep the heels on the ground and the back straight. Hold the arms out sideways, for balance. Bend the knees until the thighs are horizontal, then stand up again.
Repeat twenty times.
Purpose: a warming-up exercise.

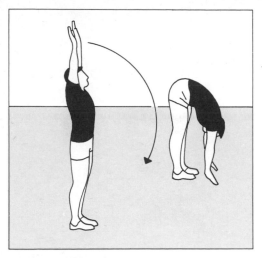

2 Toe touching
With the feet together, raise both arms upwards. Breathe in, lean forward from the hips, and touch the toes with the hands. With practice it should be possible to place the palms of both hands flat on the floor. Keep the legs straight, and do not round the back. Breathe out when standing up again.
Repeat fifteen times.
Purpose: a warming-up exercise.

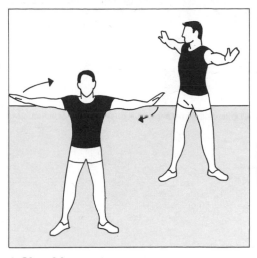

3 Shoulder turn
With the feet apart, hold the arms outstretched at shoulder height. Do not bend the arms, and do not allow the hips and legs to move. Keeping the back straight and the arms parallel to the floor, turn the head and shoulders as far as possible to the left, then to the right, in a steady movement.
Repeat thirty times.
Purpose: a warming-up exercise.

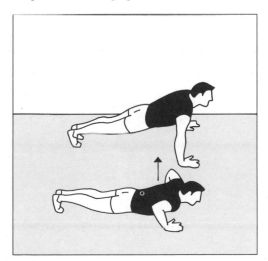

5 (and 15) Push-ups
Lean forwards, with the hands and toes on the floor, arms extended, and body straight. The hands should be about 45cm (18 inches) apart, with the fingers pointing forwards. Bend the arms so the chest touches the floor, then push up to straighten the arms.
Repeat ten times.
Purpose: to exercise the arms, chest, and shoulders.

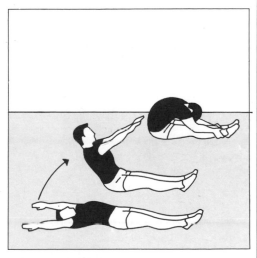

6 (and 16) Sit-ups
Lie stretched out on the back, with the arms above the head. Swing the arms upwards and forwards, and raise the body to a sitting position. Complete the movement by leaning forwards and touching the toes, trying to touch the forehead to the knees, then return to the original position.
Repeat fifteen times.
Purpose: to exercise the abdomen.

Cardiovascular and general exercises 2

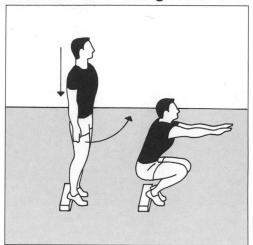

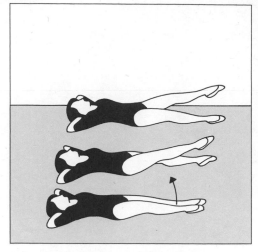

7 (and 17) Deep knee-bends

With the heels on a 5cm (two-inch) block, stand upright with the arms hanging at the sides. Keep the legs together, then bend the knees as much as possible. Swing the arms forward for balance. Keep the head up and the back straight. Stand up again and drop the arms to the sides.
Repeat twenty times.
Purpose: to exercise the hips and thighs.

8 (and 18) Alternate legs raise

Lie on the back with the hands beneath the head. Keeping both legs straight, with the toes pointed, raise one leg to about 45°, lower it, then raise the other leg. Do not bend the legs and do not lift the hips from the ground. The legs should be moved up and down as rapidly as possible.
Repeat twenty times.
Purpose: to exercise the abdomen and thighs.

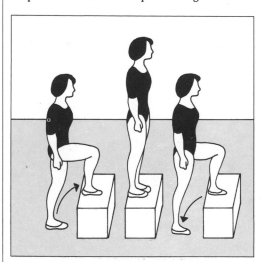

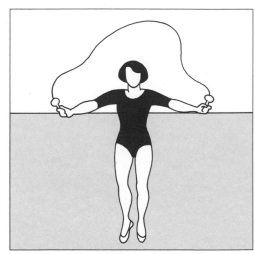

11 (and 21) Step-ups

Stand facing the seat of a chair or bench. Place the right foot on the chair, step up, and bring the left foot up beside the right. Then step down from the chair, with the right foot first. Step up and down ten times, then repeat the exercise by stepping on and off the chair or bench with the left foot first.
Repeat ten times with each leg.
Purpose: to exercise the legs, heart, and lungs.

12 (and 22) Skipping

Stand with the feet together, and hold a skipping rope in both hands, with the rope hanging behind. Swing the rope over the head and jump as it approaches the feet. Continue to swing the rope up and over the head, and jumping over it as it passes beneath the feet. Keep the head up.
Repeat fifty times.
Purpose: to exercise the legs, heart, and lungs.

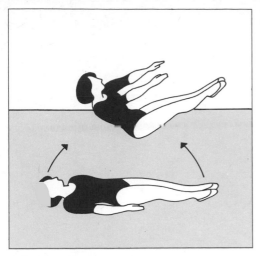

9 (and 19) Jack-knife

Lie on the back, with the arms at the sides, and palms of the hands on the floor. Raise both legs together, keeping them straight, to about 45° from the floor, and raise the shoulders and chest by the same amount. Lift the arms so that they are parallel to the legs. Hold the position for a moment, and lie back. Repeat fifteen times.

Purpose: to exercise the abdomen

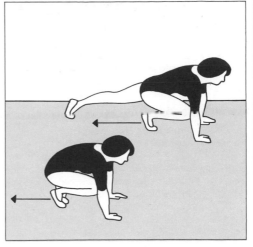

10 (and 20) Alternate leg squat thrusts

Squat, with both hands on the floor. Keep the back straight, the head up, the arms outside the knees, and the fingers spread. Stretch one leg backwards as far as possible then quickly change the position of the legs, so that the bent leg is straight, and the other is bent beneath the chest.
Repeat twenty times.

Purpose: to exercise legs, hips, heart and lungs.

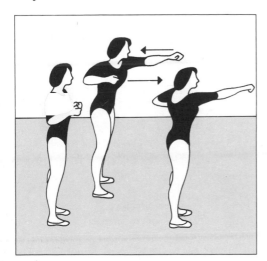

13 (and 23) Punching air

Stand with the feet apart. Hold the arms at the sides of the chest, and clench the fists. Punch forwards from the shoulder, first with the left arm, then with the right. Keep the head to the front and do not move the legs, but allow the torso to swing from the waist with each punch.
Repeat fifty times, as fast as possible.
Purpose: to exercise the shoulders and waist.

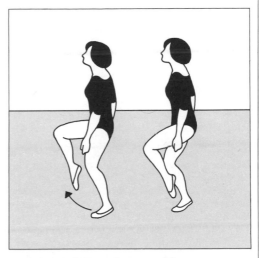

14 (and 24) Running on the spot

Stand erect, with the head up, the shoulders back, and the arms hanging down relaxed at the sides. Run on the spot, at a steady, comfortable pace. Raise the knees so that the thighs are horizontal, and keep the toes pointing down. Try to land softly on the toes, and do not jar the heels.
Repeat for a hundred steps.
Purpose: to exercise the legs, heart, and lungs.

Advanced exercises 1

For general health and physical vitality, the level of fitness attained by a person who has followed the schedules of the beginner's exercises (pp. 978-985) and the cardiovascular and general exercises (pp. 986-989) is sufficient. Once this level of fitness is reached, after about six months of regular daily exercising, it can be maintained by doing, as a minimum, the cardiovascular and general exercises three times a week.

The advanced exercises are designed for those who are not satisfied with this minimum. A person following them can go on to achieve a higher level of general fitness, and can do this using only a few basic items of gymnasium equipment.

For advanced exercises, some equipment is necessary, because the most efficent way to strengthen muscles is to make them repeatedly work against resistance. The most convenient forms of resistance are weights or dumb-bells or bar-bells. Anyone following the advanced schedule will need: a 2 metre (six-foot long) steel bar (standard bar-bell) with variable weights; two dumb-bells, with variable weights; a weight bench that has hooks and a strap at one end; a horizontal chinning bar that is at least 2.5 metres (8ft) from the floor; if possible, a set of wall bars; and a skipping rope.

With regard to the weights to use, be careful not to try to lift anything that is too heavy. The purpose of these exercises is to use muscles repeatedly, not to see how much weight can be lifted. For any one upper body exercise, use the heaviest weight that allows fifteen repetitions of the exercise to be done without discomfort.

The number of repetitions recommended for each exercise is intended as a guide, rather than a strict limit, because most people following the advanced schedule will judge from the way they feel during the exercise whether they should do more or less than the recommendations.

Finally, some essential safety precautions: **always** warm up thoroughly before starting the advanced exercises; as a minimum warm up, go through all the exercises described on pp. 978-979 and, in addition, exercise for at least five minutes by skipping or jogging; **do not** attempt the advanced exercises until the beginner's schedule (pp. 978-985) and the cardiovascular exercises (pp. 986-989) can be done without any sense of strain, either during or the day after the exercises; **do not** do any exercises that involve the use of weights if you are under fifteen years of age, because this may lead to abnormal muscular development, and may damage developing bones and joints.

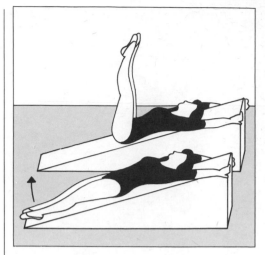

Legs raise, on angled board
Lie face-up on a bench that is inclined at about 20°, with the head at the higher end. Stretch the arms above the head and hold on to a strap, the sides of the bench, or the bar on which the bench rests. Keep the legs together, and the toes pointed. Raise the legs to a vertical position, then lower them. Repeat twenty to thirty times.
Purpose: to exercise the abdomen.

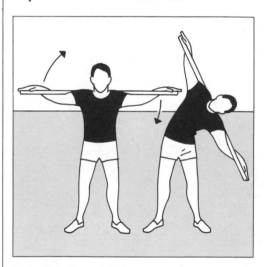

Side bends, with bar
Stand with the feet apart. Hold a six-foot steel bar, without weights, across the shoulders. Bend sideways at the waist. Do not allow the body to lean forwards or backwards, and keep the head looking to the front. Bend as far as possible one way, straighten again, then bend the other way. Repeat fifteen to twenty times.
Purpose: to exercise the waist.

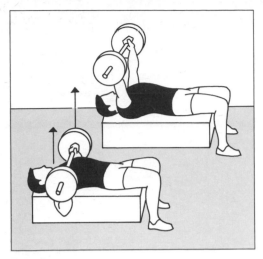

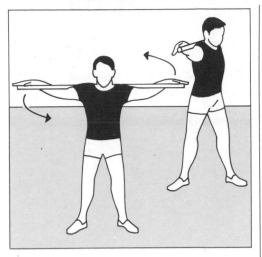

Bench press
Lie face-up on a bench, with the feet on the floor on either side. Hold a bar-bell across the upper chest. Grip the bar with both hands more than shoulder width apart. The backs of the hands should be nearest to the face. Push vertically upwards until the arms are straight, then lower to the chest.
Repeat ten to fifteen times.
Purpose: to exercise the chest and arms.

Shoulder turns, with bar
Stand with the feet apart. Hold a six-foot steel bar, without weights, across the shoulders so that it supports the arms when they are outstretched. Turn the torso, head, and arms as far as possible to the left, then to the right, in a steady movement. Do not move the legs, and keep the back straight.
Repeat fifteen to twenty times.
Purpose: to exercise the waist.

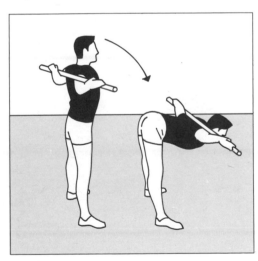

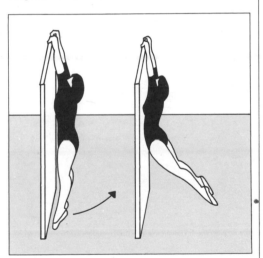

Forward bends, with bar
Stand with feet apart. Hold a six-foot steel bar, without weights, across the shoulders so that it supports the arms when they are outstretched. Bend forwards from the hips, keeping the head up, until the back is horizontal. Keep the legs and back straight, and the arms parallel to the ground.
Repeat fifteen to twenty times.
Purpose: to exercise the back, hips, and thighs.

Hanging, reverse arch
Hang with both hands from a high wall bar, face to the wall, so that the feet are clear of the ground. Lift the legs and hips backwards as far as possible, hollowing the back. The same exercise may be done from a horizontal bar, with the body hanging free.
Repeat ten to fifteen times.
Purpose: to exercise the lower back and buttocks.

Advanced exercises 2

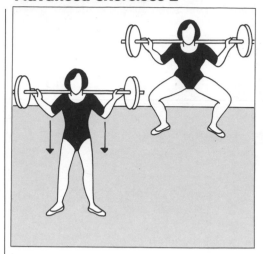

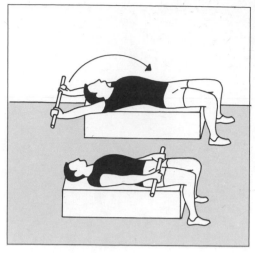

Squat

Stand with the feet apart and the toes turned out. Lift a bar-bell from a squat-rack, or from the hands of another person, on to the shoulders, behind the neck. Hold the bar-bell, and support its weight on the shoulders. Bend the legs, keeping the back straight, until the thighs are horizontal.
Repeat fifteen to twenty times.
Purpose: to exercise the hips and thighs.

Straight arm pull-over

Lie face-up on a bench, with the feet on the floor on either side. Hold a steel bar across the thighs, with the backs of the hands upwards. Lift the bar up and over the head, keeping the arms straight. Bend the hands upwards so that the tension is on the chest not the elbows.
Repeat fifteen to twenty times.
Purpose: a breathing and chest exercise.

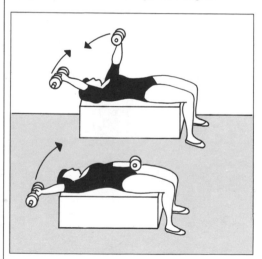

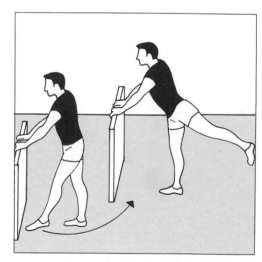

Alternate dumb-bell pull-over

Lie face-up on a bench with the feet on the floor on either side. Hold a dumb-bell in each hand, resting on the thighs, with the backs of the hands uppermost. Lift one arm up and overhead, with the arm slightly bent. As the first arm returns to the starting position, lift the other arm up and overhead. Repeat fifteen to twenty times.
Purpose: a breathing and chest exercise.

Leg back raise

Stand facing a firm horizontal support, with the heels together and the toes turned out, holding the support with both hands. Keep the toes pointed, and swing the left leg backwards as far as possible. Keep the body upright. Complete the exercise with the left leg before starting it with the right leg.
Repeat fifteen to twenty times with each leg.
Purpose: to exercise the hips and buttocks.

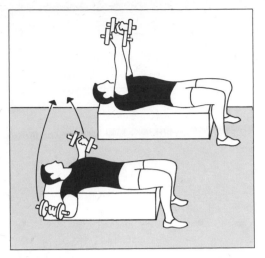

Flying exercise

Lie face-up on a bench, with the feet slightly
apart on the floor. Hold a dumb-bell in each
hand directly above the chest. Start with the
arms straight, then move them outwards and
downwards, bending the arms slightly so that
the elbows are not strained. Lower the arms
until the weights are level with the shoulders.
Repeat fifteen to twenty times.
Purpose: a breathing and arm exercise.

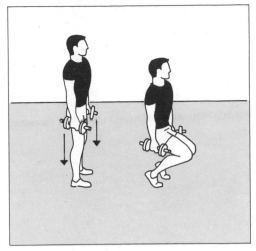

Deep knee-bends with dumb-bells

Stand with the feet slight apart. Hold a
dumb-bell in each hand, with the hands
straight down at the sides. Bend the knees
and squat down as far as possible, keeping
the arms by the sides. Keep the head up, the
legs parallel, and the back straight.
Repeat fifteen to twenty times.
*Purpose: to exercise the knees, thighs, and
hips.*

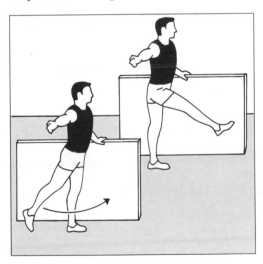

Leg forward raise

Stand sideways to a firm horizontal support,
with the heels together, and the toes turned
out, holding the support with the left hand.
Hold the right hand out for balance. Lift the
right leg forward from the hip as far as
possible, keeping the leg straight and the toes
pointed outwards. Repeat with the other leg.
Repeat fifteen to twenty times with each leg.
Purpose: to exercise the hips and thighs.

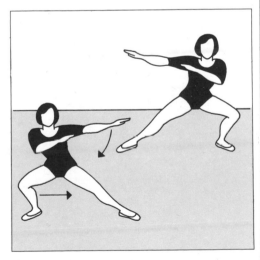

Seesaw movement

Stand with the feet wide apart, with the toes
turned outwards, and the hands by the sides.
Keep the back straight and the head up.
Bend the left knee, keeping the heels on the
ground and the right leg straight. Move both
arms to the right. Reverse the position by
bending the right knee.
Repeat ten to fifteen times on each side.
Purpose: to exercise the hips and inside thighs.

Advanced exercises 3

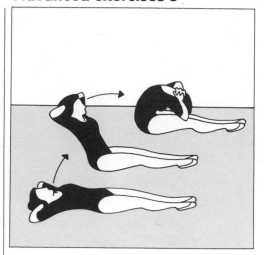

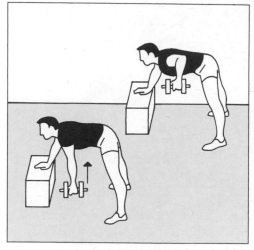

Sit-ups
Lie on the back, with the legs together, the
toes pointed, and the hands behind the head.
Sit up from this position, keeping the feet
on the ground, and lean forwards as far as
possible. The same exercise can be done on a
sloping board, with the feet held by a strap at
the top of the board.
Repeat twenty to thirty times.
Purpose: to exercise the abdomen.

One arm dumb-bell rowing
Stand with the feet apart. Lean forward, with
the legs straight, and place one hand on a
bench. Hold a dumb-bell in the other hand.
Keep the head up and the back straight.
Bend the arm to lift the dumb-bell up to the
side of the chest. Complete the exercise with
one arm before doing it with the other.
Repeat ten to fifteen times with each arm.
Purpose: to exercise the shoulders and arms.

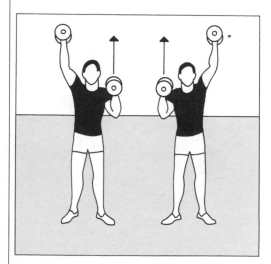

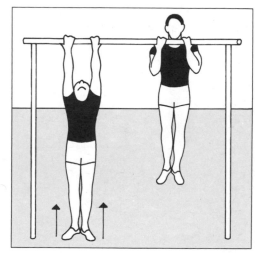

Press with dumb-bells
Stand with the feet apart. Hold a dumb-bell
in each hand, at the shoulders. Keep the back
straight and head up. Raise one arm directly
overhead, until it is straight, and then raise
the other arm while lowering the first arm to
the shoulders. Do not allow the body to lean
backwards or forwards.
Repeat ten to fifteen times.
Purpose: to exercise the shoulders and arms.

Chinning
Hang by both hands from a horizontal bar,
with the hands no more than shoulder-width
apart. Hold the bar with the backs of the
hands away from the face (undergrip). Hang
straight down, then pull up until the upper
chest touches the bar. Lower until the arms
are straight.
Repeat ten times, or more if possible.
Purpose: to exercise the shoulders and arms.

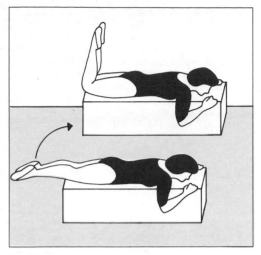

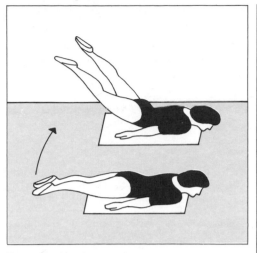

Legs curl

Lie face-down on a bench with the knees just clear of the end. Bend the legs at the knees, keeping the feet together, so that the heels touch the buttocks. Then straighten the legs to the starting position. Keep the toes pointed down for half the repetitions, then do the other half with the toes pointed up. Repeat fifty times.
Purpose: to exercise the backs of the thighs.

Face-down, legs raise

Lie face-down on the floor, with the arms close to the sides, and the hands palm downwards. Keep the legs together, and point the toes. Press down with the palms of the hands and lift both the legs and the hips as high as possible from the floor. Hold for a moment, then return to the original position. Repeat ten to fifteen times.
Purpose: to exercise the buttocks and back.

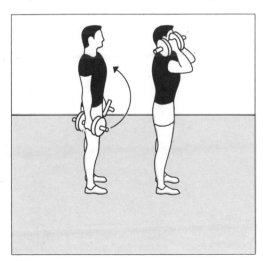

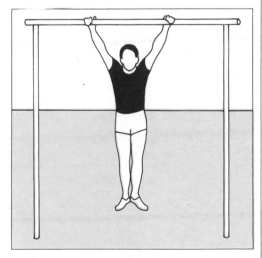

Curl

Stand upright, with the feet slightly apart. Hold a dumb-bell in each hand, with the arms hanging at the sides. Bend both arms at the elbows, turning the forearms slightly inwards, and lift the dumb-bells up to the chest. Keep the elbows close to the body throughout the exercise.
Repeat ten to fifteen times.
Purpose: to exercise the biceps muscles.

Hang on horizontal bar

It is always wise to end an exercise session by hanging from a horizontal bar to stretch and relax the joints, particularly those of the spine. Hold the bar with the backs of the hands towards the face (overgrip), the hands wide apart, and the body and legs straight. Breathe deeply.
Hang for about fifteen to thirty seconds.
Purpose: to relax, and to stretch the spine.

Exercises and sport

Anyone involved in sports get more pleasure from them, and does them better, if he or she is physically fit. The exercise schedules described as beginner's exercises and cardiovascular exercises (pp.978–989) are an excellent preparation for any sport.

Twenty-two sports are listed below, with special exercises that are particularly useful for each. If your own sport, for example scuba diving or water polo, is not listed, you will probably find that special exercises you can use are listed under the heading of a similar sport, such as swimming.

The table also offers advice about exercises for muscles that are used relatively little by the sport. These complementary exercises are important because they help to prevent uneven development, and also improve performance by exercising the muscles that counteract those used by the sport.

SPORT	SPECIAL EXERCISES	COMPLEMENTARY EXERCISES
Archery	grip exercise: squeeze a rubber ball hard in each hand; also: one arm dumb-bell rowing (p.994); shoulder turns, with bar (p.991).	bench press (p.991); push-ups (p.987).
Badminton	wrist exercise: hold a dumb-bell rod in each hand, with the forearms horizontal, and rotate the wrists; holding a dumb-bell rod like a racket, move as during a game; also: seesaw movement (p.993); skipping (p.987).	exercise the other arm; chinning (p.994); one arm dumb-bell rowing (p.994).
Basketball	squat jumps: squat down with the hands on the floor, then jump up, stretching the arms as high as possible over the head; also: squat (p.992); press with dumb-bells (p.994).	basketball exercises all muscle groups.
Canoeing	sit-ups (p.987); shoulder turns with bar (p.991); bench press (p.991); press with dumb-bells (p.994); flying exercise (p.993); chinning (p.994).	leg exercises (pp.982–983); skipping (p.988); face-down, legs raise (p.995).
Cricket	sprinting exercise: run hard for 30 metres (30 yards), lie down, do two push-ups, sprint thirty metres; also: grip exercise (*see* **Archery**); shoulder turns with bar (p.991).	exercise the other arm.
Cycling	squat (p.992); deep knee-bends with dumb-bells (p.993); legs curl (p.995); sit-ups (p.994); step-ups (p.988); leg exercises (pp.982–983).	chinning (p.994); hanging, reverse arch (p.991); shoulder turn (p.987).
Fives	wrist exercise (*see* **Badminton**); leg exercises (pp.982–983); seesaw movement (p.993).	fives exercises all muscle groups.
Golf	knee exercise: stand with feet slightly apart, and turn the hips and knees in one direction, then the other, simulating golfing movements; also: grip exercise (*see* **Archery**).	golf uses most muscle groups to a slight extent; a more vigorous, aerobic exercise is also recommended.
Hiking	thigh and hip exercise: while standing, balance a weight, such as a sandbag, on the foot, and lift the leg as high as possible, bending the knee; also: leg exercises (pp.982–983); seesaw movement (p.993).	hiking exercises all muscle groups.
Riding	thigh grip exercise: squeeze a medicine ball hard between the knees; also: wide kneebends (p.986); squat (p.992); leg parting (p.983); one arm dumb-bell rowing (p.994).	abdominal exercises (pp.984–985); back and chest exercises (pp.980–981).

SPORT	SPECIAL EXERCISES	COMPLEMENTARY EXERCISES
Rock climbing	grip exercise (*see* **Archery**); bench press (p.991); shoulder turns with bar (p.991); hanging, reverse arch (p.991); sit-ups (p.991); chinning (p.994); leg side raise (p.983); squat (p.992); seesaw movement (p.993).	rock climbing exercises all muscle groups.
Rowing	squat jumps (*see* **Basketball**); chinning (p.994); sit-ups (p.994); push-ups (p.987); skipping (p.988); running, for stamina.	shoulder raise (p.985); face-down, legs raise (p.995); leg back raise.
Rugby	pushing exercises against an immobile object; all advanced exercises (pp.990–995); weight training with professional supervision; sprinting exercises (*see* **Cricket**).	rugby exercise all muscle groups.
Running (Jogging)	leg exercises (pp.982–983); legs raise, on angled board (p.990); shoulder turns, with bar (p.991); straight arm pull-over (p.992).	running exercises all muscle groups.
Skating	ankle exercise: stand with feet slightly apart, and rock the ankles from side to side; also: deep knee-bends with dumb-bells (p.993); seesaw movement (p.993).	back and chest exercises (pp.980–981); press with dumb-bells (p.994).
Skiing	thigh strength exercise: lean the back flat against a smooth wall, with the feet together, about 0.6 metres (2ft) away, then end the legs so that the back slides down as low as possible, and push up again; adapt ankle exercise (*see* **Skating**), and knee exercise (*see* **Golf**) to the movements of skiing; also: leg exercises (pp.982-983); seesaw movement (p.993).	skiing exercises all muscle groups.
Soccer	ankle exercise (*see* **Skating**); knee exercise (*see* **Golf**); leg exercises (pp.982–983); legs curl (p.995); neck exercises (p.979); shoulder turns, with bar (p.991).	soccer exercises all muscle groups.
Squash	wrist exercise (*see* **Badminton**); leg exercises (pp.982–983); seesaw movement (p.993); skipping (p.988); sit-ups (p.994).	exercise the other arm.
Swimming	straight arm pull-over (p.992); shoulder turns, with bar (p.991); sit-ups (p.994); shoulder raise (p.985); alternate legs raise (p.988).	chinning (p.994).
Tennis	wrist exercise (*see* **Badminton**); leg exercises (pp.982–983); skipping (p.988); straight arm pull-over (p.992); hanging, reverse arch (p.991); seesaw movement (p.993).	exercise the other arm.
Volleyball	squat jumps (*see* **Basketball**); press with dumb-bells (p.994); hanging, reverse arch (p.991); straight arm pull-over (p.992).	one arm dumb-bell rowing (p.994); chinning (p.994).
Waterskiing	squat (p.992); deep knee-bends with dumb-bells (p.982); one arm dumb-bell rowing (p.994); chinning (p.994).	hanging, reverse arch (p.991); shoulder raise (p.985).

Gymnasiums and health farms

Those who can afford the time and expense involved may wish to take advantage of the facilities offered by health gymnasiums. None of the equipment and other facilities provided by gymnasiums are strictly necessary to the process of getting fit, but they can add interest and variety to your physical exercises. Two other advantages offered by good gymnasiums are constant supervision, which enables you to exercise with safety and confidence, and a congenial atmosphere. Exercising with people who share a common purpose can provide extra enjoyment and incentive.

It is necessary first of all to distinguish between the different types of gymnasiums. Training gymnasiums are essentially for athletes and other men or women who wish to develop their skills for particular athletic activities. They provide facilities for athletes to keep themselves fit throughout the year, and to train themselves for their chosen sports. Health gymnasiums provide advice, instruction and facilities for anyone who wishes to become or keep fit, whatever his or her initial physical condition. Their clients range from professional athletes to office workers who wish only to make the best use of their lunch hours.

Health gymnasiums vary widely in quality. When choosing one for yourself, you should check that it is staffed by qualified and responsible instructors. You may feel flattered to be attended by a sports celebrity, but professionally trained physiotherapists and physical educational instructors can be equally, if not more, beneficial to an unfit person. You should expect to be asked details of your medical history, and to be carefully examined before being allowed to use all the facilities. If you have not exercised for some time, you may even be advised to have a medical check-up. You will probably be asked to perform some simple exercises that are designed to raise your pulse rate to about 110 beats per minute. If your pulse rate rises excessively, this may be an indication of some physical disorder.

Different types of exercise

The accessories provided in health gymnasiums to help you exercise range from simple weights and benches to more sophisticated equipment such as pulleys and rowing machines. These accessories are appropriate for different kinds of exercises.

Isometric exercises, the simplest type, involve applying muscular strength by pulling or pushing immovable objects. The muscles are tensed and this tension is sustained for short periods of time. Because little movement is involved in these exercises, they develop static rather than dynamic strength.

Isotonic exercises involve pulling or lifting an object to a certain position and then returning it to its original position. They cause the muscles to contract as you move but, because the weight or force employed is constant, they do not exercise your muscles to the same degree throughout the exercise. The weight or force used can only be that which you can lift or pull at the weakest point in the range of motion involved, and at other points your muscles are not sufficiently strained to develop in strength. For example, when you are exercising with dumb-bells or bar-bells, you can feel your muscles being stressed only at certain points as you lift the bars.

The third type of exercise, known as isokinetic, requires more sophisticated equipment. When using this equipment, your muscles are made to work at their maximum capacity throughout the exercise. The resistance of the object against which you pull or push varies according to the effort you employ, so that the resistance is equal to the muscular force exerted throughout the exercise. The equipment itself automatically controls both the resistance and the speed at which you perform the exercise.

Isokinetic exercises can be designed for particular needs. For example, a person who is training for a particular sport can do exercises that simulate exactly the demands of this sport, and so develop precisely the muscles that are most needed. In terms of the speed with which muscular power is developed, research has shown that isokinetic exercises are the most efficient of the three different types. They are also the safest, as the effort involved is automatically regulated.

Massage

Faclities for massage may be available at health gymnasiums or sauna baths. Massage is used in physical therapy as a means of rehabilitating patients who are suffering from certain physical pains or ailments but, as a means of getting or keeping fit, its value is very limited. It stimulates the circulation, relaxes the muscles, and can relieve local pains. But massage itself, whether performed manually or with an electrical vibrating machine, cannot increase muscular strength or reduce the amount of fat on the body.

Sauna baths

Sauna baths may be attached to health gymnasiums or may exist as separate establishments. Most sauna baths are organized according to similar basic principles, although Finnish sauna baths retain their original national characteristics. They have an invigorating effect on the whole body and aid physical and mental relaxation, but their effects are temporary rather than long-term.

On entering a sauna, you first take a warm shower to wash off the superficial dirt. You then enter the dry heat room, where you sit or lie on benches while you perspire in temperatures of up to 120°C (248°F). The heat is created by stoves or by electric heaters. Your body temperature rises by about 2°C (3.6°F), and your blood vessels dilate. This causes your heart to beat faster in order to circulate more blood to the outside of your body. Your skin pores open, and the perspiration washes out particles of dirt, dead skin, and cosmetics. These are then rinsed off in a cold shower. Alternating periods in the heat room with cold showers has an especially invigorating effect.

Sauna baths provide a healthy and enjoyable means of relaxation, but the sudden rise in pulse rate can be dangerous for anyone with a weak heart. People with any heart disorder, pregnant women, and people with high or low blood pressure, should therefore avoid them.

Health farms
A health farm is a type of clinic that is attended by those who want to improve their general physical health and mental stamina. People who attend health farms rarely have any symptoms of illness: they simply feel "out of condition" and know that, with proper care and treatment, their general health will improve. Some people visit health farms to rest from the stresses of everyday life, or to obtain help for a particular problem, such as heavy drinking.

The facilities that may be offered by a health farm will usually include regular exercise sessions, hydrotherapy, massage, and physiotherapy. Hydrotherapy involves the use of warm water to stimulate the circulation and aid mental relaxation, and also of special exercises that are performed in water. Other facilities that may be offered by health farms include special relaxation classes, yoga, and biofeedback techniques. Specialized health farms may also be equipped to offer diathermy, a form of physical therapy in which the body tissues are subjected to deep heating by the use of high-frequency electromagnetic waves.

The therapies offered by health farms may be supervised by doctors, naturopaths, or osteopaths. Diet is often an important part of the treatment, and those who want to lose weight may begin their stay with a day or two with nothing to eat, apart from fluids such as fruit juices and herbal teas. One of the aims of such treatment is to flush out any poisonous toxins that the body may contain. The diet prescribed is sometimes exclusively vegetarian.

Some health farms are organized with a religious or cultural bias. Many are situated in pleasant rural surroundings, where those attending can benefit from the relaxing atmosphere and the co-operative feeling produced by a group of people who share a common aim.

Exercise for body and mind
There are a wide variety of physical exercises that are more effective as aids to mental relaxation than in developing physical fitness. They may help to improve physical balance, co-ordination, and flexibility, but usually have little effect on strength or stamina. Their value is often more psychological than physical or medical.

Eurhythmics are exercises involving the co-ordination of physical movements with rhythmical musical sounds. They emphasize the aesthetic qualities of harmonious bodily movement, and are used as a form of musical education and in the training of modern dancers. They have had a considerable influence on the development of choreography in the twentieth century.

Yoga, originally a school of ancient Hindu philosophy, emphasizes the unity of mind and body. The form of yoga that is usually practised in Western countries is Hatha Yoga, which consists of a system of postures and breathing exercises that aid physical and mental relaxation. They develop suppleness and mobility, especially in the hip joints. It is claimed that they develop the inner resources of the body, and that they can lead eventually to complete knowledge and mastery of mind and body. Further stages of yoga involve techniques of concentration and meditation. Various techniques of meditation itself have become popular in Western countries as aids to physical and mental relaxation. Many of these techniques are derived from Eastern religions, and include breathing and relaxation exercises. Transcendental Meditation, or TM, involves profound concentration for two periods each day on a specific mantra, which is a word or formula that, when chanted or spoken repetitively, can aid concentration. Meditation techniques have been used in the treatment of patients with migraine or high blood pressure, but they have no real value in developing physical fitness.

Home gymnasium equipment

When setting up a gymnasium at home, it is advisable, first of all, to have a room, or part of a room, that can be devoted to it exclusively. If space is not available, the only pieces of equipment that can be stored conveniently after use are benches and a set of weights. The advice given on this page and the next assumes that space can be spared for the equipment to be set up permanently; or, if space cannot be spared, that modifications can be made. Many different types and makes of equipment are available for setting up a home gymnasium. The equipment described here is considered to be basic, durable, easy to use, and relatively cheap. Anyone buying more elaborate equipment should get expert advice.

A set of weights should consist of at least one bar-bell rod, and at least two dumb-bell rods, with interchangeable weights. The usual weights available are 2½lb (1.1kg), 5lb (2.2kg), 10lb (4.5kg), 15lb (6.7kg), and 20lb (9kg). It is advisable to have four of the 2½lb weights and two of each of the others. The keys, sleeves, and collars are sold with the weights, usually as part of a kit.

An abdominal board, a press bench, a 3.3 metre (11 ft) gymnastic bench, mats for floor work, and a skipping rope comprise the other pieces of basic equipment.

A set of wall bars is useful for the hanging reverse arch exercise (*see* p.991), for supporting the upper end of an angled board, and if necessary for using as horizontal supports that can be held for balance while doing various leg exercises. A free-standing horizontal chinning bar that is more than 2.5 metres (8 ft) from the floor, and parallel bars that can double as a squat-rack, are also useful.

A home gymnasium with these pieces of equipment can be used for all the exercises described in this book, and for many others. This equipment is recommended as a reasonable minimum that can also constitute the nucleus of a more elaborate gymnasium as other pieces of equipment are acquired. When a person is familiar with the uses of this equipment, he or she will have enough experience to judge the value and usefulness of other pieces, depending on needs or interests. Catalogues of such equipment are available from most large suppliers of sports equipment. Some specific pieces are illustrated here, and a local gymnasium may have other pieces of equipment that can be inspected and tried.

A home gymnasium should also have some form of heating, and a wall clock, ideally with a sweep second hand.

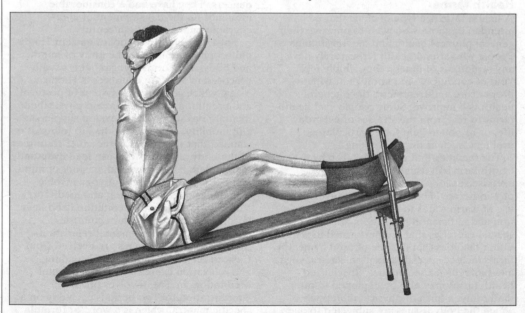

Abdominal board

The abdominal board can be used to exercise the lower abdominal muscles. The angle of the board can be adjusted according to the degree of difficulty desired. The equipment can also be used as an inclined bench for the bench press, or for flying exercises to develop the upper part of the chest. More advanced boards are available, but it is unnecessary to buy a board designed for a higher standard than you expect to achieve.

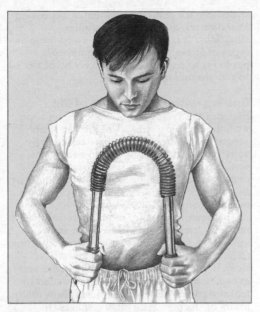

Multipurpose exerciser

This is one example of a number of similar devices that enable you to exercise several sets of muscles using the isometric principle. It is a simple piece of equipment, ideal for daily use and easy storage.

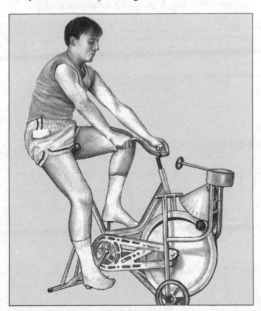

Static bicycle machine

This piece of equipment is designed to exercise the leg muscles, and stimulate the heart and lungs, improving cardiovascular efficiency. The resistance on the pedals can be gradually increased.

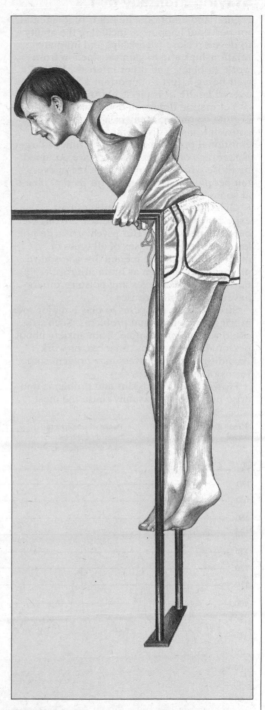

Parallel bars

The bars are used primarily for development of triceps muscles, but because this piece of equipment is usually chest high, it can be used as a rack to support a bar-bell before and after doing squats (*see* p.992).

Staying mentally fit 1

Mental and emotional health is fundamental for personal happiness, including the ability to develop close friendships and intimate relationships and to gain satisfaction from work, hobbies, and other interests. Mental well-being is just as important a factor in overall health as is physical fitness.

Yet mental illness, in one form or another, is quite common. Many of a doctor's daily consultations involve some mental or emotional problem. At any one time, a large percentage of all hospital beds are occupied by those who are mentally ill. One in every ten people needs treatment for mental illness at some time in life.

Given the right combination of past experiences and current stresses, anyone can become mentally ill. But psychiatrists do not know the specific causes of all types of mental illness. Some mental disorders have physical causes, such as brain injuries, nutritional deficiencies and poisons; others have psychological causes.

Stress, however, seems to play a major role in triggering emotional problems. Such stress could result, for example, from anxiety about personal relationships, finances, or work. Avoiding excessive stress may prevent some forms of mental illness.

However, the decisions and problems that arise unexpectedly usually cause the most stress – a sick child, an accident, a depressed friend or relative, and other similar situations. It is not possible to avoid these types of stress, so the better equipped a person is to cope, the more likely he or she is to remain mentally fit.

Coping with the stresses of life

Many of the factors that help a person cope with the ordinary stresses of life can simply involve a common-sense approach to daily activities: getting enough sleep each night; setting aside time for relaxation; avoiding overwork; discussing problems with family or friends; and cultivating a confident, positive mental attitude.

The amount of sleep required varies from person to person, and, even in the same individual, from night to night. It is important to have a steady and sufficient amount of sleep if you are to avoid chronic fatigue and exhaustion. The amount of sleep needed to feel rested and refreshed indicates how many hours of sleep an individual requires. If insufficient sleep is obtained one night, the next sleep period should be longer to make up for it. And it is better to go to bed earlier on the next night rather than to hope to wake up later on the following day.

Another major factor in promoting mental health is having a circle of relatives and

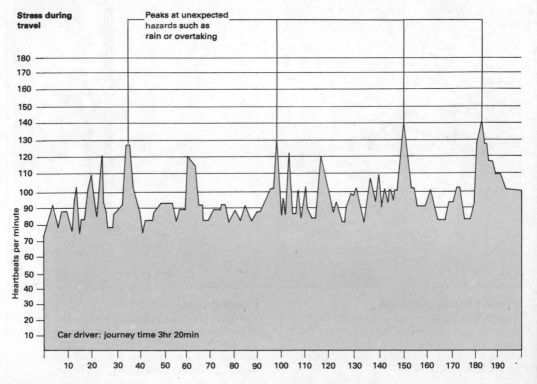

Stress during travel

Peaks at unexpected hazards such as rain or overtaking

Heartbeats per minute

Car driver: journey time 3hr 20min

friends on whom an individual can rely for psychological support or financial aid in times of trouble. The security provided by such a group can eliminate or greatly reduce anxiety about how to handle problems.

When a problem does arise, discussing it with a relative or friend is often enough to put the problem into its proper perspective. By the same token, a person can attain great satisfaction and feelings of self-esteem from supporting another in time of stress, acting as an adviser, helper, or just a good listener.

The more secure a person feels, the more likely he or she is to be mentally healthy. The foundation for emotional security is laid in childhood. Children need affection, support, understanding of their problems and fears, and a sense of being wanted in the home. Children are often troubled by ordinary fears, such as the dark, or by special circumstances, such as moving to a new house, attending a new school, witnessing an accident or other violent event, experiencing a death in the family, or having to go into hospital. Children need at least one adult on whom they feel they can rely. The child who grows up in a loving, trusting family environment has the best chance of becoming a mentally healthy adult with a confident, positive outlook on life. Such a person will in turn be well-equipped for parenthood.

Routine, boredom, and change

Developing a daily routine is an unconscious way of avoiding mental stress. Tasks done through habit cause the minimum amount of difficulty. At the same time, too much routine creates boredom, which in itself can be tiring and create stress. As with any other aspect of life, people vary widely in their need for routine in any form without realizing that they do. In fact, most people unconsciously combine routine with change and stimulation in the right proportions to maintain their own mental well-being. If the daily routine is changed, an allowance for additional rest and relaxation should be made until the initial weariness has gone. Changes in routine that are known to be unnecessary generally seem to be more tiring.

A certain amount of change from the daily routine is essential for mental well-being. But major changes can create a great deal of stress. The death of a loved one, a new job or home, marriage or divorce, even a change in diet are all sources of added stress. If several major upheavals occur within a short period, the chances of developing some type of mental, or even physical illness are greatly increased. A person experiencing such major changes should make special efforts to protect his or her mental health by getting enough rest and relaxation.

Stays level with only a few minor fluctuations

Rail passenger: 2hr 20min

Peaks at take-off and landing

Air passenger: 1hr

Heartbeats per minute

Staying mentally fit 2
Taking a holiday

For most people, holidays are the greatest change from daily routine. Some people gain the most rest and enjoyment from holidays that allow them to pursue their favourite pastimes, such as fishing, sunbathing, sailing, hiking, and other sports. Others use holiday time to see new parts of the world, shop, sample different kinds of food, and enjoy foreign cultures.

While holidays are generally beneficial to mental health, they usually require organization and travel. And this can produce varying amounts of mental stress.

Driving a car over a long distance can cause both physical and mental stress, especially if the driver attempts to meet a deadline. With air, ship, bus, or train transport available, the main cause of anxiety is arriving at the airport, harbour, or station on time. The actual travelling itself is less stressful. However, with every form of transport there may be peaks of anxiety, for example, during take-off and landing, and periods of turbulence in an aeroplane. Rail travel seems to be the most relaxing way of going from one place to another. Travel on board ship is unique in that passengers' stress levels generally change with the weather. The charts on the previous pages give some indication of the average stresses experienced on a journey of the same distance using different forms of transport.

Gaining the most benefit from a holiday requires planning and an effort to remain in a calm, unhurried state of mind. On a car journey, motorists should prepare themselves to be late if the unexpected, such as a flat tyre or traffic jam, occurs. Other travellers should be prepared to accept delays in flight, train, or bus time-tables.

Planning the details of a holiday early will eliminate the strain of handling last-minute preparations. Holidaymakers should organize their tickets, passports, visas, and room reservations well in advance and should make lists of clothing and other items needed for the journey.

People who travel by air from one time zone to another that has a difference of more than four hours will still be physically and mentally geared to the original time zone. This is called jet lag. A traveller may require several days to adjust, depending on how great is the time difference between zones. The effects of jet lag can be reduced by organizing the arrival in the new zone during the evening. Any meetings and business discussions should then take place only after a night's rest, if not sleep. If all business discussions can be arranged for times that correspond with working hours in the original "day" then little or no adaptation at all is necessary.

An alternative kind of holiday is to enjoy leisure at home in familiar holiday surroundings. Such a holiday can be used as a time for making new resolutions and for finally sorting out problems that may have seemed too difficult while other day-to-day routines and stresses were in the way.

Relieving mental tension

In the daily routine of life, it is not always easy to achieve a proper balance between work and leisure. Many people find it difficult to relax physically and mentally without making a definite effort. The thoughts of the day just ending, or worries about events to come – fears, pleasures, embarrassments and triumphs – create a state of tension that makes relaxation impossible.

There are dozens of techniques to relieve excessive tension, some from the ancient East, others from the modern West. What constitutes an effective method of relaxing depends largely on personal preference. A technique that works well for one individual might not work at all for another. Many factors enter into choosing a relaxation technique, such as the amount of time and discipline needed. Some techniques can be learned by the individual alone, others require more formal instruction.

Many people have found that various forms of meditation relieve tension. In general, meditation involves focusing on a thought, word, phrase, or object to calm the mind. Some meditation techniques also involve breathing exercises. Scientists have found that during meditation the body undergoes physical changes, such as slower heartbeat or lower blood pressure, which indicate a state of deep relaxation.

One of the more popular forms of meditation is Transcendental Meditation (TM). Those who practice TM sit quietly for 15 to 20 minutes twice each day and repeat a mantra, or word from the Hindu scriptures. TM is taught by instructors who select a personal mantra for each individual.

Some people find that simply visualizing peaceful or pleasant scenes helps relieve tension. Many books explaining other meditation and thought control techniques have been written and are widely available in bookshops and libraries.

Another relaxation technique popular in the Western world is yoga, the Hindu system of mental and physical exercise. It is wise to learn yoga from an expert instructor because many books on yoga describe some difficult yoga postures that could cause injury to a beginner.

Other Eastern systems that have been modified and adapted in the West to promote relaxation and peace of mind include some of the Japanese martial arts and the Chinese exercise, tai chi.

Because there appears to be a direct connection between mental and muscular tension, some scientists have experimented with relieving mental tension by relaxing the muscles. Using a system called Progressive Relaxation, a person alternately tenses and relaxes various muscles to become more aware of the degrees of tension and relaxation that they can achieve. A similar technique, called Autogenic Training, involves suggestions that various parts of the body are warm, heavy, and relaxed. These types of relaxation techniques can be learned from a therapist or from books available on the subject.

One of the newest relaxation techniques involves biofeedback. Researchers have found that biofeedback is useful in relaxing muscles, lowering blood pressure, and increasing the long, slow brain waves called alpha waves. Electronic sensors are placed on the skin to monitor bodily conditions, such as skin temperature, muscle tension, and brain waves. Once a person receives feedback indicating excessive tension (for example, seeing on a monitor that the brain waves have changed), he or she can direct the body to correct this condition. Because the sensitive electronic equipment involved must be calibrated carefully and the electrodes placed precisely, it is advisable that this technique be practised under the supervision of a biofeedback expert if the technique is to be successful.

Many people find inner calm and peace through sincere religious beliefs. For them, prayer and worship produce a state of profound joy and contentment that contributes greatly to their mental well-being. A strong religious faith can also help a person cope with the various crises that arise in life. Even those who do not have religious beliefs, often have some kind of faith, perhaps in a particular philosophy of life, that helps contribute to emotional stability and provides underlying mental strength.

Onset of mental problems

Everyone, on occasion, experiences the unpleasant emotions of anger, frustration, sadness, mild depression, worry, loneliness, and uncertainty. This is normal. But sometimes these feelings persist for a long time or grow more intense. This could be a sign that mental or emotional problems are developing. These feelings could stem from a specific cause, but often there seems to be no apparent reason.

Other indications of mental problems include alcoholism, drug abuse, suicidal thoughts or actions, irrational fears, sexual difficulties, obsessive thoughts, and compulsions to perform the same acts repeatedly.

Sometimes problems arise within a family that can best be remedied with outside help. These may include a troubled child, marital difficulties involving household finances, and sexual problems.

Treatment for mental problems

Mental problems may be treated with drugs, psychotherapy, or both. Some psychotherapists probe a person's past experiences to uncover connections with present feelings and behaviour. Others concentrate on changing thought patterns or behaviour without trying to establish the cause of the problem. Some people prefer individual counselling, others prefer group therapy in which the group members discuss their feelings and problems. A special type of counselling is also available for all members of the family.

People who feel in need of professional help should ask their doctor for a referral. There are also organizations, such as MIND (National Association for Mental Health) and the Samaritans, which may be able to advise on sources of help. Other organizations may be able to help with specific problems; for example, Release advises on drug problems, and Alcoholics Anonymous helps with alcoholism.

Seeking professional help

Many people benefit from discussing their problem with the family doctor and having an examination to determine whether there is an underlying physical cause. Others may seek advice from priests or ministers, many of whom have received training in family counselling. Sometimes the service of a marriage counsellor, psychiatrist, psychologist, social worker, or psychiatric nurse can provide the most help towards relieving anxiety, fear, and tension.

Schools often have access to social workers to help with the problems of children. Various organizations also run special telephone services, which are often available throughout the day and night, to advise people who need immediate help or advice with their problems.

Drugs, alcohol, and smoking

The use and abuse of "hard" and "soft" drugs, the excessive consumption of alcohol, and the smoking of cigarettes, can all have serious medical effects on the individual. The facts about addiction to each of these forms of self-indulgence are well known.

Although most addicts have a fairly clear idea of how their addiction can affect the body or the mind, very few realize that they are also a social hazard. The chart below gives an indication of the extent of alcohol and drug abuse. Both of these problems, but particularly alcoholism, are growing and placing an increasing burden on the resources of society.

Drugs

Hard drugs are socially destructive, because the people who use them are often personally and socially irresponsible. Addicts frequently commit crimes because the need to obtain expensive supplies of illegal drugs means that stealing is eventually the only way of obtaining sufficient money to buy them. Desperation may even lead to violent assault, or armed robbery.

In some countries the use of opium is still permitted. In many Western countries its use, and that of the extracts morphine and heroin, is restricted to the most carefully controlled medical prescriptions. In some countries, including the United Kingdom, the use of heroin is totally prohibited except on medical prescription.

Marijuana has been used for centuries in Eastern countries, but its unauthorised possession is an offence in the United Kingdom and many other countries. However, the drug causes little social disturbance, and virtually no violence among users. A person is unlikely to need hospitalization, although psychotherapy and psychiatric care are sometimes needed. Many people have used marijuana or other psychedelic drugs occasionally, but relatively few are regular users. Most marijuana is smuggled into the United Kingdom from the Middle East, and the people who handle the drugs are also often associated with hard drugs. Although there is no evidence to show that the use of marijuana leads directly to crime and violence, the people involved in the selling of the drug may lead a casual user onto more dangerous drugs.

Other drug-related problems are those associated with sports. "Pep" pills, usually amphetamine-based, have been used to increase stamina. They have little, if any, effect, and have occasionally proved fatal. An increasing problem in international sport is

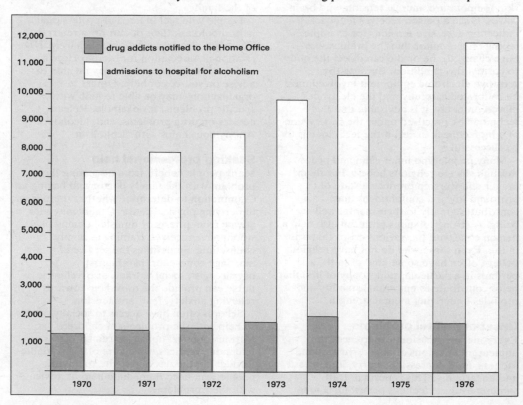

the use of anabolic steroids, drugs that increase the size and strength of muscles. Use of such drugs is now on the decline because tests can be carried out to detect steroids. If drugs are found to have been used, the athlete is banned from participation.

An increasing medical problem that is having serious, and sometimes fatal, repercussions is drugs that slightly impair a person's speed of reaction when working with moving machinery or driving a car. The use of minor tranquillizers has been associated with an increase in road traffic accidents. Antihistamines, antidepressants, and other tranquillizing drugs are known to reduce an individual's reaction time, and it is advisable for a patient who is being treated with these drugs not to drive, nor to operate any machinery, especially where the safety of others may be involved.

Another unexpected effect of the use of minor tranquillizers is an increase in the use of physical violence by some people. The drugs have a depressing effect, similar to that of alcohol, and reduce the conscious and normal social inhibitions on behaviour. Although the individual is initially calmer and better able to cope with problems, annoyance may produce an unexpected and often violent outburst, unlike the person's normal character and behaviour.

The World Health Organization tries to work through, as well as independently of, the United Nations to persuade governments to control addictive substances. So far, the W.H.O. has succeeded in controlling the growth of opium poppies in certain parts of the world.

Alcohol

Alcohol is a major social hazard. It is the most commonly abused drug in the United Kingdom. Drunken driving accounts for a large proportion of all road accidents, and it is easy to demonstrate that any driver's reflex time and ability to make decisions are greatly impaired by alcohol.

Many Middle Eastern countries have banned or restricted the sale of alcohol. In some Scandinavian countries the sale of alcohol is a state monopoly. Alcoholism in nineteenth-century England was finally reduced when the government imposed high tax levies on alcohol, and made it too expensive for many people to buy. In most countries the sale of alcohol to persons under a certain age is illegal, but drinking is usually allowed under parental supervision. In fact, there is a much lower incidence of alcoholism among the Italians and the Jews, who introduce their children to drinking at a moderate level as a part of ordinary family life.

The attitudes of different countries, societies, and religions make it difficult for a worldwide assessment to be made concerning the effect of alcohol on society. High taxes on the sale of alcohol (and tobacco) greatly benefit some governments, and offer little incentive to those same governments to reduce the sale of addictive substances even though the damaging effect on their citizens is obvious.

The effects of alcohol are not confined to drivers of vehicles. Heavy drinking can lead to violence in the home that may include baby battering or assaults on wives. Less often husbands are assaulted. In time, a marriage may break up, and children may become separated, or fostered out to relatives or placed in institutions. A person who becames an alcoholic is unable to hold down a steady job largely because of increasing unreliability and absenteeism. Throughout the United Kingdom, the number of working days lost each year because of absenteeism is immense, and the social cost of treating alcoholism is enormous.

Although the occasional use of alcohol is socially acceptable and, indeed, may help with digestion, excessive use (as with other drugs) is socially irresponsible and often legally unacceptable. It may, in fact, harm the individual's health even if there is no addiction.

Smoking

Although lung cancer is the most feared consequence of smoking (it is twenty times more likely among smokers than among non-smokers), smoking is also a destructive habit in other ways. There is a twenty-fold increase of chronic bronchitis among smokers, and many end up as respiratory cripples with emphysema. Smoking also greatly increases the risk of death from coronary heart disease. Many other serious disorders can have as their basic cause an addiction to smoking. Further details are given elsewhere in this book.

The harmful effects of smoking are not restricted to the individual but also affect other people. For instance, a pregnant woman who smokes harms her unborn child; a person who suffers from heart disease may be adversely affected by other people who smoke; and parents who die young often leave children of school age without support. Like alcohol, tobacco is one of the most easily obtainable addictive drugs. Sale of cigarettes to people below a specified age is not allowed in some countries.

Drug abuse

The abuse of drugs is an increasingly serious problem, particularly among teenagers, and should be a matter of concern for all parents. The incidence of drug use, particularly sniffing cleaning fluid, glue, and other volatile substances, is increasing among even younger children of nine or ten years of age. Drug abuse occurs throughout society and parents must not be complacent because they have provided a good home for their children.

Smoking and drinking alcohol are also serious problems among adolescents. Although these drugs are generally more socially acceptable, they are potentially as harmful as some of the less acceptable drugs.

The reasons behind drug abuse are complex. Some children take drugs out of curiosity, or because of social pressures from their friends. Others may turn to drugs as a form of escape, or to rebel against their parents or against what they consider to be an unfair society. Some children may smoke, drink alcohol, or take drugs because they think it is grown-up to do so. Once a young person has been introduced to the subculture of drug users and suppliers, it is often difficult for him or her to break away.

Amphetamines, cocaine, nicotine, LSD and other hallucinogens, and certain chemicals used in glue and some solvents are habit-forming. A person who takes such substances regularly can become psychologically dependent on them. The user feels compelled to continue taking the drug in order to maintain the state of well-being produced by it, but the drug is not essential for the physical needs of the body. When deprived of the drug, a habituated person becomes restless, irritable, and anxious. Unlike a drug addict, a person who is psychologically dependent on a drug does not experience true withdrawal symptoms.

Heroin and barbiturates are addictive. The user develops both a psychological and a physical dependence on the drug. These drugs alter the body chemistry so that the drug becomes necessary for the normal physical functioning of the body. Such physical dependence takes about six weeks of regular drug use to develop. Because of this effect on the body chemistry, an addict develops painful, physical withdrawal symptoms if the drug is discontinued suddenly. In addition to developing physical dependence, an addict also develops tolerance to the drug, so that larger doses are necessary to produce the desired effects.

Sudden withdrawal from addictive drugs produces a painful physical illness. Several hours after the last dose of heroin, an addict may develop stomach cramps, chills, nausea, diarrhoea, uncontrollable shaking, and profuse sweating. Sudden withdrawal from barbiturates is extremely dangerous, and may even be fatal. For this reason, barbiturate withdrawal should be done gradually, preferably under expert medical supervision.

Experimentation with drugs does not always lead to addiction. For example, most people who drink alcohol do not become physically dependent on it. However, psychological dependence can develop comparatively rapidly. The regular use of "soft" drugs, such as marijuana, does not necessarily result in addiction to "hard" drugs. However, experimentation with drugs must not be ignored; parents should explain to their children the dangers of even casual drug use.

Parents should establish codes of behaviour to guide their children, and should be prepared to use discipline to enforce these rules. But the parents should explain the reasons for the rules so that their children can see that they are not just arbitrary restrictions. Parents should learn how the various drugs affect the mind and body, and should explain these effects to their children. Parents should also refrain from smoking and drinking in front of children.

Drug use is less common in families where a good relationship exists between parents and children. Parents should take an active interest in their children. They should help the children with their homework and help to fill their leisure time creatively.

If parents suspect that a child is using drugs, they should try to act calmly but decisively. The sooner the parents act, the greater the likelihood of their preventing addiction. It may be difficult to determine whether or not a child is taking drugs, but there may be several indications. For example, alteration in the child's behaviour, such as apathy, furtiveness, or unusual aggressiveness; indifference to personal appearance; change in school habits, such as being late or missing school; change in work habits, such as poor homework; refusal to wear short-sleeved clothes to hide needle marks in the arms; stealing or borrowing money to pay for drugs; and being seen in the company of known drug users. Parents should be on the alert for these signs, but should also take care not to appear too authoritarian.

At the first suspicion of drug use, the parents should consult the family doctor. If the doctor is unable to deal with the problem, he or she can refer the parents to a specialist in drug problems.

Drug	Medical use	Short-term effects	Long-term effects
Alcohol	Rarely used.	Relaxation; euphoria; drowsiness; lack of co-ordination; loss of emotional control.	Habituation; liver and brain damage; obesity with excessive use; addiction with prolonged use.
Amphetamines (Dexedrine)	Relief of depression; reduction of fatigue; occasionally, for treatment of obesity.	Increased alertness; loss of appetite; insomnia; euphoria; large doses can produce hallucinations.	Habituation; irritability; restlessness; weight loss; mental disturbances.
Antidepressants (MAO inhibitors)	Treatment of depression.	Mental stimulation; elevation of mood; occasionally, trembling, insomnia, confusion, and hallucinations. MAO inhibitors may interact adversely with some foods and other drugs.	Dry mouth; blurred vision; fatigue; skin rashes; palpitations; occasionally, jaundice.
Barbiturates (Amytal; Nembutal; Seconal; phenobarbitone)	Treatment of insomnia; relief of nervous tension and epilepsy.	Intoxication; relaxation; drowsiness; lack of co-ordination; loss of emotional control; relief of anxiety; occasionally, euphoria. An overdose or a combination of barbiturates and alcohol can be fatal.	Habituation; irritability; weight loss; addiction. Severe withdrawal symptoms if the drug is suddenly discontinued.
Cocaine	Anaesthesia of the eyes, ears, or nose.	Increased alertness; reduction of fatigue; reduction of appetite; insomnia; euphoria. Large doses may cause hallucinations, convulsions, and death.	If sniffed, ulceration of the nose. Other long-term effects similar to those of amphetamines.
Hallucinogens (LSD; psilocybin; STP; DMT; mescaline)	Rarely used.	Hallucinations; lack of co-ordination; nausea; dilated pupils; irregular breathing; sometimes anxiety.	May precipitate mental disturbance in susceptible individuals. Occasionally, recurrence of original hallucinatory experience without taking further doses of the drug. May also cause chromosome damage.
Marijuana	Rarely used.	Relaxation; euphoria; alteration of time perception; lack of co-ordination. Large doses may produce hallucinations.	Long-term effects have not been definitely established. Prolonged, heavy use may lead to insomnia and depression on sudden withdrawal.
Narcotics (Opium; heroin; codeine; pethidine; methadone)	Treatment of severe pain.	Sedation; euphoria; relief of pain; lack of co-ordination; impaired mental functioning.	Constipation; loss of appetite; weight loss; temporary sterility; addiction, producing painful withdrawal symptoms on stopping use of the drug. The use of unsterilized hypodermic needles may cause severe infections.
Nicotine	None.	Mental stimulation; relaxation; relief of tension.	Cancer, particularly of the lungs; heart and blood vessel disease; bronchitis.
Tranquillizers (Benzodiazepines; phenothiazines)	Treatment of anxiety and other mental disorders.	Relaxation; relief of anxiety; general depression of mental functioning.	Drowsiness; dry mouth; blurred vision; skin rashes; tremors; occasionally, jaundice.
Miscellaneous (Amyl nitrite; antihistamines; toluene and other solvents – "glue sniffing")	None, except for antihistamines for allergies and amyl nitrite for angina.	Euphoria, lack of co-ordination; impaired mental functioning.	Variable. Some of these substances can cause liver and kidney damage.

Index

Fitness, *see* Physical fitness, Mental fitness
Flatfoot, 205
  in children, 850–851
Flatulence, 206
Flatus, 206
Fleas, 206
Flexibilitas cerea, 206
Flies, 206
Flu, *see* Influenza
Flukes, 206
Fluorescein, **206**
Fluoridation, **206,** 944–945
Fluoride, 206
Fluoroscope, 206
Flush, 207
Flutter, 207
Foetus, **207,** 747
Folic acid, 207
Folk medicine, 207
Follicle, 207
Follicle stimulating hormone, 23, **207**
Folliculitis, 207
Fomentation, *see* Poultice
Fontanelle, 207
Food poisoning, 208
  first aid for, 562
  preventing, 596
Foot, 208
  first aid for fracture of, 549
  care of, 942–943
Foot disorders, **209,** 912–913
  symptoms of, 39
Foot drop, 209
Forceps, 209
Forceps delivery, 382, **762**
Forensic medicine, 210
Foreskin, 210
Formaldehyde, 210
Formalin, 210
Formic acid, 210
Formication, 210
Fovea, 17, **210**
Fractures, **210–211, 886–887, 920–921**
  first aid for, 546–553
  at birth, 814–815
  in children, 844–845
Fragilitas ossium, 211
Framboesia, *see* Yaws
Fraternal twins, 211
Freckles, 211
Friar's balsam, 212
Friedreich's ataxia, 212
Frigidity, **212,** 417
Fröhlich's syndrome, 212
Frontal lobe, 19
Frostbite, 212–213
  first aid for, 558–559
Frozen section, 213
Frozen shoulder, **213, 898–899**
FSH, *see* Follicle stimulating hormone

Fugue, 213
Fulguration, 213
Fumigation, 213
Fungal disorders, 213–214
Funny bone, 214
Furred tongue, 214
Furuncle, *see* Boils
Furunculus, *see* Boils

G

Gall, *see* Bile
Gall bladder, 12–13, **214**
Gallstone, 214
Gamma globulin, 214
Ganglion, 215
Gangrene, **215, 922–923**
Gas gangrene, 215
Gas poisoning, 216
  first aid for, 562–565
Gastrectomy, 216
Gastric flu, 216
Gastric ulcer, 216
Gastrin, 216
Gastritis, 216
Gastroenteritis, 217
Gastroenterostomy, 217
Gastroscopy, 217
Gastrostomy, 217
Gaucher's disease, 217
Gene, 2, **217,** 237
Genetic abnormality, 218
Genetic counselling, 218–219
Genitourinary, *see* Urogenital
Genu valgum, *see* Knock-knee
Genu varum, *see* Bow-legs
Germ, 219
German measles, **219,** 380, 749, 853, **858–859**
Gigantism, 219
Gingivitis, **219–220, 898–899**
Gland, 21, **220**
Glandular fever, **220, 874–875**
Glaucoma, **220, 910–911**
Glioma, 220
Globulin, 220
Globus hystericus, 220
Glomerulonephritis, 221
Glomus tumour, 221
Glossitis, 221
Glucagon, 21, **221**
Glucose, 21, **221**
Glucose tolerance test, 222
Glycogen, 222
Glycosuria, 222
Goitre, 222
Gonorrhoea, **222–223, 874–875,** 957
Gout, **223, 912–913**
Graafian follicle, 224
Graft, 224
Grand mal, *see* Epilepsy

Granuloma inguinale, **224, 874–875**
Graves' disease, *see* Hyperthyroidism
Grawitz's tumour, *see* Hypernephroma
Greenstick fracture, 224
Grief, 224
Gripes, *see* Abdominal pain, Colic
Grippe, *see* Influenza
Gristle, *see* Cartilage
Group therapy, 225
Growing pains, **225, 858–859**
Guinea worm, 225
Gullet, 225
Gum, **225, 945**
Gumboil, 225
  treatment of, 595
Gumma, 225
Gut, *see* Intestine
Guthrie test, **225,** 767
Gynaecological disorders, 225–228
Gynaecology, 228
Gynaecomastia, 228

H

Haemachromatosis, *see* Haemochromatosis
Haemangioma, 228
Haematemesis, *see* Blood, vomiting of
Haematocolpos, 228
Haematology, 228
Haematoma, 228
Haematuria, 228
Haemochromatosis, 228
Haemodialysis, *see* Kidney dialysis
Haemoglobin, 8–9, **228,** 398
Haemoglobinuria, 229
Haemolysis, 229
Haemolytic disease of the newborn, **229, 814–815**
Haemophilia, 229
  in children, 834–835
Haemoptysis, *see* Blood, spitting of
Haemorrhage, 230
  first aid for, 516–517
  birth disorder, 812–813
Haemorrhoidal preparations, 230
Haemorrhoids, **230,** 378, 758, **898–899**
  treatment of, 586
Haemothorax, 230
Hair, 230
  ball, 858–859
  care of, 946–947
  pulling, 844–845

Marburg disease, 297
Marijuana, **297**, 1006, 1008–1009
Marrow, 297
Masochism, 298
Massage, 298, **998**
Mastectomy, 298
Mastitis, 298
Mastoid, 298
Mastoiditis, 299
Masturbation, **299**, 805, 959
by children, **846–847, 874–875**
Maxilla, 299
Measles, **299, 860–861**
Meckel's diverticulum, 299
Meconium, 299
Medical insurance, 300–301
Medical social worker, 301
Medical terms, 47–54
Medical tests, **301**, 720–723
Medicine
administering, in home, 662–663
Mediterranean anaemia, *see* Thalassaemia
Mediterranean fever, 301
Medulla, 301
Megacolon, 301
Megaloblast, 301
Megalomania, 301
Meibomian cyst, *see* Chalazion
Melaena, 301
Melancholia, *see* Depression
Melanin, 301
Melanoma, 302
Melanuria, 302
Melasma, 302
Membrane, 302
Memory, loss of, *see* Amnesia
Menarche, 302
Ménière's disease, **302, 910–911**
Meninges, 18, 302
Meningioma, 302
Meningitis, **303, 900–901**
in children, **834–835, 860–861**
Meniscus, 303
Menopause, **303–305, 900–901**, 959
Menorrhagia, 305
Menstrual problems, **305–306**, 884–885, **900–901**
in children, 876–877
Menstruation, 22–23, **306–307**, 956, 959
Mental defect, 307
Mental fitness, 1002–1005
Mental illness, **307–308, 694–697**
Mental retardation, **308–310, 696–697**

Menthol, 310
Mcprobamate, 310
Mercury, **310**, 313
Mescaline, **310,** 1008–1009
Mesentery, 310
Metabolism, 310
Metacarpal, 310
Metastasis, 112, **310**
Metatarsal, 311
Metatarsalgia, **311, 912–913,** 943
Methadone, 311
Methamphetamine, 311
Methaemoglobin, 311
Methyl alcohol, *see* Alcohol
Metropathia haemorrhagica, 311
Metrorrhagia, 311
Microbes, 311
Microcephalic, **311, 818–819**
Microsurgery, 311
Micturition, 311
Middle ear, 311
Midwife, **311,** 716
Migraine, 311–313
in children, 874–875
Miliaria, 313
Milk, **313,** 776–781
Milk of magnesia, *see* Magnesia, milk of
Milk teeth, 313
Milroy's disease, 313
Minamata disease, 313
Mineral oil, 313
Minerals, 167, **313, 966**
Miotic, 313
Mirror writing, 313
Miscarriage, **313,** 751, **888–889**
Mites, 314
Mitral valve disease, 314
Molar, 314
Mole, **314, 810–811**
Molluscum contagiosum, *see* Von Recklinghausen's disease
Molluscum fibrosum, *see* Von Recklinghausen's disease
Mongolism, *see* Down's syndrome
Moniliasis, **315, 924–925,** 957
Monoamine oxidase inhibitors, *see* MAO inhibitors
Monocyte, 315
Mononucleosis, *see* Glandular fever
Monoplegia, 316
Morbidity, 316
Morbilli, *see* Measles
Morning sickness, **316,** 376, 750
Morphine, 316
Mosquito, 316
Motion sickness, **316,** 969
first aid for, 596

Motorcycle safety, 620–621
Motoring safety, 614–619
Motor neuron disease, 317
Mountain sickness, *see* Altitude sickness
Mouth, **15, 317**
symptoms of disorders of, 27
Mouth breathing, 317
Mouth-to-mouth resuscitation, 317
in first aid, 518–519
Mouth ulcer, 317
MS, *see* Multiple sclerosis
Mucopurulent, 317
Mucous colitis, 317
Mucous membrane, 318
Mucus, 10, 15, **318**
Multipara, 318
Multiple sclerosis, **318, 900–901**
Mumps, **319, 860–861**
Münchausen's syndrome, 319
Murmur, *see* Heart murmur
Muscle, **6–7, 320**
Muscle relaxants, 320
Muscular dystrophy, 320
Mutation, 320
Mute, 320
Myalgia, 320
Myasthenia gravis, **320, 900–901**
Mycetoma, 321
Mycobacteria, 321
Mycosis, 321
Mydriatic, 321
Myelin, **321,** 327
Myelocele, 321
Myelogram, 321
Myeloid leukaemia, *see* Leukaemia
Myeloma, 321
Myocarditis, 321
Myoclonus, 322
Myoma, 322
Myopathy, 322
Myopia, *see* Shortsightedness
Myositis, 322
Myotonia congenita, 322
Myringotomy, 322
Myxoedema, *see* Hypothyroidism
Myxovirus, 322

N

Naevus, *see* Birthmark
Nail, 322
biting, 862–863
care of, 942–943
Nappy changing, 788–789
Nappy rash, **323, 836–837**
Narcoanalysis, 323

Pylorus, 394
Pyorrhoea, 394
Pyrexia, *see* Fever
Pyridoxine, 394
Pyrogen, 394
Pyrosis, *see* Heartburn

Q

Q fever, 394
Quadriceps, 394
Quadriplegia, 394
Quarantine, 394–395
Quickening, 377, **395**, 756
Quick's test, 395
Quinine, 296, **395**
Quinsy, 395
  in children, 848–849

R

Rabbit fever, 395
Rabies, 395–396
Radiation, 396
Radiation sickness, 396
Radiculitis, 396
Radiography, 397
Radiology, 397
Radiotherapy, 397
Radium, 397
Radius, 397
Rale, 397
Ranula, 397
Rash, 397
  in children, 836–837
Rauwolfia, 397
Raynaud's phenomenon, **397,**
  888–889
RBC, *see* Red blood cell
Rectal fissure, 397
Rectal prolapse, *see* Prolapse
Rectocele, 397
Rectum, 397–398
  symptoms of disorders of,
  35
Red blood cell, 8, **398**
Red eye, 398
Referred pain, 398
Reflex, 398
Regional ileitis, *see* Crohn's
  disease
Regression, 398
Regurgitation, 398
  in children, 836–837
Reiter's disease, 398–399
Relapse, 399
Relapsing fever, 399
Relaxant, 399
Remission, 399
Renal calculus, 399
Renal pelvis, 14
Renin, 399

Rennin, 399
Replacement surgery, 399
Reportable diseases, 399
Repression, 399
Reproduction, 22–23
Reproductive system, female
  symptoms of disorders of,
  36
Reproductive system, male
  symptoms of disorders of,
  37
Resection, 399
Reserpine, 399
Resolution, 399
Respiration, **10–11,** 400
Respirator, 400
Respiratory disorders, *see*
  Lung disorders
Respiratory distress syn-
  drome, **400, 816–817**
Respiratory stimulants, 400
Rest and relaxation, 954–955
Restless legs, 400
Resuscitation, 400
  in first aid, 518–523
Retardation, *see* Mental retar-
  dation
Retention, 400
Retina, **16,** 401
Retinitis, **401, 912–913**
Retinitis pigmentosa, 401
Retrobulbar neuritis, 401
Retrograde amnesia, 401
Retroversion, 401
Rhesus factor, *see* Rh factor
Rheumatic diseases, 401–402
Rheumatic fever, **402–403,**
  864–865
Rheumatism, 403
Rheumatoid arthritis, **404–**
  405, 894–895
Rh factor, 379, **405**
Rhinitis, 405
Rhinophyma, 405
Rhinoplasty, 405
Rhinorrhoea, 405
Rhonchus, *see* Rale
Rhythm method, 405
Rib, 405
  first aid for fracture of, 551
Riboflavin, **405–406,** 491
Rickets, **406, 836–837**
Rickettsia, 406
Rigor, 406
Rigor mortis, 406
Ringing ears, 406
Ringworm, 406
  in children, 864–865
Rinne's test, 407
Rio Grande fever, 407
RNA, 2
Rocky Mountain spotted
  fever, 407
Rods, 16

Rodent ulcer, **407, 926–927**
Romberg's sign, 407
Rosacea, **407, 902–903**
Roseola, **407, 848–849**
Roundworms, 408
Rubella, *see* German measles
Rubeola, 409
Running nose, 409
Rupture, 409
Ryle's tube, 409

S

Sabin's vaccine, 409
Sacroiliac, 409
Sacrum, 409
Sadism, 409
Safe period, 409
Safety, 604–629
  bicycle, 620
  car and motoring, 614–621
  hiking, 624–625
  home, 606–609
  motorcycle, 620–621
  sports, 626–629
Saint Vitus's dance, 409
Salicylate, 409
Saline, 409
Saliva, 13, **409**
Salivary glands, 12, 13, **409–**
  410
Salk vaccine, 410
Salmonella, 410
Salpingectomy, 410
Salpingitis, **410, 888–889**
Sandfly fever, 411
Saphenous vein, 411
Sarcoidosis, 411
Sarcoma, 411
Scab, 411
Scabicides, 411
Scabies, 411
  in children, 864–865
Scald, 411
  first aid for, 524–525
Scalene node biopsy, 411
Scalp, 412
Scalpel, 412
Scaphoid, 412
Scapula, 412
Scar, 412
Scarlet fever, 412
  in children, 860–861
Schick test, 412
Schistosomiasis, 412
Schizoid, 412
Schizophrenia, **413, 890–891**
School
  children's experiences in,
  807
  phobia, 866–867
Sciatica, 413
Scirrhus, 413

Stevens-Johnson syndrome, 437
Stiff neck, 437
Stiffness, 437
Stigma, 437
Stillbirth, 437
Still's disease, 437–438
Stimulant, 438
Sting, 438
  first aid for, 514–515
Stitch, 438
  first aid for, 589
Stokes-Adams attack, 438
Stomach, 12–13, **438**
  foreign body in, 588
Stomach ache, 40, **438**
Stomach disorders, 438
Stomatitis, 438
Stone, *see* Calculus
Stool, 439
Strabismus, 439
Strain, 439
  first aid for, 592–593
Strangulation, 439
Strangury, 439
Strawberry birthmark, 810–811
Streptococcus, 439
Stress, **439–440**, 1002–1003
Stress incontinence, 440
Stricture, 440
Stridor, 440
Stroke, **440–442, 926–927**
  first aid for, 573
Strongyloides, 442
Strychnine, 442
Stuffy nose, 442
Stupor, 442
Stuttering, **442, 864–865**
Stye, **442,** 662
Styptic, 442
Subacute bacterial endocarditis, 442–443
Subarachnoid haemorrhage, 443
Subconjunctival haemorrhage, 443
Subconscious, 443
Subcutaneous, 443
Subdural, 443
Sublingual gland, 443
Subluxation, 443
Submandibular gland, 443
Submucous resection, 444
Succus entericus, 444
Sudden infant death syndrome, *see* SIDS
Suffocation, 444
  first aid for, 526–527
Sugar, **444,** 964
Suicide, 444
  tendency in children, 878–879
Sulpha drugs, 445

Sulphones, 445
Sunburn, 445
  first aid for, 594
Sunstroke, 445
  first aid for, 567
Superfluous hair, 445
Suppository, 445
  use of, 664
Suppuration, 445
Suprarenal gland, *see* Adrenal gland
Surgery, 445–448
  hospital procedures for, 728–731
Suture, **448,** 729
Swab, 448
Swallowing, 448
Sweat, *see* Perspiration
Swelling, 449
Sydenham's chorea, *see* Chorea
Sympathectomy, 449
Sympathetic nervous system, 20, **449**
Symphysis, 449
Symptom, 449
Symptoms
  requiring first aid, 598–603
  index of, 24–25
Syncope, 449
Syndactyly, **449, 814–815**
Syndrome, 449
Synovitis, 449
Syphilis, 450–451
  in children, 878–879
Syringe, 451
Syringomyelia, 451
Systole, **9, 452**

T

Tabes dorsalis, 452
TAB vaccine, 452
Tachycardia, 452
Talipes, 452
Talus, 452
Tampon, 452
Tapeworms, 452
Tarsus, 452
Tartar, 453
Taste, **15, 453**
Taste bud, **15, 453**
Tay-Sachs disease, 453
TB, *see* Tuberculosis
Tears, 453
Teeth, 453
  broken, 588
  care of, 944–945
  care of baby, 795
  loss of, 914–915
Teething, 453, **795, 838–839**

Telangiectasis, 453
Temperature, 453
  of baby, 799
  taking, 660–661
Temper tantrum, **454,** 806–807, **848–849**
Temporal lobe, 19
Temporal lobe epilepsy, **191–194,** 389, **454,** 856–857, 858–859, 910–911
Tendinitis, 454
Tendon, 5, 6, **454**
Tenesmus, 454
Tennis elbow, **454, 890–891**
Tenosynovitis, 454
Teratoma, 454
Termination, **454, 751**
Testicle, *see* Testis
Testis, **22, 454**
  torsion of, in children, 866–867
  undescended, in children, 838–839
Test meal, 455
Testosterone, 22, **455**
Tetanus, 455
Tetany, 455
Tetracyclines, 456
Tetraplegia, 456
Thalamus, 18, **456**
Thalassaemia, 456
Thalidomide, 456
Thermogram, 456
Thermometer, 456
Thiamine, **457,** 491, 966–967
Thigh fracture
  first aid for, 548
Thirst, 457
Thoracic duct, 457
Thoracoplasty, 457
Thoracotomy, 457
Thorax, 457
Threadworm, 457
Throat, 10, **457**
  symptoms of disorders of, 26
Throat, lump in, 457
Throat abscess, 457
Thromboangiitis obliterans, **109, 457**
Thrombocytopenia, 457
Thrombolysis, 458
Thrombophlebitis, *see* Venous thrombosis
Thrombosis, 458
  coronary, 914–915
  venous, **486, 914–915**
Thrombus, **458, 486**
Thrush, 458
Thumb, 458
Thumb sucking, 458
Thymus, 458
Thyroidectomy, 458
Thyroid gland, **21, 459**

Vein, 8–9, **484**
Vena cava, 9, **485**
Venereal diseases, **485–486,**
957
Venerology, 486
Venipuncture, 486
Venogram, 486
Venom, 486
Venous thrombosis, **486–487,**
766, **914–915**
Ventral, 487
Ventricle
in brain, 18
in heart, 9
Vermiform appendix, 487
Vernix, 818–819
Verruca, 487
Vertebra, 4, **487–488**
Vertigo, **488,** 914–915
Vesicle, 488
Vestibulitis, *see* Labyrinthitis
Viable, 488
Vibrio, 488
Villus, 13, **489**
Vincent's angina, 489
Virilism, 489
Virus, 489
Viscera, 490
Visceroptosis, 490
Vision, *see* Eye
Vitamins, 490–492
Vitiligo, **492, 890–891**
Vitreous humour, 492
Vocal cord, 15
Voicebox, *see* Larynx
Volvulus, 492
Vomiting, 41, **493**
first aid for, 597
in children, 838–839
Von Recklinghausen's dis-
ease, 493–494
Vulva, 494

birth disorder of,
818–819
Vulvitis, 494
Vulvovaginitis, 495

W

Walking aids, 678–679
Walking problems
in children, 850–851
Warts, 495
Wasp sting, 495
first aid for, 515
Wasserman reaction, 495
Wasting, 495
Watering eyes, 495
Water on the knee, *see* Bursitis
Wax, 495
Weakness, 496
Weal, 496
Weaning, **496, 792–793**
Weight chart, 962
Weight problems, 496–498
children and, 832–833
diets for, 689–691
Welfare services, 738–741
Wen, *see* Cyst
Wheezing, 498
Whiplash injury, 498
Whipworm, *see* Worms
White blood cells, 498
Whiteleg, 499
Whooping cough, 499
in children, 462–463
Widal test, 499
Wilson's disease, 499
Wind, *see* Flatulence
Winding
babies, 782–783
first aid for, 589
Windpipe, *see* Trachea

Wisdom teeth, 499
impacted, 890–891
Witches' milk, 499
Womb, **22–23,** 306, **499**
Woolsorter's disease, 499
Worms, 499
Wound, 499. *See also* First aid
Wrist, **5, 500**
Wrist drop, 500
Writer's cramp, 500
Wryneck, 818–819

X

Xanthelasma, 500
Xanthoma, 500
X chromosome, 500
Xenophobia, 500
Xenopus test, 500
Xeroderma, 500
Xerophthalmia, 501
X-rays, **501,** 749

Y

Yaws, 501
Y chromosome, 501
Yeast, 501
Yellow fever, 501
Yellow jaundice, *see* Jaundice

Z

Zinc oxide, 502
Zip injury
first aid for, 589
Zoonosis, 502
Zygote, 502